Health, Illness, and Healing

Society, Social Context, and Self

An Anthology

Kathy Charmaz
Sonoma State University

Debora A. Paterniti
Baylor College of Medicine

New York   Oxford
OXFORD UNIVERSITY PRESS

Oxford University Press, Inc., publishes works that further Oxford University's
objective of excellence in research, scholarship, and education.

Oxford   New York
Auckland   Cape Town   Dar es Salaam   Hong Kong   Karachi
Kuala Lumpur   Madrid   Melbourne   Mexico City   Nairobi
New Delhi   Shanghai   Taipei   Toronto

With offices in
Argentina   Austria   Brazil   Chile   Czech Republic   France   Greece
Guatemala   Hungary   Italy   Japan   Poland   Portugal   Singapore
South Korea   Switzerland   Thailand   Turkey   Ukraine   Vietnam

Published by Oxford University Press, Inc.
198 Madison Avenue, New York, New York 10016
http://www.oup.com

Oxford is a registered trademark of Oxford University Press

ISBN 978-0-19-532976-6

Printed in the United States of America
on acid-free paper

In memory of
Anselm L. Strauss

Table of Contents

Section 1: Defining Health and Illness

The Problematics of Defining Health: Dilemmas and Decisions

David Mechanic

Mechanic suggests the importance of a broad definition of health in understanding health seeking and illness behaviors.

Alan Radley and Michael Billig

Radley and Billig contend that views of health and illness are inherently social and ideological rather than
being fixed and stable states and that these views
change in relation to intentions, audiences, and images
of self.

Views of Health Within Social Movements

Michael S. Goldstein

Goldstein shows how broad definitions of health and
illness generate movements that define particular attitudes and behaviors as requiring medical definition
and attention.

Deborah Lupton

Lupton discusses the implications of health promotion
strategies in the United States, Great Britain, and Australia for instilling fear and promoting public surveillance by juxtaposing "the grotesque" and "the civilized."

Section 2: The Self in Social Context

Organizational Definitions of Health and Wellness

Section 5: Social and Cultural Structures of Care

The Social and Cultural Shaping of Medical Care

importance of social support for hospitalization and illness outcomes.

Organizing Systems of Health Care

Section 6: The Social Construction of Illness: The Case of AIDS

Section 7: The Future of Health, Illness, and Healing

Acknowledgements

We would like to acknowledge our colleagues and mentors—Lyn Lofland, Virginia Olesen, and Julius Roth—whose assistance over the years has been invaluable. We also wish to thank Claude Teweles, Dawn VanDercreek, and Renée Burkhammer at Roxbury Publishing Company for their efforts in producing the book. Our reviewers gave helpful comments and raised sound questions. When our enthusiasm for an excellent piece outweighed our judgment about its appropriateness, they provided gentle correction. We thank Sharon Barnartt, Paul Benson, Anne Figert, Larry D. Hall, Janet Hankin, Allen J. LeBlanc, Judith Lorber, and Alexandra Todd.

In addition, Debora Paterniti acknowledges: students at the University of California, Davis and Yale University, who provided thoughtful feedback on some of the material in this anthology; Brad Gray's wonderful enthusiasm and rich insight into economic and political aspects of health care and services; the Houston Center for Quality of Care and Utilization Studies for resources and time to write; and Cheri and Peter Paterniti, who have been unconditionally supportive and understand a great deal about health care. ✦

About the Contributors

Emily K. Abel is associate professor of health services at the School of Public Health at the University of California, Los Angeles. She has written numerous articles in the field of gerontology and published several books and co-edited volumes about women's lives, work, and identities.

Laurie Kaye Abraham is an investigative reporter who has focused on health care. She has written about health care for the *Chicago Reporter* and expanded those articles into her book, *Mama Might Be Better Off Dead*, from which Robert Banes' story is reprinted. She has received a number of grants from foundations and individuals to pursue her research.

Hiroko Akiyama is at the University of Michigan's Institute for Social Research and Training Program in Social Research on Applied Issues of Aging. His interests include cross-cultural research on well-being, social support, intergenerational family relations, and health behaviors.

Gary L. Albrecht is professor of health policy and administration at the University of Illinois School of Public Health. He has published extensively in medical sociology and public health. His book, *The Disability Business*, won several awards including one from the medical sociology section of the American Sociological Association.

Deirdre Antonius is a post graduate research assistant with the Department of General Medicine and the Center for Health Services Research in Primary Care at the University of California, Davis Medical Center. Her primary research interests include health-related attitudes and behaviors.

Michael Billig is a social psychologist in the Department of Social Sciences, Loughborough University, United Kingdom. He has written numerous articles on rhetoric and argument and published *Ideology and Opinions: Studies in Rhetorical Psychology* and *Arguing and Thinking: A Rhetorical Approach to Social Psychology*.

Charles Bosk is professor of sociology at the University of Pennsylvania. His current research includes the social construction of suffering in families, the malpractice crisis of the late 1970s, and the relationship of ethnography and ethics in bioethics. He has written *Forgive and Remember: Managing Medical Failure*, and *All God's Mistakes: Genetic Counseling in a Pediatric Hospital*.

Theron Britt is assistant professor of English at Memphis State University. His research applies perspectives from critical theory to the fields of law, mental health, and medicine.

Robert S. Broadhead is professor of sociology at the University of Connecticut. He is the principal investigator of the Eastern Connecticut Health Outreach Project that developed the "peer-driven intervention" model to combat AIDS among intravenous drug users. He also has published works on professional socialization, social movements in the professions, and emergency care.

Phil Brown is professor and chair of the sociology department at Brown University. He has published extensively in the fields of mental illness and environmental health. He is co-author of *No Safe Place: Toxic Waste, Leukemia, and Community Action* and has recently served as chair of the medical sociology section of the American Sociological Association.

Daniel Callahan is at The Hastings Center. He has written numerous books and articles on medical ethics and health policy. He is the author of *Setting Limits: Medical Goals in an Aging Society* and *What Kind of Life: The Limits of Medical Progress*, from which his selection in this volume was excerpted.

Edward J. Callahan is a professor in the department of family practice primary care center at the University of California, Davis, Medical Center.

Maggie Callanan works as a health care consultant and does freelance writing for the federal government. She is a nurse who has specialized in care of the dying. She is a frequent public speaker on death and dying and has provided training in that field.

Miriam E. Cameron received her doctorate in nursing from the University of Minnesota. Her doctoral research explored ethical problems of people with AIDS and culminated in her book, *Living with AIDS: Experiencing Ethical Problems*, from which the selection in this volume is taken. She has also been a research fellow, has taught nursing, and has won awards in the nursing profession.

Daniel F. Chambliss is professor and chair of sociology at Hamilton College. His interests include theory, medical sociology, social psychology, and formal organizations. In addition to his ethnographic research on nursing ethics, he has written about the mundanity of excellence in Olympic sports and, recently, in teaching.

Kathy Charmaz is professor of sociology at Sonoma State University. Her book, *Good Days, Bad Days: The Self in Chronic Illness and Time*, received awards from the Society for the Study of Symbolic Interaction and the Pacific Sociological Association. She is co-editor of *The Unknown Country: Death Experiences in Australia, Britain, and the United States*.

Jeffrey Michael Clair is associate professor of sociology and Medicine at the University of Alabama, Birmingham. His interests include medical sociology, sociological practice, linguistics, and social gerontology. He has co-authored *Experiencing the Life Cycle* and edited *Sociomedical Perspectives on Patient Care*.

Chiquita Collins is assistant professor at the University of Illinois, Chicago. She received her doctorate from the University of Michigan. Her interests include demography, medical sociology, human ecology, and quantitative methods.

Peter Conrad is professor of sociology at Brandeis University. He has published widely in medical sociology, including his co-authored books—*Having Epilepsy* and *Deviance and Medicalization*. His numerous articles range from empirical analyses of health, illness, and care to policy analy-

ses. His interests include medical sociology, mental health, deviance, and qualitative research.

Juliet M. Corbin is a lecturer in the Department of Nursing, San Jose State University and co-author with Anselm Strauss of *Basics of Qualitative Research, Unending Work and Care*, and *Shaping a New Health Care System*. Their co-edited volume, *Grounded Theory in Practice*, has recently been published.

Gena Corea is an investigative reporter whose writings address issues in medicine affecting women. She is the author of *The Hidden Malpractice* and *The Mother Machine: Reproductive Technologies from Artificial Insemination to Artificial Limbs*.

Kathy Davis is associate professor in the department of Women's Studies at the University of Utrecht in the Netherlands. She is the author of *Power Under the Microscope*.

Timothy Diamond is visiting associate professor at the Institute for Health and Aging at the University of California, San Francisco while on leave from the Sociology Department at California State University, Los Angeles. He is author of *Making Gray Gold: Narratives of Nursing Home Care* and is currently working on a book on institutional ethnography.

Marcia Dunham is a physician with Kaiser Permanente in Northern California.

Joel Frader is associate professor of pediatrics and associate professor of medical ethics and humanities at Northwestern University Medical School and Children's Memorial Hospital in Chicago. He does research and teaching in medical ethics and medical sociology with special concern for issues involving children. He is also interested in ethical issues in biomedical research and innovation.

Arthur W. Frank is professor of sociology at the University of Calgary. His research includes the sociology of the body and narratives of illness. His recent book, *The Wounded Story-teller: Body, Illness and Ethics*, explores written narratives by or about people who have serious illnesses.

Michael S. Goldstein is professor in the School of Public Health at University of

California, Los Angeles. His interests include medical sociology, mental health, and collective behavior and social movements.

Audrey K. Gordon is at the Prevention Research Center of the School of Public Health at the University of Illinois, Chicago. She has long been involved in hospice work and research. She has served as a founding member of several hospices in the Chicago area.

Howard S. Gordon is assistant professor of medicine at Baylor College of Medicine. He is a general internist and health services researcher at the Houston Veterans Affairs Medical Center and the Houston Center for Quality of Care and Utilization Studies. His research has focused on outcomes assessment of hospitalized patients.

Amy Gross is a free-lance writer. She has also served as the editor of *Mirabella* magazine and has written on women's issues.

Frederic Hafferty is professor of behavioral sciences, University of Minnesota, Duluth, School of Medicine. His interests include medical sociology, occupations and professions, and socialization. He has recently written a co-authored book, *The Changing Medical Profession: An International Perspective*.

Michelle Harrison is a physician and specialist in obstetrics and gynecology. She has worked as a family practitioner and has gained a reputation for being an articulate critic of the medical care system.

Douglas D. Heckathorn is professor of sociology at the University of Connecticut and co-principal investigator of the Eastern Connecticut Health Outreach Project. He has written extensively on rational choice theory, the sociology of organizations, and social control.

David Hilfiker graduated from Yale University and the University of Minnesota Medical School. He practiced medicine as a Board Certified Family Practitioner in rural Minnesota and has worked in Washington, D.C., in two small health clinics. The selection in this anthology comes from his book *Healing the Wounds*.

David U. Himmelstein practices and teaches medicine at the Cambridge Hospital/Harvard Medical School. He and Steffie Woolhandler are co-founders of Physicians for a National Health Program and authors of the *National Health Program Book*.

John K. Iglehart is the founder and editor of *Health Affairs*, the largest circulating health policy journal in the U.S. He has been a member of the Institute of Medicine (IOM) and has served on the Governing Council for the National Academy of Sciences. He writes the "Health Policy Report" for the *New England Journal of Medicine*, and has served as the national correspondent for *NEJM* for the last fifteen years.

Dee Ito is a writer, lecturer, journalist and filmaker in New York City. She has written *The Healthy Body Handbook* and *Without Estrogen: Natural Remedies for Menopause and Beyond*. She has also written for film and television.

David A. Karp is professor and chair of sociology at Boston College. The chapter for this volume is drawn from *Speaking of Sadness: Depression, Disconnection and the Meanings of Illness*, which won the 1996 award from the Society for the Study of Symbolic Interaction.

Patricia Kelley has worked as a hospice nurse and in education for two decades. She is now an international consultant who provides training and education about death and dying, grief and bereavement, and HIV and AIDS. She is involved in the international hospice movement.

Timothy Kenny is a writer and former television newscaster. Our selection in this volume comes from his autobiographical account of having chronic fatgiue syndrome, *Living with Chronic Fatigue Syndrome: A Personal Story of the Struggle for Recovery*.

Perri Klass is a pediatrician and a prolific author of fiction and nonfiction. She has published stories and articles in *The New York Times Magazine*, *The Antioch Review*, and *Vogue*. She is the author of numerous books, including *Baby Doctor* and *A Not Entirely Benign Procedure*, from which the selection in this volume was taken.

Richard L. Kravitz is associate professor of medicine and director of the Center for Health Services Research in Primary Care at the University of California, Davis. He is a Fellow of the American College of Physicians and the Association for Health Services Research and has recently received the University of California, Davis School of Medicine Faculty Research Award.

Judith A. Levy is associate professor of health policy and administration at the University of Illinois School of Public Health. She has published works on hospice care, chronic illness, aging, and recently has conducted research on the efficacy of community-based services to end drug abuse and to reduce HIV infection.

Charles E. Lewis is a professor of medicine at the Center for Health Promotion and Disease Prevention at the University of California, Los Angeles.

Marsha Lillie-Blanton is associate director of Health Services Quality and Public Health Issues of the United States General Accounting Office (GAO). She also serves as adjunct assistant professor at The Johns Hopkins School of Public Health. She has authored and co-authored numerous reports and publications. She is the author of *Achieving Equitable Access: Studies of Health Care Issues Affecting Hispanics and African Americans*.

Deborah Lupton is associate professor in cultural studies and cultural policy and deputy director of the Centre for Cultural Risk Research at Charles Stuart University, Bathurst, Australia. She is the author of nine books including her recent co-authored volume, *Constructing Fatherhood: Discourses and Experiences*.

Karen Lyman is professor of sociology and coordinator of the Gerontology Program at Chaffey College. She won the dissertation award from the medical sociology section of the American Sociological Association and has published extensively in gerontology. Currently she is involved in developing ethical guidelines for treatment centers for Alzheimer's patients.

Nancy Mairs is an award-winning poet and acclaimed writer of several autobiographical works about living with chronic illness and disability including *Plaintext* and her recent book, *Waist-high in the World: A Life Among the Nondisabled*. She has also taught in the women's studies and writing programs at the University of Arizona.

Emily Martin is professor of anthropology at The Johns Hopkins University. She has recently written *Flexible Bodies: Tracking Immunity in American Culture from the Days of Polio to the Age of AIDS*.

Rose Marie Martinez is senior health researcher at Mathmatica Policy Research Incorporated. She has been involved in health policy and research at the international and federal levels as well as in the private sector. She was assistant director for Health Financing and Policy with the U.S. General Accounting Office (GAO). She has also lead health care research in Spain for the Regional Institute for Studies on Health and Social Welfare.

David Mechanic is director for the Institute of Health Policy at Rutgers University where he initiated the post-doctoral program in health policy. He has published extensively in medical sociology including a series of groundbreaking works on illness behavior, an early medical sociology textbook, *Medical Sociology*, and many contributions to debate and discussion in health policy.

Mark A. Mesler is associate professor of sociology at the Massachusetts College of Pharmacy and Allied Health Sciences in Boston. He received his doctorate from the University of Connecticut and has served on the faculty of several colleges and universities. He is currently conducting research in hospices on the East and West coasts.

Robert F. Murphy was late of Columbia University where he was professor of anthropology. Long a respected scholar in his field, he published numerous works in cultural anthropology, including several editions of his widely-used textbook, *Cultural and Social Anthropology*. He became known to the general public through his poignant memoir on experiencing disability, *The Body Silent*.

Vicente Navarro is professor of public health at The Johns Hopkins University. He has published numerous articles and books which critique the U.S. health care system. He is the author of *Class Struggle, the State and Medicine*. He is also the author of *Crisis, Health and Medicine: A Social Critique* and editor of *Imperialism, Health and Medicine*.

Debora A. Paterniti is assistant professor in the Department of General Medicine at Baylor College of Medicine and a Research Health Science Specialist at the Houston Center for Quality of Care and Utilization Studies, Department of Veterans Affairs. Her current research includes physician-patient decision making and expectations for care, health seeking behaviors, and identity in long-term care institutions.

Alan Radley is a social psychologist in the Department of Social Sciences at Loughborough University, United Kingdom. He has written extensively in medical sociology including *Prospects of Heart Surgery: Psychological Adjustment to Coronary By-Pass Grafting, The Body and Social Psychology*, edited *Worlds of Illness: Biographical and Cultural Perspectives in Health on Health and Disease* and serves as editor of the new journal, *Health*.

Betty Garman Robinson is at the School of Public Health at The Johns Hopkins University.

Gary Rosenthal is associate professor of medicine at Case Western Reserve University and an internist at the Cleveland Veterans Administration Medical Center. He is currently the recipient of a Career Development Award from the Department of Veterans Affairs Health Services Research and Development Service. His research interests include: measuring severity of illness and case-mix, profiling provider performance, developing patient-centered measures of care, and studying the impact of changes in heath care on patient outcomes.

Barbara Katz Rothman is professor of sociology at Baruch College. She has written widely in the field of gender on reproductive issues, including *The Tentative Preg-*

nancy: Prenatal Diagnosis and the Future of Motherhood and *In Labor: Women and Power in the Birthplace*.

Kent L. Sandstrom is assistant professor of sociology at the University of Northern Iowa. While a graduate student at the University of Minnesota, he received the Herbert Blumer Award for the best student paper from the Society for the Study of Symbolic Interaction. He has written several important papers about gay men with AIDS and currently is co-authoring a textbook, *Symbols, Selves, and Social Life: A Symbolic Interactionist Approach*, for Roxbury Publishing Company.

Sally A. Shumaker is professor and section head of social science and health policy at Wake Forest University, Baptist Medical Center. In recent years, she has served as president of the American Psychological Association's Society for the Psychological Study of Social Issues. Her interests include women's health.

Teresa Rust Smith is research associate of social science and health policy at Wake Forest University, Baptist Medical Center. Her interests include the politics of women's health.

Anselm L. Strauss was late of the University of California, San Francisco where he was professor emeritus of social and behavioral sciences. His many publications include *Mirrors and Masks, Qualitative Analysis for Social Scientists, Continual Permutations of Actions*, and co-authored works, *Awareness of Dying, Time for Dying, The Discovery of Grounded Theory, The Social Organization of Medical Work*, and *Basics of Qualitative Research*. He received career awards from the Society for the Study of Symbolic Interaction and the American Sociological Association's sections on Medical Sociology and Social Psychology.

Andrea Kidd Taylor received her doctorate in public health from The Johns Hopkins University and has since been working on staff at United Auto Worker's Health and Safety in Detroit, Michigan, as an industrial hygienist and occupational health policy consultant. She edits the UAW Health and Safety Newsletter and is a member of the Presidential Advisory Committee on Gulf War Veterans Illness and the National Advisory Committee on Occupational Safety and Health.

Alexandra Dundas Todd is professor and chair of sociology at Suffolk University in Boston. She has written extensively on health care in America, particularly on women's health and complementary medicines. Her works include: *Intimate Adversaries: Cultural Conflict Between Doctors and Women Patients* and *Double Vision: An East–West Collaboration for Coping With Cancer.*

Lois M. Verbrugge is at the Institute of Gerontology, University of Michigan. She has published widely in epidemiology. She has conducted ground-breaking research on gender differences in health and illness. Her interests include demography, disability and physical functioning in later life, and aging.

Howard Waitzkin is professor and director of the division of community medicine at the University of New Mexico. His current research focuses on how medical discourse mediates social problems related to gender, work, aging, and migration. He also studies mental health problems in primary care and health and policy issues such as access to health care and proposals for a national health program. He is co-author of *The Exploitation of Illness in a Capitalist Society* and author of *The Politics of Medical Encounters: How Patients and Doctors Deal with Social Problems.*

Rose Weitz is professor of sociology at Arizona State University and a founding member of the Sociologists' AIDS Network. She has recently served as president of Sociologists for Women in Society and has written an important textbook in medical sociology, *The Sociology of Health, Illness, and Health Care: A Critical Approach.*

Constance Williams is instructor in medicine and attending physician in geriatrics and extended care at Harvard Medical School. Her current research interests include communication between doctors and elderly patients and automobile driving behavior.

David R. Williams is associate research scientist at the Institute for Social Research at the University of Michigan. He has published widely in medical sociology in the epidemiology of race and social class differences in incidence of disease. His areas of interest also include religion, social psychology, and mental health.

Steffie Woolhandler practices and teaches medicine at the Cambridge Hospital/Harvard Medical School. She and David Himmelstein are co-founders of Physicians for a National Health Program and authors of the *National Health Program Book.*

William C. Yoels is professor of sociology at the University of Alabama, Birmingham. His interests include social psychology, urban sociology, aging, medical sociology, and rehabilitation. He has co-authored second editions of *Being Urban, Experiencing the Life Cycle, and Sociology in Everyday Life.*

Robert Zussman is associate professor of sociology at the University of Massachusetts, Amherst. His interests include cultural sociology, medical sociology, and work and labor markets. His book, *Intensive Care*, from which his selection is excerpted, won an award from the Medical Sociology Section of the American Sociological Association. ✦

Introduction

Medical sociology, or as it is also known, the sociology of health and illness, has grown and developed into a vibrant specialty since its beginnings almost five decades ago. In its early days, the field was primarily concerned with studying social organization of care, illness behavior, and empirical investigation of questions for which physicians needed answers. Much of the thrust of medical sociology consisted of a sociology *in* medicine rather than a sociology *of* medicine (Straus 1957). Physicians defined the research problems for sociologists to investigate, rather than sociologists taking the institution of medicine and its participants as research problems to study. Since then, the field has developed solid analytic and critical emphases as well. The analytic emphasis has contributed sociological concepts to the wider discipline and has been drawn upon to develop ideas and insights within medical sociology. The critical emphasis has brought medical sociology into the policy arena to critique, to consult with policymakers, and to recast and reform medical care. In addition, medical sociology has gradually widened to consider health and illness more broadly than its earlier overriding focus on the institution of medicine. In medical sociology as well as in medical care, people with illnesses received limited direct attention. Thus, for several decades, medical sociology developed as a sociology of medical care. Broadening the field to consider what health and illness mean to various participants has brought medical sociologists out of hospitals and into community clinics and homes. Experiences of health and illness in varied contexts emerge as major themes.

The sociological study of health and illness makes four central assumptions: (1) understanding health and illness requires more than biological knowledge; (2) health, illness, and healing occur within social, political, economic, and cultural structures; (3) the institution and practices of medicine themselves must be taken as objects of inquiry and critique; and (4) studying health and illness means examining the institution of medicine *and* going beyond it. Increasingly, sociologists attempt to situate issues in health care in complex social contexts in which they occur. Our anthology furthers this direction with a new twist: we examine the effects of society and social context upon the self.

Our anthology contains a wide range of works highlighting both the subjective and structural aspects of health and health care—from the microlevel perspective (self and interaction, e.g., self-awareness, self-concept, identity, individual action, interpersonal communication), the mesolevel perspective (organizational, e.g., health practitioner training, medical organizations), and the macrolevel perspective (social-structural, e.g., differences between populations, social institutions, health policy) (Brown 1995). Topics include those traditionally meaningful to medical sociologists, experiences of illness and health—an area of increasing significance over the past decade—and concerns about ethical issues and policy directions for health care.

Stories of the self in both personal narratives and in research studies illustrate how social policies and practices are played out in the lives of individuals and, in turn, how these individuals sometimes ignore, circumvent, or adapt policies and practices to fit their lives. These stories show that both patients and practitioners simultaneously are acted upon by institutional forces and are creators of their actions. By studying these stories, we widen the focus of what constitutes sociological understanding of health, illness, and healing. We situate the individual in macrosocial issues that shape medical care today, including ethical dilemmas and policy implications. Our collection locates individual experiences of health, illness, and healing within social and institutional structures. Political and organizational policies and practices define legitimate illness and appropriate treatment. These definitions directly affect individuals. Their distress may or may not fit into neat categories; institutional treatments and definitions may not validate personal experiences. Individuals' beliefs about prevention and treatment may neither be taken seriously nor acted upon. The rhythms and reasons of institutionalized practices usurp much of the individual's choice when one's very existence is contingent upon them.

The growing literature on the experience of illness is only beginning to be covered in textbooks. Our book provides more extensive coverage of this experience than other collections. In the past, the study of health and illness focused on providers and organizations, not on those for whom health and illness was immediately crucial—people who have illnesses. These persons came into sociological view only when they were patients. Issues of health and illness transcend institutionalized medicine. People are patients for only a small part of their experience with illness. As chronic illness continues to dominate the demand for medical care, the face of health and

illness changes, even if the model of how to give care does not.

We recognize the power that practitioners often have—or take—over patients. However, visible power should not obscure less visible determining forces over the type, extent, and quality of services. Power descends through the medical hierarchy but in the United States, as in many countries, physicians no longer reside at the top of it. A private entrepreneurial structure of care with considerable physician autonomy has been replaced by corporate management. Both patients and physicians are now managed. Like other practitioners, physicians have become hired hands. The medical system circumscribes practitioners' careers and care, and, likely, their commitments. Corporate ownership has resulted in explicit measures to increase profit and to reduce costs. National health services in other countries, likewise, seek ways of cutting their health service expenditures and, thus, attend to how U.S. corporations effect cuts.

At a time when individualism flourishes, empathy wanes, and the social contract between society and citizen shrinks, issues in health care take on new resonance. The social context grows even more complex when we add current medical trends to the mix: unprecedented numbers of individuals with chronic illness, the rising spectra of uncontrolled acute illness, and the reliance of sophisticated medical technology to preserve lives of frail individuals and to extend the dying process. Failure to enact legislated reorganization does not make the pressing questions of health care organization and coverage go away. Rather, problems escalate as corporations define and provide care according to cost incentives and management priorities, not the needs of people who seek care. However, most individuals remain unaware of how health policies and practices affect them until they or a family member needs help. The sociological examination of health and illness that connects self with society makes hidden policies and practices visible.

We have planned a textbook that reflects recent developments in health and illness and have designed the book specifically for teaching and learning. This volume can be adopted in medical sociology courses as well as in courses taught by medical sociologists in other disciplines and professions. It includes new areas in medical sociology—personal definitions of health and illness, the sociology of suffering, the sociology of the body, and bioethics—and devotes a section to the study of Acquired Immunodeficiency Syndrome (AIDS). Our text starts most sections with topics and dilemmas students can respond to and takes them into issues that define the field, rather than merely characterizing the field as medical sociologists know it. We offer students succinct guides for thinking about each chapter and discussion questions to elicit their personal understandings and views of the material. Thus, we aim to bridge concerns and experiences that will involve students with larger research problems of sociological study, such as learning the rules of doctoring, facing financial devastation as a result of illness, struggling through complex decisions about health, and dying of AIDS.

Personal accounts reveal how these problems concretely affect individual life. In this sense, the personal accounts and research reports throughout the book make issues in health care empirically real as well as point to their relevance to macrosocial policies and practices. These accounts demonstrate the ethical issues of practitioners and patients. They highlight dilemmas and problems. Structural issues can no longer be taken for granted. Advanced technologies present new dilemmas for the human condition and for policymakers. Our selections uncover contemporary problems beneath the surface of changes in medical organization and technologies.

Having students understand the experience of illness lays the ground work for building awareness of its significance for defining care and policy. This anthology offers structure and exemplification within a single text. The section on AIDS not only emphasizes a pressing social issue but sheds light on arguments in previous sections. Personal struggles, interpersonal negotiations, institutional definitions, organizational constraints, and political battles are highlighted and woven together in this section.

Our volume brings together a series of interesting and accessible selections about health and illness in the contemporary United States and other industrialized countries. It introduces students to sociological perspectives of illness experiences, health care training, comparative systems, alternative definitions and practices, and critical issues in medicine and policy. Our selections are recent and complement other works in the field with which these readings can be used. These readings provide varied sources of data, theoretical perspectives, and points of view for considering issues of illness and health care. A focus on the self in social contexts emphasizes the emergent character of health, illness, and healing. It underscores the serious issues that face ill persons, practitioners, organizations, and policymakers. The links between practitioners and organizations, persons and political processes, and the problems and progress developing out of these links appear as we begin to recognize the experience of self in social context and society.

References

Phil Brown. 1995. "Naming and Framing: The Social Construction of Diagnosis and Illness." *Journal of Health and Social Behavior* (extra issue):34-52.

Robert Straus. 1957. "The Nature and Status of Medical Sociology." *American Sociological Review.* 22:200-204. ✦

Section 1

Defining Health and Illness

When we are well, few of us wake up in the morning and think about our health. Each of us variably attends to health by our hygiene practices, exercise routines, and eating habits. However, our bodies mostly get our concern when we are ill. Individuals and social groups struggle with what health and illness mean. Social movements form to draw attention to, deflect attention from, or change the definitions of health and illness. In addition, various types of organizations and governments grapple with understanding health and illness to manage resources.

According to the 1947 World Health Organization (WHO) definition, "health is a state of complete physical, mental, and social well-being and not merely the absence of disease or infirmity" (Callahan 1990: 34). The United Nations developed the WHO in 1946 to address global issues relevant to health and illness. Yet the WHO operates under a definition of health that some policy makers and administrators argue is much too broad (1) to specify a pattern of resource distribution and (2) to manage individual or social agency for implementing strategies and paradigms for treatment (Doyal 1995). Such a broad definition means looking to various arenas where health, healing, and illness are negotiated—countries, governments, organizations, physician's offices, homes, and with the self. The selections in this section discuss general contexts of negotiation for defining

health and illness; they establish a framework for considering the emergent character of health and illness. Through these readings, we see that health and illness are not steady states; their qualities unfold in social arbitration.

Characterizing health and illness requires attention to competing realms of definition. At the individual level, well-being and sickness affect self-conceptions. Here, personal definitions may be easier to incorporate into one's self-concept than those imposed from external sources like medical professionals or family. Alternatively, imposed labels may ease the tension and frustration that come with an undefined problem. Health and illness also acquire meaning in interactional encounters between health care providers and patients; between patients and their families, broadly construed; between patients and organizations; and among patients, families, professionals, and organizations. In interactional encounters, definitions may depend a great deal on patterns of communication (Waitzkin 1991) and strategies for identity management (Goffman 1963). They may also depend on social locational factors like age, race, gender, and social class. Encounters connect micro-aspects of interaction with organizational realities of health and illness. Organizational definitions affect understandings of health and illness. Organizations can be institutions or social movement groups, collectivities of individuals band together to promote or to change codes of conduct, medical and social standards, and imagined courses of action. The "how's," "who's," and "what's" of health care often gain legitimacy when framed by organizational structures and standards.

Organizational standards, interactional encounters, and self-conception evolve from and create cultural ideologies of health, healing, and illness. Threads that connect self, encounters, and organizations make up the social fabric of health and health care. Yet these patterns often arise out of a limited set of possibilities determined by the economic and political circumstances of a society, social group, or individual. As you read through these selections, consider the threads that form the cultural fabric of illness and health. Think about how health and illness become defined: Who or what is the target of definition? Who does the defining? What are the factors critical to definition? What are the consequences definitions for individual selves? For social groups? For social constructions of illness and care? For what might come to constitute cultural and global standards for health and illness?

A selection by David Mechanic introduces this section. As Mechanic aptly points out, defining health and illness is difficult. Is health the absence of illness or is it the presence of a specific set of capacities? Who decides? Sociologists and others examining health and illness generally emphasize illness behaviors in their studies of health and healing. They investigate how definitions and perceptions of illness affect treatment availability and outcomes. The boundary between conceiving of one's self as healthy or ill is a fuzzy one. It requires incorporation of or reconciliation with outside definitions of self. Alan Radley and Michael Billig illustrate the complexities of self definition and health. They show how definitions of self and health are inherently linked, and how they are both inherently social. What health is emerges out of a variety of perceptions and situations, of organizational and social constraints. Michael Goldstein describes some macro-social forces that frame micro-interactions about health and illness. He identifies factors related to competing definitions of situations

and the process of medicalization. Pervasive acceptance of scientific explanations of reality influences individual and social group life. We see this most vividly with medicalization. Medicalization involves the application of a scientific, medical label to a particular social problem, as with drunk driving (Gusfield 1981), or to an individual behavior or concern, as in the case of hyperactivity or attention deficit disorder in children (Conrad and Schneider 1992).

Medicalization has even reached into the mundane aspects of everyday life and common biological processes. In the past century, medicalization of birth (Katz Rothman 1991; Martin 1992) and mental health (Barton 1987; Vallenstein 1986) transformed ordinary life circumstances to processes requiring medical intervention, and, in some cases, institutionalization. Until recently, the Diagnostic and Statistical Manual (DSM) characterized homosexuality as a psychiatric disorder (Bayer 1981). Pre-Menstrual Syndrome (PMS) (Johnson 1987), hyper-activity (Conrad and Schneider 1992), and post traumatic stress have recently evolved as disorders. Radical movements against medicalization charge medically-based definitions of behavior as means for socially controlling populations (Szasz 1970). Yet counter evidence suggests that access to care necessitates medicalization, as with chronic fatigue syndrome and post-traumatic stress disorder. Organizational and cultural battles persist over how to define life circumstance, especially as resources become scarcer. There are tensions over when to define a phenomenon as illness, so that the people and groups afflicted by it get the attention they require—as in the cases of AIDS (Kayal 1993) and sick building syndrome—and when to fight for redefinition of illness categories—as are the concerns of disabilities movements (Shapiro 1993; Zola 1985) and women's health movements and education (Amos 1993).

Although medicalization may provide access to valued and scarce resources for treatment, medical labels operate as powerful means of social control (Fox 1977; Riessman 1983). Access in one venue may mean denial of resources in another. Medical labels affect what insurance companies will pay for and what health organizations will allow health care providers to treat and how. They affect other realms of activity—legal justifications, family life, occupational opportunities—and definitions of self. Simultaneously, seemingly private issues of health and illness can get translated into public issues for the social good. Health promotion campaigns include advertisements and widespread arguments about what "ought to be" a standard for communities. Deborah Lupton examines the cultural consequences of medicalization in the public realm through health promotion campaigns. Policy makers, health care providers, and individuals learn to value particular health behaviors because these behaviors reduce the risks and costs of care. Contemporary debates about healthy behavior have translated the discretionary judgment of individuals into public mandate. Global application of public health standards, rather than health behavior patterns as individual choice, raises concern. We see this most particularly with smoking (Daykin 1993; Mullen 1987) and pregnancy (Petchesky 1987). Lupton raises the interesting question of just how far we should go in imposing a standard of health for the public good.

As we consider global definitions of health and illness for the purposes of characterizing individual care, describing organizational patterns of treatment, and outlining social values, we need also give thought to the complexities that even the broadest of definitions cannot address: the webs of connection and conflict between selves, social contexts, and societies.

References

A. Amos. 1993. "In Her Own Best Interests? Women in Health Education: A Review of the Last Fifty Years." *Health Education Journal*. 52(3): 141-150.

Walter E. Barton. 1987. *The History and the Influence of the American Psychiatric Association*. Washington, D.C.: American Psychiatric Press.

Ronald Bayer. 1981. *Homosexuality and American Psychiatry: The Politics of Diagnosis*. New York: Basic Books.

Daniel Callahan. 1990. *What Kind of Life: The Limits of Medical Progress*. Washington, D.C.: Georgetown University Press.

Peter Conrad and Joseph W. Schneider. 1992. *Deviance and Medicalization: From Badness to Sickness*. Philadelphia: Temple University Press.

N. Daykin. 1993. "Young Women and Smoking: Towards a Sociological Account." *Health Promotion International*. 8(2): 95-102.

Leslie Doyal. 1995. *What Makes Women Sick?: Gender and the Political Economy of Health*. Boston: South End Press.

Renee C. Fox. 1977. "The Medicalization and Demedicalization of American Society." *Daedalus*. 106: 9-22.

Erving Goffman. 1963. *Stigma: Notes on the Management of a Spoiled Identity*. New York: Prentice-Hall.

Joseph R. Gusfield. 1981. *The Culture of Public Problems: Drinking, Driving, and the Symbolic Order*. Chicago: University of Chicago Press.

Thomas M. Johnson. 1987. "Premenstrual Syndrome as a Western Culture-specific Disorder." *Culture, Medicine, and Psychiatry*. 11: 337-56.

Philip Kayal. 1993. *Bearing Witness: Gay Men's Health Crisis and the Politics of AIDS*. San Francisco: Westview Press.

Emily Martin. 1992. *The Woman in the Body: A Cultural Analysis of Reproduction*. Boston: Beacon Press.

Kenneth Mullen. 1987. "The Beliefs and Attitudes of a Group of Men in Mid-life Towards Tobacco Use." *Drug and Alcohol Dependence*. 20(3): 235-46.

Roselyn P. Pechesky. 1987. "Foetal Images: The Power of Visual Culture in the Politics of Reproduction." In M. Stansworth (ed.), *Reproductive Technologies: Gender, Motherhood, and Medicine*. Cambridge: Polity Press, pp. 57-80.

Catherine Kohler Riessman. 1983. "Women and Medicalization: A New Perspective." *Social Policy*. 14: 3-18.

Barbara Katz Rothman. 1991. *In Labor: Women and Power in the Birthplace*. New York: W.W. Norton.

Joseph P. Shapiro. 1993. *No Pity: People With Disabilities Forging a New Civil Rights Movement*. New York: Random.

Thomas Szasz. 1970. *Ideology and Insanity: Essays on the Psychiatric Dehumanization of Man*. New York: Doubleday.

Elliot Vallenstein. 1986. "Great and Desperate Cures: The Rise and Decline of Psychosurgery and Other Radical Treatments for Mental Illness." New York: Basic Books Inc.

Howard Waitzkin. 1991. *The Politics of Medical Encounters: How Patients and Doctors Deal With Social Problems*. New Haven: Yale University Press.

Irving K. Zola. 1985. "Depictions of Disability—Metaphor, Message and Medium in the Media: A Research and Political Agenda." *Social Science and Medicine*. 22: 5-17. ✦

The Problematics of Defining Health: Dilemmas and Decisions

1

Conceptions of Health

David Mechanic

What *counts as health? Do we recognize it only in its absence? To understand health, sociologists, epidemiologists, health service researchers, and, most particularly, medical professionals focus on illness behaviors. Still, illness, like health, is variable. Some seek help or self-treat what might appear to be minor symptoms. Others consider very few symptoms as worthy of treatment. David Mechanic points out that paths to defining illness and health are not entirely clear for patients, providers, or systems of care. Health and illness are not independent states; treatment is rarely absolute. Physicians and other health care providers struggle with many uncertainties. Patients harbor hidden agendas and undisclosed concerns. Definitions must be negotiated—with self and with medical workers in a variety of contexts. All make definitions and decisions about healing precarious.*

As you read through this selection, consider how definitions of health and illness have changed for individuals over the past few years. How might these definitions change over the life course? Subjective perceptions of health and illness states profoundly affect treatment outcomes. As you will see in the upcoming sections, epidemiological studies show varying rates of illness among different groups of people. Consider how factors like gender, class, race, and socioeconomic status affect personal definitions of health and risk of illness. Think critically about the link Mechanic provides between microconceptions of health and macrosocial structural factors.

Epidemiological studies demonstrate, in contrast, that most people have symptoms most of the time but normalize or deny them. Indeed, acute symptoms are so ubiquitous that they are impossible to measure reliably and, thus, statistical agencies will usually only count such symptoms if the respondent actually took some action in response such as self-medication or bed rest (Mechanic and Newton 1965).

In one of the classic papers in the health services field, White, Williams, and Greenberg (1961) calculated monthly prevalence and help-seeking rates from morbidity surveys in the United States and the United Kingdom. They estimated that in any given month three quarters of the population had one or more illnesses or injuries sufficiently salient to take some action. Only one in four in the population in any month sought physician care, and not all these were necessarily symptomatic. Moreover, studies of patients' presenting complaints show great overlap with untreated symptoms in the general population. Once these facts are clear, it becomes essential to inquire why patients have chosen to present their symptoms to the medical care system at the time they do, and what differentiates them from people with comparable symptoms who do not seek assistance (Balint 1957). Asking such questions about how people select themselves from a population at risk into care constitutes one aspect of the study of illness behavior, the processes in recognizing, defining, and making attributions about illness, and what to do about it (Mechanic 1986a).

Doctors of first contact see many of the same problems commonly occurring in the population, and as Kerr White observed some years ago, almost half of the patients seen at first contact may have such vague and ambiguous presentations that they cannot be given a diagnosis that fits categories covered by the International Classification of Disease (White 1970). A substantial proportion of these patients are also depressed, anxious, and fatigued, although estimates vary wildly contingent on definition and on how such assessments are made. While there are disagreements on the precise figures, there is no disagreement that most medical problems occur in a social context complicated by issues of class, race, gender, work, family, and community ties.

Physicians throughout the world are taught to approach patients through a diagnostic process in which they elicit the chief complaint, the characteristics of the present illness, past history, and family and socially relevant factors. They then are taught to do a systems review, physical examination, and other necessary investigations leading to a diagnosis (Waitzkin 1991:25-31). They pursue this process selectively, searching for a pattern that fits preconceived disease theories. Unfortunately, the route is almost never clear in advance. Deciding about the use of tests or therapeutic approaches requires unstructured problem-solving because the physician is often working at the fuzzy boundaries of medical knowledge (p. 60).

At any point in time, the practice of medicine is a mixture of theories at varying levels of confirmation and a variety of social judgements and prejudices (Mechanic 1978). Physicians seek to identify patterns of symptoms that imply definable disorder, and if they do

so successfully, and the disease theory is relatively firm, they gain abundant information on likely course and etiology and guidance for how to proceed in treatment. Physician roles substantially transcend the corpus of medical knowledge, and both patients and the societies of which they are part demand that doctors provide assistance even when knowledge is limited.

Much disease and its course are influenced by social and environmental factors, but medical practices tend to personalize such influences by focusing on their individual manifestations and consequences typically divorced from broader implications. Why this particular emphasis evolved historically may seem natural to us, but it was neither self-evident nor inevitable and it is even arguable that the approach is particularly well-fitted to much of the morbidity that doctors now treat. As Waitzkin notes,

> That this particular format should have arisen is remarkable partly because its effectiveness in improving medical conditions remains unproven. Like many other aspect of modern medicine the beneficial impact of the format on the morbidity and mortality of large populations, as well as on individual patients, is difficult or impossible to demonstrate. . . . Many of the medical encounter's most time-consuming and thus costly components . . . have never been put to the test of cost-effectiveness. . . . Why has the medical encounter's traditional format received such wide and unquestioning acceptance that it is now essentially a sacred cow? (Waitzkin 1991:33)

Waitzkin, in a contextual analysis of a sample of doctor-patient contacts, observed the numerous ways in which doctors, explicitly or inadvertently, exercised social controls as they acted on traditional ideologies relating to family, work, appropriate behavior, age expectations, and the like. As he notes,

> Through messages of ideology and social control, and through the lack of contextual criticism, health professionals subtly direct patients' actions to conform with society's dominant expectations about appropriate behavior. . . . Doctor-patient encounters become micropolitical situations that reflect and support broader

social relations, including social class and political-economic power. The participants in these encounters seldom recognize their micropolitical situation on a conscious level. (Pp. 8-9)

In the primary medical care literature, much attention is focused on the idea of the patient's hidden agenda—the "real" reason for the consultation that becomes apparent late in the transaction, if at all (Balint 1957). An alternative to the traditional approach is to give patients greater latitude to tell their stories and to explain what they expect and hope for from the encounter. As Waitzkin notes, "Most practitioners would acknowledge that the tendencies to interrupt, cut off, or otherwise redirect the patient's story during the PI [evaluation of present illness] derive at least partly from the drive to make a diagnosis. That is, a doctor wants to hear those words that are consistent with previously defined diagnostic categories. Parts of patients' stories that do not fit neatly into these categories function as unwanted strangers in medical discourse" (p. 32).

As patterns of disease have changed, and as medicine is more concerned with chronic and degenerative diseases and behavior patterns associated with morbidity, it is appropriate to re-examine optimal approaches to identifying the real problem and alternative management strategies. Such an approach, unlike the dominant medical model, makes values and moral issues more salient. The fact that they are at present implicit in most situations makes them no less important.

In many encounters a negotiation process goes on in which doctor and patient agree to focus on one or another aspect of the problem in a way that may help bring the problem into congruence with an intelligible medical definition. But things are not always easy, and despite concerted efforts to identify a meaningful problem formulation, the doctor may fail to arrive at any hypothesis that fits. Physicians get frustrated with persistent and demanding patients who pose such ambiguities and label them as neurotic, "worried wells," "hypochondriacs," or "crocks." The failure to locate a suitable hypothesis may tell us as much about the physician's models and approaches as it does about the illness behavior

of the patient, but the failure is usually externalized and in an invidious way. When confirmed medical models don't fit, one gets a heavy dose of social judgment often disguised as diagnosis. The characteristic intermixture of clinical observations with judgmental ones makes it almost impossible to separate social from technical clinical norms.

Alternative Paradigms to the Dominant Medical Model

The dominant concept of disease and the medical process of diagnostic inquiry focused on the individual, in contrast to broader systems, is not inevitable or necessarily the most efficient or effective way of promoting individual health. Diagnosticians of first contact exist in every culture because people seek a place to bring difficult problems for which they seek relief, hope, and reassurance. But the point of clinical intervention is a peculiar vantage point for viewing the production of health and disease.

At the level of populations, the notion is now commonplace that health is shaped by the material and environmental conditions of life and by the sociocultural structures that people create as much as by their genes and individual health behavior. Much of positive or damaging health-relevant behaviors arise from the routine activities and conventional patterns of everyday life, only modestly influenced by health-relevant considerations (Mechanic 1990). The flow of health outcomes from routine processes is pervasive and powerful. The instruments to promote health, thus, are quite varied, including tax policies and other financial incentives, regulation, skillful use of mass media and education. Possibilities include social policies regulating environmental and workplace risk exposures; distribution, labeling, and regulation of food, drugs, and other commodities; controls over smoking, drinking, and other high-risk behaviors; highway construction and road and vehicle safety systems; and inducements for exercise, community participation, and social integration.

Focus on the personal level reflects in part the individualistic bias of Western culture, As concern with promoting health has grown, the emphasis has overwhelmingly been on personal health habits in contrast to other levels of intervention. In considering policy options, there are at least four major possible trade-offs: between macro nonhealth interventions that promote health (education, community empowerment and mobilization, social integration, inducing personal efficacy) and more direct health initiatives; between public health efforts and general medical care; between individual preventive versus curative foci; and between primary care and more specialized types of interventions. Most resource investment in the U.S. system is inversely related to the spheres of action most likely to have the largest impact on population health.

The Idea of Health

Our thinking is enriched by the perspectives of René Dubos, a microbiologist and discoverer of the first commercially produced antibiotics. Dubos, seeking an enzyme to decompose the envelope protecting bacteria causing lobar pneumonia, turned his attention to the study of swamp soil where he began developing his appreciation for the richness of natural variability and its effects on the development of organisms. As he pursued his studies, Dubos became convinced that the "prevalence and severity of microbial diseases are conditioned more by the ways of life of the persons afflicted than by the virulence and other properties of the etiological agents" (Dubos 1965).

As Dubos engaged the study of disease and environment and the extraordinary adaptiveness of organisms to changing conditions, he became critical of exaggerated claims about the effectiveness of solving health problems solely through medicine. While himself an eminent medical scientist, he understood that health cannot be an absolute or permanent value, however careful the social and medical planning. As he eloquently explained, "Biological success in all its manifestations is a measure of fitness, and fitness requires never-ending efforts of adaptation to the total environment which is ever changing" (Dubos 1959).

There have been numerous efforts to define health both in general and psychological terms. Marie Jahoda (1958) for example, identified six primary themes recurring in definitions of positive mental health, such as positive attitudes toward self, integration of personality, autonomy, and environmental mastery. The difficulty is the lack of specificity in these criteria and their dependence on social values and social judgments that may vary widely by culture and social context. As she herself noted, "There is hardly a term in current psychological thought as vague, elusive and ambiguous as the term 'mental health' "(Jahoda 1958). Yet the effort to study health as a global concept, whatever its difficulties, is not a fool's mission.

1. A number of important disease risk factors appear to have nonspecific effects on a wide range of disease conditions and mortality; these include broad factors such as socioeconomic status, social networks and supports, and stressful life events, as well as more specific patterns of behavior such as smoking, exercise, and intimate relations (Mechanic 1982a; Syme 1986). It is conceivable that as we learn more we will be able to account for most of these influences through specific processes linked to each disease, but the nonspecific effects are robust. Moreover, the more we learn about biological processes, the more evident it becomes that while models of specific disease syndromes are pragmatic and essential for advancements, the syndromes are related and not discrete.

2. Self-reports of health status and subjective health assessments are among the best general predictors of mortality, morbidity, and use of medical care services (Ware 1986). Various studies have found that such subjective assessments are not only significantly related to objective indicators such as physician assessments, medical record data, and mortality (LaRue et al. 1979; Ferraro 1980; Eisen et al. 1980; Fillenbaum 1979), but are independent predictors of mortality controlling for objective assessments of health and known risk factors (Mossey and Shapiro 1982; Kaplan and Camacho 1983). Mossey and Shapiro (1982), in studying 3,128 noninstitutionalized elderly people, found a threefold difference in mortality over six years be-

tween those rating their health excellent and those rating it poor, which persisted when controlled for age, sex, residence, and health status indicators. Similarly, Kaplan and Camacho (1983), in a nine-year follow-up of a large California adult sample, found large differences in mortality associated with prior subjective assessments. These effects persist when controlled for baseline measures of health practices, social networks, health indicators, and psychological status. The superiority of such self-assessments over objective medical assessments is an intriguing puzzle. Idler (1992) reviewed six follow-up studies based on large probability samples that included baseline health self-assessments and objective health status measures allowing appropriate statistical analyses. These studies consistently show the influence of self-assessed health despite controls for objective health status measures.

3. There is good statistical evidence that persons can "will" their survival or death over short time spans, and that for these limited time intervals social events can be powerful predictors (Phillips and Feldman 1973; Phillips and King 1988). Moreover, relatively modest social interventions among elderly institutionalized populations show effects not only on well-being but even mortality. Langner and Rodin (1976) assessed an intervention that gave nursing home residents more choices in their everyday lives. Followup after eighteen months found that those in the intervention group experienced improved health as well as a marginal improvement in longevity relative to the comparison group (Rodin and Langner 1977; Rodin 1986).

4. There is substantial literature linking morbidity and mortality to patterns of industrialization, urbanization, migration, and acculturation (Dubos 1959, 1965; Grob 1983). Other powerful influences include schooling, patterns of marriage and divorce, religious and group affiliation, and community participation and employment patterns (Mechanic 1978, 1982a, 1988). Many of these data are either cross-sectional or aggregated in ways that make it impossible to differentiate cause and effect. But the literature in its totality is persuasive of the importance of depicting the role of broad processes by which

the measured end results occur, and of the crucial intervening variables.

The challenge to the investigator is to dissect these enormously complicated patterns in ways that retain the meaningfulness of the original observations but with rigorous research procedures and measurement that allow testing alternative explanations.

The predictive value of simple health perceptions is remarkable, but their meaning remains uncertain. A number of studies indicate that individuals in making assessments of health adopt a holistic frame of reference that is influenced by appraisals of their ability to function and the extent to which health decrements interfere (Mechanic 1978). Even when efforts are made to focus the individual's attention on the physical dimension of health, the rating reflects broader aspects of social function and not only measurable medical morbidity or lack of physical fitness. Furthermore, such assessments seem to be made typically in terms of some standard of comparison the respondent has in mind. For example, many studies have found that elderly respondents report more positive health assessments relative to objective indicators than younger adults (Maddox and Douglass 1973; Linn and Linn 1980; Friedsam and Martin 1963; Cockerham, Sharp, and Wilcox 1983). A number of researchers have suggested that elderly persons are health optimists, but this characterization simply renames rather than illuminates the issue. One possibility is that the elderly adjust their perceptions because of health expectations that have changed as they get older (Tornstam 1975). A negative consequence of such altered expectations is that individuals may neglect remediable problems because they associate such deficits with aging rather than with disease.

In one analysis, Richard Tessler and I (Tessler and Mechanic 1978) examined four diverse data sets to ascertain the relationship between various independent predictors and persons' perceptions of their own health. Included were samples of persons participating in alternative health insurance plans, a large sample of students at a major state university, a sample of men in a state prison, and a sample of persons aged forty-five to sixty-nine in a southern state. In this analysis we were concerned with factors predicting perceived health status, controlling for measures of actual health status. The need to have a measure of objective health status, as well as some other variables, directed the choice of data sets. The particular measures used for the analysis in each of the data sets are generally comparable, although they vary somewhat. It was our view, however, that the diversity of samples and variations in measures employed were an advantage in that if the same results emerge across data sets in spite of differences, we can have increased confidence in the generality of the basis processes under study.

In each data set the dependent variable is the respondent's assessment of his or her health status, and the independent predictors consist of (1) a measure of physical health status (in two data sets we had physician ratings, while in the other two we depended on reported measures of illness); (2) a measure of psychological distress; and (3) measures of age, marital status, sex, education, and race whenever they were applicable. The main concern of the analysis was to assess the degree to which psychological distress influenced people's perceptions of their health, taking into account both sociodemographic factors and some measure of "objective physical health."

For each data set we constructed a multiple regression equation in which perceived health status was regressed simultaneously against the other variables. Psychological distress was the only variable other than the measure of physical health status that retained a statistically significant standardized beta coefficient in all four data sets. As we expected, physical health status had a larger influence on perceived health than psychological distress, although this was not true in the case of the prison sample, and the betas in the sample of older people for the two predictors were fairly close. It is worthy of note, however, that the measures of physical health status made by physicians were less powerful than those based on respondent reports of illness, suggesting that the latter are influenced by a certain degree of respondent subjectivity. This finding supported our basic contention that subjective reports of illness already reflect to some extent the psychological state of the person providing the data (Mechanic 1979).

I view the self-assessment of health as an active process involving cognitive and emotional strategies typically used in assessing the self. Thus, physical symptoms are only one of the many building blocks in forming this conception. Particular symptoms may be given prominence or may be defined as peripheral to the person's judgments of self and health. The fact that young people have little serious morbidity (Haggerty 1983) provided an opportunity to examine the constituents of health appraisals in a sample of 1,193 adolescents using longitudinal data (Mechanic and Hansell 1987). If serious illness is not a major constituent of the self-appraisal, how then do young people with little chronic disease or serious morbidity form a self-appraisal of their health? In this instance we predicted that psychological well-being and competence in age-relevant areas would shape such self-conceptions.

We indeed found that adolescents who reported higher levels of school achievement and more participation in sports and other exercise assessed their health as better over a one-year period than those reporting lower achievement and less participation, controlling for self-assessed health at the beginning of the year. Other longitudinal results showed that adolescents who were initially less depressed assessed their health more positively. Our measure of common physical symptoms was associated cross-sectionally with self-assessed health, but its longitudinal effect was mediated by initial levels of self-assessed health. In short, for these adolescents health is truly a social concept that reflects psychological well-being and competence in age-appropriate activities. If we form conceptions about ourselves by observing our own behavior as Bem (1972) has suggested, then adolescents may conclude they are healthy in part because they are active and competent. Having only limited physiological feedback, they may depend on judgments of their competence and activity to appraise themselves.

If health appraisals develop in this way it becomes easier to understand why patients' presentations to physicians intermix physical symptoms, psychological distress, and psychosocial difficulties. Physicians are trained to apply a disease model that seeks discrete infirmities but patients do not typically respond to their health problems in accord with medical models. Understanding the source of these discordant definitions and how patients' conceptions are formed provides new opportunities for medical care interventions.

Illness Behavior

The study of illness behavior seeks to identify the sociocultural, psychological, and situational determinants that make people aware of symptoms, the cognitive schemata they use to interpret them, and the ways the organization and financing of services facilitate or impede varying kinds of care seeking. Illness behavior helps shape the formation and course of illness. Illness often serves a variety of social and personal objectives that have little to do with biological systems or the pathogenesis of disease. The boundaries of illness and its definitions are extraordinarily broad, and the illness process can be used to negotiate a range of cultural, social, and personal tensions. Illness behavior is one of many alternatives for coping with personal and social tensions and conflict.

There is now an extensive literature on illness behavior (Mechanic 1978, 1982b, 1983; Kleinman 1986, 1988; McHugh and Vallis 1985), and sufficient familiarity with the concept to reduce a need for general elaboration. Here I focus on just a few points continuous with the preceding discussion on health status assessment. While we take knowing about how our body feels as self-evident, such judgments are difficult because of the absence of objective guides to which we can compare our internal experiences. Because of the absence of standards, people look to their environment or popular theories for a reasonable accounting of their experiences (Leventhal 1985). People generally believe that stress elevates blood pressure, for example, and thus, hypertensives commonly believe that their blood pressure is high when they are under stress and adapt their medications accordingly. Expecting a relation between medication and symptom change, patients typically reduce prescribed medication as symptoms abate. Medication adherence requires overcoming commonly understood popular models of cause and effect.

Very popular theories are so widely shared that both patient and doctor understand the premises upon which judgments are being made. But in many instances there are no commonly accepted conceptions, or the illness models people use are influenced by subcultures or are idiosyncratic. Thus practitioners must explore the attributions and theories that help guide the patient's responses.

Illness behavior plays an intriguing role in pain response and disability, particularly in respect to back pain (Osterweis, Kleinman, and Mechanic 1987). Spitzer and Task Force (1986), in a Canadian study, found that less than 8 percent of patients complaining of back pain not supported by objective findings became chronic. We have no adequate models that can predict which of these patients will have self-limited conditions and who will become chronic. Illness behavior plays an important role, contributing to work absenteeism, use of medical services, and demands on the disability insurance system, but the precise factors, and how they influence outcomes, are difficult to specify.

There are a number of studies demonstrating that when depression occurs concurrently with acute disease, patients may attribute it to the acute disease symptoms associated with persistent depressed affect, thus prolonging the illness process (Imboden et al. 1959; Imboden et al. 1961). Such studies alert us to the fact that many patients may have difficulty interpreting the origin of symptoms when illnesses occur concomitantly. While much of the existing literature is based on the assumption that chronicity is in some sense motivated by secondary gain, the opportunities for confusion in symptom appraisal exist independently of the use of illness to achieve advantages not otherwise available.

In a study of back pain, we had an opportunity to analyze data from the United States Health and Nutrition Examination Survey (HANES) among a subsample of 2,431 respondents for whom we had both self-report data and findings from an extensive medical examination (Mechanic and Angel 1987). This allowed development of an index that depicted the extent to which reported back pain exceeded physical findings. As in other studies, we found that older patients and those reporting higher levels of psychological well-being were less likely to make invalidated complaints, controlling for age, sex, race, marital status, education, and income. Depressed mood was associated with both more complaints and more physical findings, suggesting that causal factors operated in both directions. Our most interesting finding was that the inclination of older persons to report less pain at comparable levels of physical status based on the examination was significant only among those with higher levels of psychological well-being. This supports the notion that subjective assessments of health are made in the context of comparing oneself to others. As people age, they may attribute some of their discomforts to the aging process and, thus, are more likely to normalize bodily discomforts. Persons who, in general, are experiencing a sense of well-being may feel they are doing well relative to their reference groups. Those with depressed mood are less likely to feel so.

The tendency of patients to view their health holistically, and not in terms of discrete categories, also complicates the way they seek help and express their complaints. The association between psychological and physical symptoms is widely recognized (Eastwood 1975), and psychiatric patients are large consumers of nonpsychiatric health services (Jones and Vischi 1979) relative to the population. In a study comparing a sample of psychiatric outpatients with a representative sample from the same population from which they came (Mechanic, Cleary, and Greenley 1982), we found that the psychiatric patients made 100 percent more nonpsychiatric medical care visits in the year prior to the study and 83 percent more in the year following than those in the representative sample.

There are a variety of possible explanations. One is that the excess visit rate is largely due to physical symptoms and dysfunction concomitant with psychiatric disorder. A second is that a higher propensity to seek help contributes to both becoming a psychiatric patient and to using general medical services. A third possibility is that once a person enters the psychiatric system, access to other services is easier. We developed measures that allowed us to compare the strength of these alternative explanations. Among them, the hypothesis dealing with concomitant symptoms explained the most variance, but illness behavior propensities were also important. These results suggest that patients are often unclear about the origins of their symptoms, or the appropriate attributions and help-seeking behavior. Nor are physicians always helpful in clarifying such issues.

Conclusion

The sources of health and disease in societies are broad and complex. Communities will have different rates and patterns of pathology, depending on demographic, economic and psychosocial influences that interact with the biological potentials and limitations of people (Mechanic 1986b, 1986c), and these patterns will be altered by changes in environmental ecology and social organization. The medical model offers a useful but limited perspective on the factors that affect the occurrence and course of disease and alternatives for prevention and control. The current AIDS crisis vividly reminds us of the influence of social organization and behavior on the transmission of disease and the role of social groupings and subcultures in its spread or control. From this perspective, the idea of health and its broad conceptualization is hardly unimportant. Definition and measurement are central to the challenge but to allow the easily measurable to guide our definitions of what is important and our research efforts would be exceedingly foolish.

References

Balint, M. 1957. *The Doctor, His Patient, and the Illness.* New York: International Universities Press.

Bem, D. 1972 "Self-perception theory." In Berkowitz, L. (ed.), *Advances in Experimental Social Psychology* 6. New York: Academic Press, 2-62.

Cockerham, W. C., Sharp, K., and Wilcox, J.A. 1983. "Aging and perceived health status." *Journal of Gerontology,* 38:349-55.

Dubos, R. 1965. *Man Adapting.* New Haven: Yale University Press.

———. 1959. *Mirage of Health: Utopias, Progress, and Biological Change.* New York: Harper.

Eastwood, M. R. 1975. *The Relation Between Physical and Mental Illness.* Toronto: University of Toronto Press.

Eisen, M., C. A. Donald, J. E. Ware Jr., and R. H. Brook. 1980. *Conceptualization and Measurement of Health for Children in the Health Insurance Study.* R-2312-HEW. Santa Monica, CA: Rand Corporation.

Ferraro, K. F. 1980. "Self-ratings of health among the old and the old-old." *Journal of Health and Social Behavior,* 21:377-83.

Fillenbaum, G. G. 1979. "Social context and self-assessment of health among the elderly." *Journal of Health and Social Behavior,* 20:45-51.

Friedsam, H. and H. W. Martin. 1963. "A comparison of self and physicians' ratings in an older population." *Journal of Health and Social Behavior,* 4:179-83.

Grob, G. 1983. "Disease and environment in American history." In D. Mechanic (ed.), *Handbook of Health, Health Care and the Health Professions.* New York: Free Press, 3-22.

Haggerty, R. 1983. "Epidemiology of childhood disease." In D. Mechanic (ed.), *Handbook of Health, Health Care, and the Health Professions.* New York: Free Press, 101-19.

Idler, E. 1992. "Self-assessed health in mortality: A review of studies." In S. Mares, H. Uventhal, and M. Johnson, M. (eds.), *International Review of Health Psychology.* New York: Wiley, 33-54.

Imboden, J. B., A. Canter, and L. E. Cluff. 1961. "Symptomatic recovery from medical disorder." *Journal of the American Medical Association,* 178:1182-84.

Imboden, J. B., A. Canter, L. E. Cluff, and R. W. Trever. 1959. "Brucellosis III: Psychologic aspects of delayed convalescent." *Archives of Internal Medicine,* 103:406-14.

Jahoda, M. 1958. *Current Concepts of Positive Mental Health.* New York: Basic Books.

Jones, K. and T. Vischi. 1979. "Impact of alcohol, drug abuse and mental health treatment on medical care utilization: A review of the research literature." *Medical Care,* 17:Supplement.

Kaplan, G. A. and T. Camacho. 1983. "Perceived health and mortality: A nine-year follow-up of the Human Population Laboratory cohort." *American Journal of Epidemiology,* 117:292-304.

Kleinman, A. 1988. *The Illness Narratives: Healing and the Human Condition.* New York: Basic Books.

———. 1986. *Social Origins of Distress and Disease: Depression, Neurasthenia and Pain in Modern China.* New Haven: Yale University Press.

Langner, E. J. and J. Rodin. 1976. "The effects of choice and enhanced personal responsibility for the aged: A field experience in an institutional setting." *Journal of Personality and Social Psychology,* 34:191-98.

Larue, A., L. Bank, L. Jarvik, and M. Hetland. 1979. "Health in old age: How do physicians' ratings and self-ratings compare?" *Journal of Gerontology,* 34:687-91.

Leventhal, H. 1985. "Symptoms reporting: A focus on process." In S. McHugh and T. M. Vallis, eds., *Illness Behavior: A Multidisciplinary Model.* New York: Plenum, 219-37.

Linn, B. S. and M. W. Linn. 1980. "Objective and self-assessed health in the old and the very old." *Social Science and Medicine,* 14:311-15.

Maddox, G. L. and E. B. Douglass. 1973. "Self-assessment of health: A longitudinal study of elderly subjects." *Journal of Health and Social Behavior,* 14:87-93.

McHugh, S. and T. M. Vallis. 1985. *Illness Behavior: A Multi-disciplinary Model.* New York: Plenum.

Mechanic, D. 1990. "Promoting Health," *Society,* 27:16-22.

———. 1988. "Social class and health status: An examination of underlying processes." *Conferences on Socio-economic Status and Health.* Palo Alto, CA: Henry J. Kaiser Family Foundation.

———. 1986a. "Illness behavior: An overview." In S. McHugh and T. M. Vallis (eds.), *Illness Behavior: A Multidisciplinary Model.* New York: Plenum, 101-09.

———. 1986b. "Some relationships between psychiatry and the social sciences." *British Journal of Psychiatry,* 149:548-53.

———. 1986c. "The role of social factors in health and well-being: The biopsychosocial model from a social perspective." *Integrative Psychiatry,* 4:2-11.

———. 1983. *Handbook of Health, Health Care, and the Health Professions.* New York: Free Press.

———. 1982a. "Disease, mortality, and the promotion of health." *Health Affairs,* 1:28-32.

———. 1979. "Correlates of physician utilization: Why do major multivariate studies of physical utilization find trivial psychosocial effects." *Journal of Health and Social Behavior,* 20:387-96.

——. 1978. *Medical Sociology: A Selective View,* 2d ed. New York: Free Press.

Mechanic, D. (ed.), 1982b. *Symptoms, Illness Behavior and Help-Seeking.* New Brunswick: Rutgers University Press.

Mechanic, D., and R. Angel. 1987. "Some factors associated with the report and evaluation of back pain." *Journal of Health and Social Behavior,* 28:131-39.

Mechanic, D. and S. Hansell. 1987. "Adolescent competence, psychological well-being and self-assessed physical health." *Journal of Health and Social Behavior,* 28:364-74.

Mechanic, D. and M. Newton. 1965. "Some problems in the analysis of morbidity data." *Journal of Chronic Diseases,* 18:569-80.

Mechanic, D., P. D. Cleary, and J. R. Greenley. 1982. "Distress syndromes, illness behavior, access to care and medical utilization in a defined population." *Medical Care,* 20:361-72.

Mossey, J. M. and C. Shapiro. 1982. "Self-rated health: A predictor of mortality among the elderly." *American Journal of Public Health,* 72:800-8.

Osterweis, M., A. Kleinman, and D. Mechanic (eds.). 1987. *Pain and Disability: Clinical, Behavioral and Policy Perspectives.* Committee on Pain, Disability and Chronic Illness Behavior, Institute of Medicine. Washington, D.C.: National Academy Press.

Phillips, D. and K. Feldman. 1973. "A dip in deaths before ceremonial occasions: Some new relationships between social integration and mortality." *American Sociology Review,* 38:678-96.

Phillips, D. and E. W. King. 1988. "Death takes a holiday, mortality surrounding major social occasions." *Lancet,* ii. 728-32.

Rodin, J. 1986. "Aging and health: Effects of the sense of control." *Science,* 233:1271-76.

Rodin, J. and Langner, E. J. 1977. "Long term effects of a control-relevant intervention with the institutionalized aged." *Journal of Personality and Social Psychology,* 35:897-902.

Spitzer, W. O. and Task Force. 1986. *Rapport du Groupe de Travail Quebecois sur les Aspects Cliniques des Affections Vertebrales Chez les Travailleurs.* Québec: L'Institute de Recherche en Santé et en Securité du Travail du Québec.

Syme, S. L. 1986. "Social determinants of health and disease." In Last, J. (ed.), *Maxcy-Rosenau Public Health, Health and Preventive Medicine,* 12th ed. Norwalk, CT: Appleton-Century-Crofts.

Tessler, R. C. and Mechanic, D. 1978. "Psychological Distress and Perceived Health Status." *Journal of Health and Social Behavior,* 19:254-62.

Tornstam, L. 1975. "Health and self-perception: A systems theoretical approach." *The Gerontologist,* 27:264-70.

Waitzkin, H. 1991. *The Politics of Medical Encounters: How Patients and Doctors Deal with Social Problems.* New Haven: Yale University Press.

Ware, J. E., Jr. 1986. "The assessment of health status." In L. H. Aiken and D. Mechanic. (eds.), *Applications of Social Science to Clinical Medicine and Social Policy.* New Brunswick: NJ: Rutgers University Press, 204-28.

White, K. 1970. "Evaluation of medical education and health care." In W. Lathem and A. Newberry (eds.), *Community Medicine: Research and Health Care.* New York: Appleton-Century-Crofts, 274.

White, K., F. Williams, and B. Greenberg. 1961. "The ecology of medical care." *New England Journal of Medicine,* 265:885-92.

Further Reading

David Mechanic. 1990. "Promoting Health." *Society* 27: 16-22.

Lois Verbrugge and Frank J. Ascione. 1987. "Exploring the Iceberg: Common Symptoms and How People Care for Them." *Medical Care,* 25: 539-569.

Howard Waitzkin. 1991. *The Politics of Medical Encounters: How Patients and Doctors Deal with Social Problems.* New Haven: Yale University Press.

Discussion Questions

1. What are some of the difficulties in defining health?

2. What is the difference between studying health and studying illness behaviors? How are definitions of health and illness linked?

3. What might changes in definitions in health mean for patients seeking care? for care providers? for systems of health care?

2

Accounts of Health and Illness: Dilemmas and Representations

Alan Radley
Michael Billig

Alan Radley and Michael Billig puncture the widely held assumption that people view their health as a state with discrete, relatively unchanging properties and talk about it accordingly. Instead, people construct their views of their health in relation to the identities they claim, the interactions in which they find themselves, and the social values they take for granted. People with chronic illness may attest to how healthy they are. People who are proclaimed healthy may avow that they are plagued with symptoms. Accounts of health and illness differ according to circumstances, intentions, and audiences. Health beliefs reflect more than individual experience. Views of health and illness are inherently social and ideological. By arguing that health beliefs are ideological, Radley and Billig contend that these beliefs rest on shared value judgments and value positions. Ideologies justify past actions and call for future actions. Health beliefs simultaneously reflect general themes within a culture and specific experiences, feelings, and intentions of the individual. People develop their health beliefs through social experience and adopt their group's collective representations of health beliefs and make them their own. Yet views of health and illness are taken for granted; people assume their views

represent the real, natural order of things. They make claims about health—theirs and others'. The "shoulds" and "oughts" enter in. What kind of health a person "should" have and how someone in a particular situation "ought" to feel are claims about identities and values. And these claims change as intentions and interactions change.

By looking at accounts, Radley and Billig try to offer a more dynamic view of health beliefs than either the sociological concept of social representations or the psychological concept of attitudes alone can offer. Both of these concepts become reified—treated as if fixed and stable. Such reification locks a process in time and separates it from actions that construct it and the contexts in which these actions occur. Radley and Billig urge us to look at health beliefs as accounts that arise in specific social, interactional, and experiential contexts, rather than as fixed and static objects. People draw upon social experience, and they form attitudes but they do so in response to circumstances and intentions. Both social experience and attitudes can change.

Just as accounts of health and illness differ with different intentions, they change with different images of self and others. Radley and Billig argue that these accounts are dilemmatic; people construct accounts that reflect the dilemmas they face. One-shot interviewing fosters eliciting the public account without the private dilemmas and personal concerns. The researcher's task is to go beyond the public account into the personal realm of experience. Look for how Radley and Billig juxtapose the research participant's claims to normality with the researchers'. Also think about their analysis of how people imbed public accounts in their private disclosures and insert private accounts in their public claims.

Introduction

What are individuals doing when talking about their state of health? This question forms the starting point for the present paper, which takes a fresh look at some of the issues underlying the area now commonly called 'health beliefs'. A simple answer to our opening question might be that people talk about their health in answer to inquiries about how they feel. As well as supplying information about the body, what they say also tells others about the status of the self. In this latter aspect, it is an account offered on particular occasions, a claim to be treated by others in a particular way. . . .

When researchers speak of health beliefs they usually refer to a number of issues: how people in general regard health matters as compared with medical practitioners (Blumhagen 1980), how ordinary people give lay accounts of their experiences of ill-health during their lifetime (Blaxter 1983, Williams 1990), how they think about avoiding disease (Herzlich 1973, Pill and Stott 1982) how they define health (Baumann 1961, Blaxter 1990), or how people in different sections of society hold different views about health matters (Blair 1993, Calnan 1987, d'Houtaud and Field 1984, Pierret 1993).

. . . We shall suggest that researchers shift their attention from 'beliefs' to 'accounts', in order to analyse what individuals say about health and illness. This is because people do not merely have health beliefs, as they might have eggs carried in a shopping basket. They also construct their state of health as part of their ongoing identity in relation to others, as something vital to the conduct of everyday life. This means that the accounts that are given of health and illness are more than a disclosing of a supposed internal attitude. In offering views, people are also making claims about themselves as worthy individuals, as more or less 'fit' participants in the activities of the social world. . . .

In consequence, people's health status should not be treated as a given, but attention should be paid to the ways in which they constantly construct or re-affirm their own health in different circumstances and in different relationships. In this sense, health and illness are 'imputed'. Moreover, the imputation of illness is rarely, if ever, merely an imputation of physical condition. Any shortfall in health has important implications for other areas of one's life (e.g. work, personal relationships), in terms of which people feel that they are evaluated. Accounts of health and illness are, therefore, more than descriptions of one's physical condition and more than views about what people in society

should do to avoid disease. They also articulate a person's situation in the world and, indeed, articulate that world, in which the individual will be held accountable to others.

We have made the case elsewhere that thinking about health and illness is both ideological and dilemmatic (Billig et al. 1988). It is ideological because any attempts to define what is meant by 'a healthy life' invariably involve ideological judgments (Murcott 1979). Themes relating to health and illness are crucial factors in constituting the world of inequalities, which appears as the 'real', 'natural' world. For example, beliefs about health relate directly to issues of employment and gender (Blaxter 1990). Illness, far from being merely a physical condition, is a reason for not being expected to be in paid employment, for receiving 'unearned' (but reduced) income and for being cared for by others. If ideology refers to the process by which contingent, socially constructed beliefs appear as 'natural' (Eagleton 1991), then these expectations about illness appear 'natural' and 'common-sense'. Thus, they are ideological, perpetuating and naturalising a range of social inequalities.

Moreover, common-sense thinking about health is also dilemmatic. Being ill is not a simple matter: the entitlements must be seen to be earned and impoverishment appears 'natural' (considering the circumstances). . . . Except in extreme cases (e.g. when in intensive care, having been involved in an accident), being a good patient means having to fulfil a sociologically ambivalent position. The patient must appear to be more than a patient; a display of healthiness, or normality, is also required, for the ill person to appear worthy of receiving the entitlements. If the ill person is only an ill person they will fail to warrant their special claims, as they will do so if they appear to be healthy. In this respect, the ill person is both more and less than a physically functioning body.

This means that good health is often understood in relation to illness, while being sick is comprehended in terms of the demands of the healthy. Thus, everyday notions of health and illness reflect ideological values and representations, and do so in ways which appear both dilemmatic and 'natural'. In consequence, people use health beliefs to make themselves accountable *to others* and to articulate *for others* their own position in the world. In doing so, they are taking for granted a world in which 'making an effort' or caring for the sick by women appear as 'natural' values. In this way, 'health beliefs' are always more than health beliefs.

Accounts of Health and Illness: From Representations to Rhetoric

. . . What people say about health and illness reflects not only their individual perspectives upon these matters but also the way that society constructs these issues. Therefore, the study of such social representations promises more than a description of the ideas people share about health and about illness; it also holds out the promise of seeing how, in Herzlich's terms, 'a social object takes shape for members of our society' (1973: 12), and of grasping its implications for the relationship of the individual to society.

The concept of social representations, as used by both Herzlich and Moscovici, has an important advantage over the concept of attitudes: it points towards the social nature of beliefs (Farr 1977). People do not merely have an individual stance (or attitude), they also partake of general beliefs and shared theories about the nature of the world. . . .

On the other hand, the implications of the social representation position have not always been fully developed. There has been a tendency on the part of some writers to reify the notion of 'social representations'. . . . There has been a tendency to treat a 'social representation' as if it were an existing object. Researchers have often sought to discover the 'social representation' which is presumed to lie behind individual beliefs, existing in some undefined way. In so doing they have tended to use the notion of 'social representation' in an uncritical way, which, paradoxically, resembles the ways in which 'attitude' has been uncritically used (see the criticisms of Potter and Litton 1985, McKinlay et al. 1993).

In order to avoid the dangers of reification, we here emphasise the importance of accounts. The business of producing accounts can be described as the activity of socially representing the world, for in producing an account a person tells a story about the world, and, thus, represents it (Antaki 1994, Gilbert and Abell 1983). However, the object of study need not be the social representation itself—as if a discrete social representation of health or illness necessarily exists in a simple sense. Instead, the object of study can be the activity—the social representing of the world, rather than the presumed representation. In this respect, there is an important implication. Social representing can be seen as an activity which is accomplished through accounting. As people produce their accounts so they are representing, or depicting, the world and employing ideological themes which 'naturalise' the world. Moreover, accounts are always produced in situations and they gain their meaning from the rhetorical activities of those situations (Billig 1987, 1991; Edwards and Potter 1993b). In consequence, the study of accounting involves examining how people are using beliefs and what they are doing when giving their beliefs in particular situations. In this respect, the study of health and illness beliefs is a study of activity, not of a presumed object lying behind the activity of accounting. . . .

Being, Ill but Ordinary: Issues of Accountability

Cornwell (1984), in her account of the health beliefs of a sample of families living in East London, reports that, after first agreeing to take part in the study, some individuals then wanted to withdraw. The reason they gave was that 'really their health was good', so that she would be better off seeking ill people who could tell her more than they could. They were only reassured about participating once they had been told that it was a study of 'ordinary' people, and that they would not be represented as individuals who were less healthy than the norm. This shows that talking about one's health to others—even as part of a survey—involves more than making statements pertaining to some neutral field. In talking, one is talking to someone in a context. This observation has been made many times before, when researchers have pointed to the way in which 'illness talk' is hedged around with what have variously been called warrants, concerns with blame, or efforts at legitimation (Blaxter 1993, Calnan 1987, Cornwell 1984, Dingwall 1976, Voysey 1975, Williams 1993).

The requirement to account for one's views about health is a specific as well as a general phenomenon. There is a need to pay attention to when and how people have greater or lesser need to legitimate their position in the light of what they say. Many studies of health beliefs have used 'healthy' individuals in order to tap what they see as being the views of 'ordinary' people, thus illuminating knowledge of everyday ideas about health and illness. By comparison (and by definition) studies of illness experience have often focused upon certain patient groups in order to explore the views of those who have to cope with what are often chronic or disabling diseases. These choices bracket out two features of the interview situation that ought to be discussed. One concerns the apparently stable division of the respondents into 'healthy' and 'ill' when, as has often been shown, these categories are far from watertight. The healthy have much to say about their illness experience, while the sick are often at pains to show their 'normality'. The second feature is only exceptionally discussed in the literature—the health status of the researcher (Zola 1991). While we are not told about the health status of the investigators, it is likely that they are understood as being 'healthy'. After all, by conducting the interview they are performing their employment, and, thus, they are presenting themselves implicitly as being well enough for work. In consequence, respondents with a medical diagnosis are nearly always in the position of speaking to people who are not only seen to be experts in these matters, but are also health-privileged in the interviewing relationship itself, by the very fact that the interview is taking place at all. Here again, the ideological issues are apparent, as the issues of health and illness are directly connected with those of employment and 'earning money'.

Those who are imputed as being ill, or suffering from disability, may be faced with claiming not merely to be ill or suffering from disability: they must warrant claims to be unable to work, or deny the extent of suffering and disability. To be the good patient, they must claim to recover 'normality', which a 'straightforward' presentation of their health beliefs would continue to undermine. A good example of this is presented by Dingwall (1976), who shows (in the italicised phrases in the excerpt below) how the status of ordinariness is achieved by a girl with a considerable physical deformity:

> Interviewer: Mmm. What sorts of things depress you? Girl: *Just simple everyday* things, *just* have arguments with people and *your* parents and . . . get bored with going to the same place and meeting the same people, *you know*. I just want to get away from it for a while. (Dingwall, 1976: 64, emphasis in original)

The italicised words show that the speaker is not merely talking about her special condition. The claims she makes about herself are made in relation to claims about the world in general; about 'your parents', about people in general. The speaker, in using commonplaces, assumes the hearer will recognise the world of relationships which is being represented. In this general account, the speaker inserts herself. Like anyone else, bothered by 'simple everyday things', she just wants to 'get away' from things; but, of course, her disability prevents the accomplishment of the 'normal' wish. Thus, the speaker discursively constructs a 'normal, everyday identity', in which the 'extraordinary' is made ordinary. She gives an account which warrants her special problems in ways which are not seen to be 'complaining' or asking for special treatment.

The need to legitimate one's position extends from those who consider themselves in robust health to those who are severely ill or disabled. For the healthy, illness talk carries with it the threat that one might be seen as a potential malingerer, or even a habitual complainer. For the sick, the same threat applies, although this must be balanced against the possibility that (like the girl with a disability in the above example) one will be dismissed as unfit to participate, as being essentially different from the norm.

The chronically sick may unwittingly be placed in this dilemma when asked by us (healthy, at-work interviewers) about their state of health. Their replies cannot be seen as simply the disclosure of attitudes now coloured by the light of experience that sickness has brought them. Chronic illness, in particular, places individuals in the position of having to account for themselves against the background of potential criticisms and imputed shortcomings (Anderson and Bury 1988). . . .

Williams (1993) is sensitive to these issues when he discusses the case of a widow with rheumatoid arthritis. Unable to care fully for herself — embarrassed to call upon (female) physiotherapists, and discouraged from appealing to her own sons—she is at once defensive and assertive:

> I'm not posh . . . but I'm comfortable. If anyone comes along and they don't like it . . . what can I do about it? I'm fortunate to keep it as straight as it is. If somebody's coming they take me as I am because doing too much I could cause myself a flare-up. Why should I do it to cover something up? They must come in and find me as I am day to day, which is right. (Williams 1993: 99)

According to theorists of accounts, people often offer such accounts of themselves when they feel their personal worth is being challenged (Antaki 1994, Edwards and Potter 1993a). As Voysey (1975) points out, if one is to induce the other to regard one's actions as worthy, then one must link actions to motives and intentions which are seen to be culturally appropriate, or 'normal' (Davis 1963). Not being 'posh' and 'being comfortable' are value-laden terms, as much as economic ones, just as health and illness are likewise. The speaker is justifying her situation, thereby expressing the implied appropriateness of making such justifications. She claims that she can do no more; nothing more should be expected of her; it is 'right' that others find her as she is. In this way, the tale of poverty and illness is a 'normal tale' designed to convince the hearer. The ordinary person struggles to maintain 'ordinary' standards—explaining why higher standards are impossible—and, in giving her account, she asks for allowances to be made by the younger, healthy, middle-class, at-work, professionally sympathetic listener. In this respect, the context is not a neutral locus for the reproduction of ideology, but itself is ideological.

Health beliefs are ideological in that they are sustained within a wider social discourse that shapes not just how individuals think, but how they feel they ought to think. The sick are encouraged by the healthy to redefine their misfortune in positive ways, thus avoiding embarrassment (for the healthy), while resulting in the sick being accorded attributes such as 'strength of character'. By being 'strong of character' they can be credited with being worthy to be looked after, as if too much weakness should be insupportable. If this is to be achieved, then the sick must make manifest their difficulty while showing how they either have borne it or have overcome it. An integral part of this work in discourse involves pointing up the exception, the difference, whose rhetorical removal is the demonstration of one's similarity to the norm.

The following exchange was recorded as part of an interview with a couple approximately three months after the husband had undergone surgery in order to bypass blocked coronary arteries. Although it is an account of a particular illness experience, it is also expressive of an attitude to health and how good health might be encouraged.

> Wife: 'He didn't rest as much as he should have done. There's no doubt about that. That used to bother me. He used to go out pottering about in the shed and doing things that I didn't think he should do. I can't remember anything in particular.' Husband: 'Like chopping sticks one afternoon—all afternoon, while she was at work.' Wife: 'There's no holding him when he's alright!' Husband: 'Another time I was splitting logs for an hour.' Wife: 'That was naughty too!' Husband: 'Some people would say it was too much, but I thought it was getting me better quicker. . . . And I felt that the more exercise I did the quicker I got better.' (Radley, 1988: 129)

A full analysis of this extract is not possible here, but several features can be mentioned.

(i) The husband and wife are jointly telling a tale, in order to produce a shared memory (Edwards and Middleton 1987, Billig and Edwards 1994). When the wife declares that she can't remember something, the husband takes over the story. In this way, their joint activity collectively produces the memory, which is seen to belong to both. (ii) The account of the past events is not merely an account of past time; the telling is situated in the present, and, as the husband and wife talk about themselves, so they are instantiating their relationship, which, as will be seen, is constituted through the 'natural', unequal conventions of gender relations. (iii) The account is filled with the rhetoric of morality in a discourse of justification and criticism; there are words like 'naughty', as if a moral order is being transgressed by a naughty boy (and thereby not so naughtily), so that the joint memory is also a discussion of present morality. (iv) There is ambiguity in the wife's account. The husband is 'naughty' (and, thus, not that naughty); he should not have done what he did. As such, she was right to worry. Thus, he is to be criticised (and she justified)—there's no doubt about that, she claims. (v) Yet there is doubt, because she is collaborating in telling his 'tale'; in this joint account he emerges as the victorious hero, with her, the concerned worrying female, in the background. The moral of the tale is not her worry, but that he was right: he could do things (manly things) like chopping the wood (while she goes to work, he does not claim to attempt the womanly business of housework). 'Some people would say it was too much', he claims, as if his behaviour could have been criticised. The 'some people'—the 'some critics'—include his wife. The imputed criticism of his behaviour and the imputed estimation of his (unmanly) weakness—is refuted by the tale and its moral: he did get better and the more he did the quicker this was achieved. Thus, the hero (the sensible risk-taker who chops logs) emerges trailing clouds of glory, laughing at the cautious concerns of the traditionally caring, stay-at-work wife.

The above excerpt is illustrative of the use of legitimating talk by people who are considered to be 'ill' when they are speaking to the 'healthy'. It shows how those who are approached on the grounds that they are ill make use of ideas about health to escape the confinement of this definition. If people accept the sick role too readily they run the risk of being defined by others as weak: as evading responsibilities and not fulfilling their allotted places in the social order, and, in particular, their gendered roles. When a person is dismissed as 'sick' or 'weak', then he or she has difficulty in having his or her views on other areas of life accepted by others. This is the problem faced by those regarded as being mentally (as opposed to physically) ill, when the implicit question remains whether their illness might be self-motivated. . . .

Issues of accountability are situated, rhetorical concerns. However, in accounting for oneself, speakers must do more than talk about themselves. Accountability only arises in the first place because there are general concerns of value and morality. . . .

The statements that ill (or healthy) people make to interviewers do provide information, but they also claim to depict, or represent, a wider shared reality. Establishing the legitimacy of one's actions and beliefs is a key device in this exercise. . . .

'Public' Statements and 'Private' Stories: Issues of Communication

Cornwell (1984) has made an important distinction between 'public' and 'private' accounts of health and illness. She described 'public' accounts as being those given when individuals are concerned that whatever they say will be acceptable to other people. Such talk consists of what she calls 'meanings in common social currency' which reproduce and legitimate assumptions that are shared about the social world. In this sense, they are made up of social representations, in serving to objectify and to anchor experience in the course of communicating it to others. By comparison, 'private' accounts are those that individuals give as if to people like themselves, using terms and making assumptions that are normally shared by their own group in particular. Cornwell reported that whether people gave 'public' or 'private' accounts of their illness experience depended upon the interviewer-interviewee relationship. Where the individuals felt that the exchange was one of being questioned by an expert, then 'public' accounts were rendered; where the respondents felt that they were being asked to 'tell stories', then there was a shift in control that allowed them scope to give a 'private' account.

However, there is a problem. Cornwell presented the distinction as if people, in giving 'public' or 'private' accounts were doing very different sorts of things, using very different rhetorical strategies. However, no firm criteria are offered for distinguishing between different sorts of accounts, although there is a claim that they emerge in different sorts of contexts. When interviews are formal, and relationships not well established, public accounts will be produced. When trust has been built up, speakers will relax into their private accounts, divulging more of themselves to hearers. However, if accounts are complex and intertextual (Fairclough 1993), and if the context of accounts typically involves justifications then matters may not be so simple: stories may be told when giving the formal accounts, and justifications and legitimations are still in order during the private accounts.

One of the key features of 'public' accounts is that they reflect the speaker's concern with the medical authorities, against whose criteria their statements will be judged. Therefore this kind of talk is replete with commonsense legitimations which render the speaker morally acceptable to others, whether one is healthy or whether one is ill. The following is an example of such an account, in this case given by a man, diagnosed as needing coronary bypass surgery:

> Interviewer: 'What have you been told by the hospital about your present condition?' Patient: 'Well, to quote his actual words, the doctor he said, "If my coronaries were like yours I'd have an operation as soon as I could." That's the main thing and he has told me that there is something definitely wrong.' Interviewer: 'Have you tried to find out more about either your condition or the operation from doctors or other sources?' Patient: 'Well, he was pretty—he explained himself pretty well but as a layman I can only

imagine, I can't—he hasn't gone into detail, he just said, one doctor, it wasn't Dr. R. himself, I'm not sure who it was, on the first interview before I had the catheter he did say that he'd have to open me up and I got a brief description.'

In this excerpt the man demonstrates his moral rectitude in the face of illness by recourse to the expert knowledge of the doctor. He uses 'footings', or quotations, to warrant his need for an operation (Goffman 1981). As Edwards and Potter (1993a) argue, footings are typically used in the context of justification. Moreover, in this case, he is faced with an implicit criticism on the part of the interviewer: why did he not try to find out more about his condition? He justifies himself: the doctor explained 'pretty well'; he himself is only a layman; he isn't sure who the relevant doctor was; he got a description anyway. All these are sounds of justification, in the face of implied criticism. 'Public' accounts are, for Cornwell, always grounded in the need for the speaker to claim legitimacy in the eyes of the other. The justifications are clear. However, in making the justifications, the speaker is also telling stories about what happened, what the doctors said and so on. He is not merely giving justifications, he is also telling his past, and presenting his present self.

According to Cornwell, in 'private' accounts, moral concerns 'faded into the background' (1984: 134). This kind of talk was often structured as a personal story, in which episodes of ill health were run together with descriptions of other aspects of the speaker's biography. It is these personal aspects of what people say that also make these into 'private' accounts. However, as rhetorical analysts have argued, stories are rarely 'merely' stories: in telling stories, speakers make points and draw out conclusions (or 'points') which they communicate to their hearers. In this sense, stories have arguments (Leith and Myerson 1989, Schiffrin 1985). Here is an example of what might be thought to be a private account. It is taken from an interview with the wife of a man waiting to receive coronary bypass surgery:

> Interviewer: What about later on when you learned that it was angina? Respondent: I just wondered how he would react

to it because with him being active and knocking about such a lot it was rather a frightening experience, because I'd gone to bed and I heard him (what I thought, sneeze) and I thought, well, he's not sneezing and so I came down and he was crumpled up in the corner of the settee and obviously I knew, because I had seen during my work that this was a coronary, and I told him. I said "I think you are having a coronary and I want you to stay very still because I can't help you, and get help." I knew that the phone had been vandalised in the village, so with my coat over my night dress I ran round the corner to someone that I knew had a phone, and fortunately her son-in-law was there who had some nursing experience . . .

Again a full interpretation is not possible, but several features of the extract can be mentioned. The speaker is telling a story, with little prompting from the interviewer. As such, it bears the characteristics of a 'private account'. Yet, the tale is one of justification. She portrays herself as showing wifely concern, being quickly aware that the sneeze is not really a sneeze. Her story is also one of correct behaviour: she rushes out; she knows the phone has been vandalised; she goes to an appropriate house—in short, she is not panicking. Moreover, her tale is not merely a wife's: she talks as an experienced professional. She uses 'self-footing' to substantiate the tale. She repeats words which she claimed to tell her husband: the words are those of a professional ('coronary' . . . 'I want you to stay very still'); they are not the personal words of a wife to a husband. The point is not whether or not these words were actually used: an account is to be understood as an account, and the words should be understood in terms of what they are rhetorically accomplishing (Billig and Edwards 1994). The self-footed words amplify the tale of professional competence: they enable the hearers to hear her as business-like: she uses technical terms like coronary in an emergency; she speaks to her husband as if he is a patient and she is a professional. In this respect, the private account contains its own public dimension: the private person is appearing as a public person, behaving so in

private. And in this way, she accounts for herself and her own behaviour. . . .

. . . Cornwell (1984) underlined the legitimating work done within 'public' accounts, while indicating a lesser role for moral discourses within the 'private' account. There is a danger here of attempting to show that the 'public' account, because it is to do with terms that are identified with authorities in society, is concerned with legitimation, while the 'private' account is not. This would be a mistake. There is always the possibility that 'private' stories can be used to legitimate the speaker, while 'public' statements are more like the rehearsal of widely shared, taken-for-granted beliefs, in terms of which the speaker feels relatively secure. . . .

The Everyday Life of Health Beliefs: Public and Private Encounters

At the outset of this paper we argued that health beliefs are not best considered either as individual cognitive systems nor as fragments of a shared repertoire of social representations. Either one of these options falls short of embracing the way in which people's talk about health and illness is at times contradictory, draws upon different contexts and is used as a way of framing the ongoing exchange between the individuals concerned. Regarded as dilemmatic, being healthy or being ill are not properties or states that we possess, but claims that we have to sustain against the background of competing moral demands.

The discussion of issues of legitimation and of communication allowed us to examine 'public' and 'private' accounts of health and illness in a new light. In order to do this, we treated them separately when, in fact, they often appeared together in people's accounts of illness experience. Take for example the following excerpt, in which the wife of a heart patient is talking to the interviewer, who is a woman:

Interviewer: 'Did you suggest he went to the doctor?' Respondent: 'Yes, and he wouldn't . . . He went to Scarborough and he went right grey walking up a hill and I said, "You should go to the doctor," and he said, "I'm all right," *you know how they do*, and in the end he went and they found it with the stress cardiograph . . .'

The words italicised in the passage are an appeal to the interviewer to use knowledge that the two speakers share, as women, about men. In that sense, it is an attempt to legitimate what is being told in the story by reference to ideas that are in the public realm for women. Indeed, this excerpt suggests that this kind of warranting might be an important device for introducing or maintaining 'private' accounts. That is, where the speaker can establish a common bond, perhaps with a fellow member of a minority group, then this facilitates the move towards expressive communication (Oakley 1981). In the case of both patients and spouses in the study concerned, the therapeutic possibilities flowing from being able to share experiences with others in the same position as oneself should not be underestimated (Radley 1988).

There is a more important reason why we should consider the joint appearance of 'public' and 'private' accounts of health and illness. These terms are relative, so that what is considered private depends upon what is considered public, and vice-versa. This is another way of making the case that thinking is dilemmatic, and it is necessary to ask questions about how this occurs.

If we use the shorthand terms analysed above, how is it that 'public' statements are inserted into conversations about health that are based upon 'private' talk? And by comparison, how is it that 'private' accounts are given in the course of exchanges based upon 'public' discourse? To answer these, we shall make brief references to two different contexts in which these things occur.

One is the case of families with handicapped children, as studied by Voysey (1975). She noted that the parents made use of ideologies drawn from various agencies in order to make their situation congruent with that of 'ordinary' families. In effect, their talk, which allowed them to tell their own stories, socially represented or depicted handicap in order to minimise the special features of their situation. Voysey argued that this is a case of the use of a public morality to safeguard one's private fate. Only by appearing 'normal' could the families protect themselves from the intrusions of experts or others who might otherwise inquire further into their life. Giving 'private' accounts might allow insight into one's life situation, but this might well be at the price of risking interventions that would be unwelcome. The point is not that the situation demanded one kind of talk rather than another, rather, the deployment of this ideology alongside more 'private' stories of their experiences enabled the parents to retain a degree of privacy that otherwise might have been put at risk. Thus, there appears an apparent contradiction here in the parents' use of 'public' accounts of handicap in order to minimise the penetration of the public gaze into their family life.

A second example illustrates the same point about the co-occurrence of 'public' and 'private' accounts, but this time approaches the issue from the opposite direction. In this case we are concerned with the interposing of 'private' accounts of illness into a context defined by the 'public' authority of the medical examination. Young (1989) describes an examination of an elderly Jewish university professor by a doctor, in the course of which the patient spontaneously introduces brief stories about the various parts of his body that are being attended to. The examination can be seen as 'rendering in a physical medium the estrangement of the self and the fragmentation of the body' (Young 1989: 159). The discourse of medicine serves to distance the self from the body, so that what occurs during the examination happens only to an objective entity, not to a social self. And yet, in this examination, the patient recounts against its background his experiences as an inmate of Auschwitz. These stories, Young argues, invoke the speaker as a person, and in so doing re-insert the self into the objectified and distanced body.

This is not a case of 'private' accounts supplanting medical ('public') knowledge. Personal experience is interspersed along the lines provided by the body's physical boundaries, which form the focus of the examination's inquiry. This allows for the patient's re-emergence as a figure in a story that has wider moral and ideological elements than would be commanded by a private or inner self. It also establishes the person (as patient) as more than just a physical body. That is to say, the work of these accounts allows the patient to transmute the private indignities of the medical examination into a kind of public honour. Here the 'private' account works to display a self which is then comprehended as remarkably public.

Yet, there is a further issue here, which points to the construction of accounts. Piecing together accounts leaves gaps. The account may claim a moral point in present relationships; it may represent a wider shared world; moreover, it may co-opt the past for present rhetorical purposes. Indeed, it is only by such co-option that the past becomes socially shared. However, the experiences of health and illness are not completely encompassed within accounts. There can be more just beyond the very edge of every account. And every attempt to recapture this extra element within an account will ensure something else escapes unaccounted for.

On the Edge of Accounts: Displays of Good Health

Interviews are designed to tap ideas about health, and so they produce a certain kind of data. What gets reported and analysed is what people say, so that the account becomes focal in the investigation. This is true of the issues that we have discussed in this paper. And yet, to focus upon discourse alone is to miss out on the fact that it proceeds as part of a relationship that is situated in time and place. As mentioned above, many such interviews are conducted by putative healthy interviewers with acknowledged sick individuals. Other interviewees may feel that their health status is put in jeopardy just by being questioned about it.

To sit a person in a chair and talk about their health is to place them in a restricted situation. That is, the scope they have to demonstrate their health status is narrowed, so that they must tell the interviewer about behaviours and capacities that might be shown more effectively in other ways (Radley 1993). Illness not only disrupts the usual forms of gestural display, but is also expressed through transformations in bodily style. This

mode of communication is not separated from talk, nor is it of 'mere' metaphorical significance. For example, upright posture is an aspect of bodily conduct crucial to the constitution of lived spatiality; showing that one can 'stand on one's own feet' is more than just a figurative claim (Toombs 1992). [For an extended discussion of this thesis, see Johnson (1987).]

Therefore, although health status can be communicated effectively through talk (as illustrated in the excerpts given above), this does not remove the individual from the necessity of having to *appear* a healthy (or otherwise) person in the course of the interview. This appearance cannot be contrived by talk alone, because it involves the bodily conduct of the individual who is giving the account. Because illness is often defined in terms of loss of capacity, if not bodily impairment, then the effective conduct of the interviewee is central to the communication of a picture of good health, where this is the image so desired. . . .

Briefly, the body is both a medium through which individuals can portray their health (or illness) and a topic of these portrayals (Radley 1991, 1995). This is not a pointing to signs of disease or their absence. It is an enactment which displays and thereby exemplifies conceptions of health and illness. Goffman described this as follows:

Displays don't communicate in the narrow sense of the term; they don't enunciate something through a language of symbols openly established and used solely for that purpose. They provide evidence of the actor's alignment in the situation. And displays are important insofar as alignments are. (1976: 69)

This is to see the portrayal of one's health (or illness) as a dramatic instantiation of a condition that, while it can be used as a label, must also be shown forth. In that sense, it might be taken as a fragment of a larger whole, a dramatic performance by a 'player in the world of health'. Such a display alludes to a state of being; it does not (indeed cannot) capture that world entirely. This means that the manner of what is said (which is part of the display), is partially constitutive of the imputed state of health (or illness). In that sense, it comes closer to what Shotter (1981) has called 'avowals', which are exemplifications of a way of being. Avowals, unlike reports, are best subject to tests of sincerity, not proofs of truth and falsity. The task for the interviewer is to 'see into' them, not to try to peer behind them or through them (Tormey, 1971). This is consistent with our speaking, in everyday life, of *being* healthy or *being* ill, (as social and psychological conditions), as well as whether our bodies are inscribed with the signs of pathology.

Where does this bring us in our analysis? It draws a limit to the analysis of health through verbal accounts, collected as discourse. It shows that warrants and justifications need not be wholly concerned with what is said, but with how it is being said in that particular exchange. Accounts of health and illness are more than a reporting of a mundane state of affairs, either external (what happened) or internal (as attitudes). Instead, they are expressive and constitutive of a way of being that is invoked in the telling about health and illness. This is important, as it gives to accounts a revelatory aspect that is missing if we consider them only as making distinctions between the speaker as being either this or that type of person.

Conclusion

In this paper we have argued that 'private' and 'public' accounts of health and illness are not merely contingent upon situation or relationship. It is not that in one setting or encounter people will give one kind of account, and in another they will talk about something different. Instead, accounting for health is also constitutive of the relationships in which it takes place. In the situation of the medical consultation, the patient's public worth (our healthier self) is protected through a private display of illness. In the context of everyday life, as when confronted with an inquiring interviewer, privacy is retained on the basis of a public depiction of normality and good health. What we have described elsewhere as the dilemmas and contradictions of thinking are shown to be inescapable outcomes of our

ideological context on the one hand, and our ontological situation on the other.

The above point raises one other issue on which we should make ourselves clear. This argument is not an attempt to replace bodily disease with talk of illness. Pain and associated symptoms are inescapable facts of life. What is also inescapable, however, is the necessity of appearing before others, of presenting oneself as the owner of symptoms, the bearer of this or that illness. Giving accounts is, for both experts and laypersons, part of that business of dealing with disease and its consequences.

This point having been made, we conclude that health and illness are not merely oppositional terms defining states about which individuals have discrete attitudes. Instead, these ideas have a double existence. On the one hand, they are the means by which we can maintain and define our fitness for society; on the other, they portray a world of experience that we claim for ourselves alone.

References

Anderson, R. and M. Bury, (eds) (1988) *Living with Chronic Illness: The Experience of Patients and Their Families*. London: Unwin Hyman.

Antaki, C. (1994) *Explaining and Arguing: The Social Organisation of Account*. London: Sage.

Baumann, B. (1961) "Diversities in conceptions of health and fitness," *Journal of Health and Human Behavior*, 2, 39-46.

Billig, M. (1987) *Arguing and Thinking: A Rhetorical Approach to Social Psychology*. Cambridge: Cambridge University Press.

Billig, M. (1991) *Ideology and Opinions: Studies in Rhetorical Psychology*. London: Sage.

Billig, M., S. Condor, D. Edwards, M. Gane, D. Middleton, and A. Radley. (1988) *Ideological Dilemmas: A Social Psychology of Everyday Thinking*. London: Sage.

Billig, M., and D. Edwards. (1994) "La construction sociale de la memoire." *La Recherche*, 267, 742-45.

Blair, A. (1993) "Social class and the contextualisation of illness experience." In Radley, A. (ed) *Worlds of Illness: Biographical and Cultural Perspectives on Health and Disease*. London: Routledge.

Blaxter, M. (1983) "The causes of disease: women talking," *Social Science and Medicine*, 17, 59-69.

Blaxter, M. (1990) *Health and Lifestyles*. London: Tavistock/Routledge.

Blaxter, M. (1993) "Why do the victims blame themselves?" In Radley, A. I (ed) *Worlds of Illness: Biographical and Cultural Perspectives on Health and Disease*. London: Routledge.

Blumhagen, D. (1980) "Hypertension: a folk illness with a medical name," *Culture, Medicine and Psychiatry*, 4, 197-227.

Calnan, M. (1987) *Health and Illness: The Lay Perspective*. London: Tavistock.

Cornwell, J. (1984) *Hard-Earned Lives: Accounts of Health and Illness from East London*. London: Tavistock.

d'Houtaud, A. and M. G. Field. (1984) "The image of health: variations in perception by social class in a French population," *Sociology of Health and Illness*, 6, 30-60.

Davis, F. (1963) *Passage Through Crisis: Polio Victims and their Families*. Indianapolis: Bobbs-Merrill.

Dingwall, R. (1976) *Aspects of Illness*. London: Martin Robertson.

Eagleton, T. (1991) *Ideology: An Introduction*. London: Verso.

Edwards, D. and D. Middleton. (1987) "Conversation and remembering: Bartlett revisited," *Applied Cognitive Psychology*, 1, 77-92.

Edwards, D. and J. Potter. (1993a) *Discursive Psychology*. London: Sage.

Edwards, D. and J. Potter. (1993b) "Language and causation: a discursive action model of description and attribution," *Psychological Review*, 100, 23-41.

Fairclough, N. (1993) *Discourse and Social Change*. Cambridge: Polity Press.

Farr, R.M. (1977) "Heider, Harré and Herzlich on health and illness: some observations on the structure of 'representations collectives'," *European Journal of Social Psychology*, 7, 491-504.

Gilbert, N. and P. Abell. (eds) (1983) *Accounts and Action*. Aldershot: Gower.

Goffman, E. (1976) "Gender advertisements," *Studies in the Anthropology of Visual Communication*, 3, Whole number 2.

Goffman, E. (1981) *Forms of Talk*. Oxford: Blackwell.

Herzlich, C. (1973) *Health and Illness: A Social Psychological Analysis*. (Trans. Douglas Graham), London: Academic Press.

Johnson, M. (1987) *The Body in the Mind: The Bodily Basis of Meaning, Imagination and Reason*. Chicago: Chicago University Press.

Leith, D. and G. Myerson. (1989) *The Power of Address: Explorations in Rhetoric*. London: Routledge.

McKinlay, A., J. Potter, and M. Wetherell. (1993) "Discourse analysis and social representations." In Breakwell, G. and D. Canter (eds) *Empirical Approaches to Social Representations*. Oxford University Press.

Moscovici, S. (1976) *La Psychanalyse, Son Image et Son Public*. Paris: Presses Universitaires de France.

Moscovici, S. (1984) "The phenomenon of social representations." In Farr, R. M. and S. Moscovici (eds) *Social Representations*. Cambridge: Cambridge University Press.

Murcott, A. (1979) "Health as ideology." In Atkinson, P., R. Dingwall, and A. Murcott (eds) *Prospects for the National Health*. London: Croom Helm.

Oakley, A. (1981) "Interviewing Women: a contradiction in terms." In Roberts, H. (ed) *Doing Feminist Research*. London: Routledge and Kegan Paul.

Pierret, J. (1993) "Constructing discourses about health and their social determinants." In Radley, A. (ed) *Worlds of Illness: Biographical and Cultural Perspectives of Health and Disease*. London: Routledge.

Pill, R. and N. C. H. Stott. (1982) "Concepts of illness causation and responsibility: some preliminary data from a sample of working class mothers," *Social Science and Medicine*, 16, 43-52.

Potter, J. and I. Litton. (1985) "Some problems underlying the theory of social representations," *British Journal of Social Psychology*, 24, 81-90.

Radley, A. (1988) *Prospects of Heart Surgery: Psychological Adjustment to Coronary Bypass Grafting*. New York: Springer-Verlag.

Radley, A. (1991) *The Body and Social Psychology*. New York: Springer-Verlag.

Radley, A. (1993) "The role of metaphor in adjustment to chronic illness." In Radley, A. (ed) *Worlds of Illness: Biographical and Cultural Perspectives of Health and Disease*. London: Routledge.

Radley, A. (1995) "The elusory body and social constructionist theory," *Body and Society*, 1, 3-24.

Schiffrin, D. (1985) "Everyday argument: the organisation of diversity in talk." In van Dijk, T.A. (ed) *Handbook of Discourse Analysis*. London: Academic Press.

Shotter, J. (1981) "Telling and reporting: prospective and retrospective uses of self-ascriptions." In Antaki, C. (ed) *The Psychology of Ordinary Explanations of Behaviour*. London: Academic Press.

Toombs, S.K. (1992) *The Meaning of Illness: A Phenomenological Account of the Different Perspectives of Physician and Patient*. Dordrecht: Kluwer.

Tormey, A. (1971) *The Concept of Expression: A Study in Philosophical Psychology and Aesthetics*. Princeton, N.J.: Princeton University Press.

Voysey, M. (1975) *A Constant Burden: The Reconstitution of Family Life*. London: Routledge and Kegan Paul.

Williams, G.H. (1993) "Chronic illness and the pursuit of virtue in everyday life." In Radley, A. (ed) *Worlds of Illness: Biographical and Cultural Perspectives on Health and Disease.* London: Routledge.

Williams, R. (1990) *A Protestant Legacy: Attitudes to Death and Illness among Older Aberdonians.* Oxford: Clarendon Press.

Young, K. (1989) Narrative embodiments: enclaves of the self in the realm of medicine. In Shotter J. and Gergen K. (eds) *Texts of Identity*, London: Sage.

Zola, I. K. (1991) "Bringing our bodies and ourselves back in: reflections on a past, present and future 'medical sociology'," *Journal of Health and Social Behavior*, 32, 1-16.

Further Reading

Stephen Cole and Robert Lejune. 1972. "Illness and the Legitimation of Failure." *American Sociological Review* 37: 347-356.

Jocelyn Cornwall. 1984. *Hard-earned Lives: Accounts of Health and Illness from East London.* London: Tavistock.

Arthur Frank. 1993. "The Rhetoric of Self-Change: Illness Experience as Narrative." *The Sociological Quarterly* 34: 39-52.

Discussion Questions

1. In which ways do people's accounts of their health justify and perpetuate their actions?

2. How do you assess Radley and Billig's point that health status and accounts of it affect how other people view a sick person?

3. What differences can you discern in the public and private accounts of illness among your family and friends?

3

The Origins of the Health Movement

Michael S. Goldstein

In *this selection, Michael Goldstein highlights issues of the social construction of health and illness at a macrocultural level by showing that health, illness, and social movements are not altogether unique. As the previous selections show, individual and social group definitions mediate medical ones. Goldstein acknowledges the social construction of illness and health and movements to medicalize life events. Traditionally, medicine wins out as a cultural authority. Technology and science pervade even the most mundane aspects of living. As you review this selection, consider how cultural norms and values pervade individual and social group belief systems of what health is, how illness should be addressed, and how definitions of health and illness become constructed. Consider the cultural legitimacy of social group movements that counter medicalized depictions of health and self processes.*

Goldstein explains the reasons for increasing numbers of movements determined to reconstruct definitions of health and of self. The claims of movement groups rely on the influence of past perspectives—like religion—and *the creation of new ones—like holistic health. Think about the ways these movements challenge taken-for-granted definitions provided by medical claims about social reality.*

There are no illnesses or diseases in nature. There are only conditions that society, or groups within it, have come to define as illness or disease. Sedgwick (1973: 31) put it this way: "The fracture of a . . . femur has, within the world of nature, no more significance than the snapping of an autumn leaf from its twig; and the invasion of a human organism by cholera 'germs' carries with it no more the stamp of 'illness' than does the souring of milk by other forms of bacteria." The terms *illness* and *disease* are used to describe conditions that cause death or limit functioning among humans and a few other species of animals and plants. In some cases, such as the measles and polio, there is a very high degree of consensus that the condition is best understood as an illness. In other cases, such as depression, alcoholism, or hyperkinesis (overactivity), the use of such medical terminology is hotly disputed.

These are not trivial or merely academic matters, as what we call a phenomenon often carries with it a host of implications for how we think about and react to it. Calling a problem an illness or a disease usually implies that it has "natural" causes that are best understood by scientists or practitioners conversant with science. Such problems are seen as best dealt with through "treatment" provided by physicians or other medical personnel, in medical institutions or facilities. We expect those who suffer from an illness to want to be restored to their previous level of health. Typically, this involves cooperating with medical personnel and generally seeking to "get well" as fast and as fully as possible. All of these implications of employing medical or disease terminology may appear to be obvious. Yet if we chose to view the problem in question from a moral, political, psychological, or religious point of view, a very different set of perceptions and actions might well appear warranted.

What we call the "health movement" or the "health promotion movement" has a complex relationship with an understanding of what is usually called illness or disease. In part, the movement is a logical step arising from developments in medicine; in part, it is an attempt to avoid or challenge those developments. To some degree the health movement predates the widespread successes of medicine, while in other ways it follows and reacts to those successes. This selection sets out what it means to understand our afflictions as illnesses, to medicalize them, as well as why medicalization has occurred. Then we consider how this process itself came to be seen as problematic—a grievance that ultimately generated a broad social movement, the health movement.

The Medicalization of Life

Any number of observers have described the period after World War II as being marked by the "medicalization" of a wide range of social problems and phenomena (Szasz 1970; Illich 1976; Kittrie 1971; Zola 1975; Conrad and Schneider 1980). By now, a vast and still-growing literature—largely in sociology but with offshoots in psychology, political science, history, and other fields—has documented how various conditions came to be seen as medical problems. Medicalization replaced the earlier view that these afflictions arise from choices made by individuals and groups in response to their history, values, culture, political and religious beliefs, or the material and ideological constraints imposed by outside forces. Homosexuality (Bergler 1956; Bullough 1976; Bayer 1981), mental illness (Szasz 1961; Rothman 1971; Chu and Trotter 1974), alcoholism (Jellinek 1960; Conrad and Schneider 1980), drug addiction (Musto 1973; Szasz

1974; Alexander, 1987), childhood hyperkinesis (Conrad 1975), child abuse (Pfohl 1977; Kempe et al. 1962; Gil 1970), criminal behavior, especially among juveniles (Empey 1978; Conrad and Schneider 1980), and gambling (Roscrance 1985) are all examples of phenomena that have been medicalized. In most instances, the particular behavior was first seen as simply a choice that individuals made and for which they should be held responsible. In many cases, the behavior was considered normative, at least under certain conditions. Once the behavior came to be seen as a problem, it was typically seen as a sin, best dealt with by religious authority and sanction. Later, these conditions came to be seen as crimes, and still later as diseases. Of course sin, crime, and illness are not mutually exclusive perspectives. It is possible to believe in, and act on, all of them simultaneously. . . .

The crucial role of human actors, motives, and social movements in the course of religious, legal, and political change is easily accepted by most people. These arenas, by their nature, are marked by conflict and differences. But many people have more difficulty accepting the role of human actors and social movements in that which is thought of as based upon medicine and/or science. The popular image is that developments in science lead to medical progress toward goals shared by both the afflicted and those who care for them. This image, itself an essential component of medicalization, is fundamentally at odds with the sociological perspective that sees the medicalization of any condition as a social project, a construction of reality.

The medicalization process has not restricted itself to medicalizing conditions, behaviors, and attitudes that are usually considered to deviate from the norms of society. Increasingly, the medical model has been applied to aspects of "normal" life that may or may not be problematic to people. For example, birth and death—the two experiences all human beings share—have come to be seen as medical events (Lindheim 1981). Typically, they are monitored, controlled, and certified by medical authorities. Today, social movements have arisen whose goal is to demedicalize these events. They aim to place birth and death more squarely in the hands of lay people within institutions (homes, birthing centers, hospices) removed from total domination by physicians and their agents. One tactic employed by these demedicalizing movements has been to remind us of the important role that social and political movements played in bringing about medicalization in the first place. The knowledge that medicalization took place in response to socioeconomic factors—as opposed to objective scientific knowledge—may foster or help legitimize movements aimed at reversing the process.

The medicalization of everyday life has become a major feature of western society, particularly in the United States and Canada. Every transition and development in the lives of normal individuals has been proposed as an appropriate ground for medical observation, judgment, instruction, and control. Almost every imaginable facet of child-rearing and family life—from the spacing of children to their feeding schedules, discipline, and social skills—falls under the purview of pediatricians and other therapists. Child-rearing manuals written by physicians provide the accepted standards for the behavior of both parents and children in most middle-class homes. Sexual development and behavior have also been heavily medicalized (Gagnon and Simon 1973). In every imaginable area of sexual endeavor, norms for behavior and attitudes are dealt with as matters of health and illness in sex-education classes for children and in sex manuals and sex therapy for adults. Instruction in human sexuality has gained increasing prominence in medical school curricula, and in at least one state—California—public sentiment has resulted in legislation requiring a course in the topic prior to the granting of any medical degree. The medicalization of sexuality has ranged from concern regarding norms for specific behaviors such as masturbation (Engelhardt 1974) to the classification of pornography as "healthy" or "unhealthy" by physicians (Calderone 1972).

Another example of medicalization is the way stress and situations that produce it have come under medical purview. Stress is poorly defined and understood. But since many traditional chronic and acute illnesses are statistically associated with it, stress has become known as a "cause" of illness and hence in need of medical control. Because people appear to react to similar stresses in different ways, much attention is now devoted to the internal traits that enable individuals to resist stress. Another broad example of medicalization is the increasing effort to deal with the aging of the American population as a medical problem. The development of geriatrics as a medical specialty (national exams for board certification began in 1988) has fostered the medicalization of older people's lives with a scope similar in its attention to "normal aging" to the way pediatrics deals with "normal child development."

Thus, the phenomenon of medicalization has increasingly turned from behaviors and attitudes that had been seen as deviant to behaviors and attitudes that are seen as normal. Part of this process is the specification of attitudes that are "better" than normal; ones that are believed to prevent the occurrence of deviance or illness and maximize health and "wellness." In this context, the most frequently cited definition of *health* is the one put forth by the World Health Organization: "Health is a state of complete physical, mental, and social well-being and not merely the absence of disease or infirmity" (Callahan 1973). Given the breadth of this definition, it is difficult to imagine any aspect of human life falling outside its bounds.

In 1950, when Talcott Parsons first described the "sick role," he specified, in an idealized way, the societal norms for being sick. According to this formulation, the sick individual is unable to fulfill normal social roles due to natural forces beyond his or her control. A person enters the sick role when this set of circumstances is labeled or diagnosed by an objective professional. To remain in the sick role, a person must accept that its benefits (release from one's normal obligations and receiving professional care, social support and sympathy from others) are temporary and will continue as long as the individual sincerely attempts to get well and leave the sick role. Today, the medicalization of life has reached the point that clinicians, researchers, and policy makers speak of what could be termed the "at risk role" (Baric

1969). In this role, the individual continues to perform his/her normal roles but willfully chooses to seek objective professional advice, assistance, or support to reduce the risk of future illness and/or to improve health. Fulfilling this "at risk role" is seen as highly desirable, and the expectation is that playing the role is appropriate throughout one's entire life span. Indeed, it is even possible to perceive a refusal to play the "at risk role" as an illness itself.

Recent American history is notable for the growing number of people who have accepted—in whole or in part, implicitly or explicitly—the ideas underlying the medicalization of life. Particularly notable is the equation of normalcy with health, and of self-improvement with higher levels of health or wellness. The efforts of individuals to develop these ideas and pursue them in their own lives, as well as to influence other people and the society at large, has taken the form of a social movement: the health movement.

Because *health* is such a broad and ill-defined term, it may be more appropriate to view the health movement as a useful fiction that encompasses a wide range of very real submovements, each concerned with a particular set of attitudes and behaviors. . . .

The Origins of Medicalization

Medicalization arose from the coalescing and mutual affinity of many different factors. It is impossible to assign a specific degree of importance to each, but it is feasible to describe the most important of these factors and discuss their roles in the overall process.

The Success of Science and Technology

It is probably fair to say that over the past two hundred years, science based on "rational and objective" examination of the physical world has provided western societies with their dominant framework for understanding and manipulating the world. Although the actual benefits of science and its associated technologies relative to their costs is a matter of endless debate, they have unquestionably been perceived as highly successful and beneficial for humankind for the most part. The overriding association of medicine with science and technology has placed it squarely within this dominant world-view. The benefits and prestige of modern medicine have been generally perceived as flowing from its scientific comprehension and methods. The extent to which this view is accurate—rather than fostered by the medical profession itself—is irrelevant. The perceived equation of medicine with science and rationality has provided medicine with an aura of success as well as a justification for that success. Thus, it should not be surprising to find the general public as well as various public leaders amenable when a medical perspective is put forth as a solution to serious and/or intractable problems. Science has provided the medicalization of life with a powerful intellectual and cultural basis.

The Decline of Traditional Moral Paradigms

Science replaced other systems for understanding the world and ways of handling problems. Foremost among these were traditional religious views of the universe, which were typically seen as incompatible with science. The issue here is not the actual degree of incompatibility of religious and scientific views; rather, it is their *perceived* incompatibility that influenced and fostered the medicalization process. Prescientific religious beliefs about the origin of behavior typically emphasized either the causal role of divine extraworldly forces or the absence of external constraints and the power of the individual's free will. In either case, observable, measurable, or objective influences were slighted. Deviance was viewed as arising from moral weakness or sin. Appropriate responses included prayer, pastoral guidance, moral effort, or in their absence, guilt.

From a scientific standpoint, these responses came to be seen as both ineffectual and possibly harmful. Even if objective scientific responses carried out through medicine could not effectively remedy the problems, they did claim to provide both a better understanding of why the problems existed, as well as a more humane environment for dealing with them. Punishment and guilt were not part of the medical armamentarium. This latter reason alone was often enough to justify imposing a medical view of a problem like alcoholism (Szasz 1970; Jellinek 1960). In effect, what advocates said was, "Yes, we realize alcoholism isn't a disease like polio. But by calling it a disease, at least we will be better able to care for sufferers (in hospitals as opposed to jails), provide for them (through insurance and disability coverage), and make them feel better about themselves (by calling them sick, instead of sinful)."

A similar set of arguments was used to medicalize behavior that had typically been understood using a legal or criminal approach. In this traditional moral paradigm, the norms come from political representatives, not from God. But its emphasis on free will, moral choice, and retributional punishment is similar to that of religion. In theory, the major goal of this approach was to determine, through an adversarial process, if the transgressions that the accused had allegedly committed had in fact occurred. The assumption was that the accused would attempt to refute the allegations. There would be winners and losers. As in religious paradigms, objective truth was not highly valued in this traditional paradigm. Rather, the fundamental opposition between accused and accuser required that truth be determined within sharply constrained procedures where even very germane evidence might be ruled inadmissible. As the limited effectiveness of this approach for dealing with many important problems became acutely evident, the medical perspective's nonadversarial approach (in which both the doctor and the patient have the same goal: curing the disease), its emphasis on objectivity, and its nonpunitive character seemed increasingly appealing to the public, to political leaders, and sometimes to the police and judiciary as well.

During the time of science's ascendancy in the popular mind as the ultimate paradigm, traditional religious and legal views became correspondingly constrained. Religion's constriction reached the point that attempts were even made to define healthy and unhealthy religious views and practices. Physicians in the popular media give advice about which religious beliefs and practices are appropriate for children. Other physicians have taken much more aggressive approaches with religious practices that are out of the ordinary or that offend public sensibilities. By calling some religious groups "cults" and their rituals "brainwashing," these phenomena have been reconceptualized as mental health problems (Robbins and Anthony 1982). In this case, medicalization has led to court orders permitting the abduction of adherents, followed by therapeutic "deprogramming." These examples indicate how far American society has come in only a few decades from a time when most medical institutions were themselves creations of—and dependent upon—religious groups.

The Influence of the University and the Social Sciences

The increasing role of higher education in American life over the past few decades has had a strong elective affinity with medicalization in three ways. For one, the university has been a major source for disseminating highly favorable information and attitudes about the value of science for understanding the world. For another, colleges and universities have played a major role in training and certifying students for jobs that have a strong self-interest in seeing medical definitions expanded. This will be discussed more fully later. But the influence of higher education has operated in a third way as well: through the dissemination of social science concepts that implicitly or explicitly support notions of nonresponsibility among ever-larger proportions of the population. For example, the psychoanalytic theories of Freud, the learning theories advanced by behavioral psychologists such as B. F. Skinner, and the political theories of Karl Marx would seem to have little in common. But they all specify that the sources of human thought and action lie outside of the individual, and by implication, they limit the extent to which people are seen as responsible for what happens to them. These and other theories in psychology, sociology, and economics support an intellectual understanding of deviance and problematic behavior as illnesses, with natural causes beyond the individual's control.

Not everyone in our society is afforded an equal opportunity to receive a college education and to enter a career that has a self-interest in promoting the medicalization of life. So it is not surprising that not everyone is equally accepting of medicalization. As early as the 1930s the sociologist Kingsley Davis (1938) noted that the medicalization of mental health and illness through the so called "mental hygiene" movement served to provide a cloak of objectivity for the superiority and promotion of middle-class values and behaviors. Today, many people see the university as the arbiter of what is "true" in our society. Its incorporation of a perspective that promotes medicalization, and its inclusion of degree programs for professions that depend upon medicalization, make it a powerful ally of the medicalization process. In this way social policies that have not been concerned with medicalization—such as the expansion of higher education—may contribute greatly, if indirectly, to its acceptance.

Vested Interests of Professionals

Medicalization can be described in abstract terms, but it must be carried out by very real groups of people who are motivated in some way to do so. Often the major actors in this process are groups of professionals who feel that the medicalization of a given phenomenon will lead to enhanced status, prestige, income, or autonomy for themselves. Of course, they may also feel that medicalization is the most accurate or effective way of dealing with the problem.

That professionalism and medicalization have had a mutual affinity is supported by most sociological ideas about what it means to be a professional (Freidson 1970; Berlant 1975; Larson 1977). The body of work on this idea sees established professions as occupational groups that have successfully come to monopolize some important area of endeavor. These groups have a high degree of autonomy or self-regulation, and they are able to dominate their clients and other workers. Usually professionals are able to attain and maintain these prerogatives by the (perceived) congruence between their desires as a group and those of powerful forces in society, such as the government or economic elites. The striving of occupations to increase their professional stature fosters medicalization in a number of ways. First, many occupational groups explicitly or implicitly set out to associate themselves with physicians, who are usually taken as epitomizing a fully professional group. This typically entails working in medical institutions and employing medical terminology. Second, professionals seek to maximize and regularize their payment. The existence of an extensive private and public reimbursement system for medical problems is a powerful incentive to see the problems with which they deal as medical in nature. (Health insurance, disability payments, Medicare, Medicaid and other programs reimburse only providers who deal with medical problems.) Finally, concerns such as appropriate child rearing or sexual behavior that have been medicalized over the past few decades are highly complex and ambiguous and typically lend themselves to modification only through value-laden actions. Medicalization, with its veneer of science, objectivity, and value neutrality, offers an ideal way for workers to avoid confrontations with clients or society at large.

It is noteworthy that much of the medicalization of life has occurred through the efforts not of the medical profession as a whole, but of segments of it, such as pediatricians (for example, hyperactivity), gynecologists (for example, menopause as illness), or psychiatrists. Typically, the history of the medicalization of a problem like alcoholism, child abuse, family planning, or homosexuality reveals that most physicians were originally opposed. Looking back, we typically find that individuals or small groups—often operating as part of incipient social movements—played key roles.

Medicalization as a Grievance

As a result of these medicalizing trends, we live in a society where a good life has come to be seen as a healthy life. The specific meaning of *healthy* has increasingly been dominated and determined by medically and professionally controlled images. These images, as well as their consequences, are complex. On one level, they are positive, presenting humanitarian values and the reduction in overt moralizing that comes with a medicalized perspective. Most of all, the images are optimistic. This optimism arises from the association of medicine with scientific progress.

But medicalized popular images of a healthy life have become associated with another, more negative or ambivalent set of images as well: images critical of the medicalized view of health. This set of images has come to form the basic set of grievances and discontents that underlie the health movement in its various forms. The major components of antimedical sentiment are the following:

A Questioning of Science and Technology

The cherished notion that science and technology will inevitably improve our lives has been under attack ever since the development and use of the atomic bomb. More recently, the accidents at Three Mile Island and Chernobyl, as well as the unremitting tide of pollution in our air and water, remind us that even the peaceful use of technology can be dangerous. Increasingly, we have come to see that technological progress almost always entails costs, sometimes irreparable ones. This view is well developed in medical technology itself: surgery causes injury and death, antibiotics lead to more resistant bacteria, X-rays can cause cancer, and so on. Individuals are kept alive by medical technology, even when their minds are not functioning and the quality of their lives is abysmal. Skepticism about the claims of medicine and knowledge of its possible consequences are growing. Such consequences are not only the obvious physical dangers; rather we have come to see that simply calling someone sick or diseased may have adverse consequences in itself. Since the Middle Ages, criminals have often sought to be incarcerated away from the mentally ill, lest they be tarnished with that label. Today, social science researchers have documented that the general population considers being mentally ill more stigmatizing than being a criminal (Goldstein 1979). Susan Sontag (1978) has eloquently described how having cancer results in a powerful label that personifies evil to many people. More recently, children who carry the AIDS virus have been thrown out of school and their houses burned. Medical labels can be among the most powerful we know of, with the ability to overwhelm one's identity.

Awareness of the limits and possible adverse consequences of medicine has influenced the health movement in two ways. First, the movement has an acute appreciation of the rhetoric of rejection that is at least implicit in the use of medical terminology. Second, the omnipresence of medicine's practical limits has repeatedly turned the health movement's attention toward the prevention of illness, as opposed to the restoration of health.

The Resurgence of Spiritual and Religious Paradigms

Through the early 1960s, many observers felt that religious and spiritual ways of seeing the world would inevitably decline due to the triumphs of science. Today, the folly of this view is clear. All around us we see evidence of the resilience of traditional religions as well as a resurgence of all sorts of "new" religions and spiritual phenomena as many people seek to include a spiritual dimension in their lives. This process takes many forms—from the rediscovery and revitalization of traditional religions through fundamentalist, evangelical, and charismatic influences to involvement in "new" or "exotic" religions, cults, and worship groups. The involvement of people from all strata of society, including the young and well-educated, in these events is striking. This phenomenon is complex, and its detailed examination is beyond our scope here. But it is clear that these trends have served as one of the forces shaping the health movement's sentiment against medicine and medicalization. One reason for this has been the feeling that while medical institutions and workers are involved with people at times when their spiritual needs are greatest—such as birth, suffering, and death—medicine frequently fails to deal adequately with the spiritual needs of patients. Indeed, the bureacratization and specialization of medical practice has exacerbated these trends, despite the widespread criticisms. The revitalization of spiritual paradigms has shaped the grievances of the health movement in a number of ways. By legitimizing and popularizing religious approaches, it has offered a critique of purely rationalistic approaches to health and illness. Beyond this, it has offered a range of alternative techniques such as the laying on of hands, prayer groups, and meditation for dealing with medical problems. While there is little consensus, even among adherents, as to how these approaches can actually influence bodily states, there is widespread agreement that they are powerful factors in affecting mental states as well as spiritual well-being.

Competition Between Groups of Professionals

Groups of professionals who find themselves in conflict or competition with physicians have provided many of the substantive criticisms of medicalization. Many of these groups—such as psychologists, nurses, pharmacists, and social workers—have long worked in medical settings. Yet now they find that the dominance and autonomy of physicians has become a barrier to their own attainment of power and income. In most cases, these occupational groups have fought for their own autonomy by attempting to gain independent licensure from the state, independent reimbursement from third-party payers, and independent control of their own institutions of professional education. But in order to achieve these goals, they have had to offer a rational justification for why their work need not be dominated (or at least not as fully dominated) by physicians. Thus, the professional advancement of many occupational groups has increasingly come to rest on showing that they can do things as well as and/or for less money than physicians can. They must show that tasks usually thought of as "medical" are better conceived of in some other way. In essence, these competing groups have constructed their own set of grievances against physicians and medicalization.

These interprofessional rivalries have been very influential for the broader health movement. They have helped create a wealth of detailed information that is critical of existing medical approaches and procedures. This knowledge has been utilized by many segments of the health movement in articulating their own grievances. Perhaps most important, the criticisms and alternatives presented by these professionals have helped foster a climate in which attacks on medicalization are perceived as widespread and legitimate.

The Rise of Holistic Medicine

A major influence on the health movement has been the development of a variety of alternative approaches to healing that may be subsumed under the name "holistic medicine." Although this term is defined loosely by both practitioners and commentators (Gordon 1980; Berkeley Holistic Health Center 1978; Pelletier 1977; Sobel 1979; Berliner and Salmon 1980; Guttmacher 1979; Kopelman and Maskop 1981), its frequently cited attributes include a definition of *health* as a positive state, not merely as the absence of disease; an acceptance of both a psychological and a spiritual component in the etiology and treatment of disease; a concern for the individual's own responsibility for illness and health; an emphasis on health education, self-help, and self-healing; a relationship with the physician that is relatively open, equal, and reciprocal; a concern for how the individual's health reflects the familial, social, and cultural environment; an openness toward using natural, "low-technology," and non-Western techniques whenever possible; an emphasis on physical and/or emotional contact between practitioner and client; and an acceptance of the notion that successful healing transforms the practitioner as well as the patient.

Holistic approaches to medicine have directly influenced the health movement through their emphasis on the interpenetration of mind, body, and spirit. The mind is seen as capable of directly influencing the body, not merely influencing attitudes or reactions to illness. Therefore, the individual's reaction to stressful situations is given particular attention, and emphasis is often placed upon altering these responses through techniques such as meditation, biofeedback, and social support.

Other important aspects of holistic healing that have been influential for the health movement are its concern with nutrition, which has been poorly understood and utilized by mainstream physicians; and its concern with exercise, which is utilized in a holistic context for its positive impact on the mind and temperament as well as its effects on the body. In each of these ways, holistic practitioners stress the responsibility of the individual in contributing to the origins of his/her illness, and the changes needed to bring about a cure or improvement. Recently, holistic techniques and approaches have become more acceptable to some physicians (Goldstein et al. 1987). These explicit and implicit critiques of mainstream medicine offered by holistic practitioners have contributed to the grievances expressed in the health movement.

The Shift From Acute to Chronic Illness

Since 1950, the leading causes of death in the United States have been heart disease, cancer, stroke, and accidents. This is quite a change from 1900, when infectious diseases—particularly pneumonia and tuberculosis—were most important. The diseases that threaten most American adults today are chronic. They develop slowly over many years and are usually multicausal. Although people can live with them—sometimes for many years—with varying degrees of symptoms and loss of functioning, they are largely incurable. Prevention is the most logical, effective, and efficient strategy for reducing the burden of these conditions. Mainstream biomedicine's refusal and/or inability to deal with the prevention of these conditions has been perhaps the single most important factor in creating the grievances that underlie the health movement.

In 1983, life expectancy in America was 78.3 years for women and 71.0 years for men. This represents an increase of almost 27.5 years since 1900. As life expectancy has increased, a large portion of people's lives occurs while they suffer from one or another chronic illness or disability. For example, Americans who reached age 65 in 1983 could expect to live another 17 years (Department of Health and Human Services 1985). Being sick is no longer the temporary position described by Talcott Parsons (1950) in his formulation of the "sick role." Our illnesses can become an important part of our identities. The chronicity and disability associated with these widespread illnesses, combined with the minimal impact of medicine on them, has

strengthened the grievances that foster the health movement.

Feminism and Other Social Movements

Social movements often grow out of and influence each other. Not only can the substantive demands of a movement be shaped by others, but its strategies, self-confidence, and acceptability to the public are all responsive to the successes and failures of other movements. Feminism, gay liberation, and movements for the rights of senior citizens and the disabled as well as the consumer movement, the self-help movement, and fundamentalist religious movements have all had interactive and mutually reinforcing effects upon the health movement. As part of articulating its own particular grievances, each of these movements has been led to oppose the prerogatives of professionals and experts, especially physicians. Each has come to question the value of medical techniques for bringing about the goals desired by its members. Instead, these movements have all emphasized the possibility of their adherents attaining high levels of functioning, wellness, or health in the face of adversity from the outside. While all these movements accept the existence of various medical problems, they accentuate the possibility of prevention of illness by the thoughts and actions of the members themselves.

Rather than discussing each of these movements, we focus here on one—the feminist movement—as the best-developed example of influence on the health movement. Childbirth, sexual behavior, appearance, and menopause are all women's experiences that have been medicalized. Women's decisions to work outside the home or not, be sexually active or not, and bear children or not have all been evaluated as "healthy" or not by psychiatrists and other physicians. The women's movement seeks to have women themselves evaluate these decisions, based on their own experience. Thus, symptoms of menopause—at one time considered signs of sin—were later seen as a source of neurotic behavior and eventually in the 1960s came to be redefined through the efforts of physicians and the pharmaceutical industry as a "deficiency disease" (McCrea 1983). Feminists see menopause as a normal part of a woman's life. The widely influential book *Our Bodies, Ourselves* (Boston Women's Health Collective 1976) exemplifies the attempt to demystify and deprofessionalize health-related knowledge and experience and has become a model for many in the health movement.

Changing Political Ideologies

There is no doubt that some political ideologies are more compatible with medicalization than others (Conrad 1980). Various liberal approaches to political problems share an affinity with the decriminalization of certain deviant behaviors, the increased funding of physicians through medical education and health insurance. All these foster medicalization. More conservative approaches are likely to stress enhancing personal responsibility for all sorts of problems, as well as fiscal restraint through lower taxes and government spending. These policies reinforce trends toward demedicalization. In the United States, the Reagan presidency is an example of the latter approach. The relationship of political views to medicalization is not necessarily causal, but rather mutually reinforcing. The grievances of the health movement have been supported by the temper of recent times throughout the nation.

Taken together, all these factors have created an increased understanding of health and illness that is broadly inclusive and demedicalized. This understanding of health has incorporated the various antimedical grievances and synthesized them into something positive. The grievances do not merely suggest what the movement rejects in a medically dominated view of health and illness. Rather, the movement goes beyond this to posit its own ideology and image of health, along with a full set of attitudes and behaviors. It is this demedicalized view of health that provides the core ideology of the health movement.

References

Alexander, B. 1987. The Disease and Adaptive Models of Addiction: A Framework Evaluation. *Journal of Drug Issues* 17: 47-66.

Baric, L. 1969. Recognition of the "At Risk" Role—A Means to Influence Health Behavior. *International Journal of Health Education* 12: 24-34.

Bayer, R. 1981. *Homosexuality and American Psychiatry*. New York: Basic.

Bergler, E. 1956. *Homosexuality: Disease or Way of Life?* New York: Hill and Wang.

Berkeley Holistic Health Center. 1978. *The Holistic Health Handbook*. Berkeley, CA.

Berlant, J. 1975. *Profession and Monopoly*. Berkeley: CA.

Berliner, H., and J. Salmon. 1980. The Holistic Alternative to Scientific Medicine: History and Analysis. *International Journal of Health Services* 10: 133-47.

Boston Women's Health Collective. 1976. *Our Bodies, Ourselves*. New York: Simon and Schuster.

Bullough, V. 1976. *Sexual Variances in Society and History*. New York: John Wiley & Sons.

Calderone, M. 1972. "Pornography" as a Public Health Problem. *American Journal of Public Health* 62: 374-76.

Callahan, D. 1973. The WHO Definition of "Health." *Hastings Center Report* 1: 77-87.

Chu, F., and S. Trotter. 1974. *The Madness Establishment*. New York: Grossman.

Conrad, P. 1975. The Discovery of Hyperkinesis: Notes on the Medicalization of Deviant Behavior. *Social Problems* 23: 12-21.

———. 1980. Implications of Changing Social Policy for the Medicalization of Deviance. *Contemporary Crises* 4: 195-205.

Conrad, P., and J. Schneider. 1980. *Deviance and Medicalizations, from Badness to Sickness*. St. Louis, MO: Mosby.

Davis, K. 1938. Mental Hygiene and the Class Structure. *Psychiatry* 1:55-65.

Department of Health and Human Services, Public Health Service. 1985. *Health Status of Minorities and Low Income Groups*. Washington, D.C.: Government Printing Office.

Empey, L. 1978. *American Delinquency: Its Meaning and Construction*. Homewood, IL.: Dorsey Press.

Engelhardt, H. 1974. The Disease of Masturbation: Values and the Concept of Disease. *Bulletin of the History of Medicine* 48: 234-48.

Freidson, E. 1970. *Profession of Medicine: A Study of the Sociology of Applied Knowledge*. New York: Dodd, Mead.

Gagnon, J., and W. Simon. 1973. *Sexual Conduct*. Chicago: Aldine.

Gill, D. 1970 *Violence Against Children*. Cambridge, MA.: Harvard University Press.

Goldstein, M. 1979. The Sociology of Mental Health and Illness. *Annual Review of Sociology* 5: 381-409.

Goldstein, M., C. Sutherland, D. Jaffe, and J. Wilson. 1987. Holistic Physicians and Family Practitioners: An Empirical Comparison. *Family Medicine* 19: 281-86.

Gordon, J. 1980. The Paradigm of Holistic Medicine. In *Health for the Whole Person*, edited by A. Hastings, A. Fadiman, and J. Gordon, 3-27. Boulder, CO.: Westview Press.

Guttmacher, S. 1979. Whole in Body, Mind, and Spirit: Holistic Health and the Limits of Medicine. *Hastings Center Report* 9:15-21.

Illich, I. 1976. *Medical Nemesis: The Expropriation of Health*. New York: Random House.

Jellinek, E. 1960. *The Disease Concept of Alcoholism*. Highland Park, N.J.: Hillhouse.

Kempe, C. et al. 1962. The Battered Child Syndrome. *Journal of the American Medical Association* 181: 17-24.

Kittrie, N. 1971. *The Right to be Different: Deviance and Enforced Therapy*. Baltimore, MD.: Johns Hopkins University Press.

Kopelman, L., and J. Maskop. 1981. The Holistic Health Movement: A Survey and Critique. *Journal of Medicine and Philosophy* 6: 209-35.

Larson, M. 1977. *Professionalism: A Sociological Analysis*. Berkeley: CA.

Lindheim, R. 1981. Birthing Centers and Hospices: Reclaiming Birth and Death. *Annual Review of Public Health* 2: 1-29.

McCrea, F. 1983. The Politics of Menopause: The "Discovery" of a Deficiency Disease. *Social Problems* 31: 111-23.

Musto, D. 1973. *The American Disease: Origins of Narcotic Control*. New Haven, CT.: Yale University Press.

Parsons, T. 1950. *The Social System*. New York: The Free Press.

Pelletier, K. 1977. *Mind as Healer, Mind as Slayer: A Holistic Approach to Preventing Stress Disorders*. New York: Delacorte Press.

Pfohl, S. 1977. The Discovery of Child Abuse. *Social Problems* 24: 310-23.

Robbins, T., and D. Anthony. 1979. The Sociology of Contemporary Religious Movements. *Annual Review of Sociology* 5: 75-89.

Roscrance, J. 1985. Compulsive Gambling and the Medicalization of Deviance. *Social Problems* 32: 275-84.

Rothman, D. 1971. *The Discovery of the Asylum*. Boston,: Little, Brown & Co.

Sedgwick, P. 1973. Illness—Mental and Otherwise. *Hastings Center Studies* 1: 19-40.

Sobel, David. 1979. *Ways of Health: Holistic Approaches to Ancient and Contemporary Medicine*. New York: Harcourt Brace Jovanovich.

Sontag, S. 1978. *Illness as Metaphor*. New York: Farrar, Straus & Giroux.

Szasz, T. 1961. *The Myth of Mental Illness*. New York: Harper.

———. 1970. *Ideology and Insanity*. New York: Doubleday-Anchor.

———. 1974. *Ceremonial Chemistry*. New York: Doubleday-Anchor.

Zola, I. 1975. In the Name of Health and Illness: On Some Socio-Political Consequences of Medical Influence. *Social Science and Medicine* 9: 83-87.

Further Reading

The Boston Women's Health Collective. 1976. *Our Bodies, Ourselves: A Book By and For Women*. New York: Simon and Schuster.

Peter Conrad and Joseph W. Schneider. 1992. *Deviance and Medicalization: From Badness to Sickness*. Philadelphia: Temple University Press.

Catherine Kohler Riessman. 1983. "Women and Medicalization: A New Perspective." *Social Policy* 14: 3-18.

Iriving K. Zola. 1985. "Depictions of Disability—Metaphor, Message and Medium in the Media: A Research and Political Agenda." *Social Science and Medicine* 22: 5-17.

Discussion Questions

1. What does Goldstein mean when he claims that there are no illnesses or diseases in nature?

2. What aspects of medicine and science make medical definitions of illness culturally salient?

3. How and what kinds of social forces do public interest groups rely upon to dislodge medical labels?

From *The Health Movement: Promoting Fitness in America*. Pp. 1-16. Copyright © 1992 by Twayne Publishers. Reprinted with permission of Twayne Publishers, an imprint of Simon & Schuster Macmillan. ◆

4

The Imperative of Health: Public Health and the Regulated Body

Deborah Lupton

Deborah Lupton examines conceptions of personal health that have moved from private concerns about well-being into the public realm. This selection critically investigates the targets and philosophies of health promotion campaigns. Transformation of the grotesque, inauthentic body to a civilized, authentic self underscores health promotion materials about smoking, drunk driving, beauty, and sexuality. Deviants become exemplars, whether they are villains or victims. Social space and ways of being are transformed in the name of public health. Consider aspects of your own health life subject to control by public campaigns. Think about the issues Lupton raises in this selection. What do these issues mean for the interplay between public health concerns and private lives?

The Subject in Health Promotion Campaigns

In the quest for publicizing the ill-effects of some behaviours on individual's health, certain groups have been singled out for stigmatization in health promotion campaigns. For example, Wang (1992) points out that media campaigns directed at preventing disability (including campaigns focusing on gun control and motor cycle helmet or seat-belt wearing) simultaneously stigmatize disability by

presenting it as a fate worse than death. She gives as an example an American television advertisement which showed a young woman sitting in a wheelchair with the accompanying words, "The drunk driver got one year. She was sentenced to life," which inadvertently links criminality with disablement (1992:1099). Hevey (1992) also criticizes the ways in which visual representations of disabled individuals are used to arouse concern and pity while underlining their position as members of a deviant outgroup. He argues that in advertising images, disabled people are represented as "inhabit[ing] a living social death in a bone-cage bodily oblivion which is not of their own making. Inside the advertising image they are cripples, they are handicapped, they cannot function or work" (Hevey 1992:22). The viewpoints of these "deviant" Others who are used as tragic exemplars are rarely canvassed when health promotion campaigns are designed.

AIDS education campaigns have provided copious examples of the propensity of state-sponsored health promotion to stigmatize certain social groups and bolster conservative moralistic positions towards sexual and illicit drug-using activities. One example is the notorious multi-million dollar Australian "Grim Reaper" mass media campaign, run in 1987, which used the spectral icon of death and horror-movie effects to denote the seriousness of AIDS. The campaign was subject to much publicity and media attention because of its "shock tactics" (Lupton, 1994: 53-5). The advertisement followed the attempt to frighten people into awareness of AIDS used by the British "Don't Die of Ignorance" mass media campaign run in 1986, which adopted the imagery of massive tombstones carved with the word "AIDS," erupting volcanoes and looming icebergs to emphasize to the public that AIDS threatens everyone. The "Grim Reaper" campaign was deliberately constructed to provoke shock: it was stated by a member of the government agency responsible for AIDS education that the advertisement was planned to "stop people in their tracks and make them think seriously about AIDS . . . to make it explicitly clear that AIDS has the potential to kill more Australians than

World War II" (reported in *The Age* newspaper [Melbourne], 7 April 1987).

The discourse of punishment for sexual sins is overt in these appeals to people's anxiety and fear, as is the construction of "deviant" sexualities as threats to the body public. In the United States health promotion advertising has overtly valorized marital fidelity over multiple partners (heterosexual and homosexual) in such advertisements as:

> The faithful have nothing to fear. Not everyone has to worry about AIDS. You're safe if you're in a long-term sexual relationship with someone who's just as faithful as you. And if neither of you is using needles and drugs. AIDS—It's Up to You [with accompanying photograph of two wedding rings]. (reproduced in Bolton 1992: 175)

Similarly, part of the national "America Responds to AIDS" television campaign run in 1988 featured characters such as the unfaithful husband warning the public of the dangers of such behaviour: "I was cheating [on my wife] . . . it's not worth it" (Bush and Boller, 1991:32). A British series of television advertisements depicted the scenarios of the pick-up at the disco and the enticing woman asking her dinner partner to "stay the night," to both arouse and incite fear in the audience around the dangers of "promiscuous" sexuality (Rhodes and Shaughnessy 1989). One Australian media campaign, run in 1988 and 1989, featured television advertisements showing a heterosexual couple embracing in a double bed. The camera then panned out to show many other similar couples in beds. The wording of the campaign was as follows:

> Next time you go to bed with someone, how many people will you be sleeping with? It's quite possible your partner has had several previous partners. And it's just as likely that these partners have had several partners too, and they've had partners, and so on, and so on, and so on. And any one of them could have been infected by the AIDS virus and passed it on. But you don't know. That's why you should always use a condom. Because you can never be sure just how many people you're really going to bed with.

Such fear-invoking strategies represent members of the public as apathetic, requiring stern warnings to jolt them into action. Education via campaigns is portrayed as a "weapon" in the war against disease and a "punishment" for complacency (Lupton 1994: 59-60). For example, the "Don't Die of Ignorance" campaign suggested that lack of knowledge was the only barrier to full protection against HIV infection. Posters used in Britain in 1987 proclaiming "The longer you believe AIDS only infects others, the faster it'll spread" and "AIDS: how big does it have to be before you take notice?" were direct attempts to create fear without providing accurate information or advice about how best to protect oneself (Watney 1988: 180), as was the tag-line of an American campaign "AIDS. If you think you can't get it, you're dead wrong" (van Dam 1989:145). Ironically, however, the campaigns served only to present paradoxical appeals to behaving "rationally" on the part of the viewer by invoking highly irrational emotions of terror using horror-movie style imagery (Rhodes and Shaughnessy, 1990: 57).

Sexual behavior characterized as "immoral" has thus been represented in such campaigns as dangerous not on religious or ethical grounds, but on health grounds. The moralistic approach to "deviant" or "perverse" sexual behaviours is disguised by the appeal to the preservation of the public's health. The incursion into individual's intimate sexual relationships on the part of such campaigns is legitimized by the apparent urgency of protecting the population from the AIDS epidemic. However, rather than publicizing alternative ways of engaging in sexual acts with as many partners as one likes (such as mutual masturbation instead of penetrative sex), health promotional material on HIV/AIDS has continued to privilege the strategies of monogamous relationships, "knowing" one's partner and reducing multiple sexual contacts. In stark contrast, AIDS education materials developed by community and activist groups in Britain, the United States, and Australia have largely rejected fear appeals and hints of punishment for positive and erotic representations of safer sex which demonstrate how individuals may continue to indulge and take pleasure in their sexual fantasies and desires while avoiding infection.

Another example of the type of subject constructed by health promotional discourses, this time sponsored by a drug company, is a one-page pamphlet distributed in Australian doctors' surgeries and pharmacies and supported by a billboard campaign in late 1993. One side of the pamphlet showed the photographic image of a middle-aged man, looking disconsolate, behind "bars" of floating white smoke. The text above read, "There is a way out for smokers who want to escape." Turned over, the text read in large letters, "If you have the will, we have the way," followed by:

> Congratulations! Your decision to quit smoking is the first step toward living a more healthy, smokefree life. Quitting is never easy. But now there is something which can help you achieve your goal. Simply see your doctor and ask how you can escape from your nicotine addiction and habit. Your doctor can give you the prescription to help you succeed.

The pamphlet asserts that "You will begin to feel better very quickly," as breathing will be easier, the "smoker's cough" will be lost, there will be more energy, breath will be fresher, teeth will look brighter and skin will improve and (lastly); "You will be less likely to suffer from smoking related diseases (e.g. cancer and heart diseases)." In addition, ex-smokers will be able to save money, they will smell better (as will their house), they will not have to clear up any dirty ashtrays and cigarette butts:"You will soon begin to feel proud that you have the strength and willpower to kick the smoking habit. . . . You will find your new, clean, healthy image makes you more appealing to others. . . . You will no longer feel like a social outcast." Finally, the pamphlet asserts: "You will not be affecting the health of others." This pamphlet represents smokers as lacking discipline and will-power, needful of medical help and even a prescribed drug (nicotine patches) to beat their habit. The use of the graphics (suggesting a prisoner held against his will) and the word "escape" several times, the representation of smokers as unhealthy, dirty, lacking pride in themselves, physically unappealing, outcasts and harming others' health, all work to stigmatize smokers, representing them not only as a threat to themselves but as endangering public health. It argues for the view of the subject as having a genuine, real persona, the authentic self—the non-smoker— versus the false self of the "smoker" who is controlled by the drug. There is a non-smoker behind the bars of tobacco waiting to be freed.

Recent health education campaigns have encouraged people to carry out surveillance not only on themselves, but on others. For example, in a mass media campaign against passive smoking run by the New South Wales Department of Health in late 1993, people were warned that they should police the activities of others to protect their own health. In one newspaper advertisement, an accompanying computer-enhanced photograph, cropped just above the upper lip, showed a woman's lower lip being grotesquely drawn out by a "fishing hook" made of smoke emitting from a lit cigarette, labelled not with a known brand-name but with the words "Other People's Smoke." The heading extended the "hook" metaphor: "Just because you don't smoke, it doesn't mean you're off the hook." The text went on to claim:

> Think you're a non-smoker? Think again. If you live, work or play where other people smoke, you're inhaling—like it or not. 'Other People's Smoke.' Drifting from the burning end of other people's cigarettes, it accounts for 85% of the smoke in smoke-filled rooms. And being unfiltered, it also contains far higher concentrations of poisonous chemicals. . . . Non-smokers? There'll be no such thing until we clear the air.

The advertisement thus positions all individuals as smokers, the majority albeit involuntary smokers. In one suburban Sydney newspaper this advertisement was accompanied by a full-page "advertorial" advising people to plaster "smoke-free" stickers on their front door and on their cars, remove all ashtrays and "when smokers ask you if they can smoke in your home, say you'd prefer them to smoke outside." They were encouraged to ensure that their workplace is smoke free by approaching management and to request smoke-free dining areas in restaurants that do not already have them. Readers were exhorted to remember that "you are not alone. Three out of four people are non-smokers and everybody is affected by Other People's Smoke."

While the intention to make people aware that side-stream cigarette smoke is potentially threatening to the health of both non-smokers and smokers seems an eminently reasonable goal, the manner in which the New South Wales Department of Health chose to publicize the risk is telling for its imagery and subtextual ideological stance. The rhetoric of this campaign positions the smoker as the stigmatized Other, both overtly in the slogan of "Other People's Smoke," and less overtly, in the discursive strategies used throughout. The photograph, with its distorted image of the lip being pulled towards a cigarette's lighted end, the mouth grimacing in pain and fear, vividly denotes the threat posed by the unseen "Other People." Throughout the advertisement, it is assumed that the reader, the "you" hailed by the text, is a non-smoker, one of a community of like-minded people reading the advertisement together. The language is didactic, using imperatives to exhort this non-smoking reader to take action against "Other People." The emphasis is on the non-smoker as an innocent bystander, forced to endure the health risks posed them by "Other People" and urged to join with the community, hailed as "we" and "us" (as in the "Let's"), to "clear the air." By this rhetoric, non-smokers are positioned as consorting with the Other in their own downfall by refusing to act to prevent others from smoking in their presence. The onus is placed on them to do something, to enforce their right to clean air and good health. The overall effect is to further stigmatize smokers as not only socially unacceptable, but as selfishly endangering the health of all others around them. Such individuals, the advertisement implies, must be policed by the majority of reasonable people around them, both in public and private places. Ironically, a month before the release of the campaign the *Sydney Morning Herald* newspaper published the results of a poll it had commissioned on whether Australians would allow people to smoke in their home. Of the sample surveyed, 73 percent were non-smokers, of which almost half (46 percent) agreed that they would let others smoke in their home (Carney 1993).

Critics of health promotion campaigns have pointed out how they routinely reproduce gender stereotypes evident in commercial advertising: "Women are to be seen as passive, vulnerable and sexually available, only distinguished by their youth and beauty, while men are seen as active, possessive, and masterful" (Rhodes and Shaughnessy, 1989: 27). Since the nineteenth century public health strategies have traditionally represented women as mothers, the guardians of their families' health, and by extension, that of the nation, and have targeted them for intervention as agents of regulation. So too, contemporary health promotion campaigns tend to place the emphasis of responsibility for health promotion upon women, in their roles as wives and mothers, with little concern for women's own health status or the structural constraints under which they operate (H. Rose 1990; Amos 1993). Women are expected to regulate the diet of their partners and offspring according to the dictates of health guidelines, to monitor their partner's weight and exercise habits, to ensure the cleanliness of their children, to make sure that their children are vaccinated and to desist from smoking and alcohol consumption while pregnant and even afterwards. In 1993, an Australian woman was forced to give the Family Court an undertaking that she would not smoke in the presence of her two young children following an application made to the court by the woman's former husband. The woman also had to undertake to prevent her children's exposure to any cigarette smoke. The court supported her ex-husband's actions on the ground that the children were both asthmatic (Stenberg 1993).

Media campaigns have vacillated between representing women as carers and women as the source of contagion. For example, in HIV/AIDS media campaigns women have either been represented as *femmes fatales*, seeking to tempt men into their web of infection (as in the British advertisement described earlier), or conversely as the "responsible" partner in a heterosexual relationship who is exhorted to negotiate condom use or other safe sex techniques with her partner. As one pamphlet designed for Australian women by the New South Wales Department of Health advised them: "Women can reduce their risk of HIV infection by: insisting that their male partner always uses a condom for sex. . . . Finding a way to talk about HIV and STD prevention with your partner is very important."

Health promotional campaigns have often explicitly directed their emotional appeals to incite women's anxiety around the attractiveness and youthfulness of their bodies. Several anti-smoking advertisements, for example, in Australia and Britain have attempted to manipulate young women's concern about their physical appearance or general attractiveness to frighten them into avoiding or giving up smoking. A television advertisement run by the Western Australian Department of Health in the late 1980s showed a young woman smoking, her face slowly ageing into that of an old crone. The voice-over asserted: "What good's a pretty face when you've got ugly breath?" Health advertisements advocating breast self-examination have routinely adopted the genre of soft-porn to represent the breast. Rarely is the woman depicted as ageing in such portrayals, even though the older woman is most at risk from breast cancer. Instead, the image of the breast is youthful, firm and shapely. Young, attractive women are shown caressing their breasts like *Penthouse* Pets (Wilkinson and Kitzinger 1993). Alternatively women's bodily parts have been objectified, rendered as separate, for the purposes of health promotion. Wilkinson and Kitzinger (1993: 230) describe a British breast self-examination advertisement which showed a photographed breast with dotted circles superimposed around the nipple, with the instruction "press," implying a mechanistic metaphor which ill-fits with the dominant sexualized portrayal of the female breast.

As these examples demonstrate, a dualism is routinely constructed in health promotional campaigns between the civilized and the grotesque body. The grotesque body is commonly vividly represented, often visually, as a horror of flesh-out-of-control: the beer belly, the ugly, wrinkled face, the distorted lip, the helpless, disabled body in the wheelchair, the entrapped addict. These images provide visual evidence to support a moral tale: this is what will happen to *your* body if you are not careful. In contrast, the civilized body is that which will be achieved and preserved through the regimens of health promotion, with due application of personal control and continuous attention and awareness of the potential of the body to revolt.

Throughout the health promotional literature (both commercial and government-sponsored), the implicit assumption is that the information disseminated to patients or the general public on the part of those in authority is privileged over the lay health beliefs of those not in authority. The subjects of health promotion are constructed in a similar manner to the subject of the child in the school; needing the opportunity for self-realization but also needful of training to become a citizen; capable of self-control and self-discipline but only able to fulfil their "health potential" via governmental regulation; encouraged to acquire the ability to recognize their own best interests and to be responsible for themselves (Tyler 1993: 35). Under this notion, individuals who seemingly care little for their health status because of the desire to fulfil "short-term desires" are viewed as needful of more education. More often than not, this individual is categorized as working class, or, more euphemistically, as a member of one of the "lower socio-economic groups" or "with lower educational attainment" (Better Health Commission 1986: 39). Such understandings of health-related behaviour view it as "a 'problem' that will respond to help organized in such a way as to 'correct' an incorrect perception of interpersonal relations, or to reconstruct the world view of particular subjects and their own calculation of personal capacities" (May 1993: 60). . . .

References

Amos, A. (1993) In her own best interests? Women and health education: a review of the last fifty years. *Health Education Journal*, 52(3), 141-50.

Better Health Commission. (1986) *Looking Forward to Better Health: Volume One*. Canberra: Commonwealth of Australia.

Bolton, R. (1992) AIDS and promiscuity: muddles in the models of HIV prevention. *Medical Anthropology*, 14, 145-223.

Bush, A.J. and Boller, G.W. (1991) Rethinking the role of television advertising during health crises: a rhetorical analysis of the federal AIDS campaigns. *Journal of Advertising*, 20(1), 28-37.

Carney, S. (1993) Most are tolerant of others smoking. *Sydney Morning Herald*, 9 October.

Hevey, D. (1992) *The Creatures Time Forgot: Photography and Disability Imagery*. London: Routledge.

Lupton, D. (1994) *Moral Threats and Dangerous Desires: AIDS in the News Media*. London: Taylor and Francis.

May, C. (1993) Resistance to peer group pressure: an inadequate basis for alcohol education. *Health Education Research: Theory and Practice*, 8(2), 159-65.

Rhodes, T. and Shaughnessy, R. (1989) Selling safer sex: AIDS education and advertising. *Health Promotion*, 4(1), 27-30.

Rhodes, T. and Shaughnessy, R. (1990) Compulsory screening: advertising AIDS in Britain, 1986-89. *Policy and Politics*, 18(1), 55-61.

Rose, H. (1990) Activists, gender and the community health movement. *Health Promotional International*, 5(3), 209-18.

Rose, N. (1990) *Governing the Soul: the Shaping of the Private Self*. London: Routledge.

Stenberg, M. (1993) Mother's smoking outlawed by court. *Sydney Morning Herald*, 27 July.

Tyler, D. (1993) Making better children. In Meredyth, D. and Tyler, D. (eds), *Child and Citizen: Genealogies of Schooling and Subjectivity*. Brisbane: Griffith University Institute for Cultural Policy Studies, pp. 35-60.

van Dam, C.J. (1989) AIDS: is health education the answer? *Health Policy and Planning*, 4(2), 141-7.

Wang, C. (1992) Culture, meaning and disability: injury prevention campaigns and the production of stigma. *Social Science and Medicine*, 35(9), 1093-102.

Watney, S. (1988) Visual AIDS—advertising ignorance. In Aggleton, P. and Homans, H. (eds), *Social Aspects of AIDS*. London: Falmer, pp. 177-82.

Wilkinson, S. and Kitzinger, C. (1993) Whose breast is it anyway? A feminist consideration of advice and 'treatment' for breast cancer. *Women's Studies International Forum*, 16(3), 229-38.

Further Reading

David Armstrong. 1993. "Public Health Spaces and the Fabrication of Identity." *Sociology* 27 (3): 393-410.

R. Bolton. 1992. "AIDS and Promiscuity: Muddles in the Models of HIV Prevention." *Medical Anthropology* 14: 145-223.

Ann Oakley. 1989. "Smoking in Pregnancy: Smokescreen or Risk Factor? Towards a Materialist Analysis." *Sociology of Health and Illness* 11(4): 311-35.

Bryan S. Turner. 1992. *Regulating Bodies: Essays in Medical Sociology*. London: Routledge.

Discussion Questions

1. Should health be an entirely private matter? Explain the tensions inherent in the drive to maintain public health and to value individual lifestyle and choice.

2. What are some of the problems Lupton identifies in health promotion campaigns? Can you suggest solutions to these problems?

3. Explain how public health campaigns juxtapose the grotesque and the civilized body in an attempt to bring about individual conformity. Can you think of an example of a campaign not provided in this selection that makes use of this strategy?

Section 2

The Self in Social Context

In this section, we look at individuals—both patients and practitioners—and observe how the social context of their respective experiences affects them. We begin with voices of people who experience illness. We sense their quest for knowing self, for understanding their changed bodies, and for finding a way to live with them. The autobiographical accounts reflect thoughts, feelings, and actions. These accounts depict experiences at different points in illness. They show how individuals make sense of their situations and tell their stories. The research reports compile individual narratives and tell a "collective story" (Richardson 1988) about how experience affects self-concept, identity, and action.

These selections reveal people seeking answers to fundamental questions of human value, meaning, and purpose. Both patients and practitioners attempt to construct selves in a medical system based upon acute care that is often incongruent with their needs. Serious illness and disability can render self-concept problematic and strip a patient's former existence away. Logistics of care and limitations of knowledge can undermine the development of a professional self.

The stories go beyond the public accounts that Radley and Billig rightly criticize. These stories reveal private doubts, fears, and sorrows, as well as haunting memories. Personal accounts of four exceptionally aware and articulate men and women offer insights into experiencing illness at multiple points in their respective illness careers. Their stories are tales of stigmatizing difference and of quests for control—of their health, of their lives, and of their identities.

The voice of the self deep within suffering becomes distinct in Arthur Frank's piece, "Seeing Through Pain." Suffering is part of illness, injury, and disability—often a major part. Yet for decades, medical sociologists seldom addressed suffering, nor developed a sociology of suffering. To look at suffering means looking at loss; it frequently means acknowledging and facing negative emotions. Suffering is compounded by assaults upon the self inflicted by others—directly in face-to-face interaction or through social arrangements that demean and devalue those who are different, as Robert Murphy's portrayal of a damaged self testifies.

Though suffering may occur in isolation, it still occurs within social context and is embedded in social awareness. Comparisons can be constant—chronically ill and disabled people often develop heightened awareness of interactional nuances that separate them from others. Moreover, their bodily feelings may separate them from others. Pain forces the person into subjective experience and separates self from others. As Arthur Frank reveals, pain brings us into our bodies; it brings us into the immediate present. It usurps coherence and harmony within one's body, self, and life. Pain at once separates Frank from his world and rekindles his reverence for it. Mere words cannot express what it means to be overtaken by pain. Yet through writing about learning to see through pain, Frank himself begins to build a language to express and to share it. He not only shows us how he learned to see through pain, but also provides a window on the self in pain. We feel Frank groping for resolution, searching for meaning. In contrast, Amy Gross and Dee Ito's interviewee has decreed what her experience means. She has emerged from crisis and instructs us about what she has learned about taking charge of her care. As a person who confronted crisis, this woman recounted the story of a self in action. She presents herself as a resolute person who forbade medical professionals from usurping her rights. Her stance toward her condition combined extraordinary knowledge with exceptional vigilance. Her insistence about receiving information and making treatment decisions testifies to claiming a self as well as asserting rights. Like this woman, Nancy Mairs' previous experiences within medical worlds led her to request information. Her account brings us into her diagnostic quest. By receiving a diagnosis, she shifted from a self in limbo to an identifiable one, however ominous, that can be understood.

Nancy Mairs needed to end the mystery of not knowing what her symptoms meant and, perhaps, alleviate questions that they might be mental. Like many other chronically ill people, she discounted her early symptoms and later sought medical explanations for her growing symptoms after another person commented on them. Despite noting fleeting symptoms, people usually attribute them to the least serious possible cause. Often they do so even when onset is rapid, such as during a heart attack. For Nancy Mairs, a diagnosis that decreed her difference from other adults affirmed her competence as a rational adult.

Robert F. Murphy, in contrast, had long months and years with a progressive disability. From the beginning, he knew his symptoms amounted to losses and sensed that his most devastating losses were social and psychological. Murphy once shared society's indifference toward disabled people. His sur-

prise and sorrow over having entered their ranks permeates his account. While Arthur Frank recounts feeling separated from others, Murphy reflects upon being segregated by others through difference inflicted by disability. For him, the meaning of progressive physical losses is worsened by strained interactions, stigma, and shame and subsequent feelings of diminishment. These themes resound in the emerging literature on the experience of chronic illness and disability. David Karp demonstrates how similar identity problems arise in people diagnosed with depression. Feelings of difference and questions about self-worth permeate depressed patients' consciousness.

Chronic illness and disability make prior taken-for-granted assumptions about body and self problematic. Impairment of previously taken-for-granted health and function often comes as a shock. As Kathy Charmaz points out, people do not simply resolve issues of coping with such losses once and for all. Rather, they must deal with similar issues anew as complications occur and problems compound. The trials of managing illness in daily life may alter relationships and change the self. Yet the self discovered through illness is not inevitably the damaged self that Murphy depicts, but instead it may be a transformed, more valued self.

Several resounding themes found in patients' lives echo in lives of neophyte physicians. Both novice physicians and patients hold identities that are not entirely affirmed—identities at risk of being undermined or discredited. Like many sick patients, novice physicians live in a fragmented world and are left to their own devices to make their way and to prove themselves. Questions of competence pervade the actions and interactions of both patients and novice physicians. Patients have to demonstrate personal competence. New physicians must prove professional competence. Patients may be continually called upon to prove that their symptoms are real, their requests legitimate, and their actions appropriate, given their diagnosed conditions. New physicians are called upon to identify their patients' symptoms accurately, to keep their interventions on target, and to ensure the appropriateness of how they manage the patient, staff, and medical technology and resources—all within collapsed time, often during crises. Claiming professional competence and constructing a professional self are arduous processes based on trial and error.

Novice physicians as well as patients struggle to claim an autonomous self and to establish a respected identity, and may be isolated in their quest to do so. Like patients, novice physicians also struggle within a system that fragments their experience and reduces institutional problems to individual troubles. Thus, problems inherent within the medical care system, and in medical training specifically, become transformed into personal problems and responsibilities of the individual medical student, intern, or resident. They must try to handle the complex care of chronically ill patients within a system designed for profit and predicated on acute care. Although this system may pose severe problems for neophyte physicians, profits of money, power, and prestige may accrue to them later. Unlike people with chronic illnesses and disabilities, their problems with proving competence and making their way through the medical care system likely end upon completion of training.

Until then, they try to handle their situations themselves. Perri Klass reveals the competitiveness and gamesmanship within training that can relegate patients to incidental rather than central status. And the timing and pacing of medical care contributes to this incidental status as evident in William Yoels and Jeffrey Clair's study of medical residents. Problems and crises topple upon each other for the new physician who runs from one incident to another, from one critically sick patient to another, each time hoping to see the problem clearly and hoping to solve it. As crises accrue, the novice physician's energy plummets, judgment may fail, and timing is lost. Patient problems are weighed against a backdrop of medical hierarchy and knowledge—who has it, how is it used, when does it work, and when do fatigue, inexperience, and immediacy take their toll? Do net gains in neophyte experience merit perpetuating training that fragments care and professional responsibility? However invisible the effects of the medical care system might be, both practitioners and patients' selves and situations are affected by it.

References

Laurel Richardson. 1988. "The Collective Story: Postmodernism and the Writing of Sociology." *Sociological Focus* 21: 199-208. ◆

Becoming and Being Ill

5

Seeing Through Pain

Arthur W. Frank

Arthur Frank brings us into the patient's experience as he attempts to describe being taken over by pain. Pain results in inexpressible, unshareable separation—isolation—and, in turn, isolation intensifies pain. Pain renders ill people mute and casts them out. Rather than pain being an alien intruder, Frank tells us that pain is the signal of a sick body. Frank makes pain his own though he recognizes that becoming isolated in a pain-wracked body risks losing wholeness, coherence, and connectedness. Yet focusing beyond one's body in pain can lead to finding coherence by seeing through pain's incoherence.

In this selection, Arthur Frank brings a sociological eye to his story of suffering with pain from cancer. Look for how he reveals the separation caused by suffering, a separation of words, involvement, social space, and time. Language cannot capture the inchoate incoherence of being in pain. Life becomes pain and one's body becomes isolated in pain. The mechanical order of our bodies that we define as health is lost. As the body in pain suffers a disorder, life becomes disordered. Pain catapults the person out of ordinary reality out of the routines and spaces of everyday life and immerses him or her in an alien, incoherent reality consumed by the body. Pain brings one into the body and keeps one there, but forces change in a quest for its resolution.

How doctors came to realize that I had cancer is only the institutional part of the story of becoming ill again. The medical experience has its place, but more important is what I was experiencing in my body. That story begins with pain. Medicine has not conquered pain, though it has developed the means to control pain during much of critical illness. Pain is experienced most at the beginning of illness, before physicians understand what is happening, and at the end, when the body becomes unpredictable. Since my experience happily did not reach that end, pain belongs at the beginning of my story.

Pain is the body's response to illness; it is the first thing many people associate with illness and what they fear most. Whether or not pain is the most difficult part of cancer to live through, it is probably the hardest to describe. We have plenty of words to describe specific pains: sharp, throbbing, piercing, burning, even dull. But these words do not describe the experience of pain. We lack terms to express what it means to live "in" such pain. Unable to express pain, we come to believe there is nothing to say. Silenced, we become isolated in pain, and the isolation increases the pain. Like the sick feeling that comes with the recognition of yourself as ill, there is a pain attached to being in pain.

My pain was the result of pressure exerted by the secondary tumors in my back, a pressure that became more acute when I lay down for some time. In the mornings I would wake up feeling a viselike pressure on my lower back around the kidneys. Soon the pain began to wake me at night, preventing me from sleeping. After several nights I was too tired to shake off sleep entirely, even though rest was impossible. I spent those nights in a kind of limbo between waking and dozing, always inside the pain.

My disease connected pain with night. As the tumors took over my body, pain took over my mind. Darkness compounds the isolation and loneliness of pain, for the sufferers are separated from those whose bodies lie quiet. In darkness the world of those in pain becomes unglued, incoherent.

In writing about the incoherence of pain, one risks becoming incoherent all over again. Language easily goes wrong. I could write that at night in pain I came to know illness face to face. But this metaphor distorts the experience. However much I wanted to give illness a face—to give it any kind of coherence—it is not a presence. Giving illness a face, a temptation enhanced by the dark, only muddles things further. At night I faced only myself.

When we feel ourselves being taken over by something we do not understand, the human response is to create a mythology of what threatens us. We turn pain into "it," a god, an enemy to be fought. We think pain is victimizing us, either because "it" is malevolent or because we have done something to deserve its wrath. We curse it and pray for mercy from it. But pain has no face because it is not alien. It is from myself. Pain is my body signaling that something is wrong. It is the body talking to itself, not the rumblings of an external god. Dealing with pain is not war with something outside the body; it is the body coming back to itself.

But taking pain entirely into my own body, making it too much my own, carries the danger of becoming isolated in that body. Isolation is the beginning of incoherence. When the body is healthy, it coheres, its parts work in concert and it fits into its environment. Lying down, the body finds comfort and rest. Waking, it is ready for activity. In pain the natural rhythm of rest and activity is lost, and that loss leads to further losses of plans and expectations, of a life that makes sense as a fitting together of past and future. Order breaks down, and incoherence takes its place.

At night, while others are sleeping, it is coherent to sleep, to share that rest. To be summoned out of that rest is an incoherence, a loss of the wholeness that is the natural cycle of life among others. But again my language slips. No thing summoned me from sleep. Bodily pain woke me, and the consciousness of this pain turned into the incoherence of being awake, isolated from those who slept.

Pain is thus one of the first experiences an ill person has of being cast out. To regain a sense of coherence, in which pain may have to remain a part, the ill person has to find a way back in among those he has become separated from.

When I was awake at night in pain, I could have woken Cathie [his wife]. I could have called her to witness the pain and to break the loneliness, but waking her would have violated the coherence of her natural cycle of daily life. She still worked during the day and slept at night. Her life retained the coherence mine had lost. I was outside that natural cycle. During the day I was too tired to work, during the night the hammering in my back prevented me from sleeping. I was neither daily nor nocturnal, but suspended outside the limits of either existence. I was neither functionally present nor accountably absent. I lived my life out of place.

I used to have nightmares of finding myself in a place I knew to be forbidden, without any clothes and having to get back (in dreams you never know where) without being seen. Sometimes the nightmare would become an adventure. I would half fly and half flow, silent and naked, through dark, empty alleyways. Other times I would be caught out, fumbling and immobile, for all to see. Part of the fear in such dreams is of being out of place. I was no less out of place on those nights I half sat and half lay, trying to find a position outside of the pain.

I fantasized that this pain was "just for tonight," that it was muscular stress and would be gone tomorrow. This fantasy was fueled by my fear of what might truly be wrong with me, but it was also supported by what my doctor was telling me. One night he prescribed a strong sedative, and when I awoke even from that, the nightmares that accompanied me out of sleep did give incoherence a form and a face. After that night I could no longer sustain my part of what had been my doctor's and my mutual fantasy.

But I have only half-answered the question of why I did not wake my wife. The other reason is that her sleep was the only coherence left. Although I could no longer share in others' rest, I cared for it all the more. If I could not sleep, I could still love her sleep. Disturbing it would have been the most painful thing I could do. Later, when I was very ill, I watched people out running and loved their capacity for movement, their freedom within their bodies. My hope was that they also valued what they were able to be.

I wish I could finish my story about pain with some formula I learned for dealing with it. But I never learned one. By the time I entered the hospital, the tumors had shifted or somehow changed, allowing me to lie in bed comfortably. There is probably some medical explanation for this change, but it does not interest me much. What counts is that the pain did its proper work: it forced me to get another medical opinion. By the date of the urology appointment made by my family physician, I had already had surgery and one chemotherapy treatment. Pain was the ally it is designed to be, my body's way of insisting that something must change.

Although I never discovered a formula for dealing with pain, I did manage to break through its incoherence one night before it abated. Making my way upstairs, I was stopped on the landing by the sight—the vision really—of a window. Outside the window I saw a tree, and the streetlight just beyond was casting the tree's reflection on the frosted glass. Here suddenly was beauty, found in the middle of a night that seemed to be only darkness and pain. Where we see the face of beauty, we are in our proper place, and all becomes coherent. As I looked at the window it formed a kind of haiku for me:

The streetlight behind the branches
Projects patterns
On a misted window
Do not wipe the glass
Lest others wake.

I realized that if illness has a face, it could be the beauty of that light. But I did not see the face of illness in that window any more than I had seen it in the nightmares caused by pain breaking through the sedative. The window was no myth, no metaphor. It was exactly what it was, and seeing it completely absorbed my attention. I was still in pain, but the pain had brought me to that landing, which was the only place I could be to see the beauty of that window. Coherence was restored.

But coherence does not go without saying; it requires expression. However poor my verse was, I was once again expressing myself. Pain that is inexpressible isolates us; to be mute is to be cast out from others. Whatever form our expression takes, we offer that expression to others, whether or not anyone else is there. Expression implies the presence of others, and we begin again to share in humanity. Others slept their orderly sleep, and I, in my place as they were in theirs, saw something of beauty. I remained alone, but my words put me in the presence of those others.

It is just as hard to write about the coherence I felt as it is to write about incoherence. But it does not matter if my words are not coherent. For the ill person, the attempt to communicate creates an experience of coherence. The particular words in my verse did not matter; it was my attempt at expression that created coherence. I needed the window to see the verse, and I needed the verse to place my seeing in the world of others and thus regain my place in that world.

It is easier to write of caring. I knew that others were sleeping, and I cared for their sleep; I knew there were things of beauty in the night that I cared for. These feelings made pain something I could live with. At the moment when the incoherence of illness and pain makes it seem that all you have lived for has been taken away or is about to be lost, you can find another coherence in which to live. That night the pain mattered less, not because I dissociated myself from my body, but rather because I associated myself beyond my body. Caring for Cathie's sleep or for that window gave me the coherence I needed to go on caring for myself. I had not yet been sick enough to understand all I saw in that window; only later would language catch up to experience. But at least that night I knew I was in a place I could care for.

Further Reading

Kathy Charmaz. 1991. *Good Days, Bad Days: The Self in Chronic Illness and Time.* New Brunswick: Rutgers University Press.

Oliver Sacks. 1984. "Convalescence." *A Leg to Stand On.* New York: Summit, pp. 156-161.

May Sarton. 1988. *After the Stroke: A Journal.* New York: W.W. Norton & Company.

Discussion Questions

1. What does Frank mean by incoherence and coherence?

2. Why does Frank believe that ill persons must find another coherence beyond the experience of illness and pain?

6

Mastectomy and Reconstruction

Amy Gross
Dee Ito

This woman makes strong, clear assessments of her body and her situation. From the beginning, she sought information and chose what to do. She arrived at the juncture of diagnosis armed with information and ideas about which paths to take and when to take them. Her image of herself as a strong person and her ability to rank breast cancer as a lesser life crisis than other woes made her resolute in her choices and her control over her life.

"You know what I think? Sometimes you have to tell your doctor what to do."

A woman who became very active in breast cancer research when her sister died from the disease. She herself had a mastectomy when she was thirty-eight years old, and reconstruction surgery a year and a half later. She is an exceptionally well-informed patient.

How did you discover you had breast cancer?

I had three benign tumors, right in a row, one more frightening than the other because no one knew what they were. Then I didn't have any problem for a couple of years until four years after my sister died. In 1984 I discovered a lump one night in bed—I was just brushing my hand over the sheet and I ran over this hard lump and jumped up. Fortunately I was married at the time—we had just gotten married. The next morning I went immediately to my doctor in the city—I was part of a study there because of my sister's death. And I was frightened.

Did this lump feel different from the three that you'd had biopsied?

Yes, it was harder. But my surgeon said that he didn't feel it was anything more than another benign problem, and he didn't want to biopsy me again because I had already had three biopsies on this side, and if you have too many, the scar tissue is so dense that they can't read it. He said, "Let's wait a few weeks. We'll see if there is any change, and if there is, then we'll do something."

In the meantime, I happened to attend a breast cancer symposium. One of the exhibits was Mammacare—they have these breast forms with lumps in them so you can learn to self-exam. I was standing there, and I just sort of felt one, and I thought, "It sure feels like what I have."

A couple of weeks passed, and I kept thinking there was some kind of change, that it was getting a little larger. I went to see a friend of mine who's a surgeon, and we did a transillumination procedure on it, which they don't use anymore, and we did an ultrasound, and a clear little lump showed up, about a centimeter, with very concise borders. It looked very much like a little benign tumor—on many, many malignant tumors, the borders are not as clear. This surgeon friend of mine said, "I don't know what it is, but if I were you, I'd get that thing out of there."

I suppose this is an example of being assertive about your health care: I went back to my doctor a couple of days later, and I said, "Look, I want this thing out of here. I don't care if it causes scar tissue, I want it out." So he took it out, under a local. I was, of course, awake when he was doing it, and I kept talking to him and saying, "What does it look like?" He said, "Well, it looks benign, but I . . ." He didn't give anything away in his voice, but I had to wait an awfully long time in the recovery room, and I started getting suspicious after about ten minutes. They do a frozen section, and generally they can tell right away if it's just a benign dysplasia.

When he came back, I was kind of joking and said, "Well, is it bad? Is that why you were gone so long?" And there was this long pause, and he said, "Yeah, it *is* bad." Then it was . . . Your whole life flashes in front of you. My husband wasn't with me, and my mother wasn't with me. We didn't expect this to be bad news. I had a friend with me. I think it's helpful to be with people you really love and feel very comfortable with. Not that I didn't feel comfortable with my friend, but when you have to strip away everything, you want to be either with yourself or with people who love you unconditionally. I had just watched my sister die from this a few years before, and it was frightening.

How did you decide what to do next?

He said to me, "You have several choices. You can have a double mastectomy and get rid of the whole thing. You can have a modified radical, or you can have a lumpectomy." And of course, the patient always has the opportunity to say, "Do nothing." There are a lot of people who say, "Do nothing. Just take the lump out." Which is a very dangerous kind of attitude, but some people survive that way. We all have choices.

But my decision was driven largely by what had happened to my sister and also by what I had studied about the disease. Because, don't forget, I'd had two and a half years of baptism by fire preceding my sister's death, and I had really gone into the science of it. So I already knew a whole lot. And I knew I wasn't going to take any chances. I could have had a lumpectomy, but I just wasn't into having six weeks of radiation at the time. And I really wanted to get rid of it. So I decided to have a modified radical mastectomy and to wait and make sure that I didn't have any recurrence before I had reconstruction.

I had the surgery the next morning, and then I was one of those patients who fell in the category of needing additional therapy. So I chose to have four courses of really aggressive chemotherapy. That's less than they used to do. Today, there are studies that indicate that as little as one course is a very effective dose.

The rest of it was getting fitted for a wig, spending a year without any hair, and going through the physical travails of chemotherapy—but I've been through worse things than that.

What's worse?

Oh, a divorce. Or getting a spinal anesthetic for some minor knee surgery and ending up with one of those spinal headaches—that's the worst thing I've ever had in my life. Five days of agony. At least with chemotherapy you feel sick for only maybe a day or two, like a mild flu. There's a period of six or eight hours of extreme nausea, but I just had them drug me so heavily that I'd fall asleep.

Were you in a lot of pain after the surgery?

No. The only pain I've had is, my chest has been tight, the muscle. And now, with reconstruction, you feel like there's a vise on your chest all the time—the implant's under the chest wall, the chest muscle. But it's nothing you can't cope with. It's not excruciating pain. Having grown up as a tomboy, I have a fairly high pain threshold, so . . . I don't know, but it seems to me there are a lot worse things.

I'll tell you, I feel sorry for women who are delicate creatures, because it is much harder on them. Much. You have to be a little bit tough, I'm very involved in sports, and one thing sports does for you is, you develop a certain strength and you realize there are lots of things you can overcome. In fact, maybe every woman who has breast surgery ought to go on an Outward Bound program. Maybe she'd feel better about the whole thing. I mean, there are things that are a lot worse than this! They ought to go out in the streets and look at these people lying down without anything to eat. That's a hell of a lot worse than losing a breast or having surgery. I don't have any truck with whiners at all!

How soon after surgery did you start chemo?

Right away. In fact, today they're doing studies where you start chemo before the surgery, to see if the tumor can be shrunk.

And when did you decide to have the reconstructive surgery?

About a year and a half later. I just wanted it to be easier to buy clothes and *feel* better about how I looked. I hated looking at myself. I looked horrible, I thought. I have an eye for symmetry. I like beauty. I like fashion. I like looking good, feeling good about myself. I'm thrilled I had it done.

I wanted the most minimal thing. I had the choice of doing that flap deal, where they swing the skin and muscle around from the back, but I think that's overdoing a good thing—I agree that you get a more pendulous look and all that, but I know women who had painful scars on their back. I didn't care about being a busty brunette. I just wanted to look good, to fill a bra, look evenly matched, and go on. None of this is perfect! We're not talking here about ending up with something you're born with! I had enough tissue left to do the simple implant—some people don't, and they have to use the expander. And then six months later, I had the nipple reconstruction, which is easy. They take the skin from the top or inside your thigh. And then he had to replace the original prosthesis. They do that sometimes because it gives you a better shape. I haven't had any problems, knock wood. I know that there are many botched cases, but the advice is to go to a good comprehensive cancer center, study your plastic surgeons, and don't do it unless you've seen their work. You ask them not only for pictures, but you say, "I want to see a couple of patients you've done." And if they won't show them to you, then don't use them. You wouldn't buy a car without driving it. . . .

Further Reading

Sandra Butler and Barbara Rosenblum. 1991. *Cancer in Two Voices*. San Francisco: Spinsters Book Company.

Norman Cousins. 1979. *Anatomy of an Illness as Perceived by the Patient: Reflections on Healing and Regeneration*. New York: Norton.

Lesley Fallowfield with Andrew Clark. 1991. *Breast Cancer*. London: Routledge.

Discussion Questions

1. In which ways might this woman's experience be unusual? How does she compare herself to other women with breast cancer?

2. How do you evaluate her stance toward cancer and reconstructive surgery?

3. After reading this excerpt, how would you compare this woman's self-image to her body image?

7

The Desert

Nancy Mairs

In this short excerpt, Nancy Mairs chronicles how her symptoms began to unfold. Note that her mental history allowed her to define and dismiss her physical symptoms as neurotic. Also note that her acquaintance's pronouncement that she was limping affirmed the reality of a medical problem. Yet the nature of that problem eluded Mairs perhaps far longer than it eluded her neurologist. Like many people who have esoteric diseases, the search for a diagnosis first had to rule out a life-threatening disease. When death could loom in the horizon, a long-delayed alternative diagnosis of serious, but not life-threatening disease elicits diagnostic relief.

Though Nancy Mairs' condition gave her neurologist no chance for heroism, it gave her the opportunity to learn to live with her repudiated and objectified body.

I've known there was something wrong with me for at least a year now, in the way you have of knowing something without letting yourself know you know it. At first I started to drop things from my left hand, and the fingers, after hours of typing or knitting, felt too weak to move. I began to stumble, catching the toes of my left foot on cracks I could hardly see, and my ankle turned unpredictably. No one else seemed to notice, and I have such a long history of neurotic ills that I hardly paid attention. But after we got to Tucson, when a new acquaintance and I were going out for a beer after class one night, he asked suddenly, "Have you hurt your foot?"

"No, why?" I said, startled.

"You're limping." So someone else could see it, too. Alarmed, I went the next day to the Student Health Service, where a gentle elderly doctor, after tapping me with a rubber hammer and watching me walk a straight line, immediately picked up the telephone and made an appointment for me with a neurologist.

"Can you even guess what it might be?" I asked as I pulled my socks and shoes back on.

"No," he said. I thought his reticence a little odd, but I didn't know enough to be terrified.

When Dr. Buchsbaum told me a couple of days later about the brain tumor, I tried to explain my psychological history to him. Most likely, I told him, my condition was hysterical.

"Not this time." He softened his bluntness with a smile, but it wasn't a cheerful one. "This time there's something there."

A nurse comes in with a hospital gown for me to put on. Then an orderly arrives with a wheelchair. I'm not allowed to walk anywhere. In the corridor, I ask him to stop briefly by an open door while I breathe the unfamiliar air, damp and chill and rank with greasewood. Then we go down to the basement, to a small room where seven people are waiting to give me a pneumoencephalogram. Dr. Buchsbaum has been putting this test off because it's a little risky. But the CAT scan, which will render this procedure obsolete, won't reach Tucson for another year. And the X ray, brain scan; and electroencephalogram haven't shown what's going on. So now they've got to shoot bubbles into my brain.

I need a lot of information. That's my way of countering the helpless panic that the thought of having a brain tumor triggers. Some people don't want to know anything. "Just take care of it, doc," they say. For years my father-in-law will swallow the blood-pressure medication his doctor prescribes without once asking what his blood pressure *is*. I can't achieve blissful ignorance. I once trusted an obstetrician and a pediatrician too much, and the damage to my soul has never healed. This time, I want to participate, and if necessary to balk, every step of the way.

The team assembled for the test seems to understand. They explain the procedure in detail.

"It will hurt terribly for about seven seconds," I'm told. "But you mustn't move *at all* or you'll spoil the picture and we'll have to do it again."

"Somebody better hold me then," I say, "or I might jump."

"Oh yes," says a deep voice. He must have played football. From the vantage point of the cold table I'm strapped to, he looks like Jack's giant. "That's what I'm here for."

Dr. Buchsbaum punctures an artery in my groin. I feel only pressure, no pain, having had a local anesthetic, and I've been told to look away because blood spurts up. I'm watching television. On the small black-and-white screen, the catheter inches forward, spitting little puffs of dye that burn inside me slightly. It snakes up through my neck. And then the top of my head comes off and my brain bursts in brilliant shards all over the room. The pain is unspeakable. When my vision returns, the halfback's hands are clamped under my jaw and over my skull, his ruddy face close to mine. Everyone congratulates me. We should get a good picture.

They said it would seem like the longest seven seconds of my life, and they were right. I'd rather have both my children again, prolonged labors and complicated deliveries and all, than go through that another time. Only the brain has two hemispheres, so I have to go through it another time. At the thought, I panic and start to faint.

"Put some more Valium in the IV," Dr. Buchsbaum instructs. Almost immediately, the panic symptoms abate, and I lie still, tears washing into my ears, for the second picture.

After all, nothing is there. Nothing detectable, anyway. I go home under a shroud, not literally, thank God, but figuratively. I could have a tumor too small to see yet, Dr. Buchsbaum speculates, or a "demyelinating syndrome," whatever the hell that is. He doesn't elaborate. A few months later, during a regular checkup, I ask him, "Do I have multiple sclerosis?" I'm not sure how I know to ask about MS. I may have read about it in *Parade* magazine. I'm not the kind to pore over articles in medical journals.

"Probably," he says. "But you have to have another episode for us to be sure." There's no real test for MS at this point. It's only a clinical diagnosis. But neurological events disseminated in space (at different sites in the central nervous system) and time (over a period of months or years) characterize the demyelinating syndrome labeled multiple sclerosis. I like that construction: disseminated in space and time. It sounds like the way I live.

More than a year later, when I develop a scotoma (blurred spot) in my right eye as the result of a lesion in the optic nerve, he telephones. "Well, you've got your diagnosis," he says with his habitual bluntness. "Now go back to doing whatever you were doing before I called." His point is clear and, in an odd way, reassuring. There's nothing he can do for me. Most people with MS lead productive lives, however; and of those who don't, many are hampered more by attitude than by disease. Until I have to give up my activities, perhaps many years hence, I'd best get on with them.

Why didn't he just say it was probably MS in the first place? I wonder. I'm glad to have a name for it. There are strong cultural connections, not entirely without force, between naming and power. Perhaps he was merely being prudent, not wanting to risk misdiagnosis. But as I get to know this man, I sense that his diagnoses are seldom off the mark. He knew, I think, but he simply didn't want to say. I'll encounter this reluctance in other neurologists, as well as in the medical students I teach to give neurological examinations. They want to protect their patients, they think, from the shock of knowing what a terrible disease they have. But most patients deal with the knowledge pretty well; many, like me, are relieved to have *something*, something real, not a nameless mystery. In reality doctors project their own fears onto their patients. For a neurologist, MS must be the worst possible fate, worse even than a brain tumor, since some tumors can be sliced out or blasted away with radiation or chemicals. The chance for heroic rescue is there, at least. With MS, they stare powerlessly, sometimes for decades, at inexorable degeneration. No wonder they sometimes practice denial.

Further Reading

Arnold Beisser. 1989. *Flying Without Wings: Personal Reflections on Being Disabled*. New York: Doubleday.

Sefra Kobrin Pitzele. 1985. *We Are Not Alone: Learning to Live with Chronic Illness*. New York: Workman.

Maggie Strong. 1988. *Mainstay*. Boston: Little, Brown.

Discussion Questions

1. What sense do you make of the long delay between testing and diagnosis?

2. What kinds of events propel a person to continue a diagnostic search?

3. How do you view Mairs' stance toward obtaining information?

Illness, Disability, and the Self

8

The Damaged Self

Robert F. Murphy

Disability undermines taken-for-granted aspects of self. Robert Murphy finds that his disability diminished the self he had created, the position to which he had risen, the person he had become, and the life he had accrued. Like most middle-class Americans, Murphy had never envisioned himself as disabled. Like attitudes toward death, he had viewed disability as a misfortune happening to someone else, not to himself. That misfortune stains and strains interaction for both people with disabilities and the presumably unimpaired. Murphy's hopes were symbolized by his defining the wheelchair as only a convenience in convalescence. People with disabilities often view permanent reliance on a wheelchair as a stark symbol of a diminished self and devalued status. The wheelchair is something "needed" rather than merely "used." Not surprisingly, they rely on other or no assistive devices until long past the point of safety, or they may rent a chair because rentals symbolize impermanence.

Murphy captures the perverse reversal of guilt and shame that people with disabilities routinely endure. Seldom responsible for their conditions, they are punished by having them. Other people's responses shame them for being disabled and that, in turn, elicits their guilt for being different. Murphy voices the silent agony of feeling demasculinized and being sexually limited in a society that values male initiative, control, and performance. Stigma, shame, and demasculinization all contribute to disembodiment, especially when a man loses sensation, movement, and proprioception. Murphy reveals the existential contradiction of dissociating from his body while simultaneously being imprisoned in an overriding identity as disabled. Although Murphy dissociated himself from his body, he could not dissociate himself from his disability as its continuing presence in his dreams attests. The result of these losses and contradictions? Anger. Existential anger. And then exile.

> As Gregor Samsa awoke one morning from uneasy dreams he found himself transformed in his bed into a gigantic insect. He was lying on his hard, as if it were armor-plated, back and when he lifted his head a little he could see his domelike brown belly divided into stiff arched segments. . . . What has happened to me? he thought. It was no dream.
>
> —Franz Kafka,
> The Metamorphosis

From the time my tumor was first diagnosed through my entry into wheelchair life, I had an increasing apprehension that I had lost much more than the full use of my legs. I had also lost a part of my self. It was not just that people acted differently toward me, which they did, but rather that I felt differently toward myself. I had changed in my own mind, in my self-image, and in the basic conditions of my existence. It left me feeling alone and isolated, despite strong support from family and friends; moreover, it was a change for the worse, a diminution of everything I used to be. This was particularly frightening for somebody who had clawed his way up from poverty to a position of respect. I had become a person of substance, and that substance was oozing away. It threatened everything that Yolanda and I had put together over the years. In middle age, the ground beneath me had convulsed. And I had no idea why and how this had happened.

I cannot remember ever before thinking about physical disability, except as something that happened to other, less fortunate, people. It certainly had no relevance to me. A disabled person could enter my field of vision, but my mind would fail to register him—a kind of selective blindness quite common among people of our culture. During a year that I spent in the Sahel and Sudan zones of Nigeria and Niger, a region of endemic leprosy and missing hands, feet, and noses, the plight of those people was as alien to me as were their language, culture, and circumstances. Because of this gulf, I had no empathy for them and just enough sympathy to drop coins into cups extended from the ends of stumps. A few pennies were all that it took to buy the dubious grace of almsgiving. It was a bargain, a gesture that did not assert my oneness with them, but rather my separation from them.

With the onset of my own impairment, I became almost morbidly sensitive to the social position and treatment of the disabled, and I began to notice nuances of behavior that would have gone over my head in times past. One of my earliest observations was that social relations between the disabled and the able-bodied are tense, awkward, and problematic. This is something that every handicapped person knows, but it surprised me at the time. For example, when I was in the hospital, a young woman visitor entered my room with a look of total consternation on her face. She exclaimed that she had just seen an awful sight, a girl who was missing half of her skull. I knew the girl as a very sweet, but quite retarded, teenaged patient who used to drop in on me a few times a day; we always had the same conversation. I asked my guest why the sight bothered her so much, but she couldn't tell me. She in turn asked why it didn't trouble me. After a moment's thought, I replied that I was one of "them," a notion that she rejected vehe-

mently. But why did my visitor, a poised and intelligent person, react in this way? It aroused my curiosity.

There is something quite significant in this small encounter, for it had elements of what Erving Goffman called "one of the primal scenes of sociology."[1] Borrowing the Freudian metaphor of the primal scene (the child's traumatic witnessing of the mother and father in sexual intercourse), Goffman used the phrase to mean any social confrontation of people in which there is some great flaw, such as when one of the parties has no nose. This robs the encounter of firm cultural guidelines, traumatizing it and leaving the people involved wholly uncertain about what to expect from each other. It has the potential for social calamity.

The intensely problematic character of relations between those with damaged bodies and the more-or-less unmarked cannot be shrugged off simply as a result of the latter's ineptitude, bias, stupidity, and so forth, although they do play a part. Even the best-intentioned able-bodied people have difficulty anticipating the reactions of the disabled, for interpretations are warped by the impairment. To complicate matters, the disabled also enter the social arena with a skewed perspective. Not only are their bodies altered, but their ways of thinking about themselves and about the persons and objects of the external world have become profoundly transformed. They have experienced a revolution of consciousness. They have undergone a metamorphosis.

Nobody has ever asked me what it is like to be a paraplegic—and now a quadriplegic—for this would violate all the rules of middle-class etiquette. A few have asked me what caused my condition, and, after hearing the answer, have looked as though they wished they hadn't. After all, tumors can happen to anybody—even to them. Polite manners may protect us from most such intrusions, but it is remarkable that physicians seldom ask either. They like "hard facts" obtainable through modern technology or old-fashioned jabbing with a pin and asking whether you feel it. These tests supposedly provide good, "objective" measures of neurological damage, but, like sociological questionnaires, they reduce experience to neat distinctions of black or white and ignore the broad range of ideation and emotion that always accompanies disability. The full subjective states of the patient are of little concern in the medical model of disability, which holds that the problem arises wholly from some anatomic or physiological disorder and is correctable by standard modes of therapy—drugs, surgery, radiation, or whatever. What goes on inside the patient's head is another department, and if there are signs of serious psychological malaise, he is packed off to the proper specialist. . . .

Of all the psychological syndromes associated with disabilty, the most pervasive, and the most destructive, is a radical loss of self-esteem. This sense of damage to the self, the acquisition of what Erving Goffman called a "stigma," or a "spoiled identity,"[2] grew upon me during my first months in a wheelchair, and it hit me hardest when I returned to the university in the fall of 1977. By then, I could no longer hold on to the myth that I was using a wheelchair during convalescence. I had to face the unpalatable fact that I was wedded permanently to it; it had become an indispensable extension of my body. Strangely, I also felt this as a major blow to my pride.

The damage to my ego showed most painfully in an odd and wholly irrational sense of embarrassment and lowered self-worth when I was with people on my social periphery. Most of my colleagues in the anthropology department were old friends, some even from our undergraduate years, and they generally were warm and supportive. But people from other departments and the administration were another matter. During my first semester back at the university, I attended a few lunch meetings at the Faculty Club, but I began to notice that these were strained occasions. People whom I knew did not look my way. And persons with whom I had a nodding acquaintance did not nod; they, too, were busily looking off in another direction. Others gave my wheelchair a wide berth, as if it were surrounded by a penumbra of contamination. These were not happy encounters.

My social isolation became acute during stand-up gatherings, such as receptions and cocktail parties. I discovered that I was now three-and-a-half feet tall, and most social interaction was taking place two feet above me. When speaking to a standing person, I have to crane my neck back and look upward, a position that stretches my larynx and further weakens my diminished vocal strength. Conversation in such settings has become an effort. Moreover, it was commonplace that I would be virtually ignored in a crowd for long periods, broken by short bursts of patronization. There was no escape from these intermittent attentions, for it is very difficult to maneuver a wheelchair through a crowd. My low stature and relative immobility thus made me the defenseless recipient of overtures, rather than their instigator. This is a common plaint of the motor-disabled: They have limited choice in socializing and often must wait for the others to come to them. As a consequence, I now attend only small, sit-down gatherings.

Not having yet read the literature on the sociology of disability, I did not immediately recognize the pattern of avoidance. Perhaps this was for the best, as my initial hurt and puzzlement ultimately led me to research the subject. In the meantime, I stopped going to the Faculty Club and curtailed my contacts with the university-at-large. This is not hard to do at Columbia, as each department lies within a Maginot Line, everybody is very busy, and the general social atmosphere runs from tepid to cool. None of this is surprising, for it is also the dominant ethos of New York City. On the positive side, this same general mood allows one to work in peace. They leave you alone at Columbia, and I wanted more than ever to be left alone.

Withdrawal only compounds the disabled person's subjective feelings of damage and lowered worth, sentiments that become manifest as shame and guilt. I once suggested to a housebound elderly woman that she should use a walker for going outside. "I would never do that," she replied. "I'd be ashamed to be seen." "It's not your fault that you have arthritis," I argued. I added that I used a walker, and I wasn't ashamed—this was untrue, of course, and I knew it. But why should anyone feel shame about his disability? Even more mysterious, why should anyone feel a sense of guilt? In what way could I be responsible for my physical state? It could not be attributed to smoking or drinking, the favorite whipping boys of amateur diagnosticians, and it wasn't the result of an accident, with its possibilities for lifestyle culpability, the accusation that one brought it by living dangerously. No, I didn't do a damned thing to earn my tumor, nor was there any way that I could have prevented it. But such feelings are endemic among the disabled. One young woman, who had been born without lower limbs, told me that she had felt guilt for this since childhood, as had her parents (from whom she probably acquired the guilt). Indeed, a mutuality of guilt is the very life-stuff of the paralytic's family, just as it is, on a smaller scale, central to the cohesion—and turmoil—of all modern families.

Guilt and shame are not in fact as separate as they are often represented to be. In simple form, both are said to involve an assault on the ego: Guilt is the attack of the superego, or conscience, and shame arises from the opprobrium of others. Of the two, I believe that shame is the more potent. The sociologist George Herbert Mead wrote that an individual's concept of his or her self is a reflection, or, more accurately, a refraction, as in a funhouse mirror, of the way he or she is treated by others.[3] And if a person is treated with ridicule, contempt, or aversion, then his own ego is diminished, his dignity and humanity are called into question. Shaming is an especially potent means of social control in small-scale societies, where everybody is known and behavior is highly visible, but it is less effective in complex societies like our own, where we can compartmentalize our lives and exist in relative anonymity. But a wheelchair cannot be hidden; it is brutally visible. And to the extent that the wheelchair's occupant is treated with aversion, even disdain, his sense of worth suffers. Damage to the body, then, causes diminution of the self, which is further magnified by debasement by others.

Shame and guilt are one in that both lower self-esteem and undercut the facade of dignity we present to the world. Moreover, in our culture they tend to stimulate each other. The usual formula is that a wrongful act leads to a guilty conscience; if the guilt becomes pub-

licly known, then shame must be added to the sequence, followed by punishment. There is then a causal chain that goes from wrongful act to guilt to shame to punishment. A fascinating aspect of disability is that it diametrically and completely reverses this progression, while preserving every step. The sequence of the person damaged in body goes from punishment (the impairment) to shame to guilt and, finally, to the crime. This is not a real crime but a self-delusion that lurks in our fears and fantasies, in the haunting, never-articulated question: What did I do to deserve this?

In this topsy-turvy world of reversed causality, the punishment—for this is how crippling is unconsciously apprehended—begets the crime. All of this happens despite the fact that the individual may be in no way to blame for his condition; real ability is irrelevant. . . .

There may be no such thing as Original Sin, but original guilt lurks in the dark recesses of the minds of all humans. These ashes of our first love are the basic stuff of the indefinable, unarticulated, and haunting sense that the visitation of paralysis is a form of atonement—a Draconian penance.

Paralytic disability constitutes emasculation of a more direct and total nature. For the male, the weakening and atrophy of the body threaten all the cultural values of masculinity: strength, activeness, speed, virility, stamina, and fortitude. Many disabled men, and women, try to compensate for their deficiencies by becoming involved in athletics. Paraplegics play wheelchair basketball, engage in racing, enter marathons, and do weight-lifting and many other active things. Those too old or too impaired for physical displays may instead show their competence by becoming "super-crips." Just as "super-moms" supposedly go off to work every morning, cook Cordon Bleu dinners at night, play with the kids, and then become red-hot lovers after the children are put to bed, the super-crip works harder than other people, travels extensively, goes to everything, and takes part in anything that comes along. This is how he shows the world that he is like everybody else, only better.

Becoming a super-crip, or super-mom, often depends less on the personal qualities of the individual than on very fortunate circumstances. In my own case, I was well established in my profession at the time of my disability, so my activity was just a matter of persistence. The real super-crips are those who do it all after they become impaired, like one woman who, after partial remission from totally paralytic multiple sclerosis, went on to finish college and then obtain a Ph.D. She refused to let the disease rob her of a future. There are many such people, but, like supermoms, they are still a minority. The vast majority, as we will see, are unable to conquer the formidable physical and social obstacles that confront them, and they live in the penumbra of society, condemned to lives as outsiders.

Afflictions of the spinal cord have a further devastating effect upon masculinity aside from paralysis, for they commonly produce some degree of impotence or sexual malfunction. Depending on the extent of damage to the cord, the numbed genital area sends no signals to the brain, nor do the libidinal centers of the brain get messages through to the genitalia and the physiological processes that produce erections. This can result in total and permanent impotence, sporadic impotence, or difficulty in sustaining an erection until orgasm. There are some paraplegic men, on the other hand, who can maintain an erection but are unable to achieve orgasm, even after steady intercourse of a half hour to an hour. The effects of this on the male psyche are profound. We usually think of "castration anxiety" as an Oedipal thing, but there is a sort of symbolic castration in impotence that creates a kind of existential anxiety among all men. It is no accident that impotence is a major problem in those lands where masculine values are strongest, nor was it fortuitous that the new sexual freedom in America, with its emphasis on female gratification and male performance, has yielded a bumper crop of impotent men. After all, being a man does not mean just having a penis—it means having a sexually useful one. Anything less than that is indeed a kind of castration, although I am using this lurid Freudian term primarily as a metaphor for loss of both sexual and social power.

Most forms of paraplegia and quadriplegia cause male impotence and female inability to orgasm. But paralytic women need not be aroused or experience orgasmic pleasure to engage in genital sex, and many indulge regularly in intercourse and even bear children, although by Caesarean section. Human sexuality, Freud tells us, is polymorphously perverse, meaning that the entire body is erogenous, and the joys of sex varied. Paraplegic women claim to derive psychological gratification from the sex act itself, as well as from the stimulation of other parts of their bodies and the knowledge that they are still able to give pleasure to others. They may derive less physical gratification from sex than before becoming disabled, but they are still active participants. Males have far more circumscribed anatomical limits. Other than having a surgical implant that produces a simulated erection, the man can no longer engage in genital sex. He either becomes celibate or practices oral sex—or any of the many other variations in sexual expression devised by our innovative species. Whatever the alternative, his standing as a man has been compromised far more than has been the woman's status. He has been effectively emasculated.

Even in those cases in which the paraplegic male retains potency, his stance during the sex act changes. Most must lie still on their backs during intercourse, and it is the woman who must do the mounting and thrusting. In modern America, this is an acceptable alternative position, but in some cultures it would be considered a violation of male dominance: Men are on top in society and they should be on top in sex, and that's the end of the matter. And even in the relatively liberated United States of the 1980s, the male usually takes the more active role and the position on top. But the paraplegic male, whether engaging in genital or oral sex, always takes a passive role. Most paralytic men accept this limitation, for they discover that the wells of passion are in the brain, not between the legs, and that pleasure is possible even without orgasm. One man, who had enjoyed an intensely erotic relationship with his wife before an auto accident made him paraplegic and impotent, reported that they simply continued oral sex. The wife derives complete orgasmic satisfaction and the husband achieves deep psychological pleasure, which he describes as a "mental orgasm." The sex lives of most paralyzed men, however, remain symbolic of a more general passivity and dependency that touches every aspect of their existence and is the antithesis of the male values of direction, activity, initiative, and control.

The sexual problems of the disabled are aggravated by a widespread view that they are either malignantly sexual, like libidinous dwarfs, or, more commonly, completely asexual, an attribute frequently ascribed to the elderly as well. These erroneous notions, which I suspect arise from the sexual anxieties of their holders, fail to recognize that a large majority of disabled people have the same urges as the able-bodied, and are just as competent in expressing them. Spinal cord injuries raise special problems, but motor-disabled people with cerebral palsy, the after-effects of polio, and many other conditions often can lead almost normal sex lives. That asexuality is also attributed sometimes to the blind underlines the utter irrationality of the belief. . . .

My own sense of disembodiment is somewhat akin to that of Christina, the "disembodied lady" discussed by Oliver Sacks in his book *The Man Who Mistook His Wife for a Hat.*[4] Because of an allergic reaction to an antibiotic drug, Christina lost all sense of her body—a failure of her faculty of proprioception, the delicate, subliminal feedback mechanism that tells the brain about the position, tension, and general feeling of the body and its parts. It is this "sixth sense" that allows for coordination of movement; without it, talking, walking, even standing, are virtually impossible. In similar fashion, I no longer know where my feet are, and without the low-level pain I still feel, I would hardly know I had legs. Indeed, one of the early symptoms of my malady was a tendency to lose my balance when I would take off my pants in the dark, something that happened to me often in my drinking days. Christina's troubles differ from those of the paralytic, however, for her loss has been more complete. Besides, she became disembodied while still capable of movement, and she compensated by using her eyes to coordinate her physical actions. Quadriplegics, too, must watch what they are doing, and I have spilled drinks held in my hand because my wrist had turned and my brain didn't register it. But by the time the paralytic's failure of proprioception is as complete as Christina's, the limb is no longer movable, and the condition is moot.

I have also become rather emotionally detached from my body, often referring to one of my limbs as *the* leg or *the* arm. People who help me on a regular basis have also fallen into this pattern ("I'll hold the arms and you grab the legs"), as if this depersonalization would compensate for what otherwise would be an intolerable violation of my personal space. The paralytic becomes accustomed to being lifted, rolled, pushed, pulled, and twisted, and he survives this treatment by putting emotional distance between himself and his body. Others join in this effort, and I well remember that after I came to from neurosurgery in 1976, there was a sign pinned to my sheet that read, DO NOT LIFT BY ARMS. I weakly suggested to the nurse that they print another sign saying THIS SIDE UP.

As my condition has deteriorated, I have come increasingly to look upon my body as a faulty life-support system, the only function of which is to sustain my head. It is all a bit like *Donovan's Brain*, an old science-fiction movie in which a quite nefarious brain is kept alive in a jar with mysterious wires and tubes attached to it. Murphy's brain is similarly sitting on a body that has no movement or tactile sense below the arms and shoulders, and that functions mainly to oxygenate the blood, receive nourishment, and eliminate wastes. In none of these capacities does it do a very good job. My solution to this dilemma is radical dissociation from the body, a kind of etherealization of identity. Perhaps one reason for my success in this adaptation is that I never did take much pride in my body. I am of medium height, rather scrawny, and militantly nonathletic. I was never much to look at, but that didn't bother me greatly. From boyhood onward, I cultivated my wits instead. It is a very different matter for an athletically inclined boy or a girl on the threshold of dating and courtship.

Those who have lost use of some parts of their bodies learn to cultivate the others. The blind develop acute sensitivity to sounds, and quadriplegics, who cannot handle heavy telephone directories, have a remarkable knack for remembering phone numbers. But of a more fundamental order, the quadriplegic's body can no longer speak a "silent language" in the expression of emotions or concepts too elusive for ordinary speech, for the delicate feedback loops between thought and movement have been broken. Proximity, gesture, and body-set have been muted, and the body's ability to articulate thought has been stilled. It is perhaps for this reason that writing has become almost an addiction for me, for in it thought and mind become a system, united in conjunction with the movements of my hands and the responses of the machine. Of even more profound impact on existential states, the thinking activity of the brain cannot be dissolved into motion, and the mind can no longer be lost in an internal dialogue with physical movement. This leaves one adrift in a lonely monologue, an inner soliloquy without rest or surcease, and often without subject matter. Consciousness is overtaken and devoured in contemplation, meditation, ratiocination, and reflection without end, relieved only by one's remaining movements, and sleep.

My thoughts and sense of being alive have been driven back into my brain, where I now reside. More than ever before, it is the base from which I reach out and grasp the world. Many paralytics say that they no longer feel attached to their bodies, which is another way of expressing the shattering of Merleau-Ponty's mind-body system. But it also has a few positive aspects. Just as an anthropologist gets a better perspective on his own culture through long and deep study of a radically different one, my extended sojourn in disability has given me, like it or not, a measure of estrangement far beyond the yield of any trip. I now stand somewhat apart from American culture, making me in many ways a stranger. And with this estrangement has come a greater urge to penetrate the veneer of cultural differences and reach an understanding of the underlying unity of all human experience.

My own disembodied thoughts are crude when compared with those of many people. A blind Milton painted sweeping landscapes of the heavens in *Paradise Lost*, and Beethoven crafted the Ninth Symphony despite—or perhaps because of—being deaf. And today one of the world's leading cosmologists, a Cambridge physicist named Stephen Hawking, travels through quarks and black holes in a journey across space and time to the birth of the universe. These are voyages of the mind, for Hawking has an advanced case of amyotrophic lateral sclerosis (familiarly known as Lou Gehrig's disease), which has left him with only slight movement in one hand and an inability to speak above a whisper. There are not many Miltons, Beethovens, and Hawkings, however, and their example may be small comfort to a twenty-year-old quadriplegic who has made the mistake of diving into shallow water. For most disabled people, the loss of synchrony between mind and body has few compensations. . . .

In all the years since the onset of my illness, I have never only asked, "Why me?" I feel that this is a foolish question that assumes some cosmic sense of purpose and direction in the universe that simply does not exist. My outlook is quite fatalistic, an attitude that actually predisposes me to get all the pleasure out of life that I can, while I can. Nonetheless, though I may not brood over my impairment, it is always on my mind in spoken or unspoken form, and I believe this is true of all disabled people. It is a precondition of my plans and projects, a first premise of all my thoughts. Just as my former sense of embodiment remained taken for granted, positive, and unconscious, my sense of disembodiment is problematic, negative, and conscious. My identity has lost its stable moorings and has become contingent on a physical flaw.

This consuming consciousness of handicap even invades one's dreams. When I first became disabled, I was still walking, after a fashion, and I remained perfectly normal in my dreams. But as the years passed and I lost the ability to stand or walk, a curious change occurred. In every dream I start out walking and moving freely, often in perilous places;

significantly, I am never in a wheelchair. I am climbing high on the mast of a ship in rough seas—something I did occasionally in an earlier incarnation or I am on a ladder, painting a house. But in the middle of the dream, I remember that I can't walk, at which point I falter and fall. The dream is a perfect enactment of failure of power, the realization that what most men unconsciously fear had in fact happened to me. In other dreams, I am just walking about aimlessly when suddenly I remember my disability. Sometimes I sit down, but often I just stand puzzled until I awaken, the dream dissolves, the room comes into view, and I return to the reality that my paralysis is not a transient thing—it is an awakening much like that of Gregor Samsa in Kafka's *The Metamorphosis*. But perhaps more significant than the content of my dreams is the fact that since 1978 I have never once dreamed of anything else. Even in sleep, disability keeps its tyrannical hold over the mind.

The totality of the impact of serious physical impairment on conscious thought, as well as its firm implantation in the unconscious mind, gives disability a far stronger purchase on one's sense of who and what he is than do any social roles—even key ones such as age, occupation, and ethnicity. These can be manipulated, neutralized, and suspended, and in this way can become adjusted somewhat to each other. Moreover, each role can be played before a separate audience, allowing us to lead multiple lives. One cannot, however, shelve a disability or hide it from the world. A serious disability inundates all other claims to social standing, relegating to secondary status all the attainments of life, all other social roles, even sexuality. It is not a role; it is an identity, a dominant characteristic to which all social roles must be adjusted. And just as the paralytic cannot clear his mind of his impairment, society will not let him forget it.

Given the magnitude of this assault on the self, it is understandable that another major component of the subjective life of the handicapped is anger,[5] a disposition so diffuse and subtle, so carefully managed, that I became aware of it in myself only through writing this book. The anger of the disabled takes two forms. The first is an existential anger, a pervasive bitterness at one's fate, a hoarse and futile cry of rage against fortune. It is a sentiment fueled by the self-hate generated by unconscious shame and guilt, and it bears more than casual resemblance to the anger of America's black people. And, just as among blacks, it becomes expressed in hostility toward the dominant society, then toward people of one's own kind, and finally it is turned inward into an attack on the self. It is a very destructive emotion. In my own case, I have escaped its worst ravages only because my impairment has been so slow that I have been able to adjust to it mentally, and I am old enough to know that I am just a statistic, not the victim of a divine conspiracy. I suspect, although I lack conclusive data on this, that anger is much greater among those suddenly disabled and the young, for their impairment happens too quickly to permit assimilation, and it clouds an entire lifetime.

The other kind of anger is a situational one, a reaction to frustration or to perceived poor treatment. I have a good supply of this type. A paralytic may struggle to walk and become enraged when he cannot move his leg. Or a quadriplegic may pick up a cup of coffee with stiffened hands and drop it on his lap, precipitating an angry outburst. I had to give up spaghetti because I could no longer twirl it on my fork, and dinner would end for me in a sloppy mess. This would so upset me that I would lose my appetite. Or I may try unsuccessfully for a minute or so to pick up a paper from my desk or turn a page, casual maneuvers for most but a major challenge to me, because my fingers have lost both strength and dexterity. Such frustrations happen to me, and to other paralytics, several times a day. They are minor but cumulative, and they acquire special intensity from the more generalized existential anger often lurking below the surface.

The kind and virulence of the anger of the disabled vary greatly, for each person has a different history, but I have the impression that the depth and type of disability are critical. The extent of disablement obviously influences both existential and situational rage, but anger also seems to be most intense among people with communication disorders—primarily deaf-mutes and people with cerebral palsy and certain kinds of stroke. Most of us have watched the transparent suffering of the speech-impaired as they struggle to convey meaning to their agonized listeners. It is small wonder that the deaf form tightly circumscribed little communities or that they occasionally explode into overt hostility at those who can hear and speak.

The anger of the disabled arises in the first place from their own lack of physical functions, but, as we will see, it is aggravated by their interaction with the able-bodied world. They daily suffer snub, avoidance, patronization, and occasional outright cruelty, and even when none of these occur, they sometimes imagine the affronts. But whatever the source of the grievance, the disabled have limited ways of showing it. Quadriplegics cannot stalk off in high (or low) dudgeon, nor can they even use body language. To make matters worse, as the price for normal relations, they must comfort others about their condition. They cannot show fear, sorrow, depression, sexuality, or anger, for this disturbs the able-bodied. The unsound of limb are permitted only to laugh. The rest of the emotions, including anger and the expression of hostility, must be bottled up, repressed, and allowed to simmer or be released in the backstage area of the home. This is where I let loose most of the day's frustrations and irritations, much to Yolanda's chagrin. But I never vent to her the full despair and foreboding I sometimes feel, and rarely even express it to myself. As for the rest of the world, I must sustain their faith in their own immunity by looking resolutely cheery. Have a nice day!

In summary, from my own experience and research and the work of others I have found that the four most far-reaching changes in the consciousness of the disabled are: lowered self-esteem; the invasion and occupation of thought by physical deficits; a strong undercurrent of anger; and the acquisition of a new, total, and undesirable identity. I can only liken the situation to a curious kind of "invasion of the body snatchers," in which the alien intruder and the old occupant coexist in mutual hostility in the same body. It is also a metamorphosis in the exact sense. One morning in the hospital, a nurse was washing me when she was called away by another nurse, who needed help in moving a patient. "I'll be right back," she said as she left, which all hospital denizens know is but a fond hope. She left me lying on my back without the call bell or the TV remote, the door was closed, and she was gone for a half hour. Wondering whether she had forgotten me, I tried to roll onto my side to reach the bell. But I was already quadriplegic, and, try as I might, I couldn't make it. I finally gave up and was almost immediately overcome by a claustrophobic panic, feeling trapped and immobile in my own body. I thought then of Kafka's giant bug, as it rocked from side to side, wiggling its useless legs, trying to get off its back—and I understood the story for the first time.

At the beginning of this chapter, I spoke of the feeling of aloneness, the desire to shrink from society into the inner recesses of the self, that invades the thoughts of the disabled—a feeling that I attributed in part to the deep physical tiredness that accompanies most debility and the formidable physical obstacles posed by the outside world. But we have added other elements to this urge to withdraw. The individual has also been alienated from his old, carefully nurtured, and closely guarded sense of self by a new, foreign, and unwelcome identity. And he becomes alienated from others by a double-barreled mechanism: Due to his depreciated self-image, he has a tendency to withdraw from his old associations into social isolation. And, as if in covert cooperation with this retreat, society—or at least American society—helps to wall him off.

The physical and emotional sequestering of the disabled is often dramatic. One quadriplegic man, married and the father of two children, told us that he never leaves the house and nobody visits their home, not even the friends of his children. He confessed to feelings of shame about his condition. I was struck by the similarity between that family and the one begotten by my father. Another quadriplegic we met attends college through a program that allows home study. Even though he is capable of leaving his house with help, he never does so, and instructors from the college have to meet him at his home. He is trying to break out of his shell, but he is not quite ready. Many disabled people blame their isolation on a hostile society and often they are right. But there is also that powerful pull backward into the self. It is an urge that I have felt all my life, a centripetal force that is a universal feature of the emotional makeup of our species. Our lives are built upon a constant struggle between the need to reach out to others and a contrary urge to fall back into ourselves. Among the disabled, the inward pull becomes compelling, often irresistible, outlining in stark relief a human propensity that is often perceived only dimly. . . .

The disabled have become changed in the minds of the rest of society into a kind of quasi-human. In only a few months, I had moved subtly from the center of my society to its perimeter. I had acquired a new identity that was contingent on my defects and that either compromised or radically altered my prior claims to personhood.

Endnotes

1. Erving Goffman, *Stigma: Notes on the Management of Spoiled Identity* (Englewood Cliffs, N.J.: Prentice-Hall, 1963).

2. Goffman, *Stigma*.

3. George Herbert Mead, *Mind, Self and Society* (Chicago: University of Chicago Press, 1934).

4. Oliver Sacks, *The Man Who Mistook His Wife for a Hat* (New York: Harper & Row, 1970, pp. 42-52.)

5. Jerome Siller, "Psychological Situation of the Disabled with Spinal Cord Injuries." *Rehabilitation Literature* (1969), 30:290-96.

Further Reading

Susan Browne, Debra Connors, and Nanci Stern. 1985. *With the Power of Each Breath: A Disabled Women's Anthology*. Pittsburgh: Cleis Press.

Susan Sontag. 1977. *Illness as Metaphor*. New York: Farrar, Straus and Giroux.

Irving Kenneth Zola. 1982. *Missing Pieces: A Chronicle of Living with a Disability*. Philadelphia: Temple University Press.

Discussion Questions

1. In which ways does disability undermine the self? What can be done to minimize the assault upon the self that Murphy describes?

2. How do you evaluate Murphy's portrayal of the emotional response to disability? What parallels, if any, do you discern with people with other illnesses?

3. After reading Murphy's account, how would you change such interactions?

From *The Body Silent.* Pp. 85-104. Copyright © 1990, 1987 by Robert F. Murphy. Reprinted by permission of W.W. Norton & Company, Inc. ✦

9

'Discoveries' of Self in Illness

Kathy Charmaz

In this chapter, Kathy Charmaz looks at the effects of serious chronic illness upon the self. She argues that the consequences of illness and disability are not immediately apparent to people who have them. Look for her analysis about the difference between the stability of self-concept and the flow of experiences that undermine it. She suggests that initial episodes of chronic illness often do not alter a person's self-concept because he or she looks beyond present suffering to an anticipated recovery. If so, then people learn how their chronic illnesses affect their lives and their self-concepts later when they try to manage their daily routines and responsibilities.

See how Charmaz brings an analysis of emotions into the discussion of managing illness. As ill people learn the effects of illness, they first discover their losses of function, status, and self. Such distressing discoveries can lead to turning points toward a deeper level of knowing and feeling than these people had previously experienced. Through struggle and reflection they may transcend their losses, resolve their feelings about them, and emerge with a stronger, more valued self.

Crises and losses disrupt life but may result in a changed, more valued self. Having a serious chronic illness can produce sudden crises, unexpected losses, and lasting troubles in adult life. How do chronically ill people overcome losses, resolve feelings, and make discoveries of self? Consider this statement by a young woman whose mysterious, incapacitating symptoms first appeared thirteen years before when she was in college:

Choosing to believe in myself took a lot of courage. Because what I grew up with was not supporting that in any way, shape, or form. . . . For me, illness was the gift that brought me together with myself. It was the bridge that helped me do that. So I really see illness as a very profound gift to people, if they take it. They have the choice of using it as an opportunity and they have the choice of not using it, [or] to use it as a scapegoat.

. . . [Previously] I was hiding from who I was. That was when the separation [from self] was the strongest and that was when I felt the most alone. And then what happened gradually, is that I discovered myself in little pieces. . . . I started interacting with that self that I lost so many years ago. And so I started having fun with myself again and there was somebody there—then all of a sudden, there was somebody home again. And that— that just kept building and building. My illness started a dialogue with myself that I'd lost.

This young woman's sorrow about her declining health had turned to anger when she saw both physicians and family abandoning her. For the first five years of her illness, no one knew why she got so sick. After lengthy testing, the doctors concluded that she suffered from psychosomatic symptoms. Later, a diagnosis of lupus erythematosus validated this woman's view of herself as sick but her view of herself as a valid *person* remained impaired. The seeds of change began during long nights of immobilizing fevers while she struggled alone with her symptoms. Unable to do anything but think, the fevers sparked her curiosity about her experience. Previously, she had fought against being sick. Now she flowed with it and found her long-past self. This woman's discoveries and development of self took years but resulted in a stronger, more positive self-concept.

The study of chronically ill people provides a distilled version of changes and continuities in identity construction and self-concept that occur throughout adult life and accelerate during the later years.[1] Apparent discoveries of self emerge with new demands and new exigencies. Such "discoveries" may actually reflect development of earlier selves or of latent potentials and redirection of self as ill people adapt to their altered bodies and situations. Their self-concepts also change as they realize how others view them, reinterpret their situations, revise earlier assumptions, and devise new ways of accomplishing their lives.

Some seriously ill people do not see themselves as different or their lives as changed—at least for a time. Initially, the self in the experience of pain, suffering, and exhaustion may remain an alien, unfamiliar one. Moreover, an ill person may not view this self as reflecting his or her real self (Turner 1976). Thus, experiencing serious illness may not always directly or immediately result in a changed self-concept. When it does, those changes may be subtle and slowly accrue. If so, the person's discoveries of self may occur when he or she defines striking contrasts between past and present.

Theoretical Foundations of Self

The self is both process and product and subject and object (Gecas 1982; Mead 1934; Strauss 1969). It is process because it changes in response to emergent events. The self continually unfolds as the person interacts with others, feels cultural constraints and imperatives, and evaluates self relative to experience, situation, others, and society more generally. The self is the experiencing subject who perceives and feels (Cooley 1902). Because the person internalizes the language, culture, and meanings of his or her groups, he or she can apply socially shared measures to appraise self as an object like any other object (Mead 1934). Self-appraisals reflect feelings of self-worth and are particularly vulnerable to revision downward when people do not have strong anchors to fixed and stable social institutions, communities, and other individuals.[2]

Conceptions of self as process can complement theoretical views of the self as product, i.e. an organized entity. Following Rosenberg (1979) and Turner (1976) the self-concept is a relatively stable *organization* of attributes, feelings, and identifications that the person takes as defining himself or herself. The self-concept then has boundaries, parts, and elements that are integrated through memory and habit. Because the self-concept is an organized entity, a person does not assume that all of his or her behavior, moods, actions, or experiences reflect his or her self-concept. Rather, someone takes certain behaviors, moods, actions, and experiences as reflecting his or her "real" self (Turner 1976).

The organized and stable nature of the self-concept make it resistant to change. People view and act toward themselves in consistent ways. A person's self-concept lags behind experience and images of self given in it because experience constantly changes (Charmaz 1991a; 1991b). The self-concept particularly lags when the experience is overwhelming, occurs within an alien setting, and subsequent events differ from the person's ordinary life. Such scenarios take place when sudden, catastrophic illness causes immediate hospitalization with drastic treatment procedures. These experiences feel disconnected from one's "real" life and, likely, from one's real self. Therefore, devastating changes can occur to ill people's bodies without their immediate realization of them or accounting for them within their self-concepts. When ill people persist in assuming that their "old" self is their "real" and true self, others may view them as creating fictions and denying their illnesses.

Some chronically ill people neither define illness as adversity nor themselves as sick. If they can continue to function on their own terms, then they may define themselves as "well" for lengthy periods of their illness. Their definitions of the presence or absence of illness, of its projected course and timetable, and of its meanings for everyday life shape which "discoveries" and reconstructions of self they make in illness, how they make them, and when they do so. Their definitions of their illness and its course may differ enormously from everyone else's. What looks and feels like a forthcoming positive outcome to a patient may stand as a permanent negative turning point to a practitioner. For example, Hoffman (1981) found that stroke patients assumed that they would recover while simultaneously, their hospital staff defined them as beyond help. What stands as "fact" to one may symbolize "fiction" to the other (Charmaz 1991b). Until a person tests a fictional identity in ordinary life, he or she likely refrains from redefining self (Charmaz 1991a;1991b). In the meantime as illness progresses, assumptions about present and future self can rapidly become fictions.

Developing a Fictional Identity

If ill people do not take changes caused by disease into account, they unknowingly assume that their future selves will resemble their past selves. Thus, they may experience symptoms—even serious ones—but they do not infer that the symptoms portend permanent change in body and self (Olesen 1992). Their taken-for-granted assumptions about self and social identity still remain intact despite experience.

Ill people's unwitting adoption of fictional identities indicates how changes in self-concept lag behind on-going experience. Fictional identities can reflect lack of awareness, partial knowledge, and the absence of apparent symptoms. Thus, these fictional identities are not lies, pretense, or manipulations. Instead, they derive from these people's views of their conditions and situations.

Meanings of illness and its consequences for daily life remain elusive and typically unfold rather than become immediately apparent. In their struggle to maintain their identity and continuity in their lives, ill people usually choose the most promising interpretation of their illness and prognosis (Robinson 1988). For example, a woman who had had surgery and chemotherapy for colon cancer remarked:

> I don't—I don't sit and worry about the cancer reoccurring all the time. They said that I'm a good candidate for reoccurrence and their statistics and percentages and everything. . . . But I just say their statistics can go jump in the lake because if it gets me, it gets me, but I'm not going to lay down and let it.

Access to accurate medical information does not necessarily lead to redefining self as permanently ill. Sophisticated people, as well as those lacking medical information, can misread significant signs or symptoms. Ilza

Veith (1988:17), a physician and medical historian, noted encroaching symptoms and dismissed them. She writes:

> To be sure the peculiar symptoms I had been experiencing during the last six weeks would have been reason enough to see a doctor; instead I kept on reading about them in the medical literature and felt that they simply represented symptoms of a transitory disturbance.

Whether alternative explanations are sophisticated or simplistic, awareness of one's continuing disability forces discoveries of self. The *type* of illness shapes meaning, particularly when it continues. Some illnesses, like cancer, are laden with negative social meanings, dire images, and immediate medical intervention, and thus, intrude upon daily life more forcefully than others (see also, Swanson and Chenitz 1993). An illness that has immediate consequences, produces visible markers, and forces intrusive regimens certainly affects the individual, at least in the present (Locker 1983; Peyrot, McMurray and Hedges 1987; Pinder 1988). For example, renal failure patients often suffer pronounced discomfort after undergoing dialysis. Their dialysis shunt [a surgically-created point of entry into the body to permit redirecting the blood into the dialysis machine] marks their changed health status. A dialysis regimen of three times weekly has to be reckoned with. Having renal failure would seem, by its very nature, to lead to defining self as seriously ill. If ill people take such markers of their conditions as salient now, and, moreover, predictive of the *future*, then they would define themselves as chronically ill. But that does not always occur. Despite their evident sickness, people may see those same characteristics of illness as temporary—as lasting only until the anticipated transplant, or as only disrupting part of the day or week.

Thus, how someone interprets even severe symptoms and restrictions figures as significantly as objective disease categories. Should events and others' definitions intervene forcefully, the ill person then has to do more interpretive work to make his or her reality claims stick.

Whether people define themselves as sick depends upon whether the illness remains in the foreground or in the background of their lives. An illness with invisible disabilities may remain masked to the sick person as well as to others. An illness with infrequent episodes may be dismissed. If so, then illness remains in the background of the person's life as a distant memory rather than as an approaching storm. Further, an overall life structure and specific daily routines can mask or magnify symptoms, influence ill people's meanings of their illnesses, and shape whether they lurk in the background or loom in the foreground of their lives. A 38-year-old graduate student with a heart condition had married a retired widower almost thirty years her senior. Several years before, she had suffered from frightening, intrusive heart symptoms. However, this woman's health had improved markedly after she started heart medications and lost weight. Her husband's severe emphysema and cancer had been pronounced as life-threatening when first diagnosed twelve years earlier. This student said:

I see my role as caregiver to him, and as his wife, I see that as much more problematic than my own health stuff. His health, his needs, our relationship, the fact that he may be dying and I deal with the threat of death every day.

This woman's life revolved around the conflicting demands of marriage, children, work, and graduate school. In addition, the relative control and invisibility of her symptoms kept her own illness in the background and supported her definition of herself as "well." Her husband reinforced her self-definition through his view of her as a vibrant young woman and through his increasing frailty, growing dependence and multiplying expectations of care. Her identity was a product of interaction with others as well as with self (cf. Blumer 1969; Mead 1934; Prus 1987).

This woman's interactions, actions, and attitudes masked her own condition and may have also veiled her husband's steady decline. Spouses often help their partners to keep illness in the background. Some spouses monitor symptoms, perform daily vital tasks like dressing or driving, and camouflage the ill person's increasing dependency. For many months or even years, a spouse who runs interference for the ill person can render the illness invisible and, therefore, may sustain the ill person's beliefs (as well as those of others) that he or she remains as before.

Similarly, location and timing can foster sustaining such beliefs. People who have already reduced their responsibilities and limited their living space may remain remarkably unaware of a gradual decline. As long as they can manage their immediate environment without distressing problems or disquieting realizations, any disparity between their identity claims and emerging selves narrows. Hence, these people see themselves as quite healthy despite their diagnoses (cf. Kelleher 1988; Robinson 1990).

Perhaps the most common reason why people adopt fictional identities is lack of awareness about their condition. They simply do not have sufficient information with which to gauge their situations and to measure themselves by professionals' yardsticks. Hence, exposure to a new identification or new information can cause a sudden jolt of awareness. For example, a doctor mentioned to a man that his chronic condition would require continuing care. His response was, "A *chronic* condition? Me? Ugh. No." One middle aged woman participated in a cardiac rehabilitation program. She initially was complacent about her health status since she had only had an angioplasty. The other patients were all considerably older, less able to do the exercises, and had suffered heart attacks. The attending nurse kept nagging her about her regimen. Only after learning that medical staff regarded angioplasty as equivalent to a heart attack did this woman take note of the warnings. Until then she viewed herself as someone who had a minor condition from which full recovery would follow (cf. Charmaz 1991b).

Even if someone accepts the medical definition of the illness, that individual may neither know nor follow subsequent medical prescriptions for dealing with it (cf. Conrad 1985). Limited or compartmentalized knowledge of one's condition dims awareness of its long-term consequences and fosters developing idiosyncratic meanings of illness and of what, if anything, to do about it. For example, one man whose heart condition resulted in bypass surgery averred, "I felt completely free of my problem after the surgery." He emphasized the fear of open-heart surgery of many prospective patients and volunteered to visit them the night before their surgeries. This man also kept up with technical advances in cardiac care and maintained contact with leading cardiologists in his area. He remarked:

I'm probably much more aware of what's going on with my heart and, things like that [than he had been before surgery]. I'm aware of what's happening in the field and anytime there's something mentioned about the heart, I listen to it; I know about it—you know, that no physician can double-talk me into thinking something different.

This man failed, however, to follow his regimen to the satisfaction of his cardiac rehabilitation nurse, but he saw himself as having made significant psychological adjustments and changes in lifestyle—he changed his priorities drastically. After his heart attack, his family came first. He said:

I think I learned to really enjoy myself at this point in time because you don't know if you get a tomorrow. . . . We take a different attitude, like we take vacations now, always [before] our work came first, and we never took time to enjoy our children, each other, and things like that; we were always too busy working.

A patient's firm commitment to full recovery sets into motion the conditions that others can later take as proof of denial and of claims to fictional identities. However, the patient may gain both hope and confidence through holding tight to expectations of recovery. During a crisis, the practitioner may encourage views of recovery to get the patient through it. (Of course at that time to the practitioner, "recovery" likely means living through it and to the patient it means fully regaining former function.) Norman Cousins' (1983:74-75) expectations of recovery smoothed his course through crisis:

Being free of panic at the start helped to free me of its usual aftermath of uncertainty and dread. I told Dr. Cannon that the dominant emotion, not just at the time of the attack but during the critical period was curiosity, a sense of challenge, and confidence. Every cubit of progress since the heart attack occurred served as exhilarating evidence that we were en route to recovery.

Turning Points and Lessons in Loss

Realizations about a failing body or permanent disability come when people try to live as before and find themselves unable to do so. A bad fall, incapacitating shortness of breath, profound loss of vision, or sudden lack of strength can provide vivid evidence of changes—unwelcome discoveries of self. When ill people begin to define the changes as long-term, or as permanent, they experience lessons in loss. Moreover, their unwelcome discoveries about self constitute turning points for reconstruction of self when they tie these events to their sense of identity.

Turning points often reflect more than a shift of direction of one's life—a new opportunity, or a lost one. They reflect more than discovering new information about self. Rather they also reflect emotions about self. Sudden turning points demand reappraisals of self—both of "fact" and of feeling. In these turning points, taken for granted "facts" about self are thrown open to question or entirely negated. For example, a middle-aged man with diabetes and a minor heart condition developed ulcers on his leg. After a harrowing episode in intensive care, he related the following story:

Shortly after I went in, the infection got much worse. The doctor said that he would have to amputate my leg. I could see that it wasn't improving so I could understand that—it wasn't a total surprise. But then a day passed, and another, and another, and the leg still wasn't improving. It didn't seem to be getting worse but no surgery. I said to the doctor, "What goes?" He said, "We can't amputate. Your heart isn't strong enough to withstand the surgery. We're going to have to treat you conservatively and just play it by ear." [To me with incredulousness] My heart wasn't *strong* enough? That was the first I'd heard of that—I had no conception. Oh, I knew I had a heart condition but it didn't seem very serious. No one made anything of it and it certainly didn't affect anything I did. That was the first time I realized how bad things were.

Perhaps the most telling moments and dramatic turning points occur in interaction with others. Ill people can find themselves being betrayed, stigmatized, exploited, and demeaned. Visible disability invites rude questions and remarks about difference (see also, Albrecht 1992). Invisible disability prompts accusations about failure to meet expectations. Both can result in unpleasant discoveries of self—devastating discoveries of how one looks and seems to other people. Those with visible disabilities may discover how much their illness and disability had defined others' views of them. Shock, sorrow, and shame may follow. For example, Ernest Hirsch (1977), a psychologist who had multiple sclerosis, used a wheelchair. He believed that his colleagues had hardly noticed his illness until, to his shock, he discovered that he would not be permitted to practice psychotherapy because of it.

Shock follows such an incident since it uproots one's taken for granted assumptions about self, relationships, and social location. Ill people come to terms with shock by telling and retelling the event—to self and often, to others (Charmaz 1991b). Repeated retelling makes the event real, commits the teller to a definitive point of view on it, and strengthens that view through audience affirmation. The logic of the story provides the basis for understanding, justifying, and managing the emotions experienced within the event (cf. Hochschild 1990; Sarbin 1986).

Just telling someone else a shocking diagnosis gives it a new, more obdurate, and irreversible meaning. Conversely, not dwelling upon the shocking event to self, not announcing it to others, and not mentioning it henceforth minimizes its effect, especially if one can also refrain from thinking about it. In this instance, a shocking event becomes less pinned to self. Similarly, the person grants the event less credence for defining future images of self. To the extent that others do not witness the event, or discount its significance if they do witness it, the ill person can more easily detach the event from enduring images of self.

Sorrow complicates and extends the effects of shock. When ill people experience sorrow as well as shock, they accept the social meanings of the event imposed upon them. Moreover, they mourn the lost self that those meanings implied. Here, ill people may first express shock and then experience sorrow and shame about not having realized how others actually had viewed them all along. For example, a young woman was shocked to discover that her physicians believed she was feigning symptoms. Her shock turned to sorrow when she realized that several nurses and doctors she liked and trusted shared this belief. As she relived earlier events in her mind, she saw that she had overlooked several indications of their actual view of her. Then she felt shame about not being more perceptive and about having trusted them in the first place.

Feelings of sorrow and shame linger when ill people define a negative turning point as unalterable. A person may feel a sense of self-betrayal as well as betrayal by others because he or she (a) now defines and connects earlier clues to present negative identifications (Strauss 1969), (b) shares the stigmatized images of illness, but heretofore did not apply them to self, (c) holds a stance that led to shame. Betrayal by others is felt because they have ripped away the foundations of the person's self-concept. For example, one woman with multiple sclerosis saw her doctor, who was also her closest family friend. The swimming class he recommended turned out to be for people with severe disabilities. She described herself as intermittently having "a gimp leg, but I'm certainly not a cripple!" She was humiliated that he had seen her as similar to the people in the class.

A crucial, negative event alone can elicit shame. The images of self revealed in the event evoke the shame (Cooley 1902). As Lewis (1971) and Scheff (1990) point out, shame signals a threatened bond. Here, the bond may be with another person but, moreover, can be to attachments to self. Acknowledged shame elicits the question: "What kind of person am I?"

Shame intensifies when an embarrassing private event occurs in public. The person seldom controls who witnesses it and their responses to it (Gardner 1991). Even if responses are humane, the knowledge alone that other people *know* about the event can affect the person's self-concept. An elderly woman who suffered urinary incontinence at church one day, thereafter avoided public places entirely.

Certainly turning points that ill people define as causing shock, sorrow, and shame require the greatest effort to transcend. When the discovery of self is founded in such profound loss, rebuilding a valued self takes time, effort, and typically, repeated success. Here, the person links shame to the *self* and does not simply define the *event* as embarrassing, but soon to be forgotten or to be retold with humor. Thus, this individual will need many indications of positive value to repair his or her now diminished self.

An earlier devastating turning point can later become redefined as the beginning of a stronger, better self that emerged from struggles and hardships. For example, a thirty-five-year-old man with almost complete paralysis demanded total care. His demands wore down his wife, who left. His elderly parents tried to take over his care. Seeing the toll it took on them, he reduced his demands. To his surprise, he was able to be much more physically independent than he had believed. That began a series of new achievements.

Moments of insight pierce despair and become turning points. Arnold Biesser (1988) felt helpless when poliomyelitis left him totally paralyzed. Shortly afterward, his brother suffered from a fatal disease, his stepfather had a stroke, and his mother got the flu. When the irony of it all struck him, he began to laugh and that was the turning point. He writes:

> A person can cry only so long without the tears beginning to develop a life of their own. Eventually sadness and tears offer a spurious security by themselves, with the world viewed continuously from a down position. But humor and the laughter it brings allowed me to emerge from despair into the light of day. For a moment I could see with clear eyes again and that allowed for a fresh start. (pp. 141-142)

Turning points represent gains when ill people define themselves as having learned and grown. One woman took refuge in her spiritual pursuits which she believed deepened through her harrowing experiences with illness. She said:

> In my mind, I think of myself as a wealthy person—not materially but I think of myself as a wealthy person. . . . It [illness] was like being crushed. Someone had a real good analogy—he tried to help me a lot—he'd be phoning me all the time—he said, "Life was like a vise." This lifetime was like a vise, squeezing me.

Resolution, Renewal, and Transcendence

As people learn about living with chronic illness, their first discoveries of self are ones of loss (Sarton 1988; Veith 1988). Dealing with physical loss and subsequent hardships can put relationships, commitments, and self to the test. But simultaneously, ill people may discover that their emerging selves rise to the test. Resolving feelings of loss, hurt, and betrayal takes work. Because these feelings often surface precisely when physical distress escalates, resolution can seem a monumental task. Yet resolution may develop.

Resolution allows people to see their illness and themselves from a new perspective. They reinterpret their feelings and shift their viewpoints. Their "discoveries" of self become positive and they view themselves as having grown (cf. Sandstrom 1990; Weitz 1991). Turning anger outward, for example, instead of inward shifts self-doubt and self-pity into moral outrage. During our second interview, the woman whose statement opened this chapter described a turning point that had occurred three years before. She recalled:

> I was feeling a lot of anger towards the doctors and towards the whole thing [illness, relatives]. . . . I think that's probably when I *stopped* feeling angry towards myself. . . . I think up until then I was just totally feeling angry towards myself.

I asked, "Because?" She said, "For being alive. I thought it was awful. I was always depressed; I thought I was bad. It took the doctors blaming me for me to say, "No, maybe I'm not the one screwing up here."

Like this woman, some people perceive illness as giving them back perspectives, values, or knowledge lost along the way. One man gained the tools for self-reflection. Several women felt that through coming to terms with their feelings about illness that they had resolved life-long emotional scars from growing up in alcoholic families. A twenty-three-year-old woman with multiple sclerosis said:

But another thing I get from being a child of an alcoholic is I don't feel a lot of pain . . . which is something that M.S. gave me back. The ability to pain, to have pain, and to know it's okay . . . It's [M.S.] given me back a lot of things, too, the ability to let go.

Like many others, this woman also believed that she had gained a new awareness of her control over her feelings and herself. She said:

I can change me. And that's about the only control I have left in this life. And I have control over my behavior; I don't have control over yours. Uhm, and I wish I'd known that a long time ago. And I think that M.S. has helped me [learn that].

Resolving their feelings about illness gives people a sense of strength (cf. Lewis 1985; Pitzele 1985). They believe that they have met adversity and faced it with courage (cf. Denzin 1987a; 1987b). The woman above avowed, "And I know that I'm very strong now." I asked, "What does strength mean to you?" She replied:

The ability to cope. To know that I can get out of that bed in the morning and drag myself through the day and smile. I can laugh, which again so many can't and that's sad, because there's nothing wrong with them and their bodies. Maybe they should get a disease.

The gains that are made from reaching a state of resolution may make it possible for an ill person to gradually shift into renewal[3]

and to learn to live with illness. Experiencing chronic illness may serve to strengthen and develop attributes someone already possessed. A woman who had disabling arthritis said:

It's made me real receptive to other people's handicaps or illnesses. I always ask how they are, or I try to. So it's like—to me it [illness] has pushed me in a certain direction towards more compassion.

Many people found that experiencing chronic illness gave them a deeper understanding of life and its meaning; it gave them new purposes, new values, new realizations. With that understanding came wisdom that transcended their former self. Chronic illness had both renewed and transformed them. These new discoveries of self counter past assumptions about self. A young woman spent four years feeling self-blame, guilt, and self-pity about having colitis. Friends and professionals reaffirmed her feelings of being responsible for her fate. When she changed locales and made new friends, her feelings of guilt subsided, her spirits lifted, and her illness abated. Old doubts faded and new hopes bloomed. She said, "I was surfacing." Years after her worst episode of illness, she said:

I really think that some of these bad situations [illness, abusive relationship, poverty, and isolation] . . . were utilized towards the great growth that I then went through. I feel quite wise. I feel quite emotionally stable. I feel that I am more emotionally stable than most people that I see, but I think that's come out of these great periods of instability.

Renewal brings a revised, not merely restored, self-concept (cf. Le Maistre 1985). Experiencing a sense of renewal follows allowing oneself to experience illness. Though ill people may not accept whatever stigmatized status that illness conferred upon them, these people accept themselves.

Just a few years ago, a middle-aged woman organized her life around making money—lots of it—working out, and dating. After being ill, she redefined her past life as superficial. She reflected:

It's when you love all people, that you really love yourself. . . . I used to be very different. But through being hurt and being sick and stuff, you really learn to change your ways and values. Everybody's wonderful. I've become a better person, more loving really and I've always been a distant, private person. . . . And it's a blessing in disguise somehow in finding out that I'm giving up all these other things, but that I'm getting something deeper than I could [before].

Conclusion

The path between creating fictional identities, facing illness, resolving feelings, renewing self, and transcending loss is a slippery one. What illness portends is uncertain for many chronically ill people, at least initially. Some people aim to keep their self-concepts separate from illness because they wish neither to be in the sick role nor to have others to impose stigmatized identities upon them. They may risk adopting fictional identities. By keeping sickness apart from self; however, they maintain valued images of themselves and preserve their autonomy. Although such individuals may be aware of their illnesses, their stance *does* lead them to ignore symptoms, to take risks, and to conceal their infirmities. Because of such actions, they may ultimately find themselves in spiraling crises which could leave them much sicker—a person with diabetes might go into insulin shock; someone with heart disease could end up in the emergency room with a full-blown heart attack.

Another scenario concerns people who maintain their fictions, and who insist upon maintaining them despite the lack of concurrence of their medical professionals. These patients insist that they have an *acute* illness and will prolong this definition for as long as they can—sometimes after the last shred of others' support for their hopes has long since disappeared. Yearning for recovery, waiting for signs of it, and living a diminished life changes anyone's perspective and shrinks the boundaries of and possibilities for self. This process may happen insidiously without awareness (Sacks 1984); however, when, and if the person becomes aware of it, the losses of self seem irretrievable. For example, a man who adapted to convalescence subsequently

found that he could not handle even working part-time. The shock and depression which follows cuts further into self-definition and thus, also contributes to losses of self.

Allowing illness to touch and shape the self without becoming inundated by it is a difficult balance to achieve. Ill people may be able to do so at some points but not at others. Similarly, a person may be able to accept an illness when it remains in the background of his or her life but not when it springs into the foreground.

To gain a sense of resolution and renewal, ill people need be aware of their illness and to appraise its implications for their emerging selves. Simultaneously, they retain or gain valued attributes of self that transcend illness and the identities accompanying it. To accomplish this, ill people view essential qualities of self as distinct from their bodies. Likely too, they must find value in self that transcends the usual criteria for productivity, achievement, and success. Subsequently, for many ill people, struggling to control the defining images that reconstruct the self becomes a continuous endeavor.

Acknowledgments
This paper was presented at the Qualitative Analysis Conference at Carleton University, May 22-25, 1992 in Ottawa. Thanks to Julia Allen, Joyce Bird, Mary Lou Dietz, Anna Hazan, Pat Jackson, Candee Nagle, Catherine Nelson, Robert Prus, Nancy Sciebura, and William Shaffir for their comments and encouragement.

Notes

1. This paper is drawn from a larger qualitative research project about experiencing chronic illness (see Charmaz 1991a; 1991b). The data include 120 in-depth interviews with 55 chronically ill people, 20 informal interviews with caregivers and providers, and autobiographical accounts. I conducted multiple interviews with 26 respondents and followed 16 men and women from seven years to over a decade. The strategies of grounded theory were followed with data collection and analysis proceeding simultaneously (Charmaz, 1983; 1990; Glaser, 1978; Glaser and Strauss, 1967; Strauss, 1987).

2. Sentiments are complex, strong subjective responses that congeal into consistent emotions through definition. Feelings are more diffuse, immediate sensations and intuitions, that may be redefined (Hochschild 1990).

3. Jo-anne LeMaistre views renewal as the "hard-won ability to separate yourself from your illness" (1985:143). In contrast, I view renewal as reflecting the shifts in emotions and changes in self that come from integrating illness into one's life and self without being consumed by it.

References

Albrecht, Gary L. 1992. "The Social Experience of Disability." Pp.1-18 in *Social Problems*. Edited by Craig Calhoun and George Ritzer. New York: McGraw-Hill.

Biesser, Arnold R. 1989. *Flying Without Wings: Personal Reflections on Being Disabled*. New York: Doubleday.

Blumer, Herbert. 1969. *Symbolic Interactionism*. Englewood Cliffs, NJ: Prentice-Hall.

Brooks, Nancy A., and Ronald R. Matson. 1987. "Managing Multiple Sclerosis." Pp. 73-106 in *Research in the Sociology of Health Care: The Experience and Management of Chronic Illness*.Vol. 6. Edited by Julius A. Roth and Peter Conrad. Greenwich, CT: JAI Press.

Charmaz, Kathy. 1983. "The Grounded Theory Method: An Explication and Interpretation." Pp. 109-126 in *Contemporary Field Research*. Edited by Robert M. Emerson. Boston: Little-Brown.

——. 1990. "Discovering Chronic Illness: Using Grounded Theory." *Social Science and Medicine* 30:1161-1172.

——. 1991a. "Fictional Identities and Turning Points." Pp. 71-86 in *Social Organization and Social Process: Essays in Honor of Anselm Strauss*. Edited by David R. Maines. New York: Aldine de Gruyter.

——. 1991b. *Good Days, Bad Days: The Self in Chronic Illness and Time*. New Brunswick, NJ: Rutgers University Press.

Conrad, Peter. 1985. "The Meaning of Medications: Another Look at Compliance." *Social Science and Medicine* 20:28-37.

Cooley, Charles H. 1902. *Human Nature and Social Order*. New York: Charles Scribner's Sons.

Cousins, Norman. 1983. *The Healing Heart: Antidotes to Panic and Helplessness*. New York: Avon.

Denzin, Norman K. 1987a. *The Alcoholic Self*. Beverly Hills: Sage.

——. 1987b. *The Recovering Alcoholic*. Newbury Park, CA: Sage.

Gardner, Carol Brooks. 1991. "Stigma and the Public Self: Notes on Communication, Self and Others." *Journal of Contemporary Ethnography* 20:251-262.

Gecas, Viktor. 1982. "The Self-Concept." *Annual Review of Sociology* 8:1-33.

Glaser, Barney G. 1978. *Theoretical Sensitivity*. Mill Valley, CA: The Sociology Press.

Glaser, Barney G., and Anselm L. Strauss. 1965. *Awareness of Dying*. Chicago: Aldine.

——. 1967. *The Discovery of Grounded Theory*. Chicago: Aldine.

Hirsch, Ernest. 1977. *Starting Over*. Hanover, MA: Christopher.

Hochschild, Arlie. 1990. "Ideology and Emotion Management: A Perspective and Path for Future Research." Pp.117-144 in *Research Agendas in the Sociology of Emotions*. Edited by Theodore D. Kemper. Albany, NY: State University of New York Press.

Hoffman, Joan Eakin. 1981. "Care of the Unwanted: Stroke Patients in a Canadian Hospital." Pp. 292-302 in *Health and Canadian Society*. Edited by David Coburn, Carl D'Arcy, Peter New, and George Torrance. Don Mills, Ontario: Fitzhenry and Whiteside Limited.

Kelleher, David. 1988. "Coming to Terms with Diabetes: Coping Strategies and Non-Compliance." Pp. 155-187 in *Living with Chronic Illness*. Edited by Robert Anderson and Michael Bury. London: Unwin Hyman.

LeMaistre, Joanne. 1985. *Beyond Rage: The Emotional Impact of Chronic Illness*. Oak Park, IL: Alpine Guild.

Lewis, Helen Block. 1971. *Shame and Guilt in Neurosis*. New York: International Press.

Lewis, Kathleen. 1985. *Successful Living with Chronic Illness*. Wayne, NJ: Avery.

Locker, David. 1983. *Disability and Disadvantage*. London: Tavistock.

Mead, George Herbert. 1934. *Mind, Self and Society*. Chicago: University of Chicago Press.

Olesen, Virginia L. 1992. "Extraordinary Events and Mundane Ailments." Pp. 205-220 in *Investigating Subjectivity: Research on Lived Experience*. Edited by Carolyn Ellis and Michael G. Flaherty. Newbury Park, CA: Sage.

Peyrot, Mark, James F. McMurray Jr., and Richard Hedges. 1987. "Living with Diabetes: The Role of Personal and Professional Knowledge in Symptom and Regimen Management." Pp. 107-146 in *Research in the Sociology of Health Care: The Experience and Management of Chronic Illness* Vol. 6. Edited by Julius A. Roth and Peter Conrad. Greenwich, CT: JAI Press.

Pinder, Ruth. 1988. "Striking Balances: Living with Parkinson's Disease." Pp. 67-88 in *Living with Chronic Illness*. Edited by Robert Anderson and Michael Bury. London: Unwin-Hyman.

Pitzele, Sefra Kobrin. 1985. *We Are Not Alone: Learning to Live with Chronic Illness*. New York: Workman.

Prus, Robert. 1987. "Generic Social Processes: Maximizing Conceptual Development in Ethnographic Research." *Journal of Contemporary Ethnography* 16: 250-293.

Robinson, Ian. 1988. *Multiple Sclerosis*. London: Tavistock.

——. 1990. "Personal Narratives, Social Careers and Medical Courses: Analyzing Life Trajectories in Autobiographies of People with Multiple Sclerosis." *Social Science & Medicine* 30:1173-1186.

Rosenberg, Morris. 1979. *Conceiving the Self*. New York: Basic Books.

Sacks, Oliver. 1984. *A Leg To Stand On*. New York: Summit Books.

Sandstrom, Kent L. 1990. "Confronting Deadly Disease: The Drama of Identity Construction Among Gay Men with AIDS." *Journal of Contemporary Ethnography* 19: 271-294.

Sarbin, Theodore R. 1986. "Emotion and Act: Roles and Rhetoric." Pp. 83-97 in *The Social Construction of Emotion*. Edited by Rom Harre. London: Basil Blackwell.

Sarton, May. 1988. *After the Stroke: A Journal*. New York: Norton.

Scheff, Thomas J. 1990. *Microsociology: Discourse, Emotion and Social Structure*. Chicago: University of Chicago Press.

Strauss, Anselm. 1969. *Mirrors and Masks: The Search for Identity*. Mill Valley, CA: The Sociology Press.

——. 1987. *Qualitative Analysis for Social Scientists*. Cambridge: Cambridge University Press.

Swanson, Janice M. and W. Carole Chenitz. 1993. "Regaining a Valued Self: The Process of Adaptation to Living with Genital Herpes." *Qualitative Health Research* 3: 270-297.

Turner, Ralph. 1976. "The Real Self: From Institution to Impulse." *American Journal of Sociology* 81: 989-1016.

Veith, Ilza. 1988. *Can You Hear the Clapping of One Hand?: Learning to Live with a Stroke*. Berkeley, CA: University of California Press.

Weitz, Rose. 1991. *Life with AIDS*. New Brunswick, NJ: Rutgers University Press.

Further Reading

Juliet M. Corbin and Anselm L. Strauss. 1988. *Unending Work and Care: Managing Chronic Illness at Home*. San Francisco: Jossey-Bass

Cherie Register. 1987. *Living With Chronic Illness*. New York: Free Press.

Anselm L. Straus, Juliet Corbin, Shizuko Fagerhaugh, Barney G. Glaser, David Maines, Barbara Suczek, and Carolyn Wiener. 1984. *Chronic Illness and the Quality of Life*. St. Louis: Mosby.

Discussion Questions

1. In which ways do emotions affect turning points in self-construction in illness?

2. What is the difference between constructing a fictional identity and denying one's illness? How can you separate assumptions about recovery and hope from denial of illness?

3. What similarities and differences do you find between Charmaz' analysis of the self in illness and the self in other life crises?

From *Doing Everyday Life: Ethnography as Human Lived Experience*, M. Dietz, R. Prus and W. Shaffir (eds.). Pp. 226-242. Copyright © 1994 by Kathy Charmaz. Reprinted by permission. ✦

10

Illness and Identity

David A. Karp

In this excerpt, David Karp applies the socio-logical concept of career to depression, an ill-ness marked by an ambiguous onset of symp-toms, uncertain course, and contested treat-ments. Ordinarily, we might think of a career as a chosen path that a person takes through life within an honorable profession. However, a career also can consist of a devalued, volun-tary or involuntary undertaking or life course. Having a career means that the person holds a position, engages in routine activities, takes on certain perspectives, and moves through iden-tifiable transitions. A career has both objective and subjective components. It is objective in the sense that it shapes identity in profound ways: people become identified by inhabiting it. A career provides or enforces a path, pace, and passage through life. Being identified as having depression places certain boundaries on experience. Becoming a patient in a mental hospital creates more limits. A career as a men-tal patient takes on a life of its own. In this case, the mental patient not only suffers from depression but also is subject to domination, surveillance, and loss of control. Identities as a mental patient and as a depressed person so-lidify and become public.

These public identities hold momentous im-plications for subjective consciousness. Many people feel that being identified as a depressive enlarges and extends whatever dark thoughts of difference they had held about themselves. Nonetheless some are liberated by at last find-ing a category that describes their previous in-choate feelings. Crisis forces definition of once inexplicable feelings and behavior. Crisis also forces action as it presents a turning point from which there is no exit. Depressed indi-viduals must come to terms with a changed life and continued illness.

You know, I was a mental patient. That was my identity. . . . Depression is very private. Then all of a sudden it becomes public and I was a mental patient. . . . It's no longer just my own pain. I am a men-tal patient. I am a depressive. *I am a de-pressive* (said slowly and with intensity). This is my identity. I can't separate myself from that. When people know me they'll have to know about my psychiatric his-tory, because that's who I am.

—*Female graduate student, aged 24*

At the time we spoke, Karen, whose words open this chapter, had been doing well for more than two years, but described being badly frightened by a recent two-week period during which the all-too-familiar feelings of depression had begun to reappear. Aside from the terror she felt at the prospect of be-coming sick, Karen realized that if depres-sion returned, it would mean recasting her identity yet again. After two years with noth-ing but the "normal" ups and downs of life, she had started to feel that it might be possi-ble to leave behind the mental patient iden-tity she earlier thought she never could shed. By the time of our interview, only her family and a few old friends knew of her several hos-pitalizations. Her current roommates thought of her simply as Karen, one of about eight students in the large house they shared. She told me, "No one in my life right now knows . . . I'm so eager to talk to you about it [in this interview] because I can't talk about it with people." I said, "It must be hurtful not to be able to talk about so critical a part of your biography," and Karen responded, "Yes, but I don't want to test it with people. . . . [If I told them] they might not say anything, but their perception of me would change."

Karen was willing to be interviewed be-cause I was one of those who knew about her history with depression. Years previously, while taking one of my undergraduate courses, she had confided that she was hav-ing a terrible time completing her course work. After much tentative discussion, the word depression finally entered the conversation. She seemed embarrassed by the admission until I opened my desk drawer and showed her a bottle of pills *I* was taking for depression. With this, we began to trade depression experiences and thereby formed the kind of bond felt by those who go through a common difficulty. As her undergraduate years passed, Karen came to my office periodically and during these visits we often spoke about depression. Our shared identity as depressed persons blurred the age and status distinctions that otherwise might have prevented our friendship. . . .

Like nearly everyone whom I talked with, Karen could pinpoint the beginning of her depression career. Although she described a "home filled with feelings of sadness" for as long as she could remember, it was, she said "the beginning of the ninth grade that touched off . . . ten years of depression." She elaborated with the observation, "I was always sad or upset, but I was so busy and social [that the feelings were muted]. You know, things were not doing so well at home, but at school no one knew how much of a hellhole I lived in." She described a home life that was fairly stable until her father became ill when she was a sixth grader. "When he came back from the hospital," she said, "he was very different, unstable [and] extremely violent." Till then Karen had been able to keep the misery of her home life apart from her school world, which served as a refuge. By the ninth grade, however, she "could no longer keep the two worlds separate" and in both places the same intrusive questions, feelings, and ruminations colonized her mind. Now she didn't feel safe anywhere in the world and had these relentless thoughts: "I'm miserable. [There is] such a feeling of emptiness. What the hell am I doing? What is my life all about? What is the point?" "And that," she said, "basically started it."

In the ninth grade Karen had no word for the "it" that had started. When I asked whether she recognized her pain as depression then, she replied, "Did I say this was depression [then]? Did I know [what it was]? It was pain, but I don't think I would have called it depression. I think I would have called it *my* pain." There was another factor that contributed to the anonymity of her misery and

kept her pain from having a name—Karen was determined to keep her torment hidden. She said, "I lived with that for . . . a couple of years, from the ninth grade until the eleventh grade. [I lived] with that feeling. . . . But it was all very private. I kept it quiet. It was something inside. I didn't really talk about it. I might have talked about it with some of my friends, but no one understood."

During this time, though, a subtle transformation was taking place in her thinking about "it." Previously, Karen felt that her pain came exclusively from her difficulties at home, but by the eleventh grade she was beginning to suspect that its locus might be elsewhere. She told me, "My family life might have been hell, but it was always, 'Oh [I feel this way] because my father is crazy. It's because of something outside of me.' But it was the first time I'm feeling awful about myself." By the eleventh grade Karen's new consciousness was that there was something really wrong with *her*. Now, her feelings about the pain took a critical turn when she began to say to herself, "I can't live like this. I will not survive. I will not be here. I can't live with the pain. If I have to live with the pain I will eventually kill myself." Despite such a shift in thinking Karen still succeeded in keeping things private until she experienced a very public crisis. It was, moreover, a "crash" that she understood as a major "turning point" in her identity. Here's what she said:

> My whole family life just fell apart. There was no anchor. There was no anchor. . . . [Now] I was able to label it and say it was depression when I crashed in the eleventh grade and was hospitalized. You know, in ninth grade I told you about an experience where I was conscious of feeling pain, or whatever, but no one else knew about it. . . . It is sort of like what my life is like now. I couldn't tell people about it. How can you tell people about it? What do you say? . . .

Then the interview turned to a lengthy discussion about psychiatric hospitals, doctors, and power—all of it negative. She expressed hostility toward doctors who wanted her to "open up" and toward institutional rules that seemed authoritarian and arbitrary. She said, "Psychiatrists and mental health workers have the power to decide when you are going to leave, if you're going to leave, if you can go out on a pass, if you're good, if you're not good." This first hospitalization (eventually there would be four) also started a long history with medications of all sorts. When I asked whether she was treated with medications she replied, "Yup, always medication. That's the big thing. . . . Oh my God, I've had so many. . . . I don't think they really affected me that much. By the time I left I was doing okay. Did I have these problems solved? No, [but] I had an added one. Now I felt crazy." I used Karen's observation about "feeling crazy" as a cue for asking if she had a disease. I said, "Did you now think of yourself as having an illness in the medical sense?" and her answer reflected the ambivalence and confusion I would later routinely hear when I asked this same question of others.

> I think of it less as an illness and more something that society defines. That's part of it, but then, it *is* physical. Doesn't that make it an illness? That's a question I ask myself a lot. Depression is a special case because everyone gets depressed. . . . I think that I define it as not an illness. It's a condition. When I hear the term illness I think of sickness. . . . [but] the term mental illness seems to me to be very negative, maybe because I connect it with hospitalization . . .

Before it ended, my interview with Karen covered other difficult emotional terrain, including a major suicide attempt, additional periods of hospitalization, stays in halfway houses, a traumatic college experience, failed relationships with therapists, job interviews that required lies about health history, and a personal spiritual transformation. As indicated at the outset, things had gotten better by the time of our interview and Karen believed she was pretty much past her problem with depression. She told me, "A couple of years ago, three years ago, four years ago, I would feel a need to tell people about it because I still felt depressed, because I still felt mentally ill. But now I no longer see myself in that way. I'm other things. I'm Karen the grad student. I'm Karen the one who loves to garden, the one who's interested in a lot of things. I'm not just Karen the mentally ill per-

son." Still, such optimism about being past depression was sometimes distressingly eroded by periods of bad feelings and the ever-present edge of fear that "it" might return in its full-blown, most grotesque form. . . .

A Career View of the Depression Experience

As in many areas of social life, the notion of career seems an extremely useful, sensitizing concept. In his voluminous and influential writings on work, Everett Hughes showed the value of conceptualizing career as "the moving perspective in which the person sees his life as a whole and interprets the meanings of his various attitudes, actions, and the things which happen to him."[1] Hughes' definition directs attention to the subjective aspects of the career process and the ways in which people attach evaluative meanings to the typical sequence of movements constituting their career path. Here I shall be concerned with describing the career features associated with an especially ambiguous illness—depression.

Hughes' definition also suggests that each stage,[2] juncture, or moment in a career requires a redefinition of self. The depression experience is a heuristically valuable instance for studying the intersection of careers and identities. The following data analysis illustrates that much of the depression career is caught up with assessing self, redefining self, reinterpreting past selves, and attempting to construct a future self that will "work" better. Although all careers require periodic reassessments of self, illness careers are especially characterized by critical "turning points" in identity. In his discussion of identity transformations Anselm Strauss[3] comments on the intersection of career and identity turning points:

> In transformations of identities a person becomes something other than he or she once was. Such shifts necessitate new evaluations of self and others, of events, acts, and objects. . . . Transformation of perception is irreversible; once having changed there is no going back. One can look back, but evaluate only from the

new status. . . . Certain critical incidences occur to force a person to recognize that "I am not the same as I was, as I used to be." These critical incidents constitute turning points in the onward movement of persons' careers.

. . . While there is considerable variation in the timing of events, all the respondents in this study described a process remarkably similar to the one implicit in Karen's account. Every person I interviewed moved through these identity turning points in their view of themselves and their problem with depression:

1. A period of *inchoate feelings* during which they lacked the vocabulary to label their experience as depression.

2. A phase during which they conclude that *something is really wrong with me.*

3. A *crisis stage* that thrusts them into a world of therapeutic experts.

4. A stage of *coming to grips with an illness identity* during which they theorize about the cause(s) for their difficulty and evaluate the prospects for getting beyond depression.

Each of these career moments assumes and requires redefinitions of self.

Inchoate Feelings

. . . The ages of respondents in this study range from the early twenties to the middle sixties. All these people described a period of time during which they had no vocabulary for naming their problem. Many traced feelings of emotional discomfort to ages as young as three or four, although they could not associate their feelings with something called "depression" until years later. It was typical for respondents to go for long periods of time feeling different, uncomfortable, marginal, ill-at-ease, scared, and in pain without attaching the notion of depression to their situations. A sampling of comments indicating an inchoate, obscure experience includes these:

Well, I knew I was different from other children. I should say that from a very early age it felt like I had this darkness about me. Sort of shadow of myself. And

I always had the sense that it wasn't going to go away so easily. And it was like my battle. . . . [female travel agent, aged 41]

An awareness that was more intellectual was apparent to me about my sophomore year in high school, when I'd wake up depressed and drag myself to school. . . . I didn't know that's what it was. I just knew that I had an awful hard time getting out of bed and a hard time making my bed and a hard time, you know, getting myself to school. . . . I kind of just had the feeling that something wasn't right. . . . [It was] just like a constant knot in my stomach. But I didn't think that that was anxiety. I just thought I wasn't feeling good, you know (laughing). [unemployed disabled female, aged 39].

If I think about it, I really can't pinpoint a moment [when I was aware that I was depressed]. . . . [male professor, aged 48]

Most of those reporting bad feelings from an early age could not conclude that something was "abnormal" because they had no baseline of normalcy for comparison. As might be expected, several respondents in this sample came from what they now describe as severely dysfunctional family circumstances, often characterized by alcoholism and both physical and emotional abuse. These individuals described feeling unsafe at home and often devised strategies to spend as much time as they could elsewhere. . . .

For most respondents the phase of inchoate feelings was the longest in the eventual unfolding of their illness consciousness. Particularly salient in terms of personal identity is the fact that initial definitions of their problem centered on the "structural conditions" of their lives instead of on the structure of their selves. The focus of interpretation was on the situation rather than on the self. Their emerging definition was that escape from the situation would make things right. Over and again individuals recounted fantasies of escape from their families and often from the community in which they grew up. However, initially at least, they felt trapped without a clear notion of how the situation might change.

I remember from like five, starting to subtract five from eighteen, to see how many years I have left before I could get out [of the house]. So, I would say the overwhelming feeling was that I felt powerless. I felt a lot of things early. And I felt that I was stuck in this house and these people controlled me, and there wasn't anything I could do about it, and I was stuck there. So I just started my little chart at about four and a half or five, counting when I could get out. [female baker, aged 41]

. . . A decisive juncture in the evolution of a "sickness" self-definition occurs when the circumstances individuals perceive as troubling their lives change, but mood problems persist. The persistence of problems in the absence of the putative cause requires a redefinition of what is wrong. A huge cognitive shift occurs when people come to see that the problem may be internal instead of situational; when they conclude that something is likely wrong with *them* in a manner that transcends their immediate situation.

Something Is Really Wrong with Me

In 1977, Robert Emerson and Sheldon Messinger published a paper entitled "The Micro-Politics of Trouble"[4] that analyzes the regular processes through which individuals come to see a personal difficulty as sufficiently troublesome a problem that something ought to be done about it. The materials offered in this chapter affirm the general process they describe. The process begins with a state of affairs initially "experienced as difficult, unpleasant, or unendurable."[5] At first, sufferers try an informal remedy, which sometimes works. If it doesn't, they seek another remedy. The decision that a consequential problem exists warranting a formal remedy typically follows a "recurring cycle of trouble, remedy, failure, more trouble, and a new remedy, until the trouble stops or the troubled person forsakes further efforts."[6] Here, then, is their description of the transformation from vague, inchoate feelings to a clearer sense that one is sufficiently troubled to seek a remedy.

Problems originate with the recognition that something is wrong and must be remedied. Trouble, in these terms, involves both definitional and remedial components. . . . On first apprehension

troubles often involve little more than vague unease. . . . An understanding of the problem's dimensions may only begin to emerge as the troubled person thinks about them, discusses the matter with others, and begins to implement remedial strategies.[7]

Despite the difficulties they have in naming their feelings as a problem, all of the respondents eventually conclude that something is *really wrong* with *them*. To be sure, many used identical phrases in describing their situations. The phrases "something was really wrong with me" and "I felt that I could no longer live like this" were repeated over and over. Respondents commented in nearly identical ways on the heightened feeling that "something is really wrong with me."

When it really became apparent that I was just a mess was in January of 1989. I made the decision really quickly at the end of 1988 to go to school at [names a four year college] and live with my father and my stepmother and commute. And I packed up all my stuff in my car and went. I was miserable. I cried every day. Every single day I cried. I think I went to two classes [at the new school] and lasted there only a month. I was absolutely miserable. There was a lot of different factors that were involved with it [but] I just didn't feel right. There was something wrong with me, you know. [unemployed female, aged 23]

I guess it's the fall of '90 when I had done the family therapy. I felt great about that. I was back at Harvard. My work was going okay. I loved myself. I loved my husband. Everything was great. [But] I wanted to die. I had no pleasure in anything. What finally got me [was that] I looked at the trees turning and I didn't care. I couldn't believe it. I'd be looking at this big flaming maple and I'd look at it and I'd think, "There it is, it's a maple tree. It's bright orange and red." And nothing in me was touched. At that point I went back to my therapist and said, "There's something really wrong here." [female software quality control manager, aged 31]

. . . These quotes suggest a fundamental transformation in perception and identity at this point in the evolution of a depression consciousness. Respondents now located the source of their problem as somewhere within their bodies and minds, as deep within themselves. Such a belief implies a problematic identity far more basic and immutable than those associated with social statuses. If, for example, someone has a disliked occupational identity, the possibilities for occupational change exist. If the occupational identity becomes onerous enough, it is possible to quit a job. Similarly, without minimizing the difficulties of change, we can choose to become single if married, to change from one religion to another, and, these days, even to change our sex if the motivation is great enough. However, to see oneself as somehow internally flawed poses substantially greater problems for identity change or remediation because one's whole personhood is implicated. Getting rid of a sick self poses far greater problems than dropping certain social statuses. The important point here is that the rejection of situational theories for bad feelings is a critical identity turning point. Full acceptance that one has a damaged self requires acknowledgment that "I am not the same as I was, as I used to be."

Another important dimension of the career process that becomes apparent at this point is the issue of whether to keep the problem private or to make it public, especially to family and friends. The private/public distinction was a dominant theme in respondents' talk throughout the history of their experience with depression. The question of being private or public is, of course, central to one's developing self-identification. As Peter Berger and Hansfried Kellner[8] point out in describing the "social construction of marriage" and Diane Vaughan[9] indicates in analyzing the process of "uncoupling" from a relationship, the moment a new status becomes public is a definitive one in solidifying a person's new identity. In the cases of both creating and disengaging from relationships, people are normally very careful not to make public announcements until they are certain they are ready to adopt new statuses and identities. The significance attached to public announcements of even modest shifts in life style is indicated by the considerable thought people sometimes give to making public such relatively benign decisions as going on diets or quitting cigarettes.

Decisions about "going public" are, of course, greatly magnified when the information to be imparted is negative and, in the case of emotional problems, potentially stigmatizing. As Emerson and Messinger note, the search for a remedy necessarily involves sharing information with others. Still, at this early juncture of dealing with bad feelings, most respondents elected to keep silent about their pain. . . .

Whether or not they made their feelings public, this second phase of their illness career involved the recognition that they possessed a self that was working badly in *every* situation. Although everyone continued to identify the kinds of *social* situations that had caused their bad feelings in the past and precipitated them in the present, the qualitative change at this juncture was in the locus of attention from external to internal causes. At this point respondents were struggling to live their lives in the face of debilitating pain. This stage ended, however, when efforts to control things became impossible.

At some point everyone interviewed experienced a crisis of some sort. For the majority (29) the crisis meant hospitalization. At the point of crisis, whatever their wishes might have been, they could not prevent their situation from becoming public knowledge to family, friends, and co-workers. Whether they were hospitalized or not, everyone reached a point where they felt obliged to rely on psychiatric experts to deal with their difficulty. Receiving an "official" diagnosis of depression and consequent treatment with medications greatly accelerated the need to redefine their past, present, and future in illness terms. The crisis solidified the emerging consciousness that the problem was within themselves. More than that, it was now a problem beyond their own efforts to control.

Crisis

Nearly everyone could pinpoint the precise time, situation, or set of events that moved them from the recognition that something was wrong to the realization that they were desperately sick. They could often remember in vivid detail the moment when things absolutely got out of hand.

> So I went to law school in the fall. I was at Columbia and in the best of times Columbia is a depressing place. I mean, it's a shithole. And you know, I was pretty messed up when I got there. . . . I remember Columbia was a nightmare. . . . So, I was getting to the point where I was paranoid about going to class and so someone talked to the dean and said, "Hey, you've got to do something about this guy, he's off the deep edge." [male administrator, aged 54]

> I think the significant moment was when I got stage fright in high school. There were earlier moments when I felt something was wrong. I can remember feeling real dizzy when I was on the stage in the 8th grade. But the significant moment was in high school and I was seized by just pure terror. And the fear was so horrible that I couldn't tell it to anybody. I couldn't share it. It was something beyond my ability to communicate. It was so horrible that no one could understand it. [male professor, aged 66]

. . . At the crisis point, people fully enter a therapeutic world of hospitals, mental health experts, and medications. For many, entrance into this world is simultaneous with first receiving the "official" diagnosis of depression.[10] It is difficult to overstate the critical importance of official diagnoses and labeling. The point of diagnosis was a double-edged benchmark in the illness career. On the one hand, knowing that you "have" something that doctors regard as a specific illness imposes definitional boundaries onto an array of behaviors and feelings that previously had no name. Acquiring a clear conception of what one has and having a label to attach to confounding feelings and behaviors was especially significant to those who had gone for years without being able to name their situation. To be diagnosed also suggests the possibility that the condition can be treated and that one's suffering can be diminished. At the same time, being a "depressive" places one in the devalued category of those with mental illness. On the negative side, respondents made comments like these:

> I kept going to doctor after doctor, getting like all these new terms put on me. . . . My family was dysfunctional and I was an alcoholic with an eating disorder and bulemia and depression and it was just all these labels. "Oh my God!" [unemployed female, aged 22]

> My father went to his allergy doctor who referred us to a guy who turned out to be a reasonable psychiatrist. I'll never forget. He said, "Your daughter is clinically depressed." I remember sitting in his office. He saw us on a Saturday like at six o'clock. He did us a favor. And I remember I just sat there. It was a sort of darkened office. It was the first time I ever cried in front of anybody. [female social worker, aged 38]

And on the liberating side:

> They gave me a blood test that measures the level of something in the blood, in the brain. And they pronounced me, they said, "Mr. Smith [a pseudonym], you're depressed." And I said, "Thank God," you know. I wasn't as batty as I thought. It was like the cat was out of the bag. You know? It was a breakthrough. . . . [Before that] depression wasn't in my vocabulary. . . . It was the beginning of being able to sort out a lifetime of feelings, events . . . my entire life. It was the chance for a new beginning. [male salesman, aged 30]

. . . It is impossible to consider the kinds of profound identity changes occasioned by any mental illness without paying special attention to the experience of hospitalization. It is one thing to deal alone with the demons of depression, or to privately see a psychiatrist for the problem, but once a person "shuts down" altogether and seeks asylum or is involuntarily "committed," he or she adds an institutional piece to their biography that is indelible. . . .

A few interviewees described the hospital as truly an asylum that provided relief and allowed them to "crash." Being hospitalized enabled them to give up the struggle of trying to appear and act normally. One person, in fact, described the hospital as a "wonderful place" where "I was taken care of, totally taken care of." Another was relieved "to go somewhere where I won't do anything to myself, where I can get in touch with this." Someone else explained, "I was glad to be there, definitely. It was a break from everything." Sometimes people were glad to be hospitalized since it provided dramatic and definitive evidence that something was really wrong with them when family and friends had been dismissing their complaints. More usual, though, were the responses like that of the person who said that "the experience of hospitalization was devastating to me" and the several who reported that being hospitalized made them feel like "damaged goods."

Of all the tough things associated with depression, nothing would frighten me more than hospitalization. Along with the social science ethnographies that have been done over the years describing the deplorable and dehumanizing character of mental hospitals, I have seen Frederick Wiseman's incredibly distressing documentary, *Titicutt Follies*, which portrays the brutally awful conditions in a Massachusetts State Hospital during the 1960s. No doubt things have generally improved since the years when Hollywood could portray asylums as "snake pits" run by mean-spirited, authoritarian personalities like Big Nurse in *One Flew Over the Cuckoo's Nest*. As well, the "deinstitutionalization" process beginning in the 1970s resulted in the closing of many of the country's worst hospitals. Still, recent books on the hospitalization experience[11] and the sometimes gruesome stories I heard during interviews greatly strengthen my resolve never to go into a hospital.

I found particularly chilling Sam's account. Sam was another person I first met at a depression support group. At age 58, he seemed anxious to recount what hospital treatment was like "before they even had antidepressants." I knew from our previous casual conversation and his distinctive accent that Sam had grown up in the South. During the interview I learned more about his religious upbringing. His father had been a minister and his mother, although a stern figure, "was dependable." Sam first became sick enough to be hospitalized when he was a high school senior. He remembers that after his two-month stay, "You went back with the stigma on you because people who went off their rocker went to [names a state hospital].

You know how kids are. They make jokes about crazy people. . . . The cops also knew about this and had me marked down as a crazy person from then on." However, it wasn't remembrance of his return home that startled me. I could barely listen to his description of the hospitalization itself. Although Sam did not blame anyone for his treatment, saying, "It's not that they were cruel or anything. They just didn't know." I could not imagine being a 17-year-old and living through an experience like Sam's. Here, in some detail, is what he told me.

. . . It's like suffocating [shock induced by carbon dioxide treatments]. That's the first thing they did to me. I remember thinking, "My God, they're trying to kill me for being sad." This is at [names a university hospital]. Not pleasant. . . . And I had ECT before they put you out. . . . They gave it to you straight. No anesthesia.

No anesthesia?

You lie there and they put the electrodes on your head. . . . It's like waiting to be electrocuted. I can't put it any other way. You're leaning back, looking, and they got the machine over there and they throw the switch and I don't think you feel anything or know anything. It just knocks you out instantly. But, waitin' for it. . . . I'm not a scared person. There's not too many things that I'm afraid of, but that's one. I'll admit to that. And the woman who held the electrodes had a face that Dracula would kill to get. Ooh, she looked a lot worse than Elsa Lanchester in the *Bride of Frankenstein*. I'll never forget that. And you'd see the guy next to you getting it, and the grand mal seizure, and snorting, and they'd turn blue and purple. You'd see them go by in the beds right after they had it, and believe me people looked like a drowning case. And you're next, you know. It was not good. It's pretty awful. I remember waking up and you just had been talking to some nurse or something, but you can't remember her name for the life [of you]. You wake up and see them, but you don't know what things are. And then it eventually comes back . . . "Oh yeah, it's the ceiling." And stuff starts to come back, short-term things come back. But, you know, you have to work hard for the names. [unemployed male, aged 58]

. . . Although Sam's story was the most disturbing I heard, many of the 29 people who spoke of their time in hospitals spontaneously acknowledged the extraordinary impact of the experience on the way they thought about themselves. Sometimes they were themselves shocked that they had landed in a hospital. Several mentioned that hospitalization caused them to confront for the first time just how sick they were.

I remember being put onto the floor that was probably for the worst people of the sickness, because it was one of those floors where everything was really locked up. So I guess I was in pretty bad shape. [male administrator, aged 54]

So I went to [names hospital] and I remember praying that I would get out. To me it seemed at the time as if the door would close—it was a secure facility—and I would never leave. I know I'm a basket case at this point. . . . The experience of having that severe depression, going to the hospital, and most of all being given shock treatments. . . . It made me feel . . . like damaged goods, impaired in some way that I was just not normal. It did make me feel impaired. [male professor, part-time, aged 48]

Among the identity-related comments about the hospitalization experience, one set of observations, although made by only a few individuals, caught my attention. Once in the hospital these persons surveyed their environment, both the oppressive physical character of the place and the sad shape of their fellow "inmates," many of whom seemed to them destined for an institutionalized life. However awful their condition, these respondents made a distinction between their trouble and patients who were overtly psychotic. Unlike those unfortunates, they had a choice to make, as they saw it. Either they would capitulate completely to their depression and possibly, therefore, to a life in the mental health system or they would do whatever necessary to leave the hospital as quickly as possible.

Giving up completely did have some appealing features. Full surrender meant relief from an exhausting battle and absolution from personal responsibility. One woman said, "I saw these people going back and forth [in and out of the hospital] for their whole lives [and] that I could be one [of them]. If I went in that direction, it somehow absolved me from responsibility. And I teetered on the edge for a long time. It involved a conscious decision . . . [about whether] I'm going to become a [permanent] part of the system because it's safe and where I belong.". . .

. . . It should be noted that one outstanding uniformity in the interviews was the initially strong negative reaction people had to taking drugs. One person was "leery of it" and others variously described the idea of going on medications as "revolting," "certainly not my first choice," and "embarrassing." Others elaborated on the recommendation that they begin drug therapy in ways similar to the nurse who said: "I didn't want to be told that I had something that was going to affect the rest of my life and that could only be solved by taking pills. And there was sort of a rebellion in that: 'No, I'm not like that. I don't need you and your pills.' ". . . [Respondents] held the shared feeling that taking drugs was yet another distressing indication of the severity of a problem they could not control by themselves. The concurrent events of crisis, hospitalization, and beginning a drug regimen worked synergistically to concretize and dramatize respondents' status as patients with an illness that required ongoing treatment by therapeutic experts.

Coming to Grips With an Illness Identity

Whether people are hospitalized or not, involvement with psychiatric experts and medications is the transition point to a number of simultaneous processes, all with implications for the reformulation of identity. They are (1) reconstructing and reinterpreting one's past in terms of current experiences, (2) looking for causes for one's situation, (3) constructing new theories about the nature of depression, and (4) establishing modes of coping behavior. All of these activities require judgments about the appropriate metaphors for describing one's situation. Especially critical to ongoing identity construction is whether respondents approve of illness metaphors for describing their experience. A few individuals were willing clearly to define their condition as a mental illness:

> I know I have a mental illness. I'm beginning to feel that. [But] actually, there is a real relief in that. It's a sense of "Whew! Okay, I don't have to masquerade." I mean, sure I'll masquerade with work, because, listen, I've got to get the bread and butter on the table. But I don't have to masquerade in other ways. . . . It's sort of like mentally ill people in some ways . . . are my people. There is a fair amount of really chronically mentally ill people at [names hospital where she works]. They're all on heavy-duty meds and I figure like "I know what it's like for you." I mean, I can imagine what it's like. I know some of that pain. I'm sure I don't know all of it, because, you know, I'm not that bad off, but there is sort of a sense like they could understand me and I could understand them in something that's really, really painful. [female physical therapist, aged 42]

. . . Most, however, wanted simultaneously to embrace the definition of their problem as biochemical in nature while rejecting the notion that they suffer from a "mental" illness.

> I don't see it as an illness. To me, it seems like part of myself that evolved, part of my personality. And, I mean, it sounds crazy, but it is almost like a dual personality, the happy side of me and the sad side of me. . . . [female nanny, aged 22]

> *Well, do you have an illness? What do you have?*

> I tend to think of it as a condition. I don't think of it so much an illness, although it feels like an illness sometimes. I think it's an unintegrated dimension of myself that's taken [on] kind of a life of its own, that has its own power. . . . [Unemployed female, aged 35]

. . . Adopting the view that one is victimized by a biochemically sick self constitutes a comfortable "account" for a history of difficulties and failures and absolves one of responsibility. On the negative side, however, acceptance of a victim role, while diminish-

ing a sense of personal responsibility, is also enfeebling. To be a victim of biochemical forces beyond one's control gives force to others' definition of oneself as a helpless, passive object of injury. . . .

Respondents generally fall into two broad categories regarding their hopes that they can put depression behind them. First are those who view having depression as a life condition that they will never fully defeat and second are those who believe that either they are now past the depression forever or that they can attain such a status. As might be expected, the two categories are generally formed by those who have experienced depression as an ongoing chronic thing, on the one hand, in contrast to those who have had periods of depression punctuated by wellness. The role of medications is interesting in establishing for some the idea that depression is something they can leave behind. Among the words that reappeared in comments about drugs was "miracle." Although, as noted, most of those interviewed at first took medication reluctantly, several reported that often for the first time in their lives they felt okay after a drug "kicked in." Generally, subjects were split between those who felt that while there was always the possibility of a reoccurrence, they essentially could get past depression and those who have surrendered to its inevitability and chronicity in their lives. The following comments summarize the two positions:

> I've stopped thinking, "OK I'm going to get over this depression. I'm going to finally, like, do this primal scream thing, or whatever. . . . [At one point] I did buy into [the idea] of the pursuit of happiness and the pursuit of fulfillment. I hate that word. And the mental health equivalent to finding fulfillment is to fill up the gaps inside of you and everything grows green. And that's what [psychiatry] is really striving for . . . and that's the standard life should be lived on. . . . But then I finally realized that well, maybe I'm in a desert. Maybe your landscape is green, but, you know, I'm in the Sahara and I've stopped trying to get out. . . . I'd rather cure it if I had my choice, but I don't think that is going to happen. My choice is to integrate it into my life. So, no, I don't see it going

away. I just see myself becoming, you know, better able to cope with it, more graceful about it. [female mental health worker, aged 27]

I would say that this particular period of my life is a period where I don't have the fear or feeling [that depression will reoccur]. That's why, for me at least, I'm more inclined now to take the depression as an aberration and to take me in my more expansive, expressive state as the norm. For me, maybe I'm deluding myself, the way I feel now, and it's been three years since the hospitalization and I take no medications of any kind, [is] that I may be out of the woods, so to speak. . . . At the moment I don't have a fear of reoccurrence, but I do remember having it. [male professor, part-time, aged 48]

Unfortunately, the norm is for people to have repeated bouts with depression. In this regard, the process described here has a feedback-loop quality to it. Individuals move through a crisis with all its attendant identity-altering features, come to grips with the meaning of their experience by constructing theories about causation, and then sometimes reach the point where they feel they have gone beyond the depression experience. A new episode of depression, of course, casts doubt on all the previous interpretive work and requires people to once again move through a process of sense-making and identity construction. In this way, depression is like a virus that keeps mutating since each reliving of an experience, as the philosopher Edmund Husserl tells us, is a new experience. Chronically depressed people are constantly in the throes of an illness that is tragically familiar, but always new. As such, depression often involves a life centered on a nearly continuous process of construction, destruction, and reconstruction of identities in the face of repeated problems. . . .

Notes

1. E. Hughes, *Men and Their Work* (New York: Free Press, 1958).
2. Although the notion of "stage" is difficult to avoid, I want to suggest that in much social science literature the term conveys a determinism that I find unfortunate. Stages imply that, for whatever process being described, everyone must move through them in a predictably timed sequence. Hence, I often use the terms "moment," "benchmark," or "juncture" in the depression career to suggest a process that is more fluid than the stage idea.
3. A. Strauss, "Turning points in identity." In C. Clark and H. Robboy (eds.), *Social Interaction* (New York: St. Martin's, 1992). The identity transitions described in the pages to follow bear an instructive resemblance to the idea of biographical "epiphanies" developed by Norman Denzin in a number of important books. See N. Denzin, *The Alcoholic Self* (Newbury Park, Cal.: Sage Publishing Co., 1987); N. Denzin, *Interpretive Interactionism* (Newbury Park, Cal.: Sage Publishing Co., 1989); N. Denzin, *Interpretive Biography* (Newbury Park, Cal.: Sage Publishing Co., 1989).
4. R. Emerson and S. Messinger, "The micropolitics of trouble," *Social Problems* 25 (1977): 121-133. For another formulation of the trouble idea, see the early work of Charlotte Schwartz. Schwartz's doctoral dissertation studied how 30 people who sought help at a university psychiatric service conceptualized their problem. Her interview data suggested that informants distinguished three mutually exclusive subjective states of trouble. She calls them *exigencies of living* (or momentary difficulties), *normal trouble* (ordinary trouble), and *special trouble* (serious problems). An elaboration of these categories can be found in her work entitled *Clients' Perspectives on Psychiatric Troubles in a College Setting* (unpublished doctoral dissertation, Brandeis University, 1976). See also her article with Merton Kahne entitled "The social construction of trouble and its implications for psychiatrists working in college settings," *Journal of the American College Health Asssociation* 25 (February, 1977): 194-197.
5. R. Emerson and S. Messinger, op. cit., p. 122.
6. Ibid.
7. Ibid.
8. P. Berger and H. Kellner, "Marriage and the construction of reality," *Diogenes* 46 (1964): 1-25.
9. D. Vaughan, *Uncoupling: Turning Points in Intimate Relationships* (New York: Oxford, 1986).
10. Social scientists have been critical of the meaning of psychiatric diagnoses and the processes through which they are established. For examples, see P. Brown, "Diagnostic conflict and contradiction in psychiatry," *Journal of Health and Social Behavior* 28 (1987): 37-50

and M. Rosenberg, "A symbolic interactionist view of psychosis," *Journal of Health and Social Behavior* 25 (1984): 289-302.

11. See S. Kaysen, *Girl, Interrupted* (New York: Vintage Books, 1994); N. Mairs, *Plaintext Essays* (Tucson: University of Arizona Press, 1986); L. Shiller, *The Quiet Room* (New York: Warner Books, 1994). Another recent book by Jeffrey Geller and Maxine Harris entitled *Women of the Asylum: Voices from Behind the Walls, 1840-1845* (New York: Doubleday, 1994), offers a broader historical perspective by using a variety of first-person accounts to document the plight of women committed to asylums against their will. For a look at life inside McLean's Hospital in Massachusetts see *Under Observation: Life Inside a Psychiatric Hospital* (New York: Ticknor and Fields, 1994) by Lisa Berger and Alexander Vuckovic. Vuckovic is a physician at the hospital.

Further Reading

Kat Duff. 1993. *The Alchemy of Illness*. New York: Bell Tower.

Erving Goffman. 1961. "The Moral Career of the Mental Patient." *Asylums*. Garden City, NJ: Doubleday Anchor.

Erving Goffman. 1963. *Stigma: Notes on the Management of Spoiled Identity*. Englewood Cliffs, NJ: Prentice-Hall.

Discussion Questions

1. How does Karp's depiction of the depression experience compare with that of physical illness?

2. Why does Karp assert that each stage of the depression assumes and requires redefinitions of self? Do you agree?

3. What does coming to terms with an illness identity entail? What are its implications for future identities?

11

The Body, Identity, and Self: Adapting to Impairment

Kathy Charmaz

This selection traces relationships between body and self. Chronic illness forces new relationships between body and self. A functioning body can no longer be taken for granted. Social and personal identity are concepts that link the relationships between body and self. As Kathy Charmaz points out here, the body is not the same as the self. Thoughts, images, and feelings about one's body may affect the self, and social identifications of the body often shape personal identifications. Presumably healthy people more or less assume bodily functioning and a harmony between body and self—more so when health and fitness bloom, less so when concerns about appearance and appeal flood consciousness. In contrast, that harmony between body and self becomes problematic when people are chronically ill.

This paper draws explicitly upon a symbolic interactionist perspective, which emphasizes the meanings and intentions people construct through their interactions. Prior exposure to language and gesture—social and cultural experience—is crucial in this perspective. Symbolic interactionists assume that people draw upon their experience, including their knowledge of language and gesture, as they interpret their lives and worlds. Because human beings have language, minds, and selves, we can evaluate ourselves as we would any other object in our worlds. In this perspective, we are active agents in creating our actions and in defining ourselves. Look for how the interview participants reevaluate their bodies and themselves as they experience altered bodies.

Chronically ill people, like anyone else, may observe how others view them but refuse to share that view. Here, the social identification is incongruent with the personal identification. Note the conditions under which these interview participants accepted or rejected the social identifications thrust upon them. Surely experiencing bodily feelings such as fatigue or discomfort so great that they cannot be ignored affects how individuals respond to social identifications. In keeping with the emphasis on emergent processes in symbolic interactionism, Charmaz points out that chronically ill people form identity goals in relation to their health as well as to their lives. These goals may shift and change as their experiences change and as they reinterpret their lives.

Serious chronic illness undermines earlier assumptions about bodily functioning, the relation between body and self, and sense of wholeness of body and self (cf. Bury 1982; Brody 1987; Charmaz 1991; 1994a; 1994b; Gadow 1982; Kestenbaum 1982; Monks and Frankenberg n.d.; Murphy 1987). . . .To explicate how the body, identity, and self intersect in illness, I outline *one* mode of living with impairment or loss of bodily function: adapting. By adapting, I mean altering life and self to accommodate to physical losses and to reunify body and self accordingly. Adapting implies that the individual acknowledges impairment and alters life and self in socially and personally acceptable ways. Bodily limits and social circumstances often force adapting to loss. Adapting shades into acceptance. Thus, ill people adapt when they try to accommodate and flow with the experience of illness.

Other ways of living with illness include ignoring it, minimizing it, struggling against it, reconciling self to it, and embracing it (see Charmaz 1991; Radley 1991). Through ignoring and minimizing, ill people may preserve the sense of unity between body and self that they had before illness. But constant struggle against illness makes preserving it much harder. Not only do people fight illness, but also they fight the identifications that come with it. Later, they may reconcile themselves to illness, sometimes for years. Then they tolerate it—within limits. These people acknowledge and attempt working around their illness, but they neither accept it as defining them nor do they accept others' pronouncements of whom they now should be. In contrast, embracing illness means seeking refuge in it.

People with chronic illnesses often experience all these ways of living with impairment at different times. All may be necessary and natural responses to their experience, depending on their situations. After long years of ignoring, minimizing, struggling against, and reconciling themselves to illness, they adapt as they regain a sense of wholeness, of unity of body and self in the face of loss.

Some people never adapt to impairment; others refuse to admit that they have suffered losses (see examples in Albrecht 1992; Herzlich 1973; Radley and Green 1985; 1987; Williams 1981a; 1981b). Still others adapt to their impaired bodies only long after suffering losses. Many people, however, must adapt time and again as they progressively experience failing health, whether they slowly decline or rapidly plummet during acute episodes, crises, or complications. In whatever way people live with impairment, they prefer to have certain future identities over others, although their preferences may be wholly unattainable.

Adapting to an impaired body means resolving the tension between body and self elicited by serious chronic illness. It also means defining integration and wholeness of being while experiencing loss and suffering. These meanings of adapting to an impaired body become implicit criteria for "successful" adaptation with the taken-for-granted proviso that the person also remains as independent and autonomous as possible. Hence, successful adaptation means living with illness without living solely for it. Adapting to physical loss ebbs and flows and repeats itself in similar forms as further episodes, complications, and additional illnesses occur.

Studying adaptation to loss through impairment illuminates tensions within continuing metaphors of opposition:[1] the self versus the body, struggle versus surrender, the idealized body versus the real, experienced body, social identifications versus self-definitions, objective reality versus subjective experience, struggling with versus struggling against illness, invisible disability versus obvious impairment, freedom of bodily movement versus physical constraint and dependence, and bodily control versus loss of function. Though quelled before, these tensions reemerge with each disruptive episode or with deteriorating social conditions.

Adapting to impairment consists of three major stages. First, it depends upon experiencing an altered body that in turn leads to defining impairment or loss and to making reassessments. Whether chronically ill people objectify their bodies and struggle against illness or subjectively integrate their ill bodies with self shapes whether or not they create a sense of wholeness of body and self and of their lives. Bodily appearance affects social identifications and self-definitions and, therefore, how an individual experiences an altered body. Second, assessing one's altered body, appearance to self and others, and the context of life results in changing one's future identity accordingly. Ill people make identity trade-offs, in other words, opting for one identity over another, as they weigh their situations and losses and gains. Even when forced to accept a lesser identity than previously, they often redefine their decisions as positive and find value in their restricted lives. Third, surrendering to the sick body means the end of the quest for control over illness. At this point, people open themselves to experiencing their illness; they define unity of body and self through this experience.

Theoretical Framework

This article takes a symbolic interactionist perspective on identity and draws upon philosopher Sally Gadow's (1982) clarification of the relation between body and self. Personal identity refers to the way an individual defines, locates, and differentiates self from others (see Hewitt 1992). Following Peter Burke (1980), the concept of identity implicitly takes into account the ways people *wish* to define themselves. Wishes are founded on feelings as well as thoughts. If possible, ill people usually try to turn their wishes into intentions, purposes, and actions. Thus, they are motivated to realize future identities, and are sometimes forced to acknowledge present ones. However implicitly, they form identity goals, i. e. *preferred identities* that people assume, desire, hope, or plan for (Charmaz 1987). The concept of identity goals assumes that human beings create meanings and act purposefully as they interpret their experience and interact within the world. Some people's identity goals are implicit, unstated, and understood; other people have explicit preferred identities. Like other categories of people, some individuals with chronic illnesses assume that they will realize their preferred identities; others keep a watchful eye on their future selves and emerging identities as they experience the present (see also, Radley and Green 1987).

Gadow (1982) assumes that human existence essentially means embodiment and that the self is inseparable from the body. . . .Yet, as Gadow points out, body and self, although inseparable, are not identical. The relation between body and self becomes particularly problematic for those chronically ill people who realize that they have suffered lasting bodily losses. . . .They risk becoming socially identified and self-defined exclusively by their impaired bodies (Bury 1988; Goffman 1963; Locker 1983; MacDonald 1988). Thus, chronically ill people who move beyond loss and transcend stigmatizing negative labels define themselves as much more than their bodies and as much more than an illness (Charmaz 1991).

Gadow argues that illness and aging result in loss of the original unity of body and self and provide the means of recovering it at a new level. She assumes that an original unity existed and implies that loss and recovery of unity is a single process. However, what unity means can only be defined subjectively. Some people may not have defined themselves as having experienced such unity before illness, or as only having partially experienced it. Further, with each new and often unsuspected bodily impairment, people with chronic illnesses *repeatedly* experience loss of whatever unity between body and self they had previously defined or accepted. Thus, at each point when they suffer and define loss, identity questions and identity changes can emerge or reoccur. Throughout this article, I deal with the loss of body-self unity and its recovery through acknowledging bodily experience and opening oneself to the quest for harmony between body and self.

In order to understand how loss and recovery of body-self unity occurs, we must understand ill people's meanings of their bodily experiences and the social contexts in which they occur (Fabrega and Manning 1972; Gerhardt 1979; Radley and Green 1987; Zola 1991). Such meanings arise in dialectical relation to their biographies (Bury 1982; 1988; 1991; Corbin and Strauss 1987; 1988; Dingwall 1976; Gerhardt 1989; Radley 1989; Radley and Green 1987; Williams 1984) and are mediated by their interpretations of ongoing experiences. Present meanings of the ill body and self develop from, but are not determined by, past discourses of meaning and present social identifications (Blumer 1969; Goffman 1963; Mead 1934).

As chronic illness encroaches upon life, people learn that it erodes their taken-for-granted preferred identities as well as their health. Further, they may discover that visible illness and disability can leave them with a master status and overriding stigmatized identity. Because of their physical losses, they reassess who they are and who they can become. Subsequently, they form identity goals as they try to reconstruct normal lives to whatever extent possible (Charmaz 1987; 1991). Frequently, people with chronic illnesses initially plan and expect to resume their lives unaffected by illness, or even to exceed their prior identity goals. As they test their bodies and themselves, ill people need to make identity trade-offs at certain points, or even to lower their identity goals systematically until they match their lessened capacities. At other times, they may gradually raise their hopes and progressively increase their identity goals when they meet with success. Therefore, both raised or lowered identity goals form an implicit identity hierarchy that ill people create as they adapt to bodily loss and change (Charmaz 1987)[2].

Experiencing an Altered Body

Experiencing an altered body means that people with illnesses note physical changes and diminished bodily functions (cf. Charmaz 1991; Kahane 1990; Kelly 1992; Yoshida 1993). Thus, experiencing an altered body means more than having or acquiring one. It means that these people begin to *define* bodily changes or the illness itself as real (if already diagnosed) and to account for how changes and symptoms affect daily life.[3] Distressing bodily sensations and impaired functions as well as disquieting feelings about body and self give rise to defining bodily changes. The unity of prior embodied experience has been shaken; assumptions about body and self have been jolted (see also, Olesen et al. 1990). At this point, people with illnesses compare their present body with their past body; they assess the differences between then and now, and they measure the costs and risks of ordinary activities. Before becoming ill, most people took their bodies for granted as functioning instruments or vehicles subjugated to the self. This taken-for-granted instrument becomes the yardstick against which they compare their altered bodies. A forty-one-year-old woman who had asthma described the bodily changes she experienced within the last year:

I really couldn't go for a walk, um, the way I used to, so I felt like my body had betrayed me. By that time I had, even though I hadn't really been diagnosed, I . . . knew that things that I used to do easily without any strain at all were a challenge. And so I was real aware of it. And also, probably at that time, I'd probably been running a low-grade fever for a long-time, and I knew it. . . . So I mostly felt like my body was sort of foreign territory—it was not the body that I knew.

Like others, this woman experienced her body as more than altered—she felt it was alien. Thus, she experienced a radical disruption of body and self. Experiencing this bodily alienation leads people to rethinking explicitly their previously held notions of body and self. This woman and several men with respiratory disease found that rapid weight gain accompanied plummeting physical activity. Mirror images of the body further call into question a previously taken-for-granted self. She said, "So I'm heavy—I'm heavy in a way I've never been before." Experiencing multiple bodily losses in a short period intensifies feelings of estrangement, of separation from one's past familiar body, and of loss of self. The body once viewed as a taken-for-granted possession to control and master has spun out of control. At best, the body is now a failed machine, an obstacle to be repaired, overcome, or mastered. At worst, it has become a deadly enemy or oppressor (cf. Charmaz 1980; 1994b; Gadow 1982; Herzlich 1973; Herzlich and Pierret 1984; Williams 1981a; 1981b).

When wholly unanticipated, even middle-aged people may view their bodily changes with a sense of betrayal. They may describe their past bodies as "invincible," "indestructible," and "immortal" and express regret and anger about their losses. In turn, their anger and regret intensify when ill people feel that their illnesses control them. They have lost control of their body as an object they assumed they could master. Moreover, they view themselves as overtaken by an alien force. The woman mentioned above stated:

It has probably slowed me down, and I'm very aware that I have this and if I really want to be as healthy as I can be, it's—it will control where I live; it will control what kind of work I do; it will control who I can be around—I can't be around someone who insists on wearing perfume; I can't be around anyone who smokes anything at all; I can't be around people who insist on having . . . certain kinds of chemicals.

Perhaps more destructive than the anger is the guilt and shame followed by self-abasement that ill people with failing bodies experience: guilt because they share cultural standards of ageless bodily perfection and correct appearance (cf. Glassner 1988); shame because their very existence testifies to a failure to meet these standards. Self-abasement follows and intensifies the humiliation. Robert F. Murphy (1987, p. 111) observes:

In my middle age, I had become a changeling, the lot of all disabled people. They are afflicted with a malady of the body that is translated into a cancer within the self and a disease of social relationships. They have experienced a transformation of the essential condition of their being in the world. They have become aliens, even exiles in their own lands.

For a time, people with chronic illnesses may make firm separations between their impaired bodies and their self-concepts (cf. Charmaz 1991; Register 1987; Weitz 1991). That way they can keep their illness separate from themselves and their lives. The extent to which they keep it separate and their stance about doing so is crucial. By keeping illness separate, they allay disquieting feelings about themselves and their bodies.

Struggling against illness differs from struggling with it. When people struggle *against* illness, they view their illness as the enemy with whom they must battle (cf. Charmaz 1980; 1994b). They hope to regain their past identities and to restore a now missing sense of self. Usually at this point, they can neither face nor accept more restricted lives and lesser identities than what they had before illness.

When people struggle *with* illness, they struggle to keep their bodies functioning and therefore, their lives "normal" to whatever extent possible. Hence, they do not give up. In struggling against and with illness, they try to take control over their illnesses and their bodies. Gregg Charles Fisher (1987, p. 13) describes how he and his wife struggled with chronic fatigue syndrome, implying that they learned to differentiate between body and self, despite their struggles: "Through the long years of this illness, we have had to struggle every day to cope with our affliction. As the years go by, we are more determined than ever to remain strong. The saying that time heals all wounds is true, not because wounds, like sand castles, wash away with the first tide but because in time you learn to survive your wounds."

Through struggling with illness, these people eventually integrate new bodily facts into their lives and their self-concepts (cf. Charmaz 1991; Corbin and Strauss 1987). But until they define the changes as chronic and experience their effects daily, ill people look for recovery and can keep illness and therefore their bodies at the margins of their self-concepts (Charmaz 1991; 1994a). Subsequently, they continue to objectify their bodies and distance themselves from them.[4] Not only do their bodies become objects to mend but they are also worksites in which to do it. The situation differs for people who have already struggled with bodily oddities or "psychological" quirks now redefined and legitimated as bona fide physical symptoms. Their initial diagnostic relief turns into the sobering experience of adopting their medical label and of defining what it means to them. As they do so, they may make the label their own while simultaneously objectifying their symptoms that fit the diagnostic label. The writer Nancy Mairs (1989, pp. 234-235) redefines herself and her body as a woman with multiple sclerosis but also objectifies her body:

> Now I am who I will be. A body in trouble. I've spent all these years trying alternately to repudiate and to control my wayward body, to transcend it one way or another, but MS [multiple sclerosis] rams me right back down into it. "The body," I've gotten into the habit of calling it. "The left leg is weak," I say. "There's a blurred spot in the right eye." As though it were some other entity, remote and traitorous. Or worse, as though it were inanimate, a prison of bone, the dark tower around which Childe Roland rode, withershins left, withershins right, seeking to free the fair kidnapped princess: me.

The horror of the unknown—disability and death—prompts the distancing inherent in objectification. Distancing continues as long as the person assumes that mastering his or her wayward body is necessary to make it acceptable. Relinquishing notions of mastering one's body, in contrast, allows a receptivity to bodily experience. Arthur Frank (1991, pp. 60-61) reveals the moment when he shifted from objectifying his body to embracing it as subject: "I wondered at what the body could still do for me, as diseased as I knew it must be. That day I stopped resenting 'it' for the pain I had felt and began to appreciate my body, in some ways for the first time in my life. I stopped evaluating my body and began to draw strength from it. And I recognized that this body was me."

As ill people objectify their bodies less, they are more open to attending to the cues their bodies provide. They learn how to protect their bodies and therefore are able to extend their control over their lives. For example, a woman with lupus erythematosus learned that she could work at home while she was sick. At home, she could control the temperature, light, seating, and interruptions, as well as the pacing of her tasks. When she worked at her clients' offices, she could control little of that. She said:

> But see, I've always gone to the client's place to do the work and now, when I don't feel good, I'm finding that it's much easier to do it here at the house. And then I can just do—I can just do it at night; I can do it early in the morning. Yeah it's too hard to go and sit—sometimes the chairs they make me sit on or the—and it's too cold or it's too hot, or it's just real hard. I don't have the patience I used to have. I lost that. I used to have a lot of patience; I could bear anything. I don't think I was even aware of it. But now my body tells me. I can't control my body.

Before her illness, this woman had ignored bodily discomfort. At that time, she had committed herself, not only to a demanding work and social life but also to a rigorous fitness routine. She had pushed her body to be slim, strong, and taut, as she put it, "like a jungle tiger." She had internalized and met the prevailing standards for appearance. But as she learned to listen to her body, she had to abandon those standards. Uncontainable sickness forced adopting other priorities for her body. Like this woman, other people cease to measure their body against past perfection, or past hopes of perfecting it, and begin to live with it. The sick body becomes familiar and perhaps even comfortable. This familiarity and comfort increases if treatments, regimens, or health practices seem to work. If so, the sick body becomes predictable and manageable. The ill person may feel that he or she is beginning to unify the altered body and the self. Arthur Frank (1991, p. 87) identifies this unity of body and self, "As soon as cancer happened to me, not just to anyone, it ceased

to be random. I am a bodily process, but I am also a consciousness, with a will and a history and a capacity to focus my thoughts and energies. The bodily process and the consciousness do not oppose each other; what illness teaches is their unity."

Typically, however, this unity has limits, albeit unstated, taken-for-granted limits. Ill people often believe that they have already suffered beyond tolerable limits. Thus, they see themselves as having filled their quota of human misery and earned their right to a just reprieve. They often said, "I've paid my dues [of suffering]." If so, then new, foreboding symptoms or conditions shock them. Moreover, these people experience the unpredictability of their bodies afresh as they grapple with new or intensified distress. Their uncertain lives and their frail grasp on health again takes center stage. For the past year, a middle-aged woman with multiple sclerosis had fought constant, debilitating infections. She said:

> My body is distressed, and it needs attention, and I'm working very hard to give it that . . . I really feel with MS, I have a much better hold on it, handle on the MS, much better visualization where I'll be in—what I'll do with it in five years, ten years, because I can adapt as I go along. The problem with infections is that infections going on with MS can alter the disease severely in a negative way, and so I want to get more of a handle on the infections.

After being diagnosed and experiencing her condition for over fourteen years, having multiple sclerosis with some residual disability had become familiar and manageable. This woman had had several extremely debilitating exacerbations but after each one had improved considerably. For lengthy periods, she struggled with keeping her illness contained by maintaining and protecting her body (cf. Charmaz 1991; Monks and Frankenberg, n.d.). Although she always acknowledged that her MS could take a downhill course at any time, she expected to have ups and downs. The belief that she had faced the worst before and improved, gave her hope and caused her to view her MS as predictable and manageable. The infections, however, posed grave uncertainty. She said, "The aging with the MS really doesn't bother me. Aging with chronic infections—the infections can just screw up your body in so many ways, and so I'm more frightened by that because it's unknown."

The unknowns of the past echo in the uncertainties of the present. Ten years before, this woman's MS symptoms had rapidly worsened. She had said then, "I'm just so frightened . . . by the unknowns. If I knew that this was the worst, I could deal with that. But not knowing . . . My legs are getting weaker and I'm so frightened because of the unknowns. My doctor says I may have to go into a wheelchair. That's my bottom line. I won't go into a chair."

Coping With Changes in Bodily Appearance

Having a visibly altered body provides the experiencing person, as well as family and friends, with immediate images of change. Such changes occur throughout the course of illness. I use the term "appearance" symbolically as well as literally since knowledge of loss can cast new light and force new self-images upon an individual. But not all people with serious chronic illnesses have visible symptoms and disabilities. Looking healthy can undermine a person's credibility with health practitioners. Women particularly have difficulty being taken seriously. One woman who had a recent angioplasty, angina, an old spinal injury, and bowel disease was told by two of her physicians and her pharmacist, "You don't look like you're old enough to have anything like that happen. You don't look like there could be anything wrong." Even those closest to ill people may not understand their conditions and so expect them to function as before. A middle-aged man had an automobile accident while having a heart attack. Although he sustained some injuries, afterwards, he looked healthy and fit. He lost weight, exercised, and his injuries slowly healed. Yet he had residual fatigue, occasional memory loss, emotional swings, and lethargy from his multiple medications. Because he seemed to have regained health, his losses remained masked. Subsequently, his wife lost patience with him as his business declined and he withdrew from the family. She saw him as shirking responsibility.

Relatives and friends may not be able to fathom debilitating changes in a person who shortly before had functioned with extraordinary competence. Youth and beauty render an invisible illness even more invisible. While in her early thirties, a woman's youth disguised her debilitating arthritis. Her much older boyfriend saw her as healthy and beautiful. For years, her constant complaints of pain mystified him. She could not enforce her identity claims as ill as long as she appeared healthy, pretty, and able. Because of her appearance, both her private and public identities belied how she defined her self. She said:

> I may look like I'm healthy and all this stuff and I get—all these guys start making catcalls and I'm in pain and it just seems incongruous. I go, "What are they whistling at?" I usually identify with how I *feel*, even though I go through a lot of effort to make myself look good, I still identify with how I feel. It's like being—feeling like an old person in a young person . . . It's like only an old person is entitled to have all this pain.

By four years later, this woman's disabilities had become apparent. Although she had long identified herself as in pain and disabled, she also had been accustomed to other people noting only her beauty. Being socially identified as disabled undermined her self-worth and sense of wholeness. She said:

> I think it's real embarrassing. You know, like say if someone can see that I can't walk or something, I'm all stooped over, you know, I catch a glimpse of myself in ah, like a window, it's very shocking sometimes what I see. [I asked, "In which way?" She said:] Well, I can see that, other people can see is that, you know, my leg, I can hardly walk on it. And I feel like somehow I'm not a whole person and . . . people can look at it and feel sympathetic, but they can look at you and see you as less than whole, you know. (Charmaz 1991, p. 111)

She added, "Somehow it's almost like a defect to me. And. . . , it's frightening, I guess." Five years later her disability was quite marked. Because she questioned whether she still was attractive to men, she had several affairs, which she regretted.

Ill people may evince few problems about impairment or loss of function until a hidden loss becomes visible. For example, impotency can be a problem known only to a man's wife unless the marriage dissolves. The tension between invisible disability and visible impairment becomes evident. Lesley Fallowfield and Andrew Clark (1991, p. 66) show how some British women with mastectomies rejected their altered bodies when their breast amputation was visible:

Interviewer: Can you tell me how you felt about your appearance since your operation?
Patient: Mm, that depends—I think I look OK when I'm wearing my false one, don't you? I don't think anyone could tell.
Interviewer: And without your clothes?
Patient: That's rather different—I tend not to look at myself—it upsets me that I don't look like a woman anymore.
Interviewer: What about when you're with your husband?
Patient: Oh, I don't let him see me, oh no. I couldn't. He'd be horrified. I always undress in the bathroom now.

Like the woman above, other ill people tried to reduce the effects of visible disability on their pursuits and relationships. And like her, they could then reduce the effects of it on themselves and their social identities. One man on kidney dialysis always wore long sleeves and usually a jacket to hide his dialysis shunt. Feelings about visible disability influenced both men's and women's identity goals. When men could not hide or minimize their changed appearance, they often withdrew. Hence, their identity goals plummeted. Women withdrew less but dwelt upon appearance issues in the interviews much more than men. They tried to manage their appearance to handle their feelings and to bolster their confidence. Nancy Dyson, who had a mastectomy, said:

Wearing bright colors and makeup and pulling myself together before I go out is

a way of protecting my vulnerability so people don't make assumptions. It's like camouflage. It's sort of like the camouflage is the door and I can open it or not. It is another way of having control over my disease. I choose whom I share my vulnerability with. (Donnally 1991, p. D5)

Women under fifty evinced much concern about the effects of illness on their appearance. I asked a forty-one-year-old woman with lupus erythematosus if her thoughts about her appearance had changed at all in the last five years. She replied with fervor:

I hate my body; I hate my body. Mostly because I've gained so much weight and—and then my face breaks out [lupus has a characteristic rash]. People look at you like something's wrong [with your character]. I don't hate it because it's sick; I hate it because it's ugly. . . .You're supposed to be skinny and pretty."

When changes in appearance are sudden and visible, women may define those changes as tests of their love relationships. A forty-two-year-old woman suffered a devastating reoccurrence of mixed connective tissue disease when she was pregnant three years ago. She had not had such a serious episode for eighteen years, long before she had met her husband. During that previous episode, her boyfriend had left her and her parents had ignored her. She described herself and her concerns during this second flare-up:

Oh, I was just a disheveled lump, I mean I was a disheveled lump. I'm sort of still a disheveled lump. . . . But it doesn't much matter to me [now]. . . . [T]his was a little bit of a test of me with Bob [husband]. It's like, "Here's the worst I can possibly be," you know; "I'm sick; I'm vomiting; I look like crap." And then I gained so much weight, so it's like, "Here's the worst I can be. Are you going to leave me now?" you know. "Are you going leave now? When are you going to leave? Are you going to leave next week?"

Changing Identity Goals

Bodily Changes and Identity Goals

Bodily changes prompt changing identity goals. Upward changes allow ill people to entertain possibilities and try new ventures. A successful transplant, cardiac rehabilitation program, or medical regimen means feeling better and more able. Then people reentered the worlds they left or embarked on new pursuits. They readily moved on with their lives when they had alternatives and when their identity goals throughout illness had assumed moving beyond it. Thus, these people returned to work, or if working, increased their work hours, pursued sports and hobbies, and planned to redirect their lives. Men returned to their careers. A few women started new businesses. Several men and women went back to school.

Bodily changes, including noticeable improvement, do not automatically result in changed identity goals. Emotions and social relationships influence choices and actions. When fear of failure or further sickness permeates ill people's thoughts, they proceed slowly in forming or changing their identity goals. A young married woman who had had cancer feared a recurrence. She resisted investing herself in a valued pursuit because she could not tolerate the possibility of losing it. Her husband's income allowed her to experiment with college courses and low-paying, part-time jobs. Relying solely on self led some people to measure their options, situations, and bodies carefully when they prized their autonomy. These people could not risk becoming immobilized. Paradoxically, they risked becoming social captives of their sick bodies.[5] Under these conditions, people made changes very slowly and avoided taking risks. They often needed substantial encouragement to reach for more challenging identity goals. After spells of sickness, they had difficulty imagining themselves going beyond their current situations. For example, a woman who had lupus erythematosus had wanted just to be able to work enough to remain self-supporting. Her appalling encounters with eligibility workers and social service employees resulted in her avowals never to depend on public assistance. She recounted:

I didn't think—didn't have any wide horizons. My friend Ken, he told me last year, "Bonnie, I just can see you managing a business, right?" I said, "Oh, give me a break," you know. And he even probably said it to me in February. "You know, Bonnie, you ought to open an office and blah, blah, blah." I said, "Don't even talk about it; I'm not interested in it." But it just happened. One day I had too much work and I said, "Wait a minute." So I got up, called the *Times* [local paper] and as I was walking away from the phone, I went, "What did I do?" That's the way it all happened. And my friends gave me [money] to get started in my business.

In contrast, a downward spiral, or sudden serious episode can force lowering identity goals. Ill people must either adapt because they cannot handle the lives they had—even in the recent past—or they realize that they now have a tenuous hold on managing their lives. How do they do it? What social context affects their choices?

Certainly, markedly altered bodily functioning and feeling can undermine present identities or force lowering identity goals (see, for example, Albrecht 1992; Dahlberg and Jaffe 1977; Pitzele 1985; Plough 1986). People with chronic illnesses resist lowering their goals if they believe others need them to function as before. They put their bodies and their lives at risk when they view their identity losses as too great or when they remain unaware of the extent of their physical losses. For example, several heart patients abandoned their diets and regimens after a few months because they no longer felt sick. In addition, people who recognize but cannot account for their reduced capacities tenaciously try to function. One middle-aged woman said, "It was scary at times. I didn't know what was wrong. [I was] not feeling well, and always having to push, push, push. Always behind the eight ball, always tired, always pushing against this wall of fatigue. And trying to keep up, you know."

The Social Context of Changing Identity Goals

Identities bring commitments and responsibilities. In turn, how individuals define these commitments and responsibilities in relation to other people deeply affects their identity decisions. Changing identity goals then takes into account (1) the individual's definitions, (2) significant others' views and wishes, and (3) the interactions and negotiations among them. Once chronically ill people have altered their lives to accommodate to limited identity goals, it takes substantial support to move beyond them. Given their definitions, ill people may only relinquish their identities and their accompanying identity goals when forced to do so. They may develop intricate strategies to preserve their identity goals. For years after having been immobilized by illness, a single woman had balanced her work productivity with her energy limits. When necessary, she simply took time off from work to avoid a full-blown exacerbation or to regain her energy. By carefully monitoring and maintaining her body, she could realize her overriding identity goal of remaining independent. But keeping bodily needs and identity goals in balance can prove to be arduous. Now married, this woman has two young children as well as farm animals to care for in addition to a part-time university teaching job seventy miles away. Her identities as mother, wife, and teacher supersede any illness identity and cause her to persevere beyond her bodily limits. Her children need her; she and her husband committed themselves to not using child care. The family's need for her income also tugs at her, especially since her husband lost his main job. Thus, by realizing her identities, she risks being forced to relinquish them. She compared how she handled illness when she was single with her current situation, "Going through that whole period in my life when I was real sick, I got very used to just listening to my body and how it's feeling and totally going how—by how I was feeling from day to day. And I can't really, I can't always do that now. There's sometimes when I have to push it much more than I would have before."

Before her marriage, this woman was a successful independent entrepreneur. Her autonomy combined with her control over employees' work assignments permitted her to take time-outs from work to nurture her body. More frequently, middle-class and professional men, not women, can fit their work around their bodily needs. When they can control the social context of work, they can realize and further their identity goals concerning it.

A major part of the social context revolves around spouses or partners. In long-term marriages among older couples, loyalty and attachment typically remain unquestioned although spouses may have sharp differences about health monitoring (Johnson 1985). Wives of all ages willingly saw their husbands through crises, even when marriages were shaky. Problems generally arose later as the long-term effects of illness emerged. In contrast, support from husbands and boyfriends of middle-aged and younger women was more tentative throughout illness. These men did not take over tasks as readily as wives did, and they abandoned their relationships emotionally, if not completely, more quickly than women. Women with illnesses sometimes relied on adult children, friends, and healthcare workers for emotional support and practical assistance.

Multiple crises and disabilities that cut into pivotal roles (e.g. breadwinner, sex partner) undermined middle-aged and younger spouses' support. Previously conflicted marriages may break at this point. Subsequently, taken-for-granted identities as companion and parent may also dissolve. Conflicts about identity goals may develop in strong relationships. The type of identity goal and rate and intensity with which the sick person pursues it can all become points of contention (see also Peyrot, McMurry, and Hedges 1988; Speedling 1982). A woman with multiple sclerosis wants to do volunteer work in a busy hospital; her husband feels her body cannot handle the stress. A man with heart disease waits for his health to improve; his wife believes that he is becoming an invalid and should go back to work.

Certainly age, gender, work, and marital status shape, but do not determine, the context in which chronically ill adults change identity goals. As Alan Radley (1989) states, what people with chronic illnesses adjust *with* is as important as what they adjust *to*. Their ways of changing identity goals and adapting to the changes also reflect the content of their lives and the meanings they attribute to their ongoing interactions. Money and help make an enormous difference as to how, when, and why people will or will not lower their identity goals. Single mothers often sacrificed their health for sustaining their identities as workers and parents. Money and help also affect how people feel about changing identity goals (see, for example, Albrecht 1992). Possessing sufficient funds allows older men and women to retire early, a socially acceptable disengagement for the affluent. Having financially secure spouses permits others to leave their jobs or to reduce their work hours. In short, money and help allow ill people more choices about which identity trade-offs to make and when to make them.

The social context of changing identity goals may itself change. The designated "patient," financial resources, and potential help may change and thus result in shifting identity goals. For example, one older woman with a mild heart condition felt forced to seek employment when her husband's health declined (after two heart attacks and bypass surgery) and he lost his job (and his pension) three years before his expected retirement. Two years later, however, she suffered a small stroke. Though she had little lasting impairment, she took the stroke as a warning that she had been under too much pressure. She then became the designated patient in the family. Fortuitously, her husband had become re-employed and could again support them. The move of an adult daughter back into their area also meant help with household tasks and errands. Subsequently, this woman relinquished her identity goal of being fully employed.

Identity Goals and Identity Trade-offs

Identity goals emerge and change through mediation of subjective and social meanings. Hence, ill people sacrifice some identities in favor of retaining others. Noted anthropologist Robert F. Murphy (1987) suffered from a progressive paralysis. He did not endure the professional and financial devastation common to many adults with disabilities because he could continue to work in a field in which he had already established himself. Nonetheless, he felt pressured to remain a productive scholar to validate his worth and to command his colleagues' respect. He writes about returning to teaching in a wheelchair:

My overreach beyond the limits of my body was a way of telling the academic world that I was still alive and doing what I always did. And all my feverish activities in both academia and my community were shouts to the world: "Hey it's the same old me inside this body!" These were ways of protecting the identity, for preserving that inner sense of who one is that is an individual's anchor in a transient world. (p. 81)

Feeling devalued results in weighing interactional costs and in balancing necessities against possible identity trade-offs. To the extent that these identity issues are direct and explicit, people will construct explicit identity goals. Murphy's interactions formed an unspoken yet unyielding mirror that reflected the renegotiation of his preferred identities. Because Murphy's strained interactions with acquaintances at work reduced his self-worth, he avoided meetings and receptions. He knew that he could not conduct field research so he became a textbook author. He preserved his sense of self by choosing his activities carefully and by making identity trade-offs. Murphy viewed textbook authorship as a lesser identity than ethnographer but also saw himself as "too old" for ethnographic forays, which mitigated his identity trade-off. As people shift their identity goals laterally or downward, they may relinquish what others view as the more socially valued identity. They feel their losses. They think about their lives. They assess the costs and benefits of relinquishing activities and responsibilities and, therefore, identities. When costs to their bodies and intimate relationships exceed relative gains, they give up valued identities. A middle-aged woman related:

I'd come home and I was in such pain— you have to work [on the job] seven hours but you put in eight or nine. It's very stressful. But I never succumbed to stress but once or twice. It was doable because I only worked three days a week . . . But Alan [husband] would come home and I'd be on the couch in such pain I couldn't get off, too tired to fix dinner and he was just wonderful. He'd call at work, "Well, what should I bring home tonight?" And some nights I'd cook, but not many. And so I decided, this isn't a way to live. I don't have to work . . . So it was with great regret, and not something I planned, I turned in my resignation. It's the best thing I ever did.

Concurrence from others strengthens the person's belief in having made the right choice. The woman above agreed with former associates' appraisals of her appearance. She recalled, "I went to a wine tasting that we put on a couple weeks ago . . . and some of the Board members were saying, 'Gee, you look so much better. You were all bent over; you looked terrible.' I did look awful. I need more rest; you have to pace yourself."

After making identity trade-offs, people often try to redefine their identity choices in positive ways. Similar to other kinds of decision making, they want to view their choices as sound. At this crucial point, the tension becomes apparent between acknowledging bodily limits and needs and constructing a preferred identity for those who must make significant changes of activity and direction in their lives. In order to handle their lives, they must integrate self and illness without having it consume their self-concepts. Thus, like the woman above, they may, in effect, view identity loss as identity gain. In essence then, people can move up their identity hierarchy while they move down their bodily hierarchy.

By this time, these ill people account and care for their altered bodies while viewing themselves as residing in their bodies but not as wholly defined by them. Part of redefining personal identity depends upon seeing one's self as more than one's body and the illness within it (Charmaz 1991). The woman above defined the place of illness in relation to identity:

Fibromyalgia does not define who Ellen Thomasen is. It's baggage I've got to carry along. We've all got baggage. Some of it's light and some of it's heavy. And we'd like to check it in a locker awhile. And sometimes you can do that and sometimes you can't but it's not going to stop me from going on a trip. That's the way I feel.

Simultaneously, she recognized her limitations and her need to care for her body while creating her life and facing an uncertain future. She said, "I wonder if I'm going to be able to be active with my grandchildren . . . I'm wondering—we don't know what the symptoms are going to do, you know. I plan to fight as long as I can. And by fighting—it's an attitudinal thing—it's also resting and doing the things you need to do. I don't—I've always been so active that I don't like this at all. But it's doable, you know?"

Finding the balance between struggling with illness and relinquishing identity goals permits ill people to construct valued lives. A woman with multiple sclerosis once felt deep regrets about lost chances and dashed hopes. She feared then "that having MS will affect my life in a negative way," as well as affect her husband and children seriously. Although ten years later she had relinquished some earlier dreams, she had also realized several, including traveling, which she had expected to forego. Deeply imbedded in her family life, she could now say, "I'm comfortable with who I am, where I am."

Surrendering to the Sick Body

Surrendering means to stop pushing bodily limits, to stop fighting the episode or the entire illness. The quest for control over illness ceases and the flow with the bodily experience increases. Surrender means awareness of one's ill body and a willingness and relief to flow with it (cf. Denzin 1987a; 1987b). A person ceases to struggle against illness and against a failing body at least at this specific time. Through surrendering, the person anchors bodily feelings in self. No longer does he or she ignore, gloss over, or deny these feelings and view the ill body as apart from self.

Conditions for surrender to occur include (1) relinquishing the quest for control over one's body, (2) giving up notions of victory over illness, (3) affirming, however implicitly, that one's self is tied to the sick body. Ill people may surrender and flow with the experience in the present but hope for improvement in the future. Yet they are unlikely to entertain false hopes. At this point, the person views illness as integral to subjective experience and as integrated with self (see also Le-Maistre 1985; Monks and Frankenberg n.d.).

Surrendering differs from being overtaken by illness, resigning oneself to it, or giving up (cf. Charmaz 1991; Radley and Green 1987). Being overtaken occurs without choice; surrendering is an active, intentional process. However silently and tacitly, ill people agree to surrender. When surrender is complete, the person experiences a new unity between body and self. Mark Kidel (1988, p. 18) advocates "reclaiming our illnesses as expressions of our own being," to gain authenticity. Like Arthur Frank (1991, p. 1), who views illness as "an opportunity but a dangerous one," Kidel also recognizes that doing so risks opening "ourselves to the full and unpredictable impact of the unknown" (p. 19). Hence, ill people define their experience as newly authentic when they realize that having an ill body is part of them and they allow themselves to experience it. They also may define their past ways of relating to illness as inauthentic. Several people echoed this man's view, "I was just a phony, pretending I didn't have it [kidney failure], trying to do everything everyone else did when my body was telling me I couldn't."

Surrendering also can be distinguished from becoming resigned and losing hope. Becoming resigned means yielding to illness, acquiescing to its force, or to the devalued identities attributed to it. Such resignation means accepting defeat after struggling against illness. When people give up, they lose hope and crumble inward. Passivity, depression, and debility follow. They are overtaken by illness. Under these conditions, people with chronic illnesses can become much more disabled than their physical conditions warrant. They lose interest in their regimens and, perhaps, in living. As they give up, they give in to fear and despair. In contrast, surrender means permitting oneself to let go rather than being overtaken by illness and despair.

Resisting surrender means holding on and, with advanced illness, refusing to die. Fear may propel critically ill people. When they struggle against illness and try to impose order upon it and their lives, they are unlikely to surrender during the midst of crisis. But

later, learning to live with residual disability can teach them about surrender. As Arnold Beisser (1988) acknowledges, he learned about surrender through facing defeat. Like many other men, Beisser had earlier believed, then later hoped, that his sustained effort would force change to occur and victory to prevail. Yet no amount of effort changed the fact of his disability. Beisser (1988, pp. 169-170) reflects:

> Defeated on all fronts, I had to learn how to surrender and accept what I had become, what I did not want to be.
> Learning to surrender and accept what I had not chosen gave me knowledge of a new kind of change and a new kind of experience which I had not anticipated. It was a paradoxical change.
> When I stopped struggling, working to change, and found means of accepting what I had already become, I discovered that that changed me. Rather than feeling disabled and inadequate as I anticipated that I would, I felt whole again. I experienced a sense of well-being and a fullness I had not known before. I felt at one not only with myself but with the universe.
> This was not the change that had been wrought by struggle, work and effort, but by learning not to struggle, how to give in, to stand aside and let truth emerge. It was not the tragic truth I expected at all.

For Beisser, surrender meant stripping away the fantasy of recovery, the wish for recovering former wholeness. Still, surrender allowed for being in the flow of the moment rather than wishing and waiting for a mythical future. No longer could pressing symptoms, marked disability, and progressive illness be ignored or redefined. When surrendering, illness merges with subjectivity; it *becomes* subjectivity. Surrendering to illness opens the possibility of transforming the self. By reentering the present anew and flowing with it, ill people gain fresh views of themselves and their situations. External social mandates melt away as the person gains voice from within. Subsequently, a new sense of wholeness of self can emerge.

When an individual is very sick, surrender permits unity with the diseased body. Fighting illness at this point may amount to fighting *against* oneself instead of *for* oneself. One woman struggled against Hodgkin's disease for twelve years; she resisted being constrained and defined by her illness. During her last hospitalization for a bone transplant, her last hope of recovery, she realized that her body could handle no more. At that point, she relinquished her struggle and surrendered to illness and death. How do people know when to surrender and to what to surrender? When overtaken by illness, the woman who resisted relinquishing her responsibilities said of surrendering:

> It means that I don't have—I can't control it [ill body] and [it means] to look at what it has to teach me. Just . . . let it tell me what it needs to tell me. You know, that willingness and that acceptance. . . . So it didn't come instantly, but I was willing to surrender and to look at what was going on. But it did come; it did happen. And I'm always much more at peace after I'm able to do that anyway.

Fighting for her meant fighting for control over an unwilling body. Surrender allowed her to find new integration of body and self. She disclosed, "I become more when I surrender, I mean I become more; my spirit's able to grow. And it can't do that if I'm holding on to control."

In this sense, by freeing the self from a quest for control, it becomes possible to experience the moment and to allow the boundaries of self to flow and to expand. Yet self also anchors the person to continuity with past, present, and future. And that anchor itself becomes problematic while surrendering to sickness. Another woman reflected upon this problematic relationship between body and self:

> To me it's [immersion in illness] sort of moving toward spiritual states where you do lose a sense of self and time as a release. I mean, self is a kind of bondage in a way—so it's wonderful—you move toward heaven—to not have that burden. But the other thing, of course, is that we are here. I exist as Jane so Jane comes back and wants to exist. So that's the hellish side. (Charmaz 1991, p. 104)

Conclusion

The process of adapting outlined above offers a window on unity between body and self in illness. Illness presents the possibility of developing new and deeper meanings of the relation between body and self. Such possibilities remain more hidden and implicit in ordinary adult life. But as ill people go through and emerge from crises, complications, and flare-ups, they also reenter mundane adult worlds. Meanings gained through experiencing surrender may fade and recede into the past. Yet these meanings and their accompanying feelings may be reawakened and remembered when illness progresses and health again fails.

Appearance issues affect women more heavily than men. However, compared to men, women show greater resilience in the face of illness and greater ability to adapt and flow with the experience of illness. Men more often than women take an all-or-nothing approach to identity goals. They place a higher stake in recapturing the past and with it, their past identities (cf. Charmaz 1994b). If they cannot reclaim all of their past identities, they drop the struggle. Failing to achieve their preferred identities becomes tantamount to complete failure. Under these conditions, such men give up.

How might adapting affect those whose lives are intertwined with an ill person? Whether they welcome adapting or define it as defeat depends on their views and interests. Adapting can cause havoc in the lives of people who depend on the ill person and who cannot or will not renegotiate or relinquish earlier reciprocities. If family and friends believe the proper stance toward illness is struggling against it or politely ignoring it, then they will be displeased to witness their ill person adapting to it. More likely, however, family and friends are relieved when the ill person begins to adapt. As he or she does so, earlier anger, self-pity, guilt, and blame dissipate. Adapting leads to taking responsibility for self. Hence, spouses and partners may feel much less need to monitor the ill person and to patrol his or her activities. Moreover, chronically ill people who adapt do not require their friends and family to construct a fictional present and mythical future with them. Adapting fosters candor and openness. And ultimately, surrendering to illness permits grave illness and death to be a part of life for the survivors as well as the sick person.

Adapting to impairment takes people with serious chronic illness on an odyssey of self (cf. Charmaz 1991). Their bodies become alien terrain. Their altered lives can transport them into unfamiliar worlds where they feel estranged. Furthermore, the familiar becomes strange when altered bodies pose new constraints, require careful scrutiny, and force attending to time, space, movement, and other people in new ways. By struggling *with* illness while constructing their lives, chronically ill people feel that they regain lost control over their bodies and their lives. By regaining control and coping with bodily changes, these people learn to live with their illnesses. As they do, the strange becomes familiar. Because surrendering to the sick body strips the journey of routine distractions and obstacles, conditions exist for ill persons to experience self anew and to continue the odyssey with renewed clarity and purpose. In this sense then, adapting to impairment fosters redemption and transcendence of self.[6]

Through struggle and surrender, ill people paradoxically grow more resolute in self as they adapt to impairment. They suffer bodily losses but gain themselves. Their odyssey leads them to a deeper level of awareness—of self, of situation, of their place with others. They believe in their inner strength as their bodies crumble. They transcend their bodies as they surrender control. The self is of the body yet beyond it. With this stance comes a sense of resolution and an awareness of timing. Ill people grasp when to struggle and when to flow into surrender. They grow impervious to social meanings, including being devalued. They can face the unknown without fear while remaining themselves. At this point, chronically ill people may find themselves in the ironic position of giving solace and comfort to the healthy. They gain pride in knowing that their selves have been put to test—a test of character, resourcefulness, and will. They know they gave themselves to their struggles and lived their loss with courage.

Yet the odyssey seldom remains a single journey for these chronically ill people. Frequently, they repeat their journey on the same terrain over and over and, also, find themselves transported to unplanned side trips and held captives within hostile territories as they experience setbacks, flare-ups, complications, and secondary conditions. Still they may discover that each part of their odyssey not only poses barriers, but also brings possibilities for resolution and renewal.

Notes

1. I am indebted to Margaret Purser (personal communication, 1993) for the term "continuing metaphors of opposition."

2. While completing a study of the experience of chronic illness, I found that issues about having a problematic body arose repeatedly. This study included 115 intensive interviews of fifty-five adults with serious, intrusive chronic illnesses. Sixteen of these respondents were followed longitudinally from five years to over a decade. After analyzing the earlier interviews for content about the body in illness, 25 focused interviews about the body and self were conducted (including 12 interviews with respondents from the longitudinal portion of the original study) of two to three hours in length. I also collected personal accounts of experiencing chronic illness and disability to examine them for statements about the body (see, for example, Beisser 1988; Fisher, Straus, Cheney, and Oleske 1987; Frank 1991; LeMaistre 1985; Mairs 1989; Murphy 1987; Pitzele 1985; Register 1987). Grounded theory methods provided the strategies for collecting and analyzing data (Charmaz 1995; Glaser 1978; Glaser and Strauss 1967; Strauss 1987). Consistent with the emergent character of grounded theory methods, my analysis evolved as I collected and interpreted data.

3. Olesen et al. (1990) refer to this type of self-appraisal as the self as knower because a hurting body provides significant reference points in relation to self and illness.

4. When the diagnosis is not understood, objectifying the body likely increases and intensifies if patients and families also do not understand chronicity. Then ill persons may detach themselves from their impaired bodies and even view their bodily changes as unreal (Manning 1991).

5. Physical loss can consume caregivers as well as their patients. Maggie Strong (1988, p. 254)

reveals how her husband's continued physical losses steadily consumed *her* self and body. . . . "My sorrow for Ted's hearing faded into a growing panic and rage. He was climbing right into my body. I was climbing right into his, into his sensory lobes, into his auditory cortex and he into mine. This was a gradual total body transplant in which my own self would be entirely usurped."

6. I am indebted to Norman K. Denzin (personal communication, 1993) for reminding me of the cultural myth of redemption after loss followed by transcendence of self (see also, Charmaz 1991).

References

Albrecht, Gary. 1992. "The Social Experience of Disability." Pp. 1-18 in *Social Problems*, edited by Craig Calhoun and George Ritzer. New York: McGraw-Hill.

Beisser, Arnold R. 1988. *Flying without Wings: Personal Reflections on Being Disabled*. New York: Doubleday.

Blumer, Herbert. 1969. *Symbolic Interactionism*. Englewood Cliffs, NJ: Prentice-Hall.

Brody, Howard. 1987. *Stories of Sickness*. New Haven: Yale University Press.

Burke, Peter J. 1980. "The Self: Measurements from an Interactionist Perspective." *Social Psychology Quarterly* 43:18-29.

Bury, Michael. 1982. "Chronic Illness as Biographical Disruption." *Sociology of Health & Illness* 4:167-182.

_____. 1988. "Meanings at Risk: The Experience of Arthritis." Pp. 89-116 in *Living with Chronic Illness*, edited by Robert Anderson and Michael Bury. London: Unwin Hyman.

_____. 1991. "The Sociology of Chronic Illness: A Review of Research and Prospects." *Sociology of Health & Illness* 13:452-468.

Charmaz, Kathy. 1980. *The Social Reality of Death*. Reading, MA: Addison-Wesley.

_____. 1987. "Struggling for a Self: Identity Levels of the Chronically Ill." Pp. 283-321 in *Research in the Sociology of Health Care: The Experience and Management of Chronic Illness*, Vol. 6, edited by Julius A. Roth and Peter Conrad. Greenwich, CT: JAI Press.

_____. 1991. *Good Days, Bad Days: The Self in Chronic Illness and Time*. New Brunswick, NJ: Rutgers University Press.

_____. 1994a. "Discoveries of Self in Chronic Illness." Pp. 226-242 in *Doing Everyday Life: Ethnography as Human Lived Experience*, edited by Mary Lorenz Dietz, Robert Prus, and William Shaffir. Mississauga, Ontario: Copp Clark Longman.

_____. 1994b. "Identity Dilemmas of Chronically Ill Men." *The Sociological Quarterly* 35: 269-288.

_____. 1995. "Grounded Theory." Pp. 27-49 in *Rethinking Psychology*: Vol. 2, *Rethinking Methods in Psychology*, edited by Jonathan Smith, Rom Harre, and Luk Van Langenhove. London: Sage.

Corbin, Juliet, and Anselm L. Strauss. 1987. "Accompaniments of Chronic Illness: Changes in Body, Self, Biography, and Biographical Time." Pp. 249-281 in *Research in the Sociology of Health Care: The Experience and Management of Chronic Illness*, Vol. 6, edited by Julius A. Roth and Peter Conrad. Greenwich, CT: JAI Press.

_____. 1988. *Unending Work and Care: Managing Chronic Illness at Home*. San Francisco: Jossey-Bass.

Dahlberg, Charles Clay, and Joseph Jaffe. 1977. *Stroke: A Doctor's Personal Story of His Recovery*. New York: Norton.

Denzin, Norman K. 1987a. *The Alcoholic Self*. Newbury Park, CA: Sage.

_____. 1987b. *The Recovering Alcoholic*. Newbury Park, CA: Sage.

Dingwall, Robert. 1976. *Aspects of Illness*. Oxford. Martin Robertson.

Donnally, Trish. 1991. "Healing Power of Looking Good." *San Francisco Chronicle*, July 10. D3-5.

Fabrega, Horace, Jr., and Peter K. Manning. 1972. "Disease, Illness and Deviant Careers." Pp. 93-116 in *Theoretical Perspectives on Deviance*, edited by Robert A. Scott and Jack D. Douglas. New York: Basic.

Fallowfield, Lesley, with Andrew Clark. 1991. *Breast Cancer*. London: Tavistock.

Fisher, Gregg Charles, with Stephen E. Straus, Paul R. Cheney, and James M. Oleske. 1987. *Chronic Fatigue Syndrome*. New York: Warner Books.

Frank, Arthur W. 1991. *At the Will of the Body*. Boston: Houghton Mifflin.

Gadow, Sally. 1982. "Body and Self: A Dialectic." Pp. 86-100 in *The Humanity of the Ill: Phenomenological Perspectives*, edited by Victor Kestenbaum. Knoxville: University of Tennessee Press.

Gerhardt, Uta. 1979. "Coping and Social Action: Theoretical Reconstruction of the Life-event Approach." *Sociology of Health & Illness* 1: 195-225.

Gerhardt, Uta. 1989. *Ideas About Illness*. New York: New York University Press.

Glaser, Barney G. 1978. *Theoretical Sensitivity*. Mill Valley, CA: Sociology Press.

Glaser, Barney G., and Anselm L. Strauss. 1967. *The Discovery of Grounded Theory*. Chicago: Aldine.

Glassner, Barry. 1988. *Bodies*. New York: Putnam.

_____. 1989. "Fitness and the Postmodern Self." *Journal of Health and Social Behavior* 30:180-191.

Goffman, Erving. 1963. *Stigma*. Englewood Cliffs, NJ: Prentice-Hall.

Herzlich, Claudine, and Janine Pierret. 1984. *Illness and Self in Society*. Baltimore: Johns Hopkins University Press.

Hewitt, John P. 1992. *Self and Society*. New York: Simon and Schuster.

Johnson, Colleen Leahy. 1985. "The Impact of Illness on Late-life Marriages." *Journal of Marriage and the Family* 47:165-172.

Kahane, Deborah H. 1990. *No Less a Woman*. New York: Prentice-Hall.

Kelly, Michael. 1992. "Self, Identity and Radical Surgery." *Sociology of Health & Illness* 14:390-415.

Kestenbaum, Victor. 1982. "Introduction: The Experience of Illness." Pp. 3-38 in *The Humanity of the Ill: Phenomenological Perspectives*, edited by Victor Kestenbaum. Knoxville: University of Tennessee Press.

Kidel, Mark. 1988. "Illness and Meaning." Pp. 4-21 in *The Meaning of Illness*, edited by Mark Kidel and Susan Rowe-Leete. London: Routledge.

LeMaistre, Joanne. 1985. *Beyond Rage: The Emotional Impact of Chronic Illness*. Oak Park, IL: Alpine Guild.

Locker, David. 1983. *Disability and Disadvantage: The Consequences of Chronic Illness*. London: Tavistock.

MacDonald, Lea. 1988. "The Experience of Stigma: Living with Rectal Cancer." Pp. 177-202 in *Living with Chronic Illness*, edited by Robert Anderson and Michael Bury. London: Unwin Hyman.

Mairs, Nancy. 1989. *Remembering the Bonehouse: An Erotics of Place and Space*. New York: Harper and Row.

Manning, Peter. K. 1991. "The Unreality of the Body." Paper presented at the Stone Symposium of the Society for the Study of Symbolic Interaction, University of California, San Francisco.

Mead, George Herbert. 1934. *Mind, Self and Society*. Chicago: University of Chicago Press.

Monks, Judith, and Ronald Frankenberg. n.d. "The Presentation of Self, Body and Time in the Life Stories and Illness Narratives of People with Multiple Sclerosis." Unpublished manuscript, Brunel University.

Murphy, Robert F. 1987. *The Body Silent*. New York: Henry Holt.

Olesen, Virginia, Leonard Schatzman, Nellie Droes, Diane Hatton, and Nan Chico. 1990. "The Mundane Ailment and the Physical Self: Analysis of the Social Psychology of Health and Illness." *Social Science & Medicine* 30:449-455.

Peyrot, Mark, James F. McMurry, Jr., and Richard Hedges. 1988. "Marital Adjustment to Adult Diabetes: Interpersonal Congruence and Spouse Satisfaction." *Journal of Marriage and the Family* 50:363-376.

Pitzele, Sefra Kobrin. 1985. *We Are Not Alone: Learning to Live with Chronic Illness*. New York: Workman.

Plough, Alonzo L. 1986. *Borrowed Time: Artificial Organs and the Politics of Extending Lives*. Philadelphia: Temple University Press.

Purser, Margaret. 1993. Personal Communication, 24 June.

Radley, Alan. 1989. "Style, Discourse, and Constraint in Adjustment to Chronic Illness." *Sociology of Health and Illness* 11: 230-252.

Radley, Alan. 1991. *The Body and Social Psychology*. New York: Springer-Verlag.

Radley, Alan, and Ruth Green. 1985. "Styles of Adjustment to Coronary Graft Surgery." *Social Science and Medicine* 20:461-472.

_____. 1987. "Illness as Adjustment: A Methodology and Conceptual Framework." *Sociology of Health & Illness* 9:179-206.

Register, Cherie. 1987. *Living with Chronic Illness*. New York: Free Press.

Speedling, Edward. 1982. *Heart Attack: The Family Response at Home and in the Hospital*. New York: Tavistock.

Strauss, Anselm. 1987. *Qualitative Analysis for Social Scientists*. New York: Cambridge University Press.

Strauss, Anselm L., Juliet Corbin, Shizuko Fagerhaugh, Barney G. Glaser, David Maines, Barbara Suczek, and Carolyn L. Wiener. 1984. *Chronic Illness and the Quality of Life*. 2d ed. St. Louis: Mosby.

Strong, Maggie. 1988. *Mainstay: For the Well Spouse of the Chronically Ill*. New York: Penguin.

Weitz, Rose. 1991. *Life with AIDS*. New Brunswick, NJ: Rutgers University Press.

Williams, G. 1984. "The Genesis of Chronic Illness: Narrative Reconstruction." *Sociology of Health & Illness* 6:175-200.

Williams, R. G. A. 1981a. "Logical Analysis as a Qualitative Method I: Themes in Old Age and Chronic Illness." *Sociology of Health and Illness* 3:140-164.

_____. 1981b. "Logical Analysis as a Qualitative Method II: Conflict of Ideas and the Topic of Illness." *Sociology of Health and Illness* 3:165-187.

Yoshida, Karen K. 1993. "Reshaping of Self: A Pendular Reconstruction of Self and Identity among Adults with Traumatic Spinal Cord Injury." *Sociology of Health & Illness* 15: 217-245.

Zola, Irving K. 1991. "Bringing Our Bodies and Our-
selves Back In: Reflections on a Past, Present, and
Future 'Medical Sociology.' " *Journal of Health and
Social Behavior* 32:1-16.

Further Reading

Kathy Charmaz. 1987. "Struggling for a Self: Identity
Levels of the Chronically Ill." *Research in the Sociology of Health Care: The Experience and Management
of Chronic Illness* vol. 6: 283-321, edited by J. Roth
and P. Conrad. Greenwich: JAI Press.

Sally Gadow. 1982. "Body and Self: A Dialectic." *The
Humanity of the Ill: Phenomenological Perspectives*,
edited by Victor Kestenbaum. Knoxville: University
of Tennessee Press., pp. 86-100.

Alan Radley. 1991. *The Body and Social Psychology*.
New York: Springer-Verlag.

Discussion Questions

1. Why does the issue of harmony between
   body and self remain continually problematic for chronically ill people?

2. What do you see as the difference between struggling with illness and struggling against it?

3. How would you apply the concepts from
   this selection to your life or to the lives
   of people with whom you are well ac-
   quainted?

From *The Sociological Quarterly*, Vol. 36 (No. 4). Pp. 701-
724. Copyright © 1995 by The Midwest Sociological
Society. Reprinted by permission. ✦

12

The Rigors of Kidney Dialysis for Robert Banes

Laurie Kaye Abraham

Robert Banes' story reveals the daily routine of a patient who must have dialysis or die. Robert's story tells more, however, than a saga of sickness. This chapter links the personal experience of illness to larger trends in incidence of disease and differentials by race and class in receiving care. Like anyone else with a chronic illness, Robert experiences the vicissitudes of kidney dialysis within the parameters of a life. End Stage Renal Disease (ESRD) with subsequent dialysis is not the crisis in Robert's life. Rather, it is one more crisis in a life ridden with crises born out of poverty, limited education, and lack of opportunity. For people like Robert and his wife, Jackie, disability and death are routine events. Pooled resources and shared housing with relatives help some but poverty and ill health prove to be relentless.

As you read this selection, look for places where both Robert and Tommy could have been helped, where a further slide downhill could have been prevented. Note the contrast in economic circumstances between Robert and Dr. Laing. Assess the structure and quality of treatment available to Robert.

Robert was thinking about frying some bacon for breakfast when the driver who takes him to the kidney dialysis center sounded his horn from the street. This was unusual because it was just a little after 5:30 A.M., and Robert is scheduled for a six o'clock pickup, Mondays, Wednesdays, and Fridays. Robert has known drivers to be late, sometimes by hours; he has known drivers not to show. They are rarely early.

Still sleepy, he dropped down on the couch to pull on his leather high-tops. A lamp glowed orange in one corner of the living room; otherwise, it was early-morning gray. Latrice slept next to him. Her long, brown legs stretched the length of the couch that does double-duty as her bed. She lay on top of a rust-colored throw that Jackie uses to cover the couch's thinning, stained upholstery. Jackie was already up, washing in the bathroom. Her grandmother lay still in her bed; she had not yet called for her breakfast or a morning drink of water.

The living room is substantially longer than it is wide and is divided into two main sections. The back area, where Robert sat and Latrice slept, holds Jackie's furniture, the couch and a matching love seat she brought when she, Robert, and Latrice moved in with her grandmother in 1986. A dark wood hutch, built into the back wall, is filled with pictures of the family. Some of the photos are old and tattered, their frames tarnished, but none of that seems to matter much. The pictures look as if they have been there for a long time and will remain for a long time to come. A light-colored wood bookshelf next to the hutch is overflowing with knickknacks: ceramic figurines Jackie gave to her grandmother mixed with animals made from shells (souvenirs of a craft project at a nursing home where Mrs. Jackson worked), mixed with a dozen basketball trophies that Robert won in high school and junior college.

Toward the front, outside Mrs. Jackson's bedroom door, sits a more formal-looking couch, upholstered in faded gold, that the old woman has owned since Jackie was a girl. DeMarest is an active little boy and has torn and poked through its plastic slipcover until it no longer provides much protection, but Jackie resists removing it. Her grandmother insisted on the plastic cover, and Jackie does not want her to think the family is defying her now that she cannot do anything about it. A low-slung credenza, about thirty years old, with a working radio and a broken turntable inside, is across the room from Mrs. Jackson's couch. Three color TVs are stacked together near it, although only one works.

Robert finished tying his shoes. Eyes half shut, he pushed aside a vinyl recliner the Baneses put in front of the door at night for extra security and descended the stairs that lead down to a small front porch. "Heh, Banes, I knew I'd get you today," called the driver, who has transported Robert before. Each weekday, private companies that contract with the Chicago Transit Authority take Robert and twenty-five hundred other disabled Cook County residents to medical appointments and wherever else they need to go. In the summer of 1989, there were five transportation companies working for the CTA (subsequently one of them was kicked out of the program for fraud, as another had been earlier in the year). Robert used SCR Transportation, which had the worst on-time record in the program. SCR arrived on time for about half of its rides; the rest of the time, drivers were anywhere from ten minutes to more than an hour late.[1]

Nonetheless, the ride was a blessing because the dialysis clinic is a good hour away on the bus or train. Robert would have to leave for the clinic in the dark, an unsettling proposition in a neighborhood imprisoned by nightfall. The Baneses rarely go out at night, and even at dusk, when Latrice wants to run down to her cousin's apartment less than a block away, Jackie watches her come and go from the front porch. Robert also appreciates the ride home after dialysis because sometimes he feels weak and shaky, not at all in the mood to be jostled on the bus.

As soon as Robert got into the car, he pulled a pack of cigarettes out of his jacket and lit one. "My wife doesn't know I smoke," he said. Robert tries to curry Jackie's favor with small gestures such as pretending not to smoke and buying her a box of candy when she gets mad. What Jackie wants most, though, is for him to stay away from cocaine, and that he has a harder time doing. He sometimes goes weeks, even a month or two, without using cocaine but then binges and spends every cent he can find on drugs. That leaves Jackie straining to meet her household budget, and it cannot be good for Robert's health. Robert refuses to discuss drugs with anyone but Jackie and then only if she pushes the issue.

The twenty-minute ride to Neomedica Dialysis Center, located in the most exclusive area of Chicago, had the feel of a boys' night out. The two men bantered about NBA stars they had met, gangsters the driver had chauffeured, and the high cost of dating.

"Give me some cash and I can go out, buy some drinks for the ladies," the driver boasted.

"So you can make things *happen*," Robert said with a vicarious thrill.

Robert wears a dialysis uniform of sorts: a navy and white nylon sweatsuit and a red Bulls cap. His arms are still sculpted from his basketball-playing days, but the muscles look as if they have been sanded down. All that's left are a few bulges covered by a thin layer of skin. He has lost twenty pounds in the six months since he began dialysis, a big enough drop that the clinic nutritionist said she plans to put him on a supplemental diet. On the warmest days, Robert gets cold, and when he sees a woman walk down the street in shorts and a sleeveless shirt, he often says, "I wish I had her blood." Like most dialysis patients, Robert is chronically anemic.

Neomedica's clerk calls patients back for dialysis two or three at a time, so Robert found a chair in the waiting room and turned to the *Sun-Times* sports pages. Other patients killed time with talk of the Bulls and high blood pressure pills, the Cubs and the restrictive diets patients are supposed to follow. Robert was one of the last patients left when he was summoned at 7:30. That is his regular dialysis time, but Robert gets to the clinic a little after six because he has found that the earlier the pickup, the more likely the transportation company is to be on time. When patients are late getting to Neomedica, they may wait hours to be dialyzed.

Upon hearing his name, Robert pitched his paper and walked to his recliner, past a score of patients tethered to blinking, beeping machines. Two thin plastic tubes, reddened by steady streams of blood, snaked from each of the patients' forearms. On their inner arms, dialysis patients have knots called fistulas, where doctors connect a vein and an artery to enable them to receive dialysis. The arterial tube feeds blood into the dialyzer, where a six-inch filter composed of dozens of tiny strawlike tubes draws out wastes the kidneys can no longer expel. The cleansed blood is then pumped back into patients' bodies, Without dialysis, Robert and the other patients would die within a few weeks.

Fourteen of the patients on Robert's morning shift at Neomedica are black, five are Hispanic, two are white, and one is Asian. The racial mix of the group nearly matches that of Chicago's dialysis population, though the center has fewer whites than the city as a whole.[2] Nation-wide, the incidence of kidney failure among blacks is four times that among whites.[3]

Much of that racial difference results from kidney failure caused by hypertension, a disease that usually can be controlled by medication. In other words, a significant portion of the kidney failure among blacks is largely preventable with regular care. For those who are poor, the reasons they do not receive care range from inadequate or nonexistent insurance, to a misunderstanding of the seriousness of the condition, to an inability to cope with anything other than immediate threats to their well-being. A sad mix of all three caused Jackie's father, Tommy Markham, to suffer another of the consequences of uncontrolled high blood pressure, a stroke, when he was only forty-eight.

Tommy gives only sketchy details about his youth, but he apparently had a contentious relationship with his parents, Mrs. Jackson and her first husband. He stayed behind in Mississippi when the couple moved north, to Gary, Indiana, though his young daughter, Jackie, went with them. Jackie's teenage mother had given her daughter to Mrs. Jackson to raise. After Tommy got into trouble for car theft, he moved to Chicago, where Mrs. Jackson had gone after she split from her husband. Tommy's run-ins with the law did not stop, however. The way Tommy tells it, he got fed up with a man who wrongly accused him of "going with his woman" and "beat the shit out of him." He was convicted of armed robbery and spent seven years in Illinois's Stateville Correctional Center during his twenties. (Tommy huffily denies the robbery: "I didn't rob the dude. I just beat him up. . . . He was laying there in the gangway, and peoples from the lounge ran out. They took the money off him.")

When Tommy was released in 1971, Mrs. Jackson continued to raise Jackie. He lived with his mother and ten-year-old Jackie for a few days, but Mrs. Jackson threw him out because of his "attitude," Jackie said, and he returned to the West Side's streets. He worked off and on as a bartender, butcher, and exterminator, all the while guzzling beer, whiskey, and cognac. Six feet, two inches tall, with muscle built in the prison gym and still evident today, Tommy was menacing to Jackie and, evidently, to a lot of other people. "Everybody would be scared of Tommy, Tommy, Tommy," Jackie chanted. So intimidated by her violent father was Jackie that she has fonder memories of him when he was imprisoned than when he came out. She and her grandmother took the Greyhound bus to visit him in Joliet once a year. "I remember my father giving me bottled pop and peanuts," she said. "It used to be a nice ritual for me, The prison had beautiful flower gardens and afterward we'd go shopping in Joliet."

Tommy's stroke did not come out of the blue. He knew he had high blood pressure, but he stopped taking antihypertensive medication because of its side effects—impotence, for one. His alcoholism and smoking also almost certainly contributed to the stroke. But high blood pressure does not cause any discomfort for most people, which is why doctors call it the "silent killer," and so Tommy, who generally does not look past the next day, paid no attention. "Nature will takes its course," he likes to say. And it did. The left side of his body is now paralyzed, and he spends most of his time in a wheelchair, though he can walk very slowly with the assistance of a brace and cane. As Tommy tells the Currency Exchange clerk with whom he flirts when he picks up his welfare check, "I can't run no more yards; the All-American Tom Cat done slowed down."

The casualties that high blood pressure inflicts on blacks are enormous; they suffer strokes at twice the rate of whites,[4] and there are sixty thousand excess deaths a year among blacks from hypertension-related diseases.[5] In Chicago, where the population of blacks and whites is roughly equal, there are more blacks with kidney failure caused by high blood pressure than whites with kidney failure *regardless of cause.*[6]

Hypertension does not account for all of the difference in black and white kidney-failure rates. Blacks with diabetes also lose kidneys more than whites.[7] But the main reasons that high blood pressure, diabetes, and even Robert's relatively rare focal glomerulosclerosis take a higher toll on blacks are probably similar: a third of blacks are poor, and for lack of money, or understanding, the poor easily can get shut out of medical care.

Robert was born thirty-five-years ago at what was then called the Illinois Research and Educational Hospital, part of the University of Illinois medical school complex. He still goes there for care, as an outpatient in the transplant program.

As a boy, Robert moved between the West Side apartments of his young mother and his grandmother. Fearing he would get tangled up with a gang, they sent him to Panola, Alabama, when he was seventeen to live with relatives. Panola was so small, Robert says, that "by the time you raise your hand to wave to somebody, you're out of town."

His next stop was a Tennessee community college where he studied and played basketball until he dropped out in the spring of 1975. Not long after, Robert returned to Chicago and his mother's house, located several miles away from where Robert and Jackie live today. He met Jackie at a birthday party for his mother in 1977, the same year he received the first sign that his kidneys were failing. A job physical revealed protein in his urine—a warning that his kidneys were not functioning well. A renal biopsy later that year showed the focal glomerulosclerosis.

There is no cure for focal glomerulosclerosis—it progressively scars kidneys until they are destroyed—and doctors are baffled by the disease's cause. Steroids and chemotherapy are used to slow its progress, but they may or may not work. Robert received no treatment for this potentially fatal condition. He did not even see a doctor again until four years later, in April 1981, when he showed up at Cook County Hospital's emergency room. Robert had been unusually tired for several months and had trouble keeping his food

down. When his ankles began to swell at Latrice's third birthday party, a friend drove him to the hospital. There, doctors discovered his kidneys were working at less than 5 percent of capacity.

The chairman of general medicine at Cook County Hospital, Dr. Terrence Conway, has seen hundreds of patients with advanced, untreated conditions similar to Robert's. His first experience at County came during the Vietnam War, when he was assigned to the hospital as an orderly to fulfill conscientious objector requirements. After graduating from medical school in 1976, he worked at a federally funded health clinic on the South Side, then as the medical director of another such clinic in the Cabrini-Green housing project, and in 1988, he returned to County. When Robert came there, he was near death, Dr. Conway said. "His blood pressure was high, blood clotting was not very good. His fluid was backing up, which could have caused heart failure. He probably could have gone another three weeks without one of his systems failing, but not much longer."

Why Robert waited until he was in such crisis to seek medical care is not entirely clear. In the medical record, a Cook County social worker wrote that Robert told her that he didn't have any money to pay his hospital bill. None of his short-term, minimum-wage jobs provided medical insurance to pay for diagnostic kidney studies, or medications, or follow-up visits to the doctor, and he was not consistently enrolled in Medicaid, which has very limited coverage for single adults, anyhow.

Beyond Robert's inability to pay for care is the fact that he did not seem to understand the gravity of his illness, or that medical care could have extended the life of his kidneys. Cook County's medical history for Robert says: ". . . a renal biopsy at Columbus Hospital showed focal glomerulosclerosis, but Mr. Banes neglected to continue his follow-up."

This is what Robert recalls: "I was thinking there wasn't that much wrong. I thought whatever it was might clear up on its own. They told me I had something on my kidney, but nobody told me to come back."

Patricia Barber, a nurse and clinical transplant specialist at the University of Illinois, coached Robert through his first kidney transplant in 1982. In January 1989, his body rejected the transplanted organ, and Barber was preparing him to get onto the transplant waiting list for a second time. "When patients come into Cook County with chronic renal failure and say, 'Nobody ever told me this could happen,' they're partly right. They've been told but not in a way that sticks," says Barber. "Robert was referred back for treatment, but being young and feeling well, he did not have a lot of motivation to follow through."

Then, too, people who can barely afford food and shelter may not think they have much to gain from spending scarce dollars for doctors' visits. "For someone who is poor, health care is not the highest priority," Dr. Conway said, an observation offered repeatedly by doctors and nurses who work with poor patients.

It's also possible that friends and family were not pushing Robert to go to the doctor, Dr. Conway continued. "People in Chicago's poorer neighborhoods are used to a lot of sick people around. When someone says 'Something's wrong with my kidneys,' the automatic response is not 'Well, what doctor are you going to?' When you live on the North Shore [the affluent suburbs north of Chicago], that's the first thing people ask you."

Dr. Conway also speculated that since Robert's disease is a chronic one, doctors may have told him that "there was nothing they could do," a phrase that can mean one thing to patients and another to doctors. "It sounds black-and-white, but it's not. We can't cure AIDS, but we don't say 'You're on your own. Don't come back.' We can do things to prolong life."

Doctors may face a particular challenge getting that message across to people as fatalistic as Robert and Jackie. Asked at least a half-dozen times to discuss her feelings about her family's unrelenting illness—did she think they were unusual or especially cursed? —Jackie got exasperated. "Look," she finally said, obviously hoping to close the subject, "I just say it *happens*."

The fantastic and horrid deaths that mark their daily lives feed such fatalism. Perhaps only the most stout-hearted—or delusional—

could retain a sense of control over their destiny. One day, a thirtyish-looking man spotted Jackie in a car and ran up to the side window, puckering his lips in an exaggerated kiss. "I went to school with him," Jackie said, laughing at his foolishness. Then, without skipping a beat: "They found his brother dead right up under the house, this tall building right up on the corner. I heard rumors when I was in grammar school. The kids was playing and they kept saying they smelled something foul, like dead rats, and it was his brother's body down in the sewer."

Then there is the death of Robert's beloved mother. The official version of her story is that she went out drinking with friends after work on a Friday, returned home, and passed out in the garage with the car running. The unofficial version is considerably more vivid. "She was murdered," Jackie said once. Then she corrected herself. "Carbon monoxide, that's what's on the death certificate. But [Robert and his family] say there was scratches and blood. And I've heard that she was disrobed halfway. And I remember Robert getting her bra and there was blood stains on it, so we feel like, the family felt, there was foul play somewhere."

It would be easy to dismiss this as an example of devoted children unable to face the mundane but ultimately tragic circumstances of their mother's death. And that may be all it is. But in a neighborhood where the cliché "truth is stranger than fiction" takes on pointed meaning, who knows for sure?

There has been little rigorous study of how fatalism and other accompaniments of poverty influence communication between doctors and patients, but at least one investigator of the subject found that doctors spend more time discussing diagnoses and treatments with well-educated people, resulting in a "paradoxical situation whereby patients most in need of education receive the least."[8] At the same time, blacks report more often than whites that doctors do not adequately explain the seriousness of their illnesses or how medications work.[9] Robert, for one, is often confused by doctors, but he rarely if ever asks them for more information.

Several days before he was admitted to University of Illinois Hospital because of the blood in his urine, Robert had visited a urologist at the university's outpatient clinic. He had never seen the doctor before, but Barber, the transplant nurse, made him an appointment because of the unusual bleeding. At that appointment, the doctor told him he would have to be hospitalized. He also told Robert that before he could be admitted to the hospital he would need blood tests and an ultrasound study of his kidneys.

"When am I going to have to have surgery?" Robert asked, certain of that eventuality though the doctor had not mentioned it.

"That's only if the ultrasound shows us something like a cyst, like cancer on the kidneys," the doctor said flatly.

"Don't tell me that, please," Robert pleaded. The doctor smiled sympathetically and walked out of the examining room without explaining further.

Through the open door, Robert could see but not hear the doctor conferring with a nurse who was holding a small plastic cup of blood that seemed to be Robert's.

"Don't be whispering," he said to himself. "Tell me, too."

But when the doctor returned moments later, Robert did not ask him what he had been talking about. He lay back on the examining table and offered up his arm for his blood pressure to be taken. If Robert wondered what the chances were of his having cancer, he said nothing.

Robert says he is not angry that no one effectively explained to him that his kidneys were failing. Then again, Robert does not admit that much of anything disturbs him. "I look at dialysis like a setback. Why should you get down? It just makes you sicker."

It's understandable, perhaps admirable, that Robert does not want to dwell on his illness. But Robert is so matter-of-fact and publicly emotionless about how he got sick—and even the most devoted doctors and nurses are so used to situations like Robert's—that it is easy to be lulled into taking it all for granted. Whose fault is it that Robert did not have health insurance, and that at least thirty-five million Americans are without it today?[10] What about doctors' inability to communicate to patients in a way that makes them understand their illnesses—whose fault is

that? Who is responsible for the many poor minorities who are so socially and economically isolated that they cannot take advantage of the medical system in the same way that many whites can?

No one is forced to take responsibility for these inequities. Medical ethicist Larry Churchill describes well the forces that allow the United States to remain the only industrialized country other than South Africa that does not provide at least basic health care to all of its citizens, "Access to health care is mostly contingent on having a way to pay for it, either out of one's own resources or with some form of insurance," he writes. "The essential point is that [this] allocation by price is a rationing scheme—one which we have easily accepted in health care as an extension of a basic economic philosophy, and one which largely absolves any particular person from responsibility for the results. Since no one actually decided to exclude the poor (as it is their lack of money that excludes them, not our actions) no one is responsible and no one is to blame."[11]

The morning the dialysis driver arrived early, Robert fell asleep within minutes after his blood began cycling through the dialysis machine at Neomedica. Before settling in for a nap, he covered himself with a blue bedspread he'd brought from home to ward off the chill he gets during dialysis. The elderly Hispanic woman who sat next to him had the opposite problem: she brought a small fan to cool her as she slept. Cigarette smoke curled over the backs of several of the recliners spread across the room. Some patients watched a TV that hung from the ceiling; others chatted quietly.

Dr. Gordon Lang, the medical director of Robert's facility, had begun making his rounds. With graying, curly hair, a strong-boned face, and stylish ruby-red glasses, he is quite handsome. He quickly scanned medical charts, exchanged a few words with patients, and was gone within a half-hour. Dr. Lang is also the president of Neomedica Dialysis Centers, Inc., and along with monitoring the medical care of the downtown clinic's patients, he has to oversee this expanding for-profit dialysis chain, which in 1989 included eight other Chicago-area dialysis units.

Dialysis is one of few areas of medical care dominated by for-profit providers, and it has been at the center of a nationwide debate about the costs and quality of proprietary medicine. Medicare pays dialysis units a fixed fee for each dialysis session— Neomedica currently gets $131 per treatment[12]—but exercises little control over how that money is spent. Officials at the Health Care Financing Administration, which administers Medicare, charge that, to preserve high profit margins, many centers compromise patients' care by reducing staff and shortening treatment times.[13] Such cost-cutting changes have been made at Neomedica, Dr. Lang freely admits, but he said they do not threaten patients' health. Neither, he said, do Neomedica's physician-owners earn excessive profits.

Dr. Lang founded Neomedica with another doctor when Medicare began to pay for dialysis in 1972 and today owns 14 percent[14] of the $6.7 million chain.[15] Public documents do not show how much Dr. Lang makes as the corporation's chief executive, but his job as a medical director of Robert's unit, which Dr. Lang estimated occupies him for three or four hours a week, pays well: $68,480 in 1989, according to Medicare cost reports.[16] Completely apart from what he makes for running Neomedica, he earns a monthly fee as the nephrologist for Robert and forty-five to fifty other dialysis patients.[17] For that work, Medicare pays doctors an average of $173 per patient per month, which would mean Dr. Lang earns roughly another $100,000 each year from Medicare.[18] Finally, a medical practice he maintains outside of the dialysis unit further enhanced his income. Dr. Lang will not say how much he currently makes a year, but according to the Internal Revenue Service, his taxable income in 1985 was $362,964.[19] (That figure comes from a suit Dr. Lang filed against the IRS to block the agency's attempt to recover $160,000 for alleged improper deductions he took on a ski resort condominium in Utah.)

Dr. Lang's manner with the dialysis patients at Neomedica's downtown unit was brisk and efficient if not cursory, but for Robert, at least, he is "the man." Though Robert and the other patients regularly grumble about every aspect of dialysis, little of their anger seems directed at Dr. Lang. The technicians and nurses take the brunt of it, even though it is Dr. Lang who has ultimate responsibility for the way the unit is run. . . .

Notes

1. Chicago Transit Authority, on-time performance of CTA Special Services transportation companies 1989–1991, obtained through a Freedom of Information Act request, December 1991.

2. Renal Network of Illinois, "Chicago Dialysis Population: Race within Age," special data run obtained through a Freedom of Information Act request, July 1989.

3. Committee for the Study of the Medicare-ESRD Program, Institute of Medicine, prepublication copy, *Kidney Failure and the Federal Government* (Washington, D.C., National Academy Press, 1991), p. 122.

4. National Center for Health Statistics, "Advanced Report of Final Mortality Statistics, 1989," in *Monthly Vital Statistics* 40, no. 8, suppl. 2 Hyattsville Md.: Public Health Service, 1992). The 1989 age-adjusted stroke rate for whites was 25.9 per 100,000 population, for blacks, 49.0 per 100,000.

5. Elijah Saunders, "Epidemiologic Factors in the Management of Hypertension," *Journal of the National Medical Association* 81, suppl. (April 1989): 9. The excess death rate is the number of deaths minorities would not have suffered had they died at the same rate as whites.

6. Renal Network of Illinois, "Chicago Dialysis Population: Race within Age within Zip Code, Diagnosis Hypertension," special data run obtained through Freedom of Information Act request, July 1989.

7. Committee for the Study of the Medicare ESRD Program, *Kidney Failure and the Federal Government*, p. 126.

8. D.R. Levy, "White Doctors and Black Patients: Influence of Race on the Doctor-Patient Relationship," *Pediatrics* 75, no. 4 (April 1985) 639–43.

9. Robert J. Blendon et al., "Access to Medical Care for Black and White Americans," *Journal of the American Medical Association* 261, no. 2 (13 January 1989): 278–81.

10. In 1991, 35,445,000 people were uninsured. Personal communication with Shirley Smith, Income Branch, Housing, Household, and Economic Statistics, U.S. Bureau of Census, 1993.

11. Larry R. Churchill, *Rationing Health Care in America* (Notre Dame, Ind.: University of Notre Dame Press, 1987), p. 14.

12. Medicare reimburses the average dialysis facility at a rate of $125 per treatment, but Neomedica gets a little more because of Chicago's relatively high wage-scale. Medicare only pays 80 percent of that rate; the secondary insurers—Medicaid, private insurance companies, and the special state plan—make up the difference.

13. Matthew Purdy, "Dialysis: The Profit Machine," *Philadelphia Inquirer*, reprint of series, 1988, p. 2. Bernadette Shoemaker, a federal official who oversees Medicare's End Stage Renal Disease Program, told Purdy: "We don't ask questions about how [dialysis clinics] parcel out that amount of money. We pay the [money]. It's up to the [clinics] to divvy up the amount."

14. Dr. Lang's financial interest in Neomedica was included in the Medicare cost reports Neomedica filed with Blue Cross and Blue Shield of Illinois for fiscal 1990. Judging from cost reports filed in 1988 and 1989, his percentage of the business seems to change slightly from year to year, as medical directors at other units are brought into the company.

15. Dun & Bradstreet, Inc., credit report for Neomedica, 30 June 1990.

16. Neomedica's Medicare cost reports, filed with Blue Cross and Blue Shield of Illinois for fiscal 1989.

17. In a 1992 interview, Dr. Lang told me he received the monthly Medicare payment for forty-five to fifty dialysis patients.

18. To arrive at the $100,000 estimate of Dr. Lang's payments from Medicare for outpatient dialysis at Neomedica, I multiplied the number of patients for which he said he received the monthly Medicare fee—45 to 50—by the average monthly payment per patient, $173, according to *Kidney Failure and the Federal Government*. For 45 patients, at $173 per patient per month, Dr. Lang would earn $93,420 annually from Medicare. For 50 patients at the same rate, he would earn $103,800.

19. Gordon R. Lang and Angelika Lang v. Commissioner of Internal Revenue, filed 20 August 1991.

Further Reading

Robert Anderson and Michael Bury (eds.). 1988. *Living With Chronic Illness: The Experience of Patients and Their Families*. Unwin Hyman: London.

Alonzo Plough. 1986. *Borrowed Time: Artificial Organs and Politics of Extending Lives*. Philadelphia: Temple University Press.

Anselm Strauss, Juliet Corbin, Shizuko Fagerhaugh, Barney Glaser, David Maines, Barbara Suczek, and Carolyn Wiener. 1984. *Chronic Illness and the Quality of Life*. St. Louis: Mosby.

Discussion Questions

1. If dialysis is available to all patients with ESRD, why do socioeconomic factors still matter? List the ways in which your economic circumstances would affect how you could handle the daily routines necessary with ESRD and then compare your list with what you glean about Robert's life and world.

2. How do you account for both Robert's and Dr. Laing's seeming affect about experiencing kidney disease?

3. What social policies are needed to ensure that people like Robert Banes receive adequate and timely treatment?

Illness and the Work Routine

13

A Weekend in the Life of a Medical Student

Perri Klass

Students learn about hierarchies in medical practice during medical school. Medical student training involves immersion in the world of the hospital, in medical tasks, and in routine work. Most importantly, this immersion introduces students to their place in medical hierarchy. Perri Klass, a third-year medical student, reports the trials and tribulations of being "on call" for the weekend. She recounts hospital relationships between variously skilled physicians and patients, families, and staff. Her diary-like account depicts a weekend "on call" through the perspective of a medical student. Routine rounds. Demands from superiors. Decisions about patient definition and treatment. Coping with errors and lack of sleep. Defining who is to blame for misdiagnosis. Listening to and comforting patients and their families. Klass reports learning about how medicine requires attending to the classifications and deliberations of superiors. Follow her through this process and listen to her discuss the everyday uncertainties of medical work and work performance. Pay attention to the ways Klass describes how the real work of medicine requires decision making about illness, about health, and about the limits of being a medical student.

... Internship is the first year after medical school. All internships begin in July, so in August, all the interns have been doctors for a month or so. They are just barely accustomed to writing "M.D." after their names, and they are profoundly aware of their limited experience, their limited knowledge in a profession in which it is impossible to know it all. They depend on the people above them in the hierarchy to save them from the possible results of limited experience and limited knowledge. The resident has already finished internship; he directs the team and oversees the interns. The interns and the residents together constitute the house staff. And the medical students are wetting their feet for the first time, in the hospital to learn about the hospital, to watch the interns and imagine themselves doing that job, as they will be, in a couple of years.

The resident is John McGonigle. He is quite small, thin and wiry, with curly red hair; he almost dances through the hospital, and his ironic nickname among the interns and residents is Godzilla. His style is brusque and rapid-paced; he likes to imagine his team rolling quickly along, making decisions, firing snappy insults at one another, and, if possible, making it to the cafeteria before breakfast is over. He is very fond of cheese Danish. Twenty-nine years old, this month he will put in about 130 hours a week, in a position of tremendous responsibility, and earn something over $24,000 a year.

The intern on call for the day is Phil Maxwell, a blond twenty-seven-year-old hotshot from the Midwest, open-faced, blue-eyed, and profoundly compulsive. Even among the house staff, where people proudly acknowledge themselves as type A's, Phil has the reputation of going a little too far, working a little too hard. The intern who is post-call, who has been in the hospital all night, is

Karen Newton, thirty years old; she has curly brown hair and tired brown eyes. She did research for a couple of years at the end of medical school, got an MD-PhD, and though she is respected by the house staff for the important papers which are now being published with her name on them, she is also known to be a little rusty at clinical work; all that time in the lab. The interns don't work quite as many hours as the resident this month, since they get days off now and then. Say 115 hours a week. They make about $22,000 a year.

That leaves the two medical students. They work with the interns, so one of them is post-call, and one of them is on call. The post-call student is Matthew Baxter; it is no coincidence that his name is the same as the name of one of the hospital buildings, generally referred to as "Baxterville." Matthew is to be the fourth generation of brilliant physicians in his family, and since they have been associated with this hospital for over a century, he has very little choice about where he will do his residency. Fortunately, he is an extremely reverent young man, and it has apparently never occurred to him to resent his manifest destiny. Like Karen, he has been up most of the night, preparing one of his customary superb workups on the patient he admitted, and also helping with blood drawing, errands, whatever came along. The other medical student, the one who is on call for the night to come, is more than a little like me. Her hair is pinned up in a bun, her earrings are maybe a little inappropriately large for the hospital (they sometimes clink against her stethoscope and make it hard to hear heart sounds), and she looks a little bit tense and a little bit depressed. It was, needless to say, she and not Matthew who complained of not wanting to be here. We can call her Elizabeth, which is, in fact, my middle name. The medical students are following the interns' schedule, about 115 hours a week. They are each paying $14,000 a year for the privilege.

Work rounds: this is the time for the intern who was on call to bring the team up to date on all the patients, both the old ones, who may have gotten worse overnight, and the new ones she has admitted. The team moves along the hall, pausing in front of every door for Karen to give them a few lines on the patient within.

"Mr. Harrison, definitely ruled out for an MI, spiked to a hundred three last night, I cultured him up, nothing on his chest film, might just be the flu." [Mr. Harrison has been determined not to have had a heart attack (myocardial infarction), had a temperature of 103 last night, got specimens of his blood and his urine sent to the lab to be cultured for bacteria, and has no pneumonia or other problems showing up on his chest X-ray.]

"Mrs. Kaplan, stable, awaiting placement." [Mrs. Kaplan is ready to leave the hospital but has nowhere to go, Social Service needs to find a place for her in a nursing home.]

"New admission, Mr. Russo is a sixty-six-year-old white COPDer with multiple admits here, who presented yesterday with increased DOE, admitted to juggle his meds around. He's been intubated twice in the past. . . ." [Mr. Russo is a sixty-six-year-old white man with chronic obstructive pulmonary disease who has been in this hospital many times and came in yesterday with increased dyspnea (shortness of breath) on exertion and was admitted so we could adjust his drug regimen. He has needed a breathing tube and a ventilator twice in the past. . . .]

The resident, John McGonigle, makes notes about each new patient on a new file card, updates his file cards on the old patients. He is responsible for all these people; if the intern has made a mistake, this is his first opportunity to catch it. He occasionally raps out a question, as about Mr. Harrison: "Did you look at his sputum?"

"He wasn't really bringing anything up," Karen says, not adding that she was much too busy last night to stand around waiting for someone to cough up some sputum, and then go prepare and stain slides in the lab and hunt for bugs under the microscope.

"I could check that later, if you want," offers Matthew Baxter; sputum examination is frequently a medical student job. Elizabeth feels a very slight and completely unreasonable irritation at his eager-beaver manner.

The team finishes rounds, and does indeed make it down to the cafeteria in time for breakfast; John gets his Danish and everyone else gets coffee and rather uninspiring scrambled eggs. The food is eaten quickly, and conversation is restricted to the events of the previous night on the ward.

Attending rounds: the attending is the senior physician responsible for supervising the team. He comes in every day except Sunday to hear about new admissions, teach the students, advise on complicated cases. The attending is Dr. Harry Black, a soft-spoken man with a rather distressing talent for going off on tangents, but a good and humane doctor.

Matthew Baxter presents his patient, a twenty-seven-year-old black woman who came to the hospital with a vague history of fatigue, weight loss, stomach pains—and in the emergency room, the intern examining her felt an enormously enlarged liver. So now she is in the hospital to be worked up, and Matthew runs down a list of possible diagnoses: hepatitis, other infections, malignancies. Dr. Black, after listening to the details of the case, announces that he would personally put his money on malignancy.

John McGonigle's eyes light up at this turn of phrase. "What kind?" he wants to know. He proposes a bet: is this a primary liver cancer, is it a metastasis from a gut cancer, or from a lung tumor, or from a breast tumor?

Dr. Black, who is perhaps now a little uncomfortable with this talk of betting, turns to the medical students and asks suddenly, "What other cancer commonly metastasizes to the liver, and why is it unlikely in this patient?"

Elizabeth has no idea, though she thinks quickly of a likely guess, but Matthew has been up all night reading about liver disease, and says quickly, "Melanoma, very unusual in blacks."

But John McGonigle is attached to the idea of a bet, and is in addition not unwilling to struggle a little with the attending for control of rounds, so he persists: a bottle of wine to the person who correctly names the malignancy. He himself will go for gut metastasis, and Matthew Baxter, eager to please his resident, immediately claims primary liver cancer, since some people think that is associated with the birth control pill and this patient, Mrs. Ropers, has taken the Pill in the past. Phil Maxwell, looking a little bored, says that

in that case he'll go with lung tumor, which leaves Karen and Elizabeth, the two women, with breast, and that makes everyone slightly uncomfortable. Nevertheless, John writes out a list, more than a little tickled.

The team briefly discusses one other new admission, a diabetic man named Mr. Theokratis, visiting from California, sixty years old, who seems to have had a very bad attack of his customary asthma. Karen Newton explains that though both Mr. Theokratis and his wife were a little frightened by the severity of the episode, it is something that has apparently happened many times before, and Mr. Theokratis is looking much better already this morning. "He may be ready to go home tomorrow," she adds.

Attending rounds are over and the real work of the day begins. Because it is Saturday, there are no conferences; also because it is Saturday, most tests are not available except in cases of emergency. For their investigative CAT scans, their barium swallows, their echocardiographies, their pulmonary function tests, the patients will wait for next week. The team will try to keep them stable, get them through the weekend, and where further diagnostic workups are needed, pick those workups up again in a couple of days.

Matthew Baxter goes in to get an arterial blood gas on Mr. Theokratis, to measure the amount of oxygen in his blood. Because getting blood from an artery means a much more painful needle stick than in a regular blood-drawing from a vein, some people inject a little local anesthetic into the skin of the wrist before aiming the needle directly down at the beating pulse. Matthew, however, prefers not to do this, on the perfectly reasonable grounds that it means two needle sticks instead of one, and in addition the local anesthetic can mean a little swelling in the area of the wrist, making it that much harder to hit the artery on the first try. However, Mr. Theokratis is an old veteran of arterial blood gas samples; the first thing he says when he sees the syringe is, "Get some Xylocaine, young man, or you don't come anywhere near me."

Obligingly, Matthew gets the Xylocaine, injects it, and then, sure enough, it takes him two attempts to get the needle into the artery.

When he finally hits it, and the red blood begins to spurt into the syringe, powered by the strong arterial pulse, Mr. Theokratis says sourly, "You need a little more practice, sonny." Matthew, who has after all been up almost all night, feels a sudden urge to say, well, next time you want anesthetic you can whistle for it. But instead he smiles, pulls out the needle, and presses a gauze pad over the site of the puncture with one hand, while with the other he removes the needle from the now full syringe, attaches a small rubber cap in its place, and rolls the syringe back and forth between his thumb and forefinger so the blood will mix well with the anticlotting substance in the tube. The syringe full of blood goes into a bag of ice, the pressure is applied to Mr. Theokratis's wrist for the specified five minutes, and then Matthew leaves the room, depositing the sample at the ward secretary's desk. The ward secretary calls for a transporter to come take it down to the lab.

Because it is Saturday, John McGonigle sends his postcall intern home soon after noon. Karen Newton is now free for the rest of the day and for Sunday as well; since she is neither on call nor post-call, she doesn't have to come in. This adds up to one day off every three weeks, and Karen is profoundly grateful to John for letting her out so early, increasing her daylight time out of the hospital by fifty percent. . . .

John tells Matthew Baxter that he should hurry up and write notes on all his patients and get the hell out of the hospital; he too is off Sunday. Matthew, however, is very anxious that no one should see him as unenthusiastic, or eager to leave, so he says, cheerfully, "That's fine, but I'm having a good time." He is immediately conscious that everyone listening thinks he is talking like a fool, and he blushes, then goes off to see his new patient, Mrs. Ropers. An eager-beaver medical student may impress a senior physician, too far from medical school to remember the tricks of the trade, but the house staff looks on someone who spends extra unnecessary hours in the hospital as mentally defective.

Elizabeth goes down to collect the midday printouts of lab results on the bloods drawn early that morning. As she rides up in the elevator from the basement labs, she looks over the printout, wondering whether all these numbers will ever be clear and obvious to her. Her fears about her own lack of knowledge, her inability to think sanely and straightforwardly about a set medical problem, are always part of her approach to the hospital. She is stuffed full of facts, memorized and partly remembered, from her medical school courses. She has learned a certain amount in the hospital, idiosyncratically absorbed according to her own interest in certain patients, her level of alertness on morning rounds on some particular mornings, the articulateness of the people doing the teaching.

She runs her finger across the printout, trying to convince herself that the numbers are speaking to her and she is understanding their message. So this patient's liver function tests are slightly up from yesterday, up just above the edge of normal. Does that mean anything? Probably not. Suddenly she notices something in Mr. Theokratis's results, looks again, double-checks against the list of normal lab values on the back of the printout.

When she gets off the elevator at the fifth floor, she finds Phil Maxwell, her intern, and shows him the printout, asking, almost timidly, "Doesn't it look like Mr. Theokratis is having an MI?"

Phil grabs the printout away from her and stares at it. A cardiac enzyme, creatinine phosphokinase (CPK), is sharply elevated in Mr. Theokratis's blood, and this enzyme is usually elevated right after a heart attack.

"I can't believe they didn't check this out last night in the emergency room," Phil says to Elizabeth, as the two of them hurry along the corridor to find John. "This was really careless of Karen; when you're dealing with a diabetic, you have to allow for the possibility of a painless MI, they have them all the time."

They find John, and Phil thrusts the printout at him, his finger indicating the value.

"Oh, shit!" says John McGonigle.

An hour later, Mr. Theokratis is in the intensive care unit, and Team 2 is no longer responsible for his well-being. John and Phil are arguing about what the proper course of treatment and diagnosis would have been the night before, when Mr. Theokratis showed up with his story of an asthma attack like a hundred other asthma attacks. It is not completely possible to tell, of course, whether he was really having an asthma attack, and had a heart attack maybe brought on by the strain of it, or whether his difficulty breathing was actually attributable all along to his painless heart attack. One way or another, no one thought much about a heart attack last night, since the asthma therapy seemed to make him better; his electrocardiogram was very nonspecific, and the cardiac enzyme values didn't come back from the lab until morning. John McGonigle is annoyed to have a heart attack discovered like this; he feels it looks bad for his team. . . .

Matthew Baxter is furious; he has just called down to find out the results of that arterial blood gas he drew on Mr. Theokratis, now very important to know; the intensive care unit team wants those numbers. And the blood gas lab insists they never received the sample; transport must have lost it—or maybe they dropped it and broke it and didn't want to report it. The unit team will have to draw another. The little, essentially unavoidable mistakes of dropping, losing, mislabeling, misreading which would be taken for granted in many settings can become highly charged in the hospital. The support people, the techs who draw the blood, the transporters who carry it to the lab, the lab techs who do the tests and report them, are often blamed for major medical screwups, sometimes because of small errors they have made, or genuine carelessness, and sometimes because they are an anonymous and convenient scapegoat. . . .

"Elizabeth, will you please go start a new IV on Mrs. Pinkerton," says John McGonigle. . . . Mrs. Pinkerton is a lady who everyone knows is not going to get better, and she can't feel anything most of the time, and her husband sits over you when you are trying to start an IV on her, muttering, "Oh, be careful! Oh, don't hurt her, please!" So Elizabeth collects her equipment, the IV needle, a tourniquet, alcohol swabs, tape, and goes into Mrs. Pinkerton's room. Now, Mrs. Pinkerton's is a very sad story. She has had severe and inoperable brain metastases, has gone through radiation therapy with no real improvement.

She was taken home by her devoted husband to live out her days, but she developed seizures and he had to bring her back in. Her husband haunts the hospital, spending long days by her bedside, talking to her about all the things they will do together, as soon as she is well, how they will visit their children and grandchildren out in Texas, how they will buy new curtains for the living room. Mrs. Pinkerton is kept heavily sedated, and even when she is awake, it is clear enough that she does not understand what is said to her. Sometimes she can respond to simple questions or commands, but that is about it.

"Hello, Doctor," Mr. Pinkerton says to Elizabeth, as she bustles in. Mr. Pinkerton always manages to convey the hope that maybe this time, maybe this doctor, there will be a new treatment, a new answer, a new chance.

"I need to start her IV," Elizabeth says, wrapping the tourniquet around the old woman's wasted arm. Mr. Pinkerton, as usual, hangs forward, telling Elizabeth, "Now, you will be careful, won't you, Doctor? She always had such sensitive skin."

In fact, there have been so many IVs in Mrs. Pinkerton's veins, and her blood vessels in general are so thin and tortuous, that Elizabeth simply cannot see any likely place to put the new IV. And with Mr. Pinkerton sitting so close, she feels extremely reluctant to just poke blindly. She takes off the tourniquet and goes in search of John, wishing that he were gone for the day and Phil left in charge. Phil may be intense, but he is always willing to teach. She could say to him, will you help me find a vein on Mrs. Pinkerton, and he would come and help. But John McGonigle, when she finds him, merely looks at her in exaggerated disbelief and says, "You're in your third year of medical school, you should be able to start an IV. No excuses."

So Elizabeth wheels around and goes back to Mrs. Pinkerton. . . . It takes Elizabeth four tries to get the IV going, though she frankly doubts whether any of the house staff could have done it more easily; this woman's veins are simply shot to hell. Mr. Pinkerton looks at Elizabeth reproachfully, but he manages gamely, "Thank you very much, Doctor," as she gathers up her wasted needles and leaves.

Matthew Baxter goes home, after writing a two-page progress note on his new patient, Mrs. Ropers, the woman with the big liver. The progress note is a masterpiece of diplomacy, outlining all the possibilities discussed in attending rounds without committing itself to any as more likely than another, despite Matthew's bet on liver cancer. He has also, of course, written notes on all the other patients he is following, and he is getting a little exhausted.

Even John McGonigle goes home, after one last tense conversation with the intensive care unit team about how he could ever have allowed Mr. Theokratis's MI to get by him like that. "Okay, now," John says to Phil Maxwell, "call me if you have any serious problems, but they damn well better be serious." And he goes home to what is really now only a two-and-a-half-hour evening, knowing he will give himself an extra hour or two to enjoy being out of the hospital, and then be tired tomorrow.

Elizabeth is working up her patient for the evening, a twenty-six-year-old man who speaks only Spanish, who has come into the hospital because for the last three days he has had terrible vomiting and diarrhea; he is seriously dehydrated, and the most important thing to do for him is to get some fluid into him. In the emergency room they started his IV (Elizabeth is just as glad not to be doing another one of those right away), and she has some time to find out his history. Unfortunately, her Spanish is very weak, though it is better than Phil Maxwell's; he speaks no Spanish at all, which is why he assigned her to this particular patient. She manages to find out from him how long all this has been going on, whether there has been blood in his stool (*"Hay sangre?"*) and whether there has been stomach pain (*"Hay dolor?"*), and since she knows Phil will ask about this, she attempts to find out his sexual history. After all, if he is gay, there are various intestinal parasites that can be sexually acquired which ought to be included in her list of possible diagnoses, and Phil, after all, is compulsive. Unfortunately, Elizabeth is unable to make herself understood when she asks this question (all she can manage is to ask if he has female friends—*amigas*—and he says yes, so

she asks if he has male friends—*amigos*—and he again says yes, and looks puzzled). She considers drawing pictures, then decides not to pursue it, since, after all, he could also have acquired these intestinal parasites at his home in Mexico, so the sexual history would not really make any difference. Or so she will tell Phil.

. . . Phil Maxwell by now has five admissions to work up. He examines each patient as thoroughly as possible, carefully runs his mind down a list of the things to be thought of, the things to be done, the diagnoses to be ruled out, the diagnoses to be considered. His write-ups on his patients are marvels of logical organization and clearheaded ratiocination; unfortunately, his handwriting is almost unreadable. He is feeling very pressured by what happened today with Mr. Theokratis. He would like to believe that he could never let a thing like that get by him, that Karen was truly careless last night—but he knows that in fact he could easily let a great many things get by him. . . .

He, like many of the other house staff, believes that the training he is going through is necessary and irreplaceable. You cannot learn to be a doctor if you are not left alone to care for patients. But like many of the other interns, he sometimes finds himself wondering, especially in the very early hours of the morning, when he has not slept and will not sleep, whether it is actually necessary to be left alone so very tired and so very stressed. . . .

He is not at all pleased to hear about his newest admission. The Burton family is down in the emergency room; their twenty-year-old daughter, Eleanor, is dying of bone cancer, and they have brought her into the hospital because she is suddenly worse. As on so many other hospital admissions, they fear, and maybe also hope a little, that this will be the last one. Eleanor Burton has five volumes of old hospital charts that Phil will have to look at (a less compulsive intern might just glance at the most recent volume), and her family is very used to the hospital; they will not tolerate anything they see as suboptimal care. And in addition, here is this woman, younger than himself, and she is dying of a terrible, horrible disease, one that is on Phil's own personal list of the four or five worst, the shoot-me-if-I-get-like-that diseases, a list maintained by almost all medical personnel.

. . . As he is heading out, he passes Elizabeth, who is writing up her note on Mr. Vargas. He stops . . . and asks her if she would please give Mrs. Pinkerton a dose of Dilantin, an antiseizure medication. The drug is to be given intravenously, through Mrs. Pinkerton's line, and the nurses are not allowed to give IV drugs, and it is time for the dose, and Phil cannot stay to give it. He reminds Elizabeth that Dilantin has to be given very slowly, taking the patient's blood pressure at intervals while it is being given, since it can cause a sudden drop in pressure.

Mrs. Pinkerton is not actually one of the patients Elizabeth has been following, though of course she knows about her, and she knows her husband; everyone on the ward knows Mr. Pinkerton, with his gifts of cake and flowers, his embarrassing gratitude when after all they cannot make his wife better. Elizabeth has never given any Dilantin to anyone before, but the nurse helps her draw up the correct dose and warns her once again about giving it slowly and checking the blood pressure. Elizabeth does as she is told, but, to her horror, when she checks the pressure after the third tiny increment of drug, the pressure is way down. She grabs the phone by the bed and pages Phil Maxwell, tells him what is happening, and asks him to come right away.

"Okay, calm down," Phil says. "She's DNR anyway, isn't she?"

Mr. Pinkerton had been persuaded, though he was quite reluctant to agree, that it would be madness to subject his wife to cardiopulmonary resuscitation, to a mechanical ventilator, to electric shocks to the heart. Still, Elizabeth is not prepared to see her injection of Dilantin as a mercy killing.

"Come up here," she says to Phil with a certain amount of fury in her voice. She can just imagine herself facing Mr. Pinkerton tomorrow, after injecting the Dilantin too fast and killing his wife.

So Phil comes up, Mrs. Pinkerton gets fluid and medications, her blood pressure comes back up, and she will be as alive tomorrow as she was today. Elizabeth, who is trembling from having almost killed someone, goes back to finish writing her note on Mr. Vargas, telling herself over and over that she had injected the Dilantin just as slowly as she was supposed to, there had been no way to prevent the drop in blood pressure. And there is no way to know, of course, whether she in fact pushed the drug a little too fast, whether the dose she drew up with the nurse was wrong, or whether it is just that this very weak, very sick lady has many reasons for a drop in blood pressure. It is also true that the legal status of medical students in the hospital is very unclear. Are they actually allowed to give IV drugs? Who is liable for their errors? Medical students sometimes end up doing things they aren't sure they're supposed to do simply because they are needed, the intern is frantically busy, the patient is sick. . . .

The night goes on. Mr. Vargas, who is fundamentally healthy, begins feeling much better after only a few hours of intravenous fluids. Mr. Wissel wakes up and becomes first lucid, and then somewhat deranged, shouting obscenities at the nurses. They have a standing order for tranquilizers on him, since this has happened before, and they medicate him back into his dreams. Eleanor Burton is fighting her last battle, and her parents, veterans of many stays in this hospital, are sitting in her room, though visiting hours are of course long over; the nurses know them well, and everyone feels they are entitled to be there. Up in the intensive care unit, Mr. Theokratis suffers yet another painless heart attack; this time, because he is so thoroughly monitored, everyone knows exactly what is going on, but they feel a little less superior to John McGonigle and his team, since even with all their elaborate monitoring equipment, they were unable to prevent this. Mrs. Pinkerton stares up at the ceiling, seeing nothing. And Mrs. Ropers, the woman with the liver, gets a fever.

. . . Tired as he is, Phil wants to give some thought to her liver, not the kind of cursory nonsense that went on in rounds. Phil feels that Dr. Black is allowing John McGonigle to get away with altogether too much at attending rounds; Godzilla needs to be kept in hand. This silliness about betting, for example—this would have been an excellent teaching case if Godzilla hadn't sidetracked everyone with his nonsense. It's a fascinating diagnostic question, especially in this young woman who doesn't really fit the profile for any of the malignancies. If Phil had time, he would like to read through her chart carefully, do a complete physical exam himself. But he doesn't have time, of course. And now she has a fever. He thinks about possible causes for fever, all the obvious infections, the fever mysteriously associated with malignancy—tumor fever. Then he goes back to his notes. He is still sitting at the nurses' station, writing, when John McGonigle arrives the next morning for work rounds.

On Sunday, the attending does not come in. Work rounds are quickly over, and Phil gets to go home almost immediately. John also sends Elizabeth home early; by tradition, those who are on call Saturday night get some of Sunday off. John McGonigle will manage the ward alone for that day and night.

The day is comparatively quiet, a few new admissions, none of them terribly sick. Mrs. Ropers continues to run a temperature whenever she doesn't get her Tylenol, and John is unable to find a source of infection, so he doesn't have anything to treat. Mr. Russo does not have to be intubated after all, which John views as a personal triumph; he doesn't want to lose any more patients to the intensive care unit. When he runs into the unit team, he teases them without mercy for letting Mr. Theokratis have another MI.

. . . Mrs. Pinkerton stays at her usual level, Mr. Vargas is quickly getting better. There may never be a clear answer to what caused Mr. Vargas's diarrhea; something may grow on stool culture, or it may not. In any case, John speaks only enough Spanish to conduct a very basic physical exam (*"Respire profundo!"*—Breathe deeply), so he doesn't spend any time talking to Mr. Vargas. Or to Mrs. Pinkerton, who of course doesn't talk, or to Mr. Pinkerton, who is always trying to engage him in deeply respectful conversation. Or with Eleanor Burton, a clear and obvious goner.

And now Mr. Wissel, another gorked-out old gomer. The nurses have come to tell John that Mr. Wissel is complaining again, pains in his head, pains in his stomach, his children never come to visit him. They want to know if John would give him a stronger tranquilizer, which John does. Mr. Wissel settles down uneasily. John also begins to feel uneasy about this a little while later; he recalls hearing it mentioned on rounds that Mr. Wissel has been complaining of stomach pains on and off for a couple of days. Maybe just as well to have a better look at him.

Unfortunately, between Mr. Wissel's mental state and the heavy load of tranquilizers and sedatives, it's hard for John to be sure about the abdominal exam—does this hurt? does this hurt? how about if I press here? He spends a long time going over Mr. Wissel's abdomen, and finally satisfies himself that it does in fact feel suspicious. So John calls for an emergency X ray, which also looks suspicious. He is angry at himself for medicating the patient without properly examining him, and he elects to blame this on the nurses, who he feels did not keep him properly informed. He gives Mr. Wissel's nurse a short and unpleasant lecture, the gist of which is, you may have killed this patient. The nurse, who has been a nurse for almost fifteen times as long as John has been a doctor, is not unduly upset by this; John is a notorious jerk when it comes to dealing with nurses. . . .

John's mood has not improved as he calls in the surgeons, announces to them, this is one of the guys you screwed up but good, and now he has intestinal obstruction, so you damn well better cure it.

The surgeons, though they agree that it looks like obstruction, are very reluctant to operate, pointing out that Mr. Wissel is very debilitated and that his mental function is hardly what you would call intact.

Suddenly John McGonigle is in a fury. "Now, listen to me," he almost shouts at the surgeons. "This guy *walked* into this hospital. Do you hear me, he walked in, he was okay except for some little plumbing problem, and then the asshole surgeons got hold of him and since then it's been urinary tract infection and wound infection and pneumonia and bedsores and all the rest, and you can goddam well take him to surgery and try to help him out." John rather enjoys a good fit of anger;

he has never been particularly interested in Mr. Wissel before. . . .

John is impatient with paperwork, and when he sends down a tube of Mr. Wissel's blood to the blood bank so that they can match it with some blood to transfuse during surgery, he neglects to stamp up all the proper forms and labels that have to go to the blood bank. A surgeon calls, an hour later, to tell John rather gleefully that the blood bank has thrown away the improperly labeled tube and John will have to draw more blood. The blood bank is extremely picky about this, since giving someone blood that was meant for another patient could easily be fatal; unless all the stamps and identification numbers are there, no blood is matched. Cursing, John draws more blood, then asks a nurse to stamp and label the tube. The nurses do not generally like John, who is none too polite with them, but they are on his side in the matter of Mr. Wissel, whom they rather like, so no one minds helping out with the blood.

After that, it's a quiet night, no new admissions after eleven o'clock; John writes up short notes (no one is going to criticize *him*, after all) and gets a reasonable amount of sleep.

On Monday morning, just as work rounds are beginning, Eleanor Burton dies. Phil Maxwell, the intern who admitted her, finds himself awkwardly trying to comfort her parents, who are torn between relief that her miseries are over, and the grief they are finally letting out about her entire illness.

"Listen," says John McGonigle, "we've gotta start rounds. Call up their usual doc, Shlepperman, and get him over here. He's the one they need to see."

Phil Maxwell, who is, after all, from the Midwest, begins paging through the hospital phone book, looking for Shlepperman. Elizabeth waits until John is out of hearing, and then suggests, "I think the name is actually Klepperman." Phil finds the name, pages Dr. Klepperman, grateful that he doesn't have to go back in to the Burtons himself.

The week has begun, and morning rounds are brisk and efficient. Matthew Baxter is eager to get to work on establishing the diagnosis on Mrs. Ropers. Karen Newton, knowing she is on call today, has the wound-up,

tensed look of someone who is prepared not to relax for thirty-six hours. John McGonigle leads them all rapidly through the corridors, demonstrating his idea of how things ought to be done: see how smoothly things go when *I'm* on call? Phil Maxwell and Elizabeth are happy in the position of people with a good night's sleep behind them and the prospect of another tonight; true only one day out of every three.

Mr. Wissel is in the recovery room, after his surgery. His condition is tenuous. Mrs. Pinkerton is staring at the ceiling. Her condition is stable. Mr. Vargas is almost completely better, even feeling a little hungry today. Mr. Russo is also much better, moving steadily toward leaving the hospital; he will not stay out for long, of course, but he looks forward to going home. Mr. Theokratis, up in the unit, is doing amazingly well; he still refuses to believe he had even one heart attack, and he laughs at the doctors when they try to tell him that he will have to take special care of his heart from now on. Eleanor Burton is dead; her medical history is resolved, and her story is ended. And Mrs. Ropers is lying in bed, spiking her mysterious temperatures, with her mysterious big liver. Her medical history is only beginning.

Further Reading

Lisa Belkin. 1993. *First, Do No Harm*. New York: Fawcet Crest.

Renee C. Fox. 1957. "Training for Uncertainty." *The Student Physician: Introductory Studies in the Sociology of Medical Education*, edited by R. Merton, G. Reader, and P. Kendall. pp. 207-241. Cambridge: Harvard University Press.

Melvin Konner. 1987. *Becoming a Doctor: A Journey of Initiation in Medical School*. New York: Viking.

Discussion Questions

1. How does hierarchy affect the responsibilities and decision making of health care workers?

2. Give a specific example from Klass' account of how medical students, interns, and residents deal with uncertainty in medical diagnosis and treatment.

3. Describe some of the ways that work hierarchy and uncertainty affect patient care.

14

Never Enough Time: How Medical Residents Manage a Scarce Resource

William C. Yoels
Jeffrey Michael Clair

Time: a valuable medical resource. Significant to patients in how their physicians manage health care. Important to medical residents and physicians in their control over medical work. Medical residents seldom feel a sense of control over their work schedule. Its parameters are determined by patient illness and organized principally by nurses or medical superiors. William Yoels and Jeffrey Clair discuss how medical residents learn to manage time during their residency training. In previous readings, you have witnessed the significance of time in chronically ill individuals' definitions of self. During training, the element of time affects residents' views of patients, their treatment of patients, and their relations with coworkers. It forces residents to doctor together, sharing patients and their treatments. Time constraints often pit the requirements and desires of residents against the needs and wishes of patients. As medical care changes under systems of managed care and other forms of organization, time becomes a critical element for both treatment of patients and organizational finance. Learning to take less time has always been a central focus of resident subculture; the skill renders control over work.

. . . This article focuses on the management of time, a scarce resource. We report how medical residents in an outpatient clinic experience the time contingencies of their work setting, particularly, how they seek to control the work process. We analyze how residents learn about time management over the course of their residency and how they seek to control time when conducting examinations, dealing with other residents, and responding to their appointment schedules. Finally, we examine time as both a subjective experience and an axis of social organization. . . .

Setting and Method

The qualitative data presented below are part of a larger study of doctor-new patient encounters. They were generated during a twenty-two month period, primarily through field observations. At times they were supplemented by our participation in doctor-patient medical encounters and interviews with physicians treating adult patients in an ambulatory medical resident clinic housed in a Division of General Internal Medicine at a major university medical center.

The patients at this clinic were primarily non-White (80%) and female (55%). Patients' ages ranged from 20 to 95, with a mean age of 57.3 years and a standard deviation of 19.6. The clinic patient population was not representative of the general population in terms of socioeconomic status (SES), being disproportionately of lower income and education. More specifically, the median per capita annual household income was roughly $3,300 and the mean years of education was 9.3, with over 60% of the population having less than a high school diploma. Most of this population was uninsured or on Medicaid.

Throughout the study period, we worked with 150 house staff, that is, about 50 postgraduate year 1s (PGY1s), 50 PGY2s, and 50 PGY3s, as well as 24 different attendings (supervising physicians). Essentially, every medical resident at some point throughout the year served as a house staff physician in the clinic.

The resident house staff in the clinic were primarily male (76%) and White (89%), with most in the traditional (66%) as opposed to a primary care (34%) training track program. Primary care resident training involved more emphasis on community preceptorships, exposure to a greater variety of medical disciplines, and result in more outpatient rather than inpatient training, although even here, the actual number of hours per year spent in outpatient care was still a very small portion of the total number of hours worked. Physician age in this clinic was a virtual constant with 84 of the physicians between 26 and 30.

In this clinic, appointments were scheduled 48 weeks of each year, with nine half-day clinics each week. During the study period, we were able to cover approximately half of the scheduled clinics. During each day of clinical coverage, all patient appointments were stratified by a new patient status. Patients were considered new if it was their first time to the clinic or, for those who had been to the clinic before, it was their first time meeting the doctor, as in the case of a PGY1 taking over a patient from a recently departed PGY3. All new patients were entered into a sampling universe and the first new patient who kept a scheduled appointment was approached for enrollment into the study.

Entering a patient into this study and following them through their visit involved approximately 2 hours. Our remaining 2 hours or so were spent hanging around with physicians and nurses between their various duties at the nursing station and in the physician conference room. We actually sat in on 173 doctor-patient encounters involving 88 different residents. Approximately 25% of the residents were randomly selected for in-depth interviews, covering broader issues of their residency experience. . . .

We wanted to be just another part of the setting and wore white lab coats with our names and titles indicated to help us to blend in. As our relationships became well established, our obvious strategy was to be purely observers and as unobtrusive as possible. The possibility of remaining detached, however, was made problematic by physicians, patients, caregivers, and at times, oneself. As far as the health care and service providers were concerned, it was implicit that we were sympathetic to their concerns, otherwise we would not be in the clinic for such an extended period of time. This is further evidenced by the fact that we spent many hours around the nursing station, joining doctors during medical encounters, delivering a message to a doctor, helping a nurse locate someone, answering an occasional telephone, sitting around in the conference room, sharing food, coffee, opinions, and a reciprocal obligation to pass time in general. . . .

Managing a Scarce Resource

As a humanly created object, time can be interpreted in a variety of ways related to the usages to which it will be put (as the pragmatists well knew, see Blumer 1969; Mead 1932,1934; Shalin 1992). Controlling time was an ongoing concern evidenced in many ways as residents responded to their work setting. The desire for free time, or more exactly, time that one controls rather than is controlled by, was a central dimension of the residents' subculture. In the following section, we examine how residents were socialized to deal with time. Next, we focus on the organizational context of the clinic and how the issue of patients' waiting time operated as a differentiating medium for clinic personnel. Finally, we discuss how residents managed time while conducting examinations, dealing with other residents, and manipulating the appointments schedule.

Learning to Take Less Time

Interviews with residents indicate structurally distinctive responses to time as they progressed through the residency program, although we should note here that our comparisons are cross-sectional rather than longitudinal in nature. The question of how much time is an appropriate amount to spend with patients is an important dilemma first-year interns experience. They know, of course, that in terms of ideal practice, the answer should be "as long as is required." Given the reality of the time constraints imposed by 70- to 100-hour workweeks, however, they soon learned that this was an inappropriate answer in terms of organizational expectations. One PGY1 cogently remarked on this issue:

> Today we had a lecture on malpractice. And they said that one of the main reasons that people sued wasn't because they were maligned, or that something went wrong, or there was negligence. It was more because they were angry at the doctor, and their chief complaint was that the doctor didn't spend enough time with them and explain things to them. And if they train us to be just as efficient as possible, so we can get out at 5:00 . . . well then they're training us to . . . they're setting us up for malpractice in the future, I think.

This same intern also commented about the rushed pace of work by noting that:

> I think I felt less so until they told me they thought I was staying too late. And then when I started realizing that, yeah, I probably shouldn't be staying 'til 8:00 or 10:00 every night, especially on a regular night, and knowing that I'd have to be on call the next night or in a couple nights . . . and, so then I started paying attention, like oh God, this took 5 minutes, this took 10 minutes.

Interestingly, this comment also reflected the dynamics of collegial mentorship wherein managing scarce time was a vehicle through which they (i.e., attending physicians, PGY2s, and PGY3s) provided suggestions on how interns should conduct themselves. We will elaborate on this issue in a later section of the article. We want to note here, however, that such suggestions provided an anticipatory socialization foundation for interns.

Another intern also expressed anticipations of future residency experiences involving time management by stating:

> I think in your intern year, because you're like the worker . . . you do the work, and the residents supervise. So, you know, you're rushed. . . . You're rushed a lot . . . whereas probably in the second and third year, I don't think it's gonna be that bad.

One adjustment interns learned to make was to work more quickly. In the words of another PGY1, to "really push yourself to be fast and get things done and not spend a whole lot of extra time just talking to people or something . . . Or else you'd end up being here until 9 at night or something."

Interns were concerned with time available for doing everything, such as examining patients, dictating charts, writing up the orders for medications, and so on. During that first year they learned that "there's always . . . more to do in a given day . . . than there's hours for it if you just go at a normal pace." In response to such pressures, interns tried to "knock off little pieces of it at the time. And, uh, it doesn't do anybody any good to get all stressed about it."

The crucial break in the residency occurred between the first year as an intern and the last 2 years of residency. The internship involved mandatory supervision by attending physicians, which was an optional form of consultation during the last 2 years. Although PGY2s had more autonomy than did interns, they still worked closely with attending physicians. In addition, PGY2s and 3s were responsible for monitoring the work of other team members such as interns and medical students under their supervision. PGY2s, as one resident noted, "have a lot more autonomy, and technically the attendings are supposed to give you a little more looser reign, in terms of decisions in patient care."

By the second year, time pressures had become so much a part of the taken-for-granted, "background expectations," that, according to one PGY2, they could be seen as simply

> part of being a doctor. I think that we're just very limited a lot of times. I mean . . . it's become so much a part of my routine that I don't even think about it any more that we're probably kind of pressed for time.

Patient care loads in the second and third years led residents to a much more selective attentiveness to time constraints:

> As a resident you have more patient responsibilities but you don't follow them in quite the detail as when you're an intern. . . . As a resident, you have interns working for you who are following the patients. And you kind of . . . you watch the big picture. You try to pay attention to details but you can't do it to the same

depth as the interns. Because, you know, you may have two interns working for you and each one has 7 patients. And so, and then . . . you're responsible for all 14 of those patients. But, you have interns working under you and carrying out plans. And you have to monitor them. But you probably can't watch the patients as closely as the intern does because you have twice as many patients. (PGY2)

The phrase, "you watch the big picture," captures aspects of residents' changing orientation to time over the residency. Through their felt pressures to do everything, interns were so caught up in the trees, the thick details of medical care, that they lost sight of the forest, they had not yet developed the ability to look for patterns or interrelationships between things. Nor had they developed the ability confidently to differentiate between what was important and unimportant. They were so immersed in the challenge of working fast to coordinate diverse and innumerable tasks that they had not yet figured out the rhythm of medical work, the underlying beat, if you will, orchestrating the tempo of the individual steps or activities (Fine 1990; Snow and Brissett 1986). In the second and third years they learned to grasp the underlying rhythm, or structure of residency tasks, thereby modulating the speed or tempo of their work through more efficient organization. Such an adjustment involved a process of what we would call *mental targeting*, in which they learned not only to work quickly but in a more focused, integrative manner as well. In this regard, a PGY3 noted that

the main thing I try to remember—I guess, advice for other people is . . . that sometimes when people are particularly rushed, they become more inefficient instead of what they need to do, is be more efficient. I guess my technique is to try to just remember to deal with only one thing at a time. To try to maybe make a list mentally or even on paper of what things I have to do. And then just write them in the order that they need to be done, with the most pressing things first and then uh—and then the other, you know, kind of rank them and get to things as I'm able to do in that manner.

Perhaps the most critical distinction between PGY1s, PGY2s, and PGY3s involved the acknowledgment by the latter that they did not have the time to learn everything. At this point, they had also achieved a kind of humility about the interrelationships between time available, diagnostic uncertainty, and the upper limits of medical knowledge. Their interest had shifted from "doing everything" to learning as much as possible within those parameters. As one PGY3 cogently stated:

On my service right now, I probably have 15 patients, and you know, maybe half of them I know what they have . . . maybe a quarter of those I'm actively pursuing an answer, the other quarter have been pursued as far as we can pursue them. We just don't know any more. . . . So, I think there a lot of unknowns in medicine and you work real hard. But, to me there's nothing better. To me it's the most fascinating thing in the world. You could spend 12 hours a day reading a textbook and never learn everything.

As PGY2s and 3s moved through the residency program, the interns' dilemma of how much time to spend with patients ceased to be an issue of major concern. In this regard, a PGY3 noted a transformation in his attitudes toward patients:

I think I've gone through kind of a cycle of—depending on your immediate level of tiredness and whether or not you've had conflict with the patient—I think that you go through a period of where you feel like there's an adversarial relationship between yourself and the patient where, you know, the patient's just one more thing piled on for you to do. And, uh, and their complaints, you know, become a problem. You don't wanna, you know, you don't wanna deal with 'em. You don't like to hear, you know, the headaches and . . . all the little complaints. And then I think . . . at least as I've come around, I kind of just, I don't know, I just kind of accept that as the way—the way life is. . . . That's part of being a doctor, and that, you know, dealing with the complaint is, uh, necessary.

It would seem that residents saw patients as the enemy prior to realizing that the ability to control the amount of time spent with the patient was what power was all about. By their third year they had reached a deeper understanding of this important point. As we will see in our discussion of how residents dealt with the appointments, schedules, and examinations, controlling time spent with patients was critical for generating free time for oneself within the limits of the residency program.

It would be a mistake, however, to see this professional socialization process as a linear one with residents progressing from feeling rushed and out of control to feeling *in* control of time. Rather, residents came to accept scarce time as a given, yet they were amenable to personal modification within the structural constraints of the residency program.

Deflecting Time Complaints onto Nurses

The issue of patients waiting to see residents beyond what the nurses saw as reasonable waiting times was a source of organizational conflict between nurses and residents. In their efforts to carve out "time slices" (Fine 1990) for themselves, residents sometimes attended to other things prior to seeing waiting patients. Sometimes they did other things while waiting for tests to be run or X-rays to be taken instead of seeing waiting patients. From the nurses' point of view, doctors who rushed through exams or made patients wait too long were not practicing good health care, and they often discussed such doctors among themselves in very negative terms.

When a nurse was asked if patients ever complained about time spent waiting for residents, she responded that "they do to the nurses all the time." She explained that she "tells them to tell the doctors, but they never do." Nurses, then, played a very interesting role in clinic social structure. As the first persons to check-in and examine the patients through recording their weights and taking blood pressure readings, they functioned as a kind of safety-valve, siphoning off patient anger before it ever got to the point of exploding at the residents. Of course, the status and power differentials between these low-income, minority patients and residents made the nurses a much safer and less risky target for displaying such anger. The end result,

however, was the exacerbation of a sense of annoyance on the part of the nurses toward the residents. In one vivid illustration of this phenomenon, two nurses were discussing a patient who was just seen by a PGY3:

> The patient told the resident that he [the patient] had not been waiting long; in fact, according to one of the nurses, the patient told the resident that he had just driven up to the clinic. The nurse takes real offense at this and says something to the effect that "the patient doesn't know what he's talking about because he's been here for quite some time and they [the nurses] couldn't locate the resident." The other nurse reponds by saying that the patient was just trying to be cordial and let the resident off the hook by acting like he's not angry about having to wait a long time. The first nurse replies by saying that "he ain't gonna get off the hook, cause that's how we work around here," meaning we tell it like it is, especially when patients are waiting a long time. She adds once again that the patient doesn't know what he's talking about. (Fieldnotes)

Patients' reluctance to vent their anger about time delays directly at residents was an instance of a larger posture of differential deference toward doctors compared to nurses. Issues of power, authority, and expertise, as defined by patients, were clearly at play here (see also Schwartz 1975). The end result was an additional source of frustration for nurses and an intensified sense of relative deprivation vis-à-vis doctors. One form this took was an annoyance on the nurses' part at occasionally having to spend considerable time—in one instance, 30 minutes—unsuccessfully cajoling patients to do something. Shortly thereafter, she claimed, the resident entered, asked the patient to do the same thing, and the patient immediately complied!

Controlling Examination Time

Trying to carve out some time slices confronted residents with a central dilemma of having to present themselves to patients as caring and interested in their problems, which they generally were. On many occasions, however, they would have preferred to be elsewhere, such as on the wards, doing more challenging, interesting work, or perhaps getting relief from 70-hour workweeks by relaxing in the clinic's conference room or having collegial conversation at the nurses station. This dilemma was greatly reduced by the fact that patients, especially the indigent patients seen here, rarely picked up on the subtler cues of interaction with doctors and did not possess the knowledge to know whether medical corners were being cut. Although overall, patient satisfaction with clinic residents, as expressed in our postencounter interviews, was quite high, time was often associated with instances of expressed patient dissatisfaction. When patients felt that they were being rushed, or that not enough time had been spent on their problem, they were likely to voice that concern.

In terms of doctors examining patients, engaging in what Strauss et al. (1985) have called *body work*, it is important to recall Thompson's (1984) cogent remark that "the interview is the one thing which distinguishes medicine from veterinary surgery. Despite being the cornerstone of medical practice, it is often seen as a tiresome interface between the doctor and the disease" (p. 87). Moreover, observers such as Waitzkin (1991) have documented through detailed conversational analyses of doctor-patient transcripts how the psychological, emotional, and social features of patients' lives are by-passed or marginalized as a result of the reigning biomedical diagnostic model's emphasis on physically based, bodily symptoms. Waitzkin (1991) failed to emphasize, however, the extent to which the doctor's sense of time as a scarce resource also is clearly operant here. Part of the seductive appeal of the biomedical model for its practitioners, we would argue, is the way it maximizes physician control over the time agenda by immediately orienting discussion to issues that are regulated by physicians in their role as technical experts. Physicians are thus in a position to establish and, more importantly, control the social rhythm of the encounter (Fine 1990).

Feeling pressured, residents focused on what is most easily decipherable, controllable, and amenable to management—that is, bodily symptoms. Moving into areas of greater causal uncertainty, such as the psychosocial realm, struck residents as an area where they felt lacking in both training and diagnostic competence. In addition, from the residents' perspective, exploring such patient *life worlds* (Mishler 1984), also ran the risk of opening the exam up to patient involvement in an almost unbounded manner. Although humanistic approaches to medicine strongly encourage doctors to do just that (see, e.g., American Board of Internal Medicine 1991; Hendrie and Lloyd 1991), such recommendations often pose serious challenges to doctors' abilities to control the time agenda of the examination.

Few of the examinations we observed in the clinic over the 2 years involved extended treatments of the psychosocial aspects of patients' lives. One graphic illustration of how this issue was treated concerns the first-time visit of a Vietnam combat veteran:

> The patient has suffered war wounds including major facial disfigurement. Early in the exam the doctor comments on the patient's war wounds and says that he must have taken quite a while to get over that. The patient takes an audible breath, hesitates, and then states that he had to come to terms with it as part of life, reflecting his personal, emotional responses to the event, in short the meanings of the wounds for him. The resident immediately cuts him short by saying, "I meant physically." The examination then proceeded along the rather narrow tracks "constructed" by the biomedical diagnostic model. (Fieldnotes)

During an interview with a PGY3, he was quick to point out that he was aware that the physicians were, in a sense, under siege because of poor communication skills. He stated:

> People say we do the medicine part, but we miss the psychosocial aspects of patient care. People who say that usually aren't physicians. They don't know what we've gone through. They don't know how much time we're spending taking care of the patients. And people who say those things don't realize that I do—think of patients all the time; think of patients when you're driving in—going to work; thinking of patients when you're watch-

ing TV, pondering what's going on. They don't realize that you spend that much time. And they think that you leave medicine at 5:00 and you go home and you lead your own life. And, you just don't do that.

As the previous two quotes suggest, in many ways the control of time also was a proxy variable for limiting the emotional demands on doctors. Patients expect doctors not only to provide physical explanations for their problems, but a lessening of their "disease" and anxiety as well. As one of our colleagues from medicine commented in this regard, "You can't tell a patient that they can't have any more of your emotional life. You can say, however, that 'I don't have any more time.'"

On several occasions, when we approached residents about observing the exam, we were told, "I'd rather you not join me today, I don't have much time." The act of being observed may have led to their feeling obliged to deal with the patient's psychosocial life, which then lengthened the exam time. Many residents considered psychosocial questions peripheral to their technical concerns, even though they fall under the mandates of the American Board of Internal Medicine (1991) and the standards developed by faculty attending physicians in their Division of General Medicine. So, "I don't have much time," then, suggests they would rather not attend to questions they would otherwise feel free to skip if a sociologist were not in the room.

The medical examination, like any social situation, involved persons interpreting what they were experiencing and making judgments about courses of action. This situation presented residents with a host of decisions concerning how much time to devote to particular aspects of the examination format. It involved the patient's statement of their chief complaint, the residents taking a history of the present illness, and the resident's review of the patient's past medical history. The traditional approach also involved obtaining a social history and a family medical history, reviewing the major organ systems, and finally, performing the actual physical examination. Within each of these categories, judg-

ments had to be made continuously about the seriousness of the patient's problem and how much time ought to be devoted to specific sections of the examination. As noted earlier, observers such as Waitzkin (1991) have powerfully documented how the examination format is driven by the biomedical model.

Residents could quickly establish the rhythm of the examination at its inception. By communicating either verbally, through frequent interruptions, or nonverbally, through pauses to look at the medical records for a while without making any eye contact with the patient, they showed how receptive they were to patient input. Such pauses, as Snow and Brissett (1986) have aptly noted, establish the *parameters of action* for social encounters. Moreover, the decision to read the patient's medical record before entering the room and beginning the examination, or to read it while in the presence of the patient, also involved an assessment on the resident's part about saving time by doing it during the examination. Success at controlling the patient's verbal "production line" was a topic which occasioned humorous comments from residents as they talked among themselves:

> Two PGYI s are talking about an attending physician at another hospital who has a reputation for keeping the wards full, which is why one of them is so tired and busy. A PGY2 joins the conversation and they talk about being MOD (medical officer of the day) in another clinic. The PGY2 says that he writes the whole time while the patient is talking and then when the patient is done, he looks up and says "Sorry, I didn't hear what you were saying. I was writing. Here's your prescription." Everyone laughs. Another PGY2 who is mentioned as someone who is especially skilled at such tactics happens to stop by and she adds that "if you let the patients talk, you'll be there the whole day." (Fieldnotes)

In a similar vein, an attending physician was talking with a PGY2 resident about patients in another clinic and all the problems such patients presented:

> The attending says that when you ask them what's bothering them, they go into

a detailed, lengthy discussion of all their problems. She feels like saying that she only has time to deal with one problem and "You've only got 5 minutes, buddy!" (Fieldnotes)

Another PGY2 resident during an interview summed things up this way:

If you let patients and families, they will talk your ear off. A lot of times you just don't want to spend the time, I mean you don't really have the time or your time could be spent more efficiently, so you have to learn how to cut the conversation down. Especially during an admit, I've learned only to get what's important. I know that I have to be sensitive and be objective enough to make sure I don't overlook something critical, but for the most part, a lot of what they have to say is irrelevant.

One area of the examination in particular, the actual physical examination, presented a number of opportunities for controlling the length of the exam. The issue of patients' undressing, for example, could be done in a number of ways ranging from the most time-consuming to least: The resident could leave the room while the patient completely undressed and donned a gown (although even here, the resident could still use that time to attend to other business while waiting for the patient); the patient could undress in front of the resident while laying on the examining table under a sheet; the patient might only remove part of his or her clothing and, if body modesty was an issue, the exposed part being covered with a sheet; and finally, the patient could be examined with his or her clothing on, while listening to the lungs, for example, through his or her clothing. Of course, variations depending on the urgency of the patient's condition were also central here, but the residents' time agenda and sense of being rushed was at times at play as well.

The ultimate way in which residents responded to the issue of scarce time with regard to patients could be seen in their efforts to make themselves scarce. Part of learning the ropes as a resident involved knowing when and when not to be somewhere. An attending physician informed a PGY1 just starting the residency that the key to figuring

out the hospital is to "make yourself scarce around 6 p.m., after rounds, because it gets real hectic then."

Another more subtle tactic was devised by a PGY3 who never wore his white lab coat in the outpatient clinic. Instead he wore a shirt and tie with his stethoscope draped around his neck, a clear symbolic announcement that he was still a doctor despite the absence of the lab coat. This costume as a strategy for making oneself scarce is captured in the following incident taken from fieldnotes:

A PGY1 received a call in the outpatient clinic from one of his patients at another hospital, I couldn't tell which. He got off the phone and complained to the PGY3 [referred to above] about his patients calling him all the time. The PGY3 looked at him in mock disbelief and asked, "How do they know your name?" (Fieldnotes)

Because this PGY3 never wore his lab coat, it made it more difficult for his patients to remember his name.

Using Other Residents for Time Shortcuts

Time also operated as an object that both integrated and differentiated clinic personnel. It bonded residents through their mutual empathy over common concerns about schedules and appointments. Residents' collective responses to time constraints also enhanced their doctoring together (Freidson 1975), their sharing of knowledge and tasks. It also operated as a differentiating medium by placing residents in conflict with the nurse coordinator over scheduling issues. Time patients spent waiting to see residents in the clinic pitted nurses against doctors, as nurses adopted a sympathetic posture vis-á-vis patients.

The integrative dimensions of time as a factor promoting resident bonding could be seen in the frequent comments about not having enough time to read medical journal articles or to attend various on-campus medical conferences. As a result, residents frequently consulted one another about information presented in such sources. On occasion, residents who were friendly with one another offered to switch schedules based on conflicts over weekend, holiday, and vacation assignments. Work also was informally redistributed within the clinic by residents offering to share patient loads with one another. In one instance, a PGY3 told the nurse coordinator that he "feels real bad about having so few patients today" whereas Dr. Kranther (a friend of his) had so many. He told her that he was willing to take some of the other resident's walk-in patients.

Other instances of doctoring together often involved the situation of mentoring, where lower level residents asked more advanced ones for advice about what procedures to perform, what drugs to prescribe, and so on.

> In one instance a PGY1 asks a PGY3 for advice about which tests to run on a female patient, something having to do with ovaries and secretions. He tells the PGY3 that he meant to read a general medicine article on it, but didn't have the time. (Fieldnotes)

> During an interview a PGY2 expresses this practice stating: "You know, reading the literature is clearly the best way to go about learning things. But, at this point, I just haven't had time to really sit down and look things up in as much detail as I would like." Whereas talking to attendings and talking to residents it is taken care of.

Asking other residents for advice was thus a much quicker way of gathering information compared to reading journal articles (especially ones that must be read in the library) or displaying a lack of knowledge to an attending physician. Exchanges such as these also reinforced the status of higher level residents as experts vis-á-vis lower ranking ones, while simultaneously promoting a mutually shared sense of membership in the resident subculture.

Manipulating the Time Schedule

Other aspects of residents' responses to scarce time could be seen in the backstage (Goffman 1959; Scott 1990) regions of the clinic, off-limits to patients, where they dealt with the externally imposed conditions related to the scheduling of appointments. Scheduling issues were among the most central of residents' concerns. This issue often created conflicts with the clinic's nurse coor-

dinator, who was responsible for administering the schedules created by the university's central appointments office. She was in an awkward situation of *status inconsistency* because she occupied a position of much lower societal prestige than the residents but had final say over scheduling.

> In a conversation about scheduling issues, 3 PGY3s are real agitated that they are never consulted about their schedules. One PGY3 says that one of the other residents should take it up with the nurse coordinator. That resident responds by saying that he did that last week and she told him to "suck it up." (Fieldnotes)

The nurse coordinator occupied a major stress point in the clinic's social structure. She had to serve as liaison between the clinic's secretary, four other clinic nurses, residents, attending physicians, a lab technician, admitting receptionists in the front office, and patients. If any problems developed in the system, the proverbial buck stopped at her desk.

On first entering the outpatient clinic, the residents immediately checked out the appointment schedule. Numerous comments would be made about whether the schedule was heavy or light. More importantly, patient cancellations could be the occasion for the expression of pleasure, as witnessed by the following fieldnote excerpt:

> A PGY1 arrives and looking at his appointment sheet immediately lets out a cry of joy. He says something like "Great." A PGY2 is nearby and the PGY1 says to him, "Give me five." They slap each other's raised hand, much like a football player after scoring a touchdown! As he walks away, the PGY2 asks him what's going on and the PGY1 says, "My first appointment canceled."

This incident nicely captures an ongoing attitude of residents, also described in detail by Mizrahi (1986). Such a practice maximized residents' control of their own time and also freed them from what they saw as rather routine, unchallenging work, especially in contrast to the more dramatic features of acute care experienced on the inpatient hospital wards. We should indicate here that enthusiastic comments about patient cancellations were typically made about patients in general, rather than about specific patients. Even with heavy patient loads and time constraints, residents generally treated patients in humane, respectful ways. As we described earlier, however, residents' time concerns made themselves felt in a variety of subtle ways vis-á-vis patient care.

An additional dilemma faced by residents was the awareness that they must see patients to learn medicine by actually doing it. The outpatient clinic, however, often became a place where residents hoped for time, either for themselves or to better handle ward-related work. One resident was even candid enough to admit that "sometimes you see patients as the enemy the first year . . . just because it's taking up all of your time."

Residents displayed ambivalence about this conflict between free time for themselves and the desire to both see and give quality care for outpatients. In talking to a PGY3 about a patient who was scheduled at 9:40 a.m. but still hadn't arrived by 10:20 a.m., it was mentioned that his 9:40 did not look like he would show. He responded by saying, "Well, not to sound too jaded, but I hope so."

Humor about patient cancellations was another way to neutralize the ambivalence and tension residents experienced between the cross-pressures of free time for themselves and the desire to present a self that cared about patients. Jokes allowed for the distancing of self from the possibly socially unacceptable sentiment being expressed, by presenting that sentiment in a comical, nonserious way:

A PGY2 enters the clinic and, as he heads to the counter where the appointment sheets are placed, I say to him that I have good news for him. I had placed an envelope on his appointment sheets with some information about our research project. He had not seen the envelope yet nor did he know what I meant by good news. His immediate, instantaneous response to my comment, however, was a joking statement, "You mean none of my patients showed up!" We all laugh. (Fieldnotes)

Additional conflicts occurred as a result of demands imposed by the scheduling of patients, which hindered residents' desires to further their education by attending noontime medical conferences. When medical examinations spilled over into the lunch hour, patients came to be redefined as obstacles to residents' development as doctors, rather than opportunities for the learning of medicine and the practicing of humane patient care.

The desire for free time, or more exactly, time that they control rather than are controlled by, was so deeply rooted in the subculture of residents that in almost 2 years in this clinic we noticed only one occasion where an enthusiastic reference by residents to patients not showing up was treated negatively by another resident. This was a revealing incident because it highlighted the learning dimension of residents' work with patients as well as the important learning taking place between PGY3 and PGY2 residents:

A PGY2 comes in, looks at his appointment sheet, and, glancing at the sheet next to him, says "Why can't that ever happen to me?" I know by now that he's talking about the other resident having lots of cancellations, even though he hasn't said that. A PGY3 is standing nearby and since he can't see what the PGY2 is looking at, he says, "What do you mean?" The PGY2 then says "He's got three cancellations today. Why can't that ever happen to me?" The PGY3 immediately says, "You wouldn't want that to happen. How are you ever going to learn anything? Are you going to go home and read about the patients in the textbook?" The PGY2 is somewhat startled by this response and says, somewhat sheepishly, "Yeah" and lets the conversation drift. I'm real startled by this interchange as well, since it's really the first time that I've heard a resident respond negatively to another resident's positive reactions to appointment cancellations. (Fieldnotes)

Time as a *symbolic construct*, that is, an object that can take on varied meanings depending on the usages to which it will be put, also could be seen in how residents quickly "sized up" an appointment in terms of how long the exam would take. The symbolic importance of patients' medical records was a significant part of such an assessment. The thickness of these records, often referred to as *PTCAs* (positive thick chart anomalies), was often used as a short-hand reference for the time involved in a possibly lengthy examination. In talking with a PGY2 about his workload, for example, he mentioned that he's "so busy that he doesn't have time for the bathroom." He then mentioned that the clinic in another hospital is "really something." When asked for further clarification of what he meant by that phrase, he said that the "medical records are huge" and held up his fingers several inches apart. Another, more graphic, illustration of this point came from our fieldnotes:

> A PGY2, carrying a stack of thick medical records, enters the conference room where residents congregate and also consult with attendings (supervising physicians). One of the attendings looks up in disbelief as if to say, "Am I going to have to discuss this patient with you?" The PGY2 accurately assessing the attending's "headset," jokingly responds by saying something to the effect of "Don't worry, they're not for you." The attending then sighs in relief.

Two features of residents' work in this clinic related to the scheduling of patients were especially salient in understanding their desire to control time. First, there was the issue of the amount of time allocated to new versus returning patients. The university's central appointments office allotted 1 hour for new patients and 20 minutes for returning patients. Residents had some control over when to schedule returning patients, but none over new ones. They felt that it took considerably more than 20 minutes to do a good job with returning patients. As a result, it was easy to feel pressured in such situations, especially when their schedule for that day consisted of numerous returning patients.

New patients, by contrast, although having 1 hour allotted for the examination, presented a dilemma of another sort, namely, the issue of continuity of care. Residents generally wanted to do a good job with patients and they realized that entailed following patients over a considerable period of time. Because

this was a 3-year residency program that was the maximum time residents could spend with any one patient. They were continually frustrated, then, when new patients were scheduled late in their residency program because they knew at the outset that they could spend only a small amount of time with such patients. In fact, we witnessed new patients being assigned to third-year residents as late as April when they are slated to permanently leave the program in late June!

From the residents' point of view, having new patients and the 1 hour allotted for their exams did enable them to carve out chunks of free time if the exam was done quickly. As one PGY2 commented, one reason he liked having new patient appointments was that often he could simply "order an x-ray and send them home with some [pain reliever]." Such time-saving options usually were not possible within the tighter constraints of the 20-minute returning patient exams

Conclusion

We have examined how time operates as a significant object in the lives of residents working in a university-based outpatient clinic. We discussed how residents differed in their responses to scarce time over the course of the residency by focusing on their efforts to control time when conducting examinations, dealing with other residents, and responding to the scheduling of appointments. Finally, we examined the multidimensional features of time as it affected the social organization of a clinic.

Residents in this clinic experienced considerable ambivalence from the numerous cross-pressures and competing demands on their time. They wanted to learn medicine by actually seeing patients, but wanted time for themselves as well. Moreover, sometimes clinic patients became an obstacle to their education by preventing them from attending noon conferences. The pressures and exciting intellectual challenges of acute care work on the hospital wards, coupled with the small number of hours actually spent in outpatient work, made residents far more attentive to the demands of the wards. Having to continuously juggle time demands, they responded by trying to "snatch it" from wherever they could, which at times resulted in examinations conducted in an "express train" mode of operation. Finally, their desire for continuity of care with patients was sometimes frustrated by externally imposed schedules.

An important issue that emerges here concerns the difficulties doctors experience in trying to practice what they see as good medicine under such cross-pressures. Having spent a considerable part of their professional socialization as residents learning how to maneuver around time constraints, on entering private practice, residents find that they still confront structural constraints on their time (see Hassle factor 1991). Their considerably higher income along with the greater ability to choose their own patients and establish continuity of care makes such constraints more bearable.

Expenses connected with maintaining private practices will force physicians to carry high patient loads where they probably will devote little more than 15 minutes or so to the examination, with only about 1 minute, on the average, spent actually giving information to their patients (see Waitzkin 1991, 286). Given such patient loads, patients will likely spend considerable amounts of time waiting in reception areas for appointments to take place, a phenomenon that "often is an unpleasant reminder that as individuals we must play according to other people's rules" (Snow and Brissett 1986, 11). We might speculate that residents will probably progress from hoping that patients "won't show" for outpatient clinic appointments during their residency, to hoping they will show, but not talk too much (i.e., take too much time), once they are in private practice.

As we have noted, through the hegemony of the reigning biomedical model, residents are not trained to devote much time to patients' psychosocial problems, and time constraints reinforce such an avoidance. Research indicates, however, that about 30% of the patients visiting primary care doctors have such problems to an extent worthy of physicians' attention, and as many as 85% have some degree of psychological distress (see Bertakis, Ruter, and Putman 1991). Pa-

tients' high levels of dissatisfaction with the current medical system (see Blendon 1989), along with considerable numbers of Americans seeking nontraditional or "alternative" forms of health care, suggest that many patients experience these structural constraints. These patients conclude that medicine is failing to meet their health care expectations and "vote with their bodies," so to speak, for other options.

Residents' efforts to control scarce time is an issue with broad theoretical implications. Residents here seem much more constrained by external pressures than those interviewed by Finlay et al. (1990) in a Veterans Administration outpatient clinic. It might be argued that in a number of the strategies described here residents are displaying features of the "alienated labor" of the industrial workers so ably described by Blauner (1964). Time is a key aspect of this phenomenon:

> Basic to the feeling-tone of alienated labor is a heightened awareness of time. Instead of losing himself in a timeless present, the alienated actor is detached and preoccupied with thoughts and images of a future time period when the work will be over and done with. This differs, of course, from the craftsmen's image of the future appearance of his product, which serves as a model for his immersion in the present. (p. 155)

To the extent that residents experience their work in the outpatient clinic in such terms, they resemble workers manning an automobile assembly line or running a machine in a textile plant. The imposition of externally controlled schedules is a common ingredient in all these settings, although residents differ greatly from industrial workers in their ability more directly to control the tempo of the *machine*, which in this case might be viewed metaphorically as the *conveyor belt* of scheduled patient appointments. In response to such restrictive environments, as sociology would lead us to expect, industrial workers have created alternative definitions of the workplace in which they collectively, informally establish a restriction of output quotas (see Ditton 1979; Pavalko 1988; Roy 1959). It is important, then, that the more visible trappings of medical residents' professional status not blind us to the more practical, work-related features of their lives over which they continuously strive to gain control, much like workers everywhere.

References

American Board of Internal Medicine. 1991. *Guide to the awareness and evaluation of humanistic qualities in the internist, 1991-1995.* Philadelphia: American Board of Internal Medicine.

Bertakis, K., D. Ruter. and S. Putman. 1991. The relationship of physician medical interview style to patient satisfaction. *Journal of Family Practice* 32:175-81.

Blauner, R. 1964. *Alienation and freedom.* Chicago: University of Chicago Press.

Blendon, R. 1989. Three systems: A comparative survey. *Health Management Quarterly* 11:2-10.

Blumer, H. 1969. *Symbolic interactionism.* Englewood Cliffs, NJ: Prentice-Hall.

Ditton, J. 1979. Baking time. *Sociological Review* 27:157-67.

Fine, G. 1990. Organizational time: Temporal demands and the experience of work in restaurant kitchens. *Social Forces* 69:95-114.

Finlay, W., E. Mutran, R. Zeitler, and C. Randall. 1990. Queues and care: How medical residents organize their work in a busy clinic. *Journal of Health and Social Behavior* 31:292-305.

Freidson, E. 1975. *Doctoring together.* New York: Elsevier-Holland.

Goffman, E. 1959. *The presentation of self in everyday life.* New York: Anchor.

Hassle factor survey: Your answers. 1991. Editorial. *MD Magazine,* May, pp. 57-60.

Hendrie, H., and C. Lloyd, eds. 1991. *Educating competent and humane physicians.* Bloomington: Indiana University Press.

Mead, G. 1932. *Philosophy of the present.* Chicago: University of Chicago Press.

———. 1934. *Mind, self, and society.* Chicago: University of Chicago Press.

Mishler, E. 1984. *The discourse of medicine.* Norwood, NJ: Ablex.

Mizrahi, T. 1986. *Getting rid of patients.* New Brunswick, NJ: Rutgers University Press.

Pavalko. R. 1988. *Sociology of occupations and professions.* Itasca, IL: F E. Peacock.

Roy, D. 1959. Banana time: Job satisfaction and informal interaction. *Human Organization* 18:427-42.

Schwartz, B. 1975. *Queing and waiting.* Chicago: University of Chicago Press.

Scott, R. 1990. *Domination and the arts of resistance.* New Haven, CT: Yale University Press.

Shalin, D. 1992. Critical theory and the pragmatist challenge. *American Journal of Sociology* 98:237-79.

Snow, R., and D. Brissett 1986. Pauses: Explorations in social rhythm. *Symbolic Interaction* 9:1-18.

Starr, P. 1982. *The Social Transformation of American Medicine.* New York: Basic Books.

Strauss, A., S. Fagerhaus, B. Suczek, and C. Wiener. 1985. *Social organization of medical work.* Chicago: University of Chicago Press.

Thompson, J. 1984. Communicating with patients. In *The experience of illness,* edited by R. Fitzpatrick, J. Hinton, S. Newman, G. Scambler, and J. Thompson, 87-108. New York: Tavistock.

Waitzkin, H. 1991. *The politics of medical encounters.* New Haven, CT, Yale University Press.

Author's Note: This research was supported in part by grants from the University of Alabama Hospital Continuous Innovations in Patient Care Program (Richard Allman and Jeffrey Michael Clair) and the AARP Andrus Foundation (Jeffrey Michael Clair, Principal Investigator). We would like to thank Peter and Patti Adler, the anonymous reviewers, Richard Allman, Patricia Baker, Mary Harvey, David Karp, Kenneth Wilson, and Michael Wrigley, the editors, and three anonymous reviewers, for their comments on an earlier draft of this article. *Journal of Contemporary Ethnography,* Vol. 23 No. 2, July 1994 185-213.

Further Reading

Howard Becker, Anselm Strauss, Everett Hughes, and Blanche Geer. 1992 [1961]. *Boys in White: Student Culture in Medical School.* Chicago: University of Chicago Press.

William Finlay, Elizabeth J. Mutran, Rodney R. Zeitler, and Christina S. Randall. 1990. "Ques and Care: How Residents Organize Their Work in a Busy Clinic." *Journal of Health and Social Behavior* 31: 292-305.

Eliot Freidson. 1975. *Doctoring Together: A Study of Professional Social Control.* New York: Elsevier.

Jack Haas and William Shaffir. 1987. *Becoming Doctors: The Adoption of a Cloak of Competence.* Greenwich: JAI Press.

Discussion Questions

1. Explain how time as a medical resource differs for patients and medical residents.

2. How does "doctoring together" serve as a strategy for managing time?

3. In what ways might changes in the organization of health care alter the significance of time for both physicians and patients?

Section 3

Caretaking and Caregiving Relationships

In 1951, Talcott Parsons proposed a concept of physician-patient roles that is integral to what social scientists, health services researchers, and physicians call the "medical model" of health care. According to Parsons, individuals who were ill adopted a "sick role," which exempted them from usual responsibilities and obligated them to seek and to follow medical direction. As individuals surrendered control over their everyday life and medical decisions, they became passive patients dependent upon the active intervention of medical experts. Physicians, as trained professionals, thus took control in restoring patients to a healthy state. As you read the selections in this section, consider the assumptions inherent in Parsons' concept of illness and health. Think about contemporary changes in health and illness and about the experiences of illness from the previous section that make Parsons' characterization of health seeking and caretaking seem dated.

In addition to the assumption that active professionals provide expert care to unsophisticated passive patients, the medical model also assumes the following:

1. The unit of care is the atomized individual patient who is separated and isolated from family, culture, and social context.

2. The basic relationship is the professional-patient dyad characterized by private, confidential consultations that result in rapid interventions and positive treatment outcomes.

3. Medical expertise legitimizes a rigid hierarchical order of status, authority, and control.

4. Patients' ill health makes them emotionally fragile, while professionals remain composed and in control.

5. The professional's technical competence earns the patient's trust, respect, and gratitude.

6. Professional ethics require serving the patient's best interest, instead of the professional's.

7. Patients bring their problems to the professional's workshop, rather than the professional treating patients in their homes.

Thus, the medical model fosters concentration on narrow medical problems, providing fragmented care, and limited understanding of how patients' life circumstances can undermine medical objectives.

Sociologists who have examined caretaking relationships have discovered numerous problems for both patients and providers with the traditional medical model of care and treatment. Few individuals can abdicate all responsibilities in search of health, especially since much of contemporary illness is

145

chronic and persistent rather than acute and temporary (Strauss and Corbin 1988). The medical model of care fails to account for chronic illnesses that, to date, cannot be "cured." With more advanced medical technologies, specialized training, and healthier diet and exercise habits, illness and healing now take different forms than what Parsons assumed in his concept of the sick role (Parsons 1951).

The medical model of care established rigid relationships for both physicians and patients that are now unrealistic for illness and healing. Yet, many aspects of the sick role concept affect contemporary physician training, medical practice, and physician-patient relationships. Medical students, like practiced physicians, have difficulty with ambiguity (Fox 1957). A cloak of competence acquired early in their medical training makes it hard to admit uncertainty about diagnosis and healing (Haas and Shaffir 1987). Frederic Hafferty shows us how student physicians learn to adopt rigid professional roles in spite of experiences in medical school that could teach them otherwise. In the early years of medical training, mastering how to be a good professional overshadows concerns about patient health and caretaking. In Hafferty's selection, we see medical students talk about their conception of a "good patient," and we discover their sentiments toward those who are not. Good patients, students assume, follow the rules dictated to them by their practitioners.

Like the student physicians Hafferty interviews, practitioners criticize patients who do not comply with treatment regimen, often failing to consider broader reasons for patients' noncompliance than defiance of medical advice (Conrad 1985; Zola 1986). Howard Waitzkin and his coauthors provide some insight into physicians' potential to overlook illness contexts in office visits with elderly patients. Here, we gain insight into the social circumstances physicians avoid, and perhaps ignore, in the name of caretaking. Other sociologists have shown that this phenomenon is not unique to older patients (Fisher and Todd 1990; Mishler 1990). Patients sometimes have difficulty following medical advice. Their difficulty comes not from direct disobedience but from trying to manage illness and health against a complicated backdrop of life events. That phy-

sicians do not listen to patients when they discuss life circumstances that shape their illness and care raises some interesting questions about medical professionals' training and perspectives on illness and healing.

Compared with reports from citizens in other industrialized countries, U.S. citizens claim less satisfaction with American health care services and physicians. David Himmelstein and Steffie Woolhandler provide large-scale survey data indicating that Canadian citizens are more satisfied with their medical services and practitioners than U.S. citizens are. American dissatisfaction with practitioners and services may lie, in part, in patients' unmet expectations for care in their relationships with medical professionals. Richard Kravitz and his coauthors investigate patients' unmet expectations for care in physician visits. Patients come to physicians with ideas about their illness and about how a course of treatment might proceed. When physicians fail to acknowledge patients' concerns, they believe that their physicians neglect their health care needs. What should we expect when we visit a physician? This selection suggests that patients may be unwilling to recognize physicians' uncertainties about medical diagnosis and treatment, and that articulation of these uncertainties by health providers may increase patients' unmet expectations for care.

Parsons' concept also neglects care that occurs outside of institutional settings. Rigid models of medical care underestimate the significant informal, unpaid care by family, friends, and neighbors. Informal caregiving involves invisible labor. Informal labor means making everyday visits and running errands, cooking meals and caring for the body, escorting to medical and other appointments, and deciding how care should proceed. In general, women do the bulk of informal caregiving, providing everyday care to ailing family members and, sometimes, intensive long-term care for those who are chronically and terminally ill (Finch and Groves 1982; Olesen 1989). During the early eighties, AIDS activists organized diverse groups to provide informal in-home care for people living with AIDS and HIV (Shilts 1987). Informal caregiving relieves individuals and health care systems of enormous care burdens.

Informal labor is voluntary, but individual costs can be high. Emily Abel's study provides insight into effects of long-term caring on the lives of caregivers. Through the voices of caregivers, Abel shows us how this group of informal laborers manages a balance between the safety and autonomy of frail elders against the demands informal caregiving places on their own emotions. Informal caregivers, caught in mundane aspects of daily care, have scarce opportunity or resources to learn about and to consider alternative arrangements for care. The best interests of caregivers may supercede the sick person's needs. The sick person's needs may also overwhelm the caregiver's capacities. As the sick person's health deteriorates, problems arise about decisions for appropriate care and who gets to make them.

Patient autonomy means the ability to make decisions on one's behalf. Social scientists and ethicists have long been concerned with issues of patient autonomy—caretaking institutions have not. Karen Lyman recognizes conflict in exercise of autonomy when it meets with institutional barriers and routine work. Institutional standards of work, although directed at caring for patients, often do so at the expense of patients' own perspectives and understandings of their care needs. Timothy Diamond, a sociologist and nursing assistant, gives a rich account of what it means to be a caretaker in a nursing home. He describes the daily routine of institutional work characterized by patients' deficiencies. Embedded in this routine, he discovers, however, that standard organizational charting procedures fail to show the invisible work of nursing staff. As a nursing assistant, Diamond notices that caretaking is much more than what gets charted. It involves emotional labor; it requires coping with unexpected occurrences; it involves caregiving while in the context of caretaking.

As we will see in the next section, structural and professional road blocks create individual and interactional barriers between physicians and patients. Consider the relationships embedded in the American system of health care—relationships framed by medical models of acute care, and by social and institutional oversight regarding invisible aspects of care. What happens when patients grow frustrated from not being heard or understood by physicians and other health care providers? Think about hidden aspects and intricacies of care. How might we deal with issues of autonomy and control over the direction of care? As you read the selections in this section, consider struggles over care and concern for legitimacy—by both patients and care providers—in defining health and the courses of illness and healing.

References

Peter Conrad. 1985. "The Meaning of Medications: Another Look at Compliance. *Social Science and Medicine* 20:29-37.

Janet Finch and Dulcie Groves. 1982. "By Women for Women: Caring for the Frail Elderly." *Women's Studies International Forum* 5:10-15.

Sue Fisher and Alexandra Dundas Todd. 1990. *The Social Organization of Doctor-Patient Communication.* Norwood: Ablex.

Renee C. Fox. 1957. "Training for Uncertainty." In *The Student Physician*, R. Merton, G. Reader, and P. Kendall, eds. Cambridge: Harvard University Press, pp. 207-241.

Erving Goffman. 1961. "The Medical Model and Mental Hospitalization: Some Notes on the Vicissitudes of the Tinkering Trades." *Asylums.* Garden City: Anchor Books.

Jack Haas and William Shaffir. 1987. *Becoming Doctors: The Adoption of a Cloak of Competence.* Greenwich, CT: JAI Press.

Elliot Mishler. 1990. "The Struggle Between the Voice of Medicine and the Voice of the Life World." In *The Sociology of Health and Illness*, P. Conrad and R. Kern, eds. New York: St. Martin's Press, pp. 295-307.

Virginia L. Olesen. 1989. "Caregiving, Ethical and Informal: Emerging Challenges in the Sociology of Health and Illness." *Journal of Health and Social Behavior* 30:1-10.

Talcott Parsons. 1951. *The Social System.* New York: The Free Press.

Randy Shilts. 1987. *And the Band Played On.* New York: St. Martin's.

Anselm Strauss and Juliet Corbin. 1988. *Shaping a New Health Care System.* San Francisco: Jossey-Bass.

Irving K. Zola. 1986. "Medicine as an Institution of Social Control." In *The Sociology of Health and Illness*, P. Conrad and R. Kern, eds. New York: St. Martin's Press, pp. 379-390. ✦

Patients and Caregivers

15

Respect, Satisfaction, and Health Care: Canada and the U.S.

David U. Himmelstein
Steffie Woolhandler

Comparatively, the United States and Canada spend the first and second largest proportion of their Gross Domestic Products (GDP) on health care expenditures. Even though the United States allocates a larger percentage of its resources to health than Canada, the Canadian health care system rates higher among its consumers. Canadians have greater regard for the medical profession than U.S. citizens. Patients are more satisfied with health services than are patients in the United States. As respect and satisfaction in Canada increases, frustration and disapproval of the health care system in the United States builds among patients and practitioners. Take a look at the differences depicted in these graphs. Make a list of the reasons why these discrepancies in respect and satisfaction might be so great.

Figure 15-1
Applicants Per Medical School Place
U.S. Versus Canada

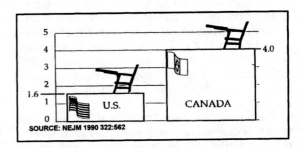

SOURCE: NEJM 1990 322:562

During the 1980s the number of people applying to medical school in the U.S. declined dramatically (though applications appear to be rebounding in the early 1990s), while Canada experienced no such decline. Medicine remains a popular and respected profession in Canada. Polls indicate that Canadian physicians believe that the national health program has improved the health of the population, and provides a good practice environment and lifestyle for physicians. In contrast, physician dissatisfaction has increased dramatically in the U.S. over the past 20 years.

Part of the U.S.–Canada differential in medical school applicants is due to the far lower tuition charged by Canadian schools. The Canadian government has recognized that the cost of medical education is an integral part of the overall costs of medical care. It has chosen to subsidize medical schools and keep tuition low (about $2000 per year) rather than bearing the costs retrospectively through higher physicians' incomes required to pay back medical school loans.

The Harris polling organization surveyed random samples of the population in each of ten industrialized nations. Canadians were most satisfied with their care, while America trailed all other nations.

Figure 15-2
Satisfaction With Health Care in Ten Nations,1990

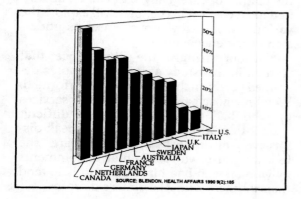

Further Reading

Arnold Bennett and Orvill Adams (eds.). 1993. *Looking North for Health: What We Can Learn From Canada's Health Care System*. San Francisco: Jossey-Bass.

David S. Brody, Suzanne M. Miller, Caryn E. Lerman, David G. Smith, Carlos G. Lazaro, and Mindy J. Blum. 1989. "The Relationship Between Patients' Satisfaction with Their Physicians and Perceptions about Interventions They Desired and Received." *Medical Care* 27: 1027-35.

Laurence Graig. 1993. *Health of Nations*, 2nd ed. Washington, DC: Congressional Quarterly Inc.

Discussion Questions

1. Given that the United States and Canada comparatively allocate the greatest percentage of their Gross-Domestic Product to health expenditures, why might the differences depicted here exist?

2. What are some of the factors you believe determine satisfaction with health care systems and providers?

3. How might trends in respect and satisfaction in the United States be reversed?

16

The Caregivers' Perspective

Emily K. Abel

Much of the literature on aging emphasizes the strains of caring for an elder. We have a hierarchy of care in the United States—care for a long-term spouse is obligatory, care for a demented parent admirable, care for a developmentally disabled adult child, necessary. But care for an aged aunt or a neighbor is either saintly or suspect. The long, thin hierarchy of care goes straight down the generations. The extent of responsibility women now take for elders with frail health is relatively new historically—people died more quickly much younger in the early part of this century. As the women in Emily Abel's research show, a sense of responsibility for the health and safety of elders easily conflicts with concern for their autonomy and quality of life.

Abel provides an important corrective to the concept of "caregiver burden" embraced by gerontologists. Like some earlier works, Abel finds that a strong bond overrides the burden, love outweighs the loss. For these caregivers, protecting dignity meant maintaining pretense. Otherwise failing memory, loss of function, and dependence might become visible and mortifying. Caregivers learn new ways to cope with emotions, though not without difficulty and often without professional validation. Look carefully at these caregivers' statements and think how you might assess the strains and rewards of caregiving.

When we hear women talk about the experience of caring for elderly parents, it is clear that caregiving does not conform to the classic distinction between instrumental tasks and affective relations. Caregivers try to provide love as well as labor, "caring about" while "caring for" (Graham 1983; Ungerson 1983). . . . Researchers frequently define caregivers in terms of the tasks they fulfill because tasks are the feature of caregiving that can be quantified most easily. This chapter will explore the various ways caregivers themselves understand their endeavors.

Not surprisingly, the importance that women in this study accorded to chores depended partly on the amount they performed. Women whose parents required few services or who had delegated the most difficult chores to paid helpers tended to speak dismissively of the tasks involved in care. The following are two representative comments by women who had hired aides to help tend their mothers with Alzheimer's disease:

> The direct care isn't really anything. Anyone can dress, give medication. What is the big deal? That is physical. The hardest thing is talking to someone who no longer can respond, where there is no reaching with one another.
>   That's the part that really hurts. The instrumental kinds of things—finding places and buying her things—that's not what I find so difficult about caring for her. What I find the difficult part is coming to terms with the course of a human being's life at this point.

Women without onerous practical responsibilities occasionally saw helping with household tasks as a way to escape what they considered the more emotionally demanding aspects of care. One woman described visits to her mother's home: "I start cleaning her house the minute I go there, making food, cooking things in her refrigerator, making the food that's rotting away. I'm not my best self. I find that I do things rather than talk to her." Women who cared for seriously impaired parents with little outside assistance were far more likely to focus on concrete tasks. One of the five women living alone with parents reported, "My day is filled up with little chores—non stop, no break until the night, when I fall asleep in front of the television." A second woman, interviewed a few weeks after the death of her father, described the daily grind in a similar way: "A typical day was complete drudgery, from the time I got up in the morning until I went to bed."

Nevertheless, even women whose days were consumed by a range of chores stressed other aspects of the caregiving experience. When asked to estimate the number of hours they devoted to caregiving tasks, most women responded that it would be impossible to make such a calculation, explaining that they remained preoccupied with their parents' well-being even when not actually rendering instrumental assistance. In their eyes, caregiving was a boundless, all-encompassing activity, rather than a clearly demarcated set of discrete tasks. The dominant element in caregiving was their overall sense of responsibility for their parents' lives, not particular chores.

Responsibility

Because the phrase "filial responsibility" appears frequently in the writings of policy analysts, it is important to understand how caregivers themselves defined this term. When some women said that they felt responsible for their parents, they meant that they had taken charge of decisions affecting their parents' lives. Some still were pondering decisions they had made months and occasionally years before, and they used the interviews as opportunities to reassess their choices.

But the meaning of responsibility typically extended much farther. Once women had begun to make decisions on their parents' behalf, they felt accountable not just for the consequences of these decisions but for virtually every aspect of their parents' lives. Several believed that they should be able to protect their parents from all physical harm. Two, for example, viewed themselves as culpable when their parents hurt themselves in falls, although they acknowledged that they could not possibly have prevented such mishaps. One woman, interviewed a few months after she and her husband had moved into her mother's house, remarked: "I felt really bad one day. I came home from work, and she'd gone in her bedroom, and I heard her fall down. It was such a shock because I thought, if I'm living here, I can protect her from this. It was so shocking to just hear her fall, and I was 20 feet away, just in the next room and not be able to do anything." Three

others faulted themselves for not having been able to halt or at least slow the progress of their parents' disease. A woman whose mother suffered from episodes of depression stated:

> When she goes to the hospital, I seem to think there should have been something I could have done to stop that from happening—that I should have better control of the situation; I should have called the doctor sooner; I should have gotten her more medicine; I should have told the other doctors to stay out of things; I should have been able to help her more, somehow.

. . . Several women considered themselves answerable for any deficiencies in medical or social service programs they arranged. And in some cases the daughters' sense of responsibility encompassed their parents' emotional as well as physical well-being. Although their parents suffered from intractable physical or mental health problems and had experienced losses that could not be repaired, the daughters believed that they should be able to make their parents happy.

How can we account for the overwhelming sense of responsibility these women felt? Nancy Chodorow argues that because women in this society fail to differentiate themselves from others, they often assume responsibility even for events they could not possibly control (Chodorow 1974). According to Elaine M. Brody (1985), women caring for aging parents measure themselves against the all-embracing care they received as children. Hilary Graham (1985:35) offers a very different explanation. Women consider themselves responsible for anything that befalls the recipients of their care because caregiving is defined as a private endeavor. In the absence of governmental responsibility for care of dependents, "experiences become personalized with problems seen as self-inflicted and failures seen as a cause for self-recrimination and blame."

The chasm between women's overriding sense of responsibility and their ultimate powerlessness is one of the major difficulties caregivers experienced. One woman recalled: "In the beginning, I cried every night. Because you feel so powerless to do anything.

And I think that's the worst thing, to see a person who's been very active, very personable, and all of a sudden, right in front of your eyes, they're just totally deteriorating." Policymakers frequently exhort adult children to display greater responsibility toward their aging parents. We will see, however, that the women in this study frequently expressed a desire to do just the opposite—to reduce their sense of involvement in their parents' lives and lower their expectations of what they could accomplish.

Dignity

Daughters also refused to define caregiving as a series of concrete chores because their primary objective was to preserve their parents' dignity. In a study of daughters caring for aging parents, Barbara Bowers (1990:279) concluded that women "conceptualized their caregiving work in terms of purpose, rather than tasks. The adult daughters . . . placed a priority on protective care (protecting or preserving the parent's sense of self and the parent-child relationship). This was especially true when their parents had either a mild or moderate form of dementia." This analysis illuminates the experiences of the women I interviewed. . . . Many women had their own reasons for seeking to protect their parents' individuality and self image. Some also invoked the authority of experts to support their definitions of good care. Books and lectures counseled them to preserve their parents' sense of competence and uniqueness and not compel them to confront their disabilities. The women interpreted this injunction in various ways.

When parents suffered little or no mental impairment, daughters defined their goal as respecting their parents' autonomy and encouraging them to remain in control of their lives. Thus, although some caregivers tried to protect their parents from all hazards, others deferred to their parents' judgment and refrained from intervening, even when the parents placed themselves in dangerous situations.

When dementia progressed, women found it more difficult to view their parents as self-governing and to leave major decisions in their hands. The daughters thus increasingly

viewed their mission as pretending that nothing had changed. One woman who spoke emphatically about the need to respect her mother's dignity explained that this meant preventing her mother from realizing that she had lost control over decisions affecting her life: "I let her think she had made the decision, or that she was taking care of herself. I don't ever let her feel that she couldn't survive if she wasn't here with me. To some people, that would be a comfort, but not to someone like my mother. If she could really come back and look and see, it would be the worst thing in the world." The daughters tried to conceal other changes in their parents' status. Women whose parents had been professionals sought to create the illusion that the parents continued to command the respect they previously had enjoyed. One woman was pleased when an aide was willing to cater to her father's professional pride, despite his severely impaired mental capacities: "This man makes an effort to be sensitive, and he is very willing to say, 'Yes, sir,' and 'Doctor this' and 'Doctor that,' kind of play to my father's authoritarianism." Another woman asserted: "My mother had been on the faculty at the university. I didn't want her ever to know that she is losing her memory, which she is; that she is losing her hearing, which she is; because her conception of herself is someone still on the faculty. I won't allow her to see that anything is wrong."

Women caring for mothers who had been housewives encouraged their mothers to believe that they still could make valuable contributions to household services. One woman discussed her mother's visits to her house:

Part of what I try and do when she's here is make sure that I have accumulated things she can do so she feels useful. For example, I may just leave a pile of laundry totally unfolded, because that's something she can do and do easily. Last time she came, I was trying to iron, and she insisted she wanted to iron, so I let her, and she ironed. I will let her do whatever I feel she can do. Sometimes it interferes because it's not exactly what I had planned to do that day, but that's the way it is.

When this woman returned from the hospital after a serious illness, she worked to foster the pretence that her mother could care for her in meaningful ways:

> By the time I came home, I could cope with her trying to take care of me. She could bring me a cup of coffee and she could bring me some food, because I made sure everything was prepared. She had the feeling she was helping because I set it up, knowing what she could do, and I think that helped her. I could just as well have gotten up and gotten a drink as have her bring me a drink, but she felt better because she was bringing me the drinks.

But women not only tried to prevent their parents from acknowledging their disabilities. Those who believed that the disease had ravaged their parents' sense of personhood viewed themselves as guardians of the people they remembered. One woman recalled a ritual she conducted during the two years she tended her mother, who suffered from Alzheimer's disease: "I kissed her goodnight every night, but it was never returned. I always felt like I'm just doing it because when she was herself, she liked that."

. . . Two women asserted that caregiving was a means of expressing loyalty to the mothers they had known. Said one:

> I loved my mother a lot when I was growing up. . . . When her memory went so poor, I realized that I really loved the lady she was. This is a different lady. This is not the mother that was, this is someone else. I can't really say that I love this person that is now, but what I do love is the memory of the person that was before, and because of that love, I have a tremendous sense of obligation to her, and I'll take care of her till the day she dies. Sometimes there's guilt involved because I don't love her in the way that I did. And sometimes I'm sad about it because I really remember the way that she was, and that's a curse and a blessing, at the same time.

The other commented: "I try to validate some of the things she tried to raise, ideals in me, things that she tried to teach us as we were growing up, that it was important to care about other people." By acting in accordance with the ideals her mother had sought to instill in her, this woman reaffirmed her bond with a mother she feared she had lost.

Finally, daughters viewed themselves as promoting their parents' self-respect when they helped their parents conceal evidence of physical frailty. . . . A key reason some women hired aides was that they did not want their parents to be compelled to reveal the extent of their physical impairments to their daughters. In addition, many daughters did not insist that their parents use walkers or wheelchairs, even when their parents had serious problems with ambulation. In a society that places a high value on independence, weakness of any kind is considered shameful; caregivers promote the dignity of recipients by hiding all signs of dependence.

Medical Diagnosis

In trying to foster their parents' dignity, the daughters in this study were following one line of advice frequently offered to caregivers. But daughters of parents with dementia also received a contradictory message—to define their relatives in terms of their diseases. Such popular advice books as *The 36-Hour Day* (Mace and Rabins 1981) stress the importance of viewing the behavior of demented adults as symptoms of disease rather than as deliberate acts. Women whose parents suffered from some form of dementia thus faced a problem that has been common since the rise of scientific medicine at the end of the nineteenth century and the new understanding of disease specificity. To what extent should patients be viewed as a configuration of symptoms and to what extent as whole and unique individuals? Because a diagnosis of dementia can call into question an individual's sense of self, this issue emerges in particularly urgent form for their caregivers. This section thus will focus on women caring for parents with dementia.

Diagnosis typically follows an evaluation by a physician. In most cases, family members initiate the process of obtaining an evaluation. One daughter in this study, however, had not even considered the possibility of dementia until she saw her mother's insurance form and learned that her mother had sought a consultation for memory loss.

Obtaining the diagnosis marked a turning point for many women. Three who had hoped that their parents had problems that could be treated (such as depression or alcohol or drug-induced dementia) were shocked to learn that their parents were suffering from an irreversible form of dementia. The reactions of two others revealed the stigma attached to Alzheimer's disease; they stated that they were relieved to learn that their parents had other types of dementia, although there still was no possibility of a cure.

But the precise designation was less important than learning that something was the matter. Although the diagnosis often confirmed daughters' worst fears, it also could be a source of reassurance. One woman explained why she and her siblings had insisted that their mother receive an evaluation:

> We suspected, and we didn't think we had a right to suspect without a professional opinion. . . . We used to swap stories of "guess what mother did now?" and it wasn't cruel. [The diagnosis] reconfirms that it's not you, because sometimes when you're in with someone who's not dealing with things properly, you begin to feel: "Was it me? Did I hear that? I don't believe she said that."

A second woman also initially had considered it improper to question her mother's mental capacities: "We just didn't know what was going on. She would say things that were strange, and I thought, 'My mama has really been very bright and now . . . .' I didn't say the word stupid, but you get the idea. I really thought that was not the respectable thing to say because it was my mother." Once their parents were labeled sick, women could trust their own instincts, make sense of their parents' behavior, and consider the best way to provide care.

After receiving a diagnosis, most women tried to learn more about the nature of their parents' impairments, seeking information from books, friends, support groups, and professionals. As their knowledge grew, many increasingly interpreted behavior in light of the disease. Some began to associate their parents with other victims of dementia. In answer to questions about their own parents, they discussed adults with dementia in general, occasionally referring to "them" or "these people." One woman lamented her in-

ability to spend more time talking with her mother "because this is what an Alzheimer's disease patient needs." Another woman explained why she had found the right aide for her father: "She is aware of how to take care of Alzheimer's people. It would be a real problem for some if they didn't understand Alzheimer's disease and the nature of it and how people are when they have that disease. She knows never to confront my dad head on, that there are other ways of getting him to do what you want." The women also used their new understanding to develop techniques for dealing with their parents themselves. One woman explained how she coped with her father's repetitive questions:

> His memory is so poor that he'll ask me the same questions over again, like, "What are you doing in your life now?" and "Do you have a job?" So I have to answer him a lot. And one thing I feel proud of myself is that, because I understand his situation, I don't put a lot of energy into answering the questions, I mean I just say the same thing over and over again. . . . I don't expect him to understand. I just answer it so he'll get the answer at that moment, but I don't expect him to remember five minutes later, and I expect it to come up again and again and again.

Another woman realized that, because her mother had the same disease as members of a day care center she observed, the daughter could learn techniques from the center staff:

> I learned so much about what must be the fright or the fear that the old people feel, the threat at the loss, even if they don't know what they're losing or what they lost. There's something that's so interesting that happens. If there's stress in the room, they pick it up like children. And what I saw at the day care center were the workers always touching the people. They give them a hug, or a pat, or hold their hand, or a kiss. Lovely, lovely. And I've learned to do that with my mother. When she's real agitated or upset, if I just sit down and put my arm around her, she calms right down.

Several women also claimed that information about the genesis of behaviors helped them to gain greater control over their own emotions. Thus one woman reported:

> We always viewed my mother as somewhat crazy and tried to get her to see a psychiatrist, but to have it be a clear dementia in some ways makes it easier to relate to her. Even though some of the things she does it's hard not to take personally, it's clearly not personal and doesn't have anything to do with who I am. . . . My coping mechanism had always been to distance myself, but there was always some doubt that maybe that was invalid, it always got to me eventually. This way, it's objective, so there is no way it could get to me.

When caregivers learned that their parents' actions were unintentional, some of their anger faded. One woman recalled:

> I took [my mother] to the doctor and he's the one that told me about the book, *The 36-Hour Day.* I went and got that book, I read it from cover to cover. And after I read that book, I started to understand some of the things that were happening to me. I started to understand why it is when she calls me and I would have her come here that she would want to go home again. It was because she felt totally uncomfortable, she wasn't in surroundings that she's used to, she would forget where rooms were. Just all these things started to come together, and I started to understand. . . .

Not all women found it . . . easy to translate information about dementia into appropriate emotional responses. Arlie Russell Hochschild (1975:289) has coined the phrase "feeling rules" to describe rules that "define what we should feel in various circumstances." An understanding of the relationship between parental behavior and disease processes convinced women that they should not be angry; but many acknowledged the difficulty of conforming their feelings to the knowledge they had gained. Looking back on the two years she spent caring for her mother, one woman stated: "I wish it hadn't upset me. I wish that I could have coped with it. I wish I could have just said, 'She can't help it,' and that was that, but I couldn't. I couldn't do it." Another woman noted that it was "hard to

put insights into practice." Nevertheless, a medical label did help women gain at least some of the emotional distance they considered critical.

Caregivers also noted the importance of learning what to expect. A diagnosis of dementia leaves many questions unanswered: How rapidly will the disease progress? What symptoms will emerge? To what extent will the individual's disease follow the widely recognized stages? Nevertheless, most women believed that the diagnosis dispelled some of the uncertainty surrounding their parents' care and enabled them to make preparations for the future. One woman remarked: "At the hospital, there was a wonderful doctor, and he said: 'Watch for these signs. When you come to pick her up and she has to brush her hair or brush her teeth, she's beginning to deteriorate. And then watch for her doing this and wandering off and not being able to get home.' So we watched for all the signs to come." Because many women insisted that their parents' illness had caught them by surprise, their ability to make plans gave them a sense of greater control over their lives.

Finally, women who attached a medical label to their parents found it easier to consult physicians about a broad range of issues. Aside from prescribing medications to control agitation, there was little that medical science could do in most cases. Physicians could neither cure the disease nor slow its progress. As one woman said, "You can't put the mind back." Nevertheless, many women sought guidance from physicians for problems that required human, not technical solutions. Women invoked physician recommendations to explain such varied steps as consulting a psychiatrist, joining a support group, enrolling their parents in day care centers, bringing their parents to live in the same city as themselves, and hiring aides and attendants.

But it is important to note that the comments of several women revealed that women were motivated less by trust in professional judgment than by their desire to use physicians to bolster their own authority. They sought professional advice in order to justify actions they already had decided were correct. Asked whether she had considered placing her father in a nursing home, one woman responded:

I don't think he's quite ready yet, and I don't want to move him until he really is, because I think once the move is made, that will be it, that will be where he'll remain. And I just feel that right now, it's just much more pleasant for him to be where be is. This is why I think I've been so insistent on finding one of these geriatric assessment services and doing the tests again, to try to get someone else to say to me, "He's not ready to go yet. He's not ready to move yet." I just wanted to put that burden, that responsibility on someone else. I'm halfway through one of these assessments, and they agree that he should stay where he is for now. And I'm relieved to hear them say that. I would like to keep him where he is as long as I can.

. . . Several other women relied on doctors in order to avoid conflicts with their parents. . . . Caregivers often must assert authority over parents and prevent them from engaging in certain activities traditionally considered basic to adulthood in our society. When physicians recommended that parents stop driving or managing their own money, the daughters were relieved of responsibility for the decision. And one woman used a consultation with a physician to puncture her brother's denial about their father's condition:

My brother kept insisting that my father's just having anxiety attacks. So I made my brother go to the doctor with my father. And he sat and watched how his father could not remember to do three things that the doctor had told him to do and how he couldn't do things properly. And he watched the whole process, and then he was willing to accept the fact that he was really sick, that there was something wrong with him. Then my brother was willing to set up a conservatorship.

In short, a diagnostic label served women in various ways—enabling them to muster resources for dealing with their parents' problems, helping them develop techniques for coping with bizarre or troublesome behavior, permitting them to gain critical emotional distance from their parents, and enabling them to rely on the authority of physicians.

Nevertheless, the women in this study resisted reducing their parents to a set of symptoms. If they "watched for all the signs to come," they also continued to respond to their parents as individuals. One woman commented:

I've just realized that there are things [my mother] can't grasp. My dad set up a trust in his will when he was ill, and I explained it to her so many times over so many months, and she still doesn't understand it. My husband finally just said, "Listen, let's just tell her it's just complicated legal stuff and you're never going to understand it, and just don't worry about it. Your husband took good care of you, and you don't need to worry about any of it." But my first impulse is always to treat her the way I've always treated her. I still try and get her preferences for things. She can't try on anything in stores anymore, it's just too hard, so I just charge everything and take it home so she can try it on. I kind of say, "Well, which one do you think looks better on you, and which colors do you like best?" I'd also like to ask her advice. I think in matters of the heart she probably could still advise me. She just can't balance her checkbook very well.

As this woman struggled to accept the fact that her mother's mental capacities had diminished, she remained attentive to her mother's wishes and sought to convince herself that her mother still possessed wisdom. Another woman described her determination not to treat her mother like every other victim of Alzheimer's disease, even as the progression of the disease threatened to destroy her mother's uniqueness:

What I find difficult is trying to figure out what's best for her, which is what a parent does for a small child, but there are many more clear directives for a parent than there are in this situation. And it's hard to separate what I would want for me in that situation [from how she might] choose for herself in a former time or now. We are dealing with a person that is different from the person that I know how to make choices for. I can't easily say that my mother would like this, this, and this, based on what she appears to want, because she can't communicate. . . . I was clear that I wanted her to have as much of her own furniture in her place around her as possible, because furniture was a big part of her life, and she loved antiques, and she got her self worth from her surroundings. There was a three-week delay in getting her furniture to where she was staying, and she'd forgotten it all. . . .

Jaber F. Gubrium and Robert L. Lynott (1987:271) argue that medical assessments of demented adults serve to construct as well as detect disease. Once evaluations have been conducted, caregivers tend to "see impairment everywhere." But a study by Betty Risteen Hasselkus (1988) suggests that family members are less easily swayed by medical labels. The caregivers she interviewed occasionally used their special knowledge of elderly relatives to cast doubt on their diagnoses. A few women I spoke to pointed to faculties their parents retained in order to question a medical diagnosis. One expressed doubts about whether her mother actually had Alzheimer's disease because she still could play the violin so well. Some who accepted the diagnosis nevertheless argued that certain behaviors experts attributed to disease actually were exaggerations of lifelong personality traits. The comments of one woman illustrate the difficulty of determining which behaviors should be attributed to a disease and which to a parent's distinctive personality:

When my mother's brother was visiting, my father had no idea who this man was, but he was quite indignant that this strange man had come to visit. My mother left the car lights on in the car, and my uncle said, "Give me the keys and I will go and turn them off," but my father said no. He told my mother that she had to go out, that she was the one who left them on, and she was going to have to turn them off. This kind of behavior was a side of him always, but it was not always so naked in front of my uncle. He would not have been totally unconscious about it. He would have veiled it in the past. But he never was a good person to get along with. It's hard to tell now when his personality is deteriorating. It is very difficult to tell whether or not it is the crankiness they talk about or the nasti-

ness related to Alzheimer's disease or if it is just him.

A second woman noted that as long as she could remember, her mother had had angry outbursts, although they now seemed to take an exaggerated form. A third was uncertain that even more aberrant behavior could be classified as a disease symptom:

The first hint that she was sick was an incident that clearly had a paranoid element because she imagined helicopters landing in her yard. But the distinction was very difficult, because she always had crazy-making behavior. For example, she changed her will and gave all her money to Harvard. It always was hard to know how much was her craziness, which always was there, and how much was a definable diagnosis. . . . She does very inappropriate things. For example, she'll say in a loud voice: "There's Helen. Don't talk to Helen; she has nothing going on upstairs." It's embarrassing. What's so funny is she might have said the same thing toned down six levels when she was more coherent. She used to say obviously embarrassing things in the middle of large groups. So in that sense it is just an exaggeration of how she is or was.

Many women also asserted that their parents' personalities transcended the disease. One woman explained why she enjoyed the time she spent with her father: "He's real sweet, he's not like sometimes Alzheimer's people get, kind of angry. He was a real sweet person to begin with, and he's still really nice. I mean, to me, he's fun, and even with his Alzheimer's, he'll say really funny things." Finally, rather than assuming that the disease had transformed their parents' personalities, three women reassessed their prior view of their parents in light of the changes that had occurred. "It's as if I've been fooled all these years," one said.

Women who emphasized their parents' uniqueness tended to be less impressed by advice books than others. One, for example, had little praise for *The 36-Hour Day*:

There's nothing human about it. The discussions about how you pick a place are all very instrumental, and none of it deals with the concerns about how you know what's good for a person. Nobody has described to me what would be the impact on me of walking for the very first time into a nursing home, the impact of seeing these very old women who were sitting and kind of nodding. I would see *my* mother in every single one of the women, and it's very hard.

Some women considered other types of professional expertise equally irrelevant. One mentioned that her husband had suggested that she consult a geriatric specialist to give her guidance about the way to care for her father. She explained why she had demurred: "We're dealing with a uniquely strong personality." Women also gained the confidence to override physicians' advice by relying on their own intimate knowledge of their parents. Some argued that physicians, acting on the basis of universalistic knowledge, missed unique aspects of their parents' experiences. Thus one woman scoffed at a physician who recommended that she give her mother a sense of security by imposing routines on her mother's life, "My mother never has lived by routines." The recommendation most commonly rejected was that parents be placed in nursing homes. Virtually all women in the study were staunchly opposed to institutionalization. One woman who did accept a physician's counsel to put her mother in a home told an unusually harrowing story:

My husband started getting terrible pains, just unbearable pains, and we went for months to doctors. They all said, "Your husband has terrible headaches because your mama is living with you." Finally, we went to a neurologist for my mother, and he examined her and took a CAT scan and he gave us the verdict that she had Alzheimer's. He said, "Let me tell you what that means." I will never forget those words. He said to me: "You have to put your mama in a nursing home because if you don't your marriage is at risk. Your husband is suffering very much. It's going to destroy your marriage. . . ." We ended up putting my mom in a nursing home about ten minutes away. I went to see her every day, and I couldn't bear seeing my mama in the situation they had her in. . . . I'll never forgive myself for letting her go there, but I was so desperate

and my husband was getting worse. A few months later he collapsed, and then he found out that it was a brain tumor, and he had twelve and one-half hour surgery and we almost lost him. . . . The worst thing I ever did was to put her in a nursing home and not let her stay with me anymore. I was given advice by professional people that I respected. . . .

During a period of enormous stress, she had allowed the judgment of physicians and other professionals to prevail, disregarding her own knowledge about both her husband and her mother. She bitterly regretted acquiescing in professional expertise and remained convinced of the importance of personalized, as opposed to scientific, knowledge.

Role Reversal

If caregivers of persons with dementia viewed their parents simultaneously as disease victims and unique individuals, they also referred to their parents as both adults and children. A cardinal principle of gerontology is that the elderly should not be considered children; despite any disabilities they may experience, they should be accorded all the rights and privileges of other adults in our society. But Karen Lyman (1988) found that at least some staff in adult day care centers for dementia patients violate this principle; believing that demented adults degenerate by regressing to the level of young children, the staff members she observed routinely infantilized their patients. From a study of 15 women caring for frail elderly parents, Lucy Rose Fischer (1986:165) reported: "All but one of the daughters declared specifically that they had experienced a role reversal."

In this study as well, women labeled their relationships as "role reversal," said "I'm the parent now," and described the "childlike" qualities of their parents. Women used such phrases to signify that their parents depended on them for care. One commented: "The day that he couldn't find his way to my house in his car was when I felt like I had really lost my father. It was almost like a dying of my father. And it was sort of like all of a sudden, I'm the big one now, and he's the little one, and I've got to take care of him.

Women who were mothers themselves reported that certain caregiving activities—tucking their parents in at night, bathing them, and hiring sitters—were reminiscent of their experiences as mothers of small children: "A couple of years ago, my mother was in the hospital, and she kept climbing out of bed and would fall. It was very difficult. I had to tell them it was O.K. to tie her down. That was so hard for me. I remembered having to make similar decisions when my child was young. Something just has to be done. I immediately went into that mode." Women without children were convinced that they would be better equipped to give directions and make decisions if they had raised children. One said:

My sister told me that when she was visiting here that she just went back to her days of having a toddler and treated Mom very much in the same way. She'd say, "Well, it's time for your bath now," and "Dinner's ready." Because she's raised a child, that's a posture she's more familiar with. For me, this has been a little harder because I haven't had any kids. I wonder if you find that women who have had children, if it's easier for them somehow.

Defining parents with dementia as children also may have enabled the women to deny some of the emotions the experience of care provoked. One woman stated: "The problems may just be me and my reactions to things. If I can try and keep the attitude that she's really just a little girl who needs to be treated gently and lovingly, then I kind of have fun with it. But if I expect her to be an adult and fend for herself, then it's much harder."

Nevertheless, all the women I interviewed emphasized the vast differences between caring for children and aging parents. Instead of fostering growth and development, they witnessed deterioration:

When my mother first came to live with me, I thought: "Oh, this isn't going to be difficult. I can manage this, I've raised six kids." I kept seeing the relationship in terms of that, she acted very much like a 3- or 4-year-old. And, goodness, I had six children, ten grandchildren, and so I could handle this. And it wasn't the same, because with children you know they're going to grow, and you know there's a future, and with this you know it's the opposite.

Caring for the elderly also lacks familiar milestones; thus, although caregivers typically have an enormous investment in providing good care, they have few ways of evaluating their work:

You expect small children to show progress. If small children don't show progress, then you really have to take steps to see what's wrong with them. The difference is that here there is no progress, there's only a slow deterioration, almost an invisible deterioration, but I know it's there. It's very different from taking care of kids. If you're doing a good job with kids, they move along, they progress, their world expands. My mother's world is contracting.

Women also pointed out that, although parents seek to produce socially acceptable children (see Ruddick 1982), they were not trying to mold their aging parents.

But the major reason women did not confuse parent care with child care is that . . . caregiving often revived powerful elements of the original parent-child relationship; several women reported that the emotional relationship with their parents remained unchanged. The term "role reversal" thus can be considered more an indication of women's discomfort at the inversion of responsibilities than an expression of their belief that they actually had traded places with their parents (see Brody 1985).

Reciprocity

It often is assumed that care for elderly parents is rooted in reciprocity—children repay parents for the care they received when young (see Bulmer 1987; Qureshi and Walker 1989; Ungerson 1987). The notion of reciprocity meshes with social exchange theory (Blau 1964). As Tamara Hareven (1987:73) writes, "The classic exchange along the life course is that between parents and children, based on parents' expectation of old age support in return for their investment in childbearing."

Six women in this study explained their motivation in terms of filial gratitude. Said one, "She was there for me, I'll be there for her." Another woman felt an obligation to repay her mother for services the daughter received when she already was an adult:

> She made me go back to college after I had graduated to become a teacher because I didn't take my education courses, and she came an hour and a half train ride to take care of my kids in the morning so I could go to school. It was three different trains for her. In snow and sleet, she carried food, and she cleaned my house and my windows and everything while I was in school, so I really owe her. I wanted to pay her back.

But, just as adult children do not simply reverse roles when caring for parents, so most women I interviewed did not perceive themselves as giving payment for services rendered. As noted, all discussed the enormous differences between parent care and care for children. Moreover, eight stated that they were rendering care in spite of rather than because of their treatment as children. They claimed that their parents either had given them insufficient love or had entrusted their care to outsiders, such as nannies or governesses. One woman mused, "My brother says to me, 'She was so awful to you, why are you so interested in taking such good care of her now?' and I can't really answer that."

Most women also did not believe that their parents had a special right to care because of the services they had rendered their own parents. The great majority asserted that they were the first in their families to care for elderly parents. And, just as some women said that they cared for their parents despite the poor care they had received as children, so some women claimed that their parents' treatment of their own parents constituted a negative, rather than a positive, model. One woman explained why she brought her mother with her when she moved across the country:

> We were originally from southern Germany, and my mother cared for her mother. By the time we emigrated from Germany, which was in the spring of [19]38, very late, my grandma had had a stroke, and my mother left her behind, and she ended up in a concentration camp, and she was killed, as far as we know. It was

something my mother never talked about. But I certainly don't want to treat my mother the way she treated her mother.

Nor did women believe that they could expect payment in the form of services from their own children when they themselves grew old. Although two women asserted that they were setting an example for their children, most were far less sanguine about their future. All the childless women expressed fears that they would have no one to care for them in old age. Most mothers shared these fears, either because they had sons rather than daughters or because they were convinced that all young people had rejected an ethic of care. "We're the last generation to provide this care," one woman asserted.

By emphasizing the reciprocal nature of caregiving, we miss its essential meaning. The notion of reciprocity rests on the assumption that individuals view each other as instrumental resources for discrete tasks, coming together primarily to exchange specific goods and services (see Glenn 1987; see Hartsock 1983). By contrast, writers such as Nancy Chodorow (1974) and Carol Gilligan (1982) argue that women experience themselves as embedded in social relationships and derive their sense of identity from such relationships. According to most women I spoke with, caregiving flowed from a sense of connection to their parents, not from a desire to repay services previously rendered or to make an investment in their own futures.

Appreciation

Partly because these women did not view themselves as either returning services or accumulating credit for their own old age, they believed that their care deserved appreciation. One woman who recently had moved with her husband into her mother's house was dismayed to discover how desperately she sought thanks:

> I think people have told her that it's good for the kids, that we won't have to pay rent, that we'll be able to save money. So I think in some ways she didn't see that it was a sacrifice for us. . . . One day she could tell I was just upset, I was kind of

banging dishes around when I was cleaning up, and it's terrible, she was saying, "Well, if you don't want to be here, you don't have to be." It was strange for me, because I realized I wanted her to be grateful, I wanted her to appreciate the sacrifice I was making. It sounds terrible. She just kind of said, "If you don't want to live here, you can leave." She's never brought it up again, but it's like she was doing us a favor. I don't like that in myself, that I want her to be grateful. I feel like a real jerk to want her to be grateful, to just kind of acknowledge that this isn't all fun and games and that I was happy with the life I had before, that I liked my privacy and my freedom, and it's a sacrifice.

A woman caring for a father also revealed an intense desire for appreciation:

Once he said to me, after we had a very good day together, he said, "Thank you for everything." I cried all the way home. It touched me, because he doesn't say thank you and sometimes I don't believe that he's aware of what's happening. Just having him say that meant that he was aware, that he appreciated it. It was such a nice thing that it moved me to tears, it doesn't happen often. In fact I even had talked to a close friend of mine, "If once he'd say thank you, if he'd say thank you just once, I would feel somewhat that he was cognizant of what was going on." And it was several days after that, that he said that. So it was very poignant. It was striking at the time he said that, although he has no idea that he has turned my life absolutely upside down, that he's caused such an upheaval and disturbance to my life.

These women were not alone in receiving less gratitude than they wanted. The great majority of women in the study complained of inadequate appreciation. Some explained that, because their parents suffered from dementia, they had little conception of what was being done for them. As we have seen, some women also took pains to conceal their contributions in order to foster their parents' self-image. In addition, women noted that their parents resented their dependency and resisted all offers of help; they could not show gratitude for services that were being rendered over their objections. Finally, some women believed that their parents simply

took their daughters' efforts for granted. One woman commented:

I keep expecting her to see that it's too much for me, that's what I'd like. My aunt and uncle do that. They fuss and fume and take care of me and say, "This is just too much for you." But the more I do for mother, the more she seems to expect. I'd like even a little concern that I'm doing too much. One day I was lugging all these groceries up the stairs, and she looked at me and said, "Smile when I smile at you." Every time you look at her she smiles, and she wants a smile back. And I didn't smile. I said, "I'm tired," and her response was, "Well, sit down." She thinks it's that easy, you just sit down. But it's not that easy.

A second woman voiced a similar complaint: "From time to time she expresses her appreciation, but on the whole I think she expects it. She expects me to be there for her. I think she does appreciate what my husband does, and she says thank you to him. I think she thinks I'm her daughter, and I should just be there for her. Women like these tended to interpret their parents' failure to appreciate their efforts as evidence of their own worthlessness in their parents' eyes.

Responses to Care

When women assessed their responses to caregiving, they agreed that stress was a major component. I have noted that stress consumes much of the attention of students of informal caregiving. Comments about stress also were constant refrains in the interviews I conducted with caregivers. As Allan Young (1980:133) writes: " 'Stress' and ancillary concepts such as 'coping' have permeated everyday discourse. . . . Information on stress is now widely available to lay audiences . . . through frequent articles in mass circulation magazines, self-help books, television programs, lectures, and pharmaceutical advertising for vitamins and sleep preparations." Although the women were not asked directly about the stresses of caregiving, nine volunteered that they had consulted therapists to help cope with the problems of caregiving, and another commented that she was considering doing so. Twenty-four women also were members of support groups, where they discussed the strains involved in rendering care. Several women attributed physical problems to stress. Three stated that the stress of caregiving created fatigue, and three others claimed that it contributed to eating problems. Four women believed that stress had precipitated even more serious health problems, including chronic back pain and cancer. Two additional women wondered if stress had exacerbated their difficulties with infertility. Women who lived apart from their parents described physical symptoms that occurred either while visiting their parents or after returning home. One woman, for example, remarked:

> I had a bad experience a couple of months ago. Boy, it taught me a lesson. I thought my mother would enjoy going to the arboretum. They had a special spring show of flowers, and I wanted to see them myself. The only problem is that it was 50 minutes in the car. I didn't realize that I couldn't sit in the car with her for 50 minutes. She talked on and on, and she says the same things over and over and over again. What happens to me when I am stressed out or anxious is I get very sleepy. I almost couldn't make it home. There were times on the freeway coming back where I thought, "If I don't pull over and take a nap, I'm going to fall asleep." If she drove, I would have said, "Please drive." I really almost couldn't make it. I'd never gotten that bad before. I got her home and I sat in the car and took a little nap before I came back home, which was only another ten minutes. I realized I can't do that anymore.

Another woman noted: "I find the day is better if I visit mother in the morning and then go about my business, and then I come home refreshed. But the majority of days I go toward the end of the day, and then I come home beaten because it takes a lot out of me. I normally am very organized, but I am not then. I drive very carefully because I'm just not all there." A woman interviewed a few days after institutionalizing a mother with whom she had lived for two years reported:

> When I woke up, I thought, oh, another day, and when I went to bed it was the same thing. All day I could keep busy, coping, but at night it was terrible. It got to the point where I was not myself anymore. One of my daughters said, "You were just driving a car with empty," and that's the way I felt. Any little thing that happened was a major catastrophe to me, and I'm not that way. I'm an easy-going person. Usually I'm not a worrier, but I couldn't relax. I was becoming uptight, neurotic. I felt someone else was coming inside and controlling me.

But, if stress was a key concern of women in this study, most insisted that it did not define their experience of caregiving. When asked how life would be different without the responsibility of care, one woman caring for her mother responded:

> I think I could plan more trips. I like to travel. I could think about moving away, which I would never do now, moving to a quieter, simpler community. I guess I'd eventually feel less burdened. But I also think that I'd miss her very much, and her presence and all the cherished moments that you have. All the family occasions and the times you want to share with a parent, that you want them to be there to see and be a part of.

Another commented: "I'd have a lot more free time and a lot more freedom of movement. I think I'd feel a lot more carefree. But, you know, it's like this is thinking back to the past, because in the future, if I'm not caring for her it means that she's not well enough for me to care for her anymore, and so I'm sure there's going to be a lot more sadness mixed in with it." And a third remarked: "It would be one less responsibility but also one less joy. I am just lucky to have her." To women such as these, a one-sided focus on the problems of caregiving denied the value of their parents' lives. They viewed caregiving as the inevitable consequence of having elderly parents and an expression of their attachment to their parents. As a result, it was a privilege as well as a burden.

When asked if caregiving offered satisfactions, a few women laughed dismissively. One angrily retorted, "You don't expect rewards for caring for your mother." Nevertheless, most women identified at least some gratifications from caregiving. Although many women said that they felt uncertain about how best to proceed when they first assumed caregiving responsibilities, four said that caregiving eventually provided them with an opportunity to display competence. Several women also took pride in making an important difference in their parents' lives. A woman who was interviewed shortly after she placed her mother in a nursing home assessed her contribution this way:

> I think I helped her just to retain her dignity a little longer, just to hang onto it a little bit. She was always a very dignified lady. It's sort of like seeing your mother stripped naked when they don't care for themselves. Their clothes are dirty; they have this look on their face of total rejection. It's like seeing them standing there naked. So I was able to, in a way, clothe her for two years.

If some women had grandiose expectations about what they could accomplish, this woman believed that she had fulfilled her desire to foster her mother's self-respect. In addition, caregiving enabled women to reaffirm their sense of themselves as good people. For example: "I don't know if I would be doing all this if I didn't get some sense that I'm helping and that I'm worthwhile for doing it, that I'm a good person, that I'm someone that can be relied on." Some women asserted that caregiving was a humanizing experience. Said one, "You gain a lot of wisdom and insight and compassion for other people's suffering and problems." Another commented: "I've always been very religious all my life, but I've always had a very wonderful life. I haven't had any massive burdens or catastrophes, just your normal things that happen in life. But because of this problem with my mother, I've had to search and realize what my faith means to me. I look at it like this was mother's final gift to me."

Conclusion

This chapter suggests that many of the concepts commonly used to describe caregiving fail to capture the experience of women engaged in this activity. Rather than perceiving caregiving as a series of chores, the women I interviewed emphasized their over-all responsibility for their parents' lives and their determination to foster their parents' self-respect. Although several spoke in terms of role reversal and reciprocity, these terms did not adequately describe the way most daughters defined their endeavor. And, despite their emphasis on the strains that caregiving generated, the majority of women resisted viewing caregiving solely in terms of stress and burdens. This chapter also demonstrates the complexities of women's relationship to professional expertise. Although some daughters whose parents suffered from dementia believed that the jurisdiction of physicians extended very broadly, most did not simply relinquish authority. Instead, they used professional opinion to enhance their own authority over their parents. Because they viewed their parents as unique individuals rather than simply victims of disease, they retained faith in their own ability to determine how care should be rendered.

References

Blau, P. 1964. *Exchange in Social Life.* New York: John Wiley.

Bowers, B. 1990. "Family Perceptions of Care in a Nursing Home." In *Circles of Care: Work and Identity in Women's Lives,* ed. E.K. Abel and M.K. Nelson, pp. 278-89. Albany: State University of New York Press.

Brody, E.M. 1985. "Parent Care as a Normative Family Stress." *The Gerontologist* 25(1):19-28.

Bulmer, M. 1987. *The Social Basis of Community Care.* London: Allen & Unwin.

Chodorow, N. 1974. "Family Structures and Feminine Personality." In *Woman, Culture and Society,* ed. M.Z. Rosaldo and L. Lamphere, pp. 43-66. Stanford: Stanford University Press.

Fischer, L.R. 1986. *Linked Lives: Adult Daughters and Their Mothers.* New York: Harper & Row.

Gilligan, C. 1982. *In a Different Voice: Psychological Theory and Women's Development.* Cambridge: Harvard University Press.

Glenn, E.N. 1987. "Gender and the Family." In *Analyzing Gender: A Handbook of Social Science Research,* ed. B.B. Hess and M.M. Ferree, pp. 348-80. Newbury Park, CA: Sage.

Graham, H. 1983. "Caring: A Labour of Love." In *A Labour of Love: Women, Work and Caring,* eds. J. Finch and D. Groves, pp. 13-30. London: Routledge and Kegan Paul.

——. 1985. "Providers, Negotiators, and Mediators: Womena as the Hidden Carers." In *Women, Health and Healing: Toward a New Perspective*, ed. E. Lewin and V. Olesen, pp. 25-52. New York:Tavistock.

Gubrium, J.F., and R.J. Lynott. 1987. "Measurement and Interpretation of Burden in the Alzheimer's Disease Experience." *Journal of Aging Studies* 1(3):265-85.

Hareven, T.K. 1987. "The Dynamics of Kin in an Industrial Community." In *Families and Work*, ed. N. Gerstel and H.E. Gross, pp. 55-83. Philadelphia: Temple University Press.

Hartsock, N.C.M. 1983. *Money, Sex and Power: Toward a Feminist Historical Materialism*. Boston: Northeastern University Press.

Hasselkus, B.R. 1988. "Meaning in Family Caregiving: Perspectives on Caregiver/Professional Relationships." *The Gerontologist* 28(5):686-91.

Hochschild, A.R. 1975. "The Sociology of Feeling and Emotion: Selected Possibilities." In *Another Voice: Feminist Perspectives on Social Life and Social Science*, ed. M. Millman and R.M. Kanter, pp. 280-307. Garden City, NY: Anchor Press/Doubleday.

Lyman, K.A. 1988. "Infantilization of Elders: Day Care for Alzheimer's Disease Victims." *Research in the Sociology of Health Care* 7:71-103.

Mace, N.L., and P.V. Rabins. 1981. *The 36-Hour Day: A Family Guide to Caring for Persons with Alzheimer's Disease, Related Dementing Illnesses, and Memory Loss in Later Life*. Baltimore: Johns Hopkins University Press.

Qureshi, H., and A. Walker. 1989. *The Caring Relationship: Elderly People and Their Families*. Philadelphia: Temple University Press.

Ruddick, S. 1982. "Maternal Thinking." In *Rethinking the Family: Some Feminist Questions*, ed. B. Thorne, pp. 76-94. New York: Longman.

Ungerson, C. 1983. "Women and Caring: Skills, Tasks and Taboos." In *The Public and the Private*, ed. E. Gamarnikow et al., pp. 62-77. London: Heinemann.

——. 1987. *Policy Is Personal: Sex, Gender, and Informal Care*. London: Tavistock.

Young, A. 1980. "The Discourse on Stress and the Reproduction of Conventional Knowledge." *Social Science and Medicine*, 14B:133-46.

Further Reading

Elaine Brody. 1990. *Women in the Middle: Their Parent-care Years*. New York: Springer.

Jay Mancini (ed.). 1989. *Aging Parents and Adult Children*. Lexington, MA: Lexington Books.

Sarah Matthews. 1988. "The Burdens of Parent Care: A Critical Evaluation of Recent Findings." *Journal of Aging Studies* 2: 158-165.

Discussion Questions

1. What are the positive consequences of caregiving for these women?

2. How is care for elders viewed in your family? For spouses? Children with physical, mental, or addiction problems?

3. How might structural issues in the medical care system affect the caregiving process?

17

Care and Control: Managing Stress by Medicalizing Deviance

Karen Lyman

Control emerges as a major theme in the following chapter. Who has it? How does it shape interaction? Control is not solely an issue of patient behavior. Staff views of patients and of how to manage them narrow the range of actions that staff take toward patients. Such views reduce uncertainty and, therefore, shape staff decisions. They control a view of their patients and views of how to manage them. Seeing Alzheimer's disease as continuous decline therefore allows and necessitates intrusions into patients' lives. This view attributes patients' problems as emanating from inside them and therefore minimizes seeing problems as resulting from the vicissitudes of growing old in an uncaring society or in the losses of autonomy, adult status, and identity. With "control," predictability increases and moral questioning decreases about whether staff act in the best interests of clients. Their autonomy steadily erodes.

Karen Lyman shows how external demands such as assessments of "levels of severity" are taken as objective facts describing concrete realities. Staff assume that clients' overt behavior problems validate an objective level of severity. Note how Lyman questions their assumption. Look for her argument that these behavior problems may be produced by the setting with its structure of relations and actions. Despite staff skepticism about procedures, they control program activities, knowledge and meanings, that in turn justify control over cli-

ents and treatment. Clients lose control and lapse in to child-like status. Staff directives, deceptions, distinctions about clients' cognitive functioning and social distance from them further enhance their control. See how the medical model of care fosters and reinforces these forms of staff control. Think about Lyman's suggestions as to how a social model might differ and consider the difficulties programs and people face when they subscribe to a social model in a system of medical dominance.

A staff meeting at Inland is devoted to a discussion of an article on "The Agitated Patient," after several unsettling incidents this week. The discussion focuses on "What sets people off." In particular, people are trying to figure out how to handle Gus. He chased Randy, the driver, threatening to "get a gun and shoot you!" Wendy, the program manager at Inland, has worked as a nurse's aide with other "agitated" people, but she never felt frightened, as she is by Gus. Wendy observes, "What's scary about Gus is that he's still young [perhaps sixty-five] and he's strong!"

Valerie, one of the program aides who is very gentle with people, and usually confident of her effectiveness, adds a note of uncertainty: "He always carries in a bag of stuff, wears a coat; you never know." Cindy is a program aide who has had experience as a nurse's aide in a long-term care facility: "I read his chart. Didn't they rule out Alzheimer's?" Wendy answers: "They're not sure what it is. . . . He's not on medication either, so. . ."

Much of the stress associated with dementia care is explained by the "uncertainty" involved in providing care for people with dementing illnesses. For many people, disease progression does not conform to predictable patterns of progressive "stages" of decline. And many are unpredictable, sometimes threatening, in their response to assistance from care providers. . . .

Assessing 'Level of Severity'

To cope with the uncertainty surrounding dementing illness, caregivers rely upon biomedical "knowledge" of people with dementia: that they will inevitably regress to a childlike state of dependency. Troublesome behavior is to be expected, and when it is found, it is explained by the medicalization of deviance. Examples drawn from notes entered in two patient information records at Bayview reveal the service providers' definition of deviance and how it might be managed: "Abigail—Strong stubborn streak. . ." "Bertha—Sit with at meals. Emotional at times, severely emotional, inappropriate demands, child-like behavior. Needs consistent approach. Sneaks food at times from others. . . ."

Similar entries are found in "progress notes" written in patient information records at Coast. The state requires periodic assessment of "problems," concerning safety, cognitive decline, or behavior problems such as "agitation." But for the day-care staff at Coast, "problems" most often centered around someone being uncooperative with the staff's plans and activities. The people with the most entries for "problems" were those described as "restless," "won't participate in the group," "requires distraction," and the like.

One medical procedure found in all eight dementia care centers is rooted in the biomedical model of dementia. Initial assessments and periodic reassessments of the "level of severity" of clients are required by the State Department of Aging for all eight Alzheimer's Day Care and Resource Centers (ADCRCs). The mission for the ADCRCs is to provide care for people with "moderate" to "severe" impairment. Standardized assessment procedures are to be followed, employing instruments such as the Mini Mental State Exam (MMSE) and scales measuring the Activities of Daily Living (ADL) and Independent Activities of Daily Living (IADL).

As in most human services occupations where staff eschew paperwork, the assessment procedures often were viewed as an intrusion into the "real" work of day care. Some staff also were skeptical of the procedures. As one program director observed, "I do it; it's required by the state. But it's so rare that somebody follows a 'stage' . . . that I think it's worthless." But seldom was there concern expressed about the impact on older adults when they are labeled (sometimes inappropriately) "moderately" or "severely" impaired.

On occasion I overheard lucid clients express concern about "failing the test," or whether or not this might mean they would have to leave the program. It is ironic that depression as a result of this labeling process then may be identified as a "personality change" in the next reassessment. These iatrogenic consequences of the assessments generally were not considered by staff, because of the circular reasoning of attributing trouble to disease progression.

The MMSE is a thirty-item test designed to assess the level of cognitive impairment (Folstein, Folstein, and McHugh 1975). Questions are asked of the people with dementia to assess immediate recall, short-term memory, language impairment, and other cognitive functioning. The ADL and IADL are assessments of the person's self-care abilities and self-sufficiency, based on questions asked of caregivers.

The ADCRCs are required by the state to determine an overall summary rating identifying the "level of severity" or stage of dementia for each client. Reassessments are to be conducted at six-month intervals or whenever a significant change in the person has been observed. The construction of this rating reveals some aspects of medicalized deviance.

The "level of severity" rating includes five categories of troublesome behavior: agitation, combativeness, wandering, communication problems, and personality change. These are commonly used medical labels for behavior problems associated with dementing illnesses (see Mace 1987). "Agitation" refers to restlessness, repetitive behavior, pacing, wringing hands, and the like. "Combativeness" refers to angry outbursts and destructiveness. "Wandering" denotes leaving without permission or supervision but sometimes overlaps the restlessness/pacing component of "agitation," if someone is "wandering around" a lot. "Communication problems" refer to garbled speech, incomplete sentences, and other difficulties in making one's needs known. And "personality change" denotes becoming withdrawn, depressed, or violent, by comparison with previous personality traits. The extent of each of these behavior problems is assigned a rating of "light," "moderate," or "severe" to connect these behaviors to degree of impairment. These ratings contribute to the overall level of severity rating, which includes ADL and IADL scores.

It is clear that in these ratings, troublesome behavior is equated with level of impairment. Gubrium and Lynott (1987) have cautioned against this assumption of the "equivalence" of impairment and trouble, to which I would add that this analysis ignores the relational and treatment context of "trouble" by attributing it to a disease stage. Since this aspect of medicalization is required of ADCRC staff in order to receive funding from the state, the result is twofold: day caregivers expect people to cause trouble as the disease progresses, and when it occurs, they "know" its origin. This knowledge provides a comforting explanation for stress in caregiving and a rationalization for "managing behavior problems" to manage stress.

In some day care centers, the assessments of impairment are reified; the numerical ratings are interpreted as objective measures of decline. For example, at Bayview, the program with the most medical features (a day health care program), the results of a reassessment of cognitive decline using the MMSE were objectified by a staff member: "Let's see how she did. She's changed!" The medical model underlying day-care work at Bayview resulted in the staff's easy acceptance of the legitimacy and objectivity of these assessments.

At other day care centers, some staff expressed skepticism about the validity and reliability of the assessments, as well as about the staff's role in administering the instruments. For example, the director in one program quite openly indicated the arbitrary and subjective quality of the required assessments, just prior to administering the MMSE to one client: "I'm going to do a Mini Mental on Maggie. It'll be a zero, but I've got to do it. . . . We get to cheat for people who can't speak—not cheat, really, but we give them a zero. I hate the Mini Mental; I don't think it says anything."

This director candidly discussed the motivation for assigning a particular score on the MMSE, which had little to do with an objective assessment of client functioning. A high score is "better for the clients but worse for us," he explained, because a population of high-scoring "lightly impaired" people does not qualify for the state ADCRC funding. The need for continued funding and the need to protect staff from the demands of too many "heavy care" clients resulted in manipulation of the overall Level of Severity Rating: "They make it look very objective but it's really very subjective. The majority I label 'moderate' [so the program meets the state requirement of serving a certain percentage of moderate to severely impaired clients]. You need the 'lights' to keep your sanity." This day-care director's candid description of the ways in which funding affects assessment illustrates a "sociology of diagnosis" (Brown 1987, 1990), the political economy and social construction of diagnoses that are driven by reimbursement formulas and other social-cultural factors.

While some staff were skeptical about the validity and reliability of the dementia stage assessments, nonetheless, the concept of stagelike disease progression was used as an explanation for trouble and as a rationalization for control over clients in each of the eight day care centers, to a greater extent in some than in others. The "level of severity" assessments contributed to these disease constructions, whether or not they furthered any understanding of disease progression.

The belief in disease-stage progression is advantageous for staff as an information resource, "knowledge" that provides the staff more certainty in their understanding of a very ambiguous medical condition. Also, if the workers are unable to manage troublesome behavior such as "anxiety," "agitation," "combativeness," and "wandering," the biomedical model offers an explanation in terms of the "stage" of the illness, which allows care providers to save face. Staff comments overheard on various occasions illustrate these rationalizations: a person cannot be managed because "she's paranoid now." Another cannot be managed because "she's at a point in her illness. . ."

The prevailing view of trouble in dementia caregiving describes a one-way relationship, stressful only for staff because of their clients' "level of impairment." In fact, once the label "Alzheimer's" or "senile dementia" is applied, even normal, reasonable behavior may be interpreted in terms of disease progression (Gubrium 1987; Smithers 1977). In dementia day-care programs, a poignant irony is that the clients' "behavior problems" as well as other sources of stress for the staff often are rooted in the caregiving relationship or the structure of the care setting. These modifiable conditions are overlooked, however, when all problems are viewed through the lens of the medical model.

Attributing trouble to the increasing severity of dementia, and the assumption of inevitable regression to a childlike state of dependency, helps staff members to cope with stressful work by rationalizing increasing control over clients. And so, the assessment of dementia, a supposedly objective medical procedure, sets the stage for medical control in the caregiving relationship.

Infantilization: The Medical Model of Care

To manage stress in caring for elderly persons with dementia, most often control is carried out and rationalized through the process of infantilization, treating older adults as if they were children (Lyman 1988). Disease progression is conceptualized as a "regression" to a childlike state of dependency and normative violations. For example, in one day care center's training manual for in-home respite caregivers, a section on "typical" Alzheimer's behavior contains four examples, all of which are of either incontinence or innocent but inappropriate sexual behavior.

The structure of day care is borrowed from the child daycare model, and few opportunities are provided in most day care centers to continue meaningful adult activity. Many staff-client interactions involve staff treating their elders like children—"for their own good." For example, the program director at Beach City described dementia in terms of "a regression in developmental stages." At Coast, the director said the program was "too

childish" for people with mild dementia, but appropriate for people who were "moderately impaired." Staff in both of these programs at times referred to and treated clients as children. At Beach City, one worker referred to the clients as "the kids." At Coast, a worker was frustrated by one client who followed her around, "like a kid you can't get rid of." A coworker at this site rewarded one client for being "a good boy" during the MMSE reassessment by offering him a lollipop.

A number of props associated with the care of children are used in caring for older adults who are cognitively impaired. For example, in one day-care program's packet of information for family caregivers, four of the eleven "tips" included reference to products designed for infants: baby gates, baby safety knobs, baby toys, baby cups with covers. The use of these props contributes to the image of older adults as childlike.

Infantilization is a strategy employed to cope with the stress of dementia care. The demands of caregiving may be eased by conceptualizing the one cared for as being childlike rather than an elder. First, much of dementia caregiving is basic custodial work: dirty work and legwork. Personal care and routine supervision are elevated to "therapy" if infantilization is viewed as part of the medical "treatment" of people who have Alzheimer's. Second, basic custodial work is made simpler if staff legitimately can "take over" in a playful manner, as one might with children who cannot complete self-care tasks. In this example from Bayview, the program director engaged in play with a client to ease the embarrassment of toileting.

> Susan is an R.N. by training, who is a very warm, affectionate companion to the people enrolled in her program. She participates with her staff in toileting and other personal care, when she is free from administrative responsibilities. She has developed a special relationship with Andrea, who can be difficult at times. She takes Andrea to the toilet, asking if she has to "pee pee," then playfully encourages Andrea to pretend that she is Susan's mom ("spank, spank"), and then assumes the adult role again: "Do you need help wiping?"

Third, staff members increase their control over working conditions and minimize some of the emotion work associated with dementia care, to the extent that they "know" what to expect and what to do. Thus, when persons with dementia "go downhill," this is taken as evidence of an "Alzheimer's disease stage." Gubrium (1987) explains this process as "ordering" the disorderly aspects of caregiving, so that dementia makes sense to caregivers.

Infantilization transforms the uncertainty concerning the nature of self-deterioration into something stereotypically familiar and manageable: older people decline to a child-like state in which it is appropriate to expect very little of them and to control their behavior. And so, dementia caregivers increase their sense of control over the conditions of their work by exercising control over their clients.

Infantilization may benefit staff, but quality of care suffers. Research in other settings has found that unnecessary control by service providers exacerbates impairment. "Excess disabilities" may result from a "highly redundant environment" in which service providers "take over" activities clients could manage themselves (Brody et al. 1971; Chappell 1978; Kielhofner 1983). Treating older adults with dementia as if they are children denies recognition of the older adult self, the person who is still inside, who has developed a lifetime of skills and who still has worth as an individual. Staff may very well provide for the physical security and comfort of clients they view as childlike. They are unable to meet people's emotional needs, however, if they deny the painful reality that their clients are older adults who live daily with cognitive impairment and who often are fully aware of frightening changes within themselves and depressing changes within their intimate and social relationships.

Social Control

In addition to the demands and uncertainties in caring for people with dementia, there are many stressful conditions in the organization of the work and the workplace. For service providers, many of the working conditions that contribute to the stress of demen-

tia care may seem to be unchangeable. For example, the staff may feel powerless to override agency policies or remodel the facility. As a result, workers may compensate for powerlessness in regard to the structure of the agency or facility by establishing a power relationship in caregiving. Control over clients is rationalized by medical labels and typifications and organized as medical authority necessary "for their own good," in caring for persons with dementing illnesses.

Six methods of control are employed by staff to cope with their stress. Most are methods typically employed with children. These forms of caregiving for older adults with dementia are part of an underlying strategy of infantilization common in dementia day care.

The first form of control is by *directives*, whereby clients are simply told what to do: "Let's sit down and relax!" These kinds of "Sit down" orders sometimes are successful, in persuading clients to stay in group activities or to refrain from leaving the building, but most often this form of control is unsuccessful. And so, frustrations for staff increase as clients disobey their commands.

The second form of control is by *deception*. For example, at Coast there were several inconveniences in the physical environment, which the staff managed by lying to clients. One bathroom was located outside in an unfenced area, requiring staff to accompany clients for their safety. Also, the office was an open space with no privacy, so it was difficult for the secretary to work when clients persisted in asking to use the phone. Staff often resorted to deception to minimize inconvenience and interruption, telling clients that "the bathroom [or telephone] is out of order; can you wait a few minutes?" Tales frequently told and retold among coworkers at Coast attributed the success of this strategy to short-term memory loss: "They forget" that the out-of-order explanation had been offered many times. . . .

The third method of control has been referred to by Conrad and Schneider (1980) as *careful coercion*, persuasive methods used in lieu of restraints to control mental patients. These methods also are among those commonly used with children. Their transference to dementia care is symbolized by the "day care" designation and is part of the process of infantilization.

In dementia care, careful coercion includes calculated compliments ("You're *so* good at that!") or requests for help intended to persuade clients to "choose" an activity. These strategies do seem successful, at times, in drawing people into group activity and boosting morale. For example, during exercise at Coast, Sarah, the program manager, successfully encouraged several people to "lead" the group.

> Sarah was an energetic, articulate Hispanic woman in her thirties, whose enthusiasm and physical energy were contagious. She asked clients to suggest exercises that the others could do: "How about an exercise, Ryan! Just one you can do from your chair!" Ryan is a slim, attractive, usually upbeat man in his seventies, a former nuclear physicist who often is on the go, looking for the next activity.
>
> Ryan: I suggest that we do this way and this way and then somersaults!!
>
> Sarah: Oh Ryan! How about something a little easier!
>
> Ryan dramatically simplifies his original suggestion: "Well . . . wiggle one toe. Now put it down and wiggle the other one. . . ."

It may not matter that these situations are staged and somewhat manipulative, if the end result is a boost for the sagging self-esteem of people suffering from cognitive impairment. Happy campers make for an easier day, both for staff and clients. However, there is a kind of dehumanization and distancing that occurs in some exchanges in which a client becomes an object of humor for the staff while being persuaded to participate in an activity. During the same exercise session at Coast this was apparent:

> Then Sarah asks Maggie to show the group an exercise. The standing joke for the staff is that she always goes to the center of the group, and she always does the same exercise, a very simple ordinary motion. Coworkers make eye contact, waiting for the inevitable repetition of this pattern. This may be staged for my benefit, or just as an inside joke for the staff.

> Maggie goes to the center of the circle, but she says: Well, I've shown you before!
>
> Sarah: Well, we'll give it a try. It's kind of hard, but we'll do it. Let's stand up and join Maggie. How many should we do?
>
> Maggie: However many you want.
>
> Sarah: How about ten. . . . Great! Let's give her a hand!
>
> Coworkers roll their eyes or share a chuckle over this favorite joke. Maggie may or may not know that she is being "a good sport."

Careful coercion also includes distraction to dissuade clients from an intended choice. Distraction, like deception, is predicated on a dementia typification, the assumption that these people, like children, will quickly forget the previous self-directed activity. Sometimes staff are surprised to find that distraction does not work, because the dementia typification was faulty: "He remembered!" But distraction often is successful.

Another form of careful coercion is "behavior modification," a term used to refer to a process of rewarding people who are coerced successfully by compliments, requests for help, or distraction. For example, at Coast the staff persisted in trying to persuade Marge, the woman who often looked as if she were about to cry, to join activity groups. Marge was almost constantly in motion; she preferred pacing or one-on-one attention from the staff. The behavior modification strategy was to offer her attention as a reward if she joined an activity group: "Someone is waiting there to give you a hug!"

This strategy rarely worked. When I asked Marge about the benefits of joining the group, she replied in a flat monotone: "It doesn't do that for me." Although the staff received little reinforcement for their behavior modification efforts with this client, the strategy was continued. In dementia care, where often nothing "works," behavior modification at least specifies whose behavior is to be changed and maintains the authority of the staff.

The fourth method of control is the most extreme: *pharmacological restraints*. According to client files from the eight day care centers, 20 to 40 percent of the clients are prescribed psychoactive drugs, administered at the discretion of the day-care staff (under a nurse's supervision) when prescribed "prn" (as required). Clients who are particularly troublesome often are "managed" by drugs, as illustrated by the case of Judy at Inland. Judy was seen by staff as very demanding because she pushed people, was unpredictable in her moods, and loudly demanded attention at inconvenient times. One staff member discussed with a sense of relief the possibility of pharmacological restraints: "She has had her medication today so she doesn't seem as bad. Her husband wasn't giving it to her. . . . Now we have permission to give it to her here too, if she's getting anxiety-ed out in the afternoon."

Ironically, when medication is used as a means of control, the "agitation" it was intended to manage often increases, resulting in greater demands on the staff. An illustration from Coast:

> Marge, the woman constantly in motion, has been prescribed mild tranquilizers, sometimes several in combination. These are supposed to be "calmer downers," according to the nurse, but obviously have the opposite effect on Marge. Penny, the nurse, recommends hospitalizing Marge to conduct a proper evaluation, to bring down the dosage or withdraw her from tranquilizers. Instead, the psychiatrist just substitutes one drug for another. Part of the problem is that Medicare will not cover hospitalization for this adjustment in medications. . . .

Even though the use of pharmacological restraints sometimes is self-defeating for the staff, as well as inappropriate treatment for the client, medication for troublesome clients is favored. Prescription drugs offer a sense of control for staff, as they attempt to manage the unpredictable, uncertain aspects of dementia care. Even if they "don't work," there is less of a sense of failure for staff than if clients "don't respond" to other efforts. If medication "has no effect," the explanation can be medicalized without taking it personally: inadequate dose, change in metabolism, disease progression. However, if medication or other restraints escalate the troublesome behavior they were intended to control, the outcome may be a cycle of control by restraints (Gubrium 1975; Mace 1987; Pynos and Stacey 1986), which increases the demands of the work for care providers.

The fifth method of control is *segregation by competence*. Dementia day care is a place where misbehavior is expected, explained, and managed within biomedical definitions of impairment. When people with dementia are "typed," as they are more in some programs than in others, they are assigned places in the facility on the basis of presumed levels of impairment. The practice of segregation by competence defines the separate places of staff and clients, as well as more- and less-impaired clients. . . .

At Valley, located in a remodeled house, some clients were taken "to the back room" when staff perceived that some of the "higher functioning" people would be "bothered" by their presence. This practice was viewed as benefiting the "higher" people without hurting the "lower" ones, who were thought to be less aware of the distinction. The view was that the "higher functioning" people were not simply intolerant of the misbehavior of their peers, but were experiencing a kind of anticipatory stigma as they observed people "farther along" than they were. And so, segregation by competence at Valley was sometimes practiced to control the misbehavior of people with more severe impairment, but more commonly it was used to ease the emotional burden of dementia on those who were less impaired. . . .

Segregation by competence is rationalized as necessary because of what the staff "know" about dementia, impairment, disease progression, and the potential for misbehavior. "Knowing one's place" is part of this staff knowledge, knowing what is required in caring for people with dementing illnesses.

A sixth method of control is the use of facility design features to isolate troublesome clients or discourage wanderers: *environmental control.*

Social Distance

In addition to exercising control over clients to manage stress, some Alzheimer's daycare staff become more distant and detached. Service providers are present, but not "there." This coping mechanism prevents staff from meeting the basic emotional security needs of their clients, while it may offer care providers a sense of control in facing the emotional demands of Alzheimer's care.

In research in long-term care settings, Asuman Kiyak and Eva Kahana have identified marginality and distancing by staff who experience stress in working with older adults. Whether they leave or stay, the lack of commitment of dissatisfied marginal workers reduces quality of care for clients (Kiyak and Kahana 1983). The links between staff stress and client care also are revealed by several indicators on Maslach's Burnout Inventory: emotional exhaustion, diminished sense of personal competence, and depersonalized detached relationships (Maslach and Jackson 1981). Burnout involves what might be called emotional absenteeism, a form of social distance that prevents high-quality care.

In several of the day-care programs included in this study, characteristics of burnout that inhibit quality of care were observed regularly. When demands were too high, when there seemed to be very little control over working conditions, and when social support was lacking, client care suffered: a client's request or apparent need for assistance was ignored; people were isolated from the group or ridiculed.

At Inland the staff ratio often was 1:10, because more privileged coworkers stayed "in back" in their offices rather than providing direct care "on the floor." The staff ratio was even worse when one of the two "floor staff" had to spend time one-on-one with clients they referred to as "heavy care," or take someone to the bathroom. As in many stressful occupations, humor relieves the tension. But for Cindy, a self-described "burned out" program aide, people with dementia sometimes became the object of insensitive ridicule, as in this example:

> Verne is in a wheelchair. He is generally cheerful and cooperative, kids around a lot, and is easy to care for. But recently Verne has had "prostate trouble," requiring frequent assistance in toileting. Often his requests have turned out to be false alarms; he has not been able to urinate at all, or much, when he is taken to the toilet. Each trip to the bathroom is not only an undesirable task for Cindy, but an interruption that requires leaving just one program aide in charge of the group. After a number of these requests on a particularly stressful day, Cindy began to loudly discuss Verne's prostate and urination problems in front of the entire group, apparently hoping to embarrass him so that he would not ask to go to the bathroom unless it was absolutely necessary. However, it is unclear to a patient who has this problem whether or not the urge to urinate is a false alarm; it is a very uncomfortable condition. At one point Cindy raised her voice and said, "I'm announcing to the world that Verne has to GO!!!". . . .

In dementia care, barriers at times are erected between workers and their stigmatized clients by avoiding meaningful conversation. Gubrium (1975) has observed administrators in a residential facility greet people with impersonal pleasantries "in passing," avoiding personal contact. Similarly, I have observed staff who dismiss or gloss over the emotional concerns of clients, as if to "move people along" and get out of the conversation without really talking with the person. Some staff members are skillful at and interested in what I would call "dementia talk," a laborious process of reflective listening to decode the personal concerns expressed by people with language impairment. But many rely upon moving people along, whenever clients begin to talk about ambiguous or personal concerns. I have heard these examples of moving people along, by various service providers in conversations initiated by people with dementia: "Oh, I see. . ." "Oh, I know. . ." "OK, I'll check on that."

This form of staff-client interaction offers superficial contact while maintaining distance. Staff stress is minimized by this strategy, but at the same time, the self-identity and emotional needs of people with dementia are ignored.

Staff Stress and Quality of Care in a Nonmedical Program

North Oaks was housed in a special day-care wing of an attractive rehabilitation hospital. But inside the doors of "the unit," this day-care program clearly was nonmedical. Staff job descriptions and the division of labor were nonspecialized. Rehabilitation aides all performed the same caregiving duties, along with one lead person who was an acting program manager.

At North Oaks there was little evidence of the medical model in caregiving. In fact, this center stood in opposition to the medical model, in stated philosophy as well as in its program activities. Catherine, the program manager, was a free spirit who had years of experience in hospital administration before moving to northern California. Alzheimer's care was a second career—and a first love. She was passionate about preserving "individual dignity" and creating a "safe place," a refuge from the "mass hatred" some people with dementia experience with their "loved ones."

> I feel really proud about this unit. . . . There's not much "acting out" or whatever you want to call it here. People say when they come in that this is a "calm" unit. That's a compliment. . . . Anything goes here. We don't use "no," or we try not to. If someone feels they need to get out of here, we get out with them.

The stated and apparent program goal at North Oaks was socioemotional: to "be with them," as opposed to more specific therapeutic goals. Catherine adamantly rejected the expectation that Alzheimer's day care include "cognitive stimulation," viewing this with disdain as meaningless and frustrating both for staff and clients: "Some people *think* they know what Alzheimer's is. They try to teach them things, ask them trivia questions, say: 'Do you remember?'. . . A lot of things people say are 'activities' are just junk."

At North Oaks staff frequently referred to their work in terms of investing emotional "energy" with their clients. Dementia typifications and medical authority seldom were observed, except by one staff member whose termination was discussed by the program manager. Most client troubles were attributed to relational problems, not simply the dementing illness. As one staff member said, "People think 'agitation' is inevitable, but it's

because they're depressed about how they're being *treated!*"

The staff at North Oaks clearly articulated and practiced a nonmedical model in their relationship with clients, emphasizing emotional connectedness, autonomy (within the boundaries of safety and physical security), and affirmation of self-identity. Staff encouraged people with dementia to express their frustration and anguish, and people were told, in many ways, "Whatever you do here is okay."

This type of relationship was of mutual benefit. The staff received reinforcement in the form of "success" in "calming" people and expressed confidence in their knowledge of "what works" in dementia care. In fact, providing high-quality care often became a source of stress management, as well as stress. This outcome illustrates the interconnections between "uplifts" and "hassles" (Kanner et al. 1981); the same caregiving experience may produce both. An example from field notes illustrates this reciprocal quality of caregiving.

> Catherine told me that one client was more "anxious" now because of his wife's recent plans to institutionalize him and the increasing distance he felt from her. She had not discussed her plans with him but he "sensed" this, according to Catherine.
> At one point, the man angrily grabbed a staff member's wrist in an attempt to leave. She was able to calm him by engaging in what I would call "dementia talk," decoding his incomplete sentences and coming to an understanding and affirmation of his feelings. He was visibly relaxed after this incident. The staff member later expressed a sense of accomplishment in managing the situation.

While the avoidance of the medical model in caregiving at North Oaks may be seen as advantageous to both staff and clients, the nonmedical program structure was a disadvantage for staff. Work-related stress was high at North Oaks largely because the demands of providing quality care were not understood or supported by the hospital administration and its policies. The staff felt impotent in arguing their case for improving the staff/client ratio, which was a primary source of staff stress. The director and program manager developed a "weighting scale," documenting the need for more staff because of frequent one-on-one care with dependent and troubled clients; however, the administration ignored this well-developed argument. Two directors came and went during the course of my fieldwork at North Oaks, largely because of unsupportive institutional policies.

One explanation for the difficulties faced by day-care staff at North Oaks is that this nonmedical program was not given legitimacy within the power structure of the larger medical facility. The new director, who quit less than six months after she was hired, expressed her frustration in being excluded from the management team meetings and not being supported by her boss. She was "fed up" with the fact that her superior had no real interest in knowing what the work was like: she "just looks at the numbers." The director continued to do as much as possible for her staff, because "I worry about them." For example, she was "selective" in admissions despite the pressure to increase the census. Describing her own work-related stress, the director said: "I've been here four months. It feels like a lifetime. If it weren't for the people, the caregivers, and the staff . . . some days . . . I'd quit." One month later, this director did resign.

An interview with the director of a day health-care (medical) program in the same rehabilitation facility revealed some striking differences in the institutional status of the two programs and in the level of staff stress in each. The adult day-health director had worked in both programs and said she could easily contrast the Alzheimer's unit with her program:

> With Alzheimer's they depend on your energy. I can leave my people from the adult day health in charge. . . . The expectation for the [Alzheimer's] workers is tremendous. They don't have a break, no time to be a little lower. There you always have to be at the same level of energy. . . . So much depends on them; they work so hard and what do they get back? I think they should work part-time and get enough salary to live on. . . . You have to be an outstanding person to do Alzheimer's work [and do a decent job]. Here in Adult Day Health—quite frankly you don't have to be outstanding to do a good job. With a little direction, clients will do it themselves.

It is clear that the staff in the Alzheimer's day-care program would fare better in the context of the larger rehabilitation facility if the program had more medical features. If they continue to operate outside the hospital power structure, staff stress will remain high because of unsupportive institutional policies. Yet staff avoidance of the medical model in their relationship with clients is a primary condition for the high quality of care in this program. According to one worker, "Most people want to be here; they don't want to go home." This does not seem to be a self-promotional exaggeration, although it refutes the almost universally accepted generalization that "people with dementia are restless in the afternoon." This is a place I found very appealing, as a temporary member, even in the afternoon. I personally would entrust this program with the care of a loved one.

Conclusion

The medical model of caregiving presents a paradox: it may relieve staff stress, but it impairs quality of care. Infantilization and other aspects of the medical model produce a relationship of control and distance in dementia care. Disease typifications become overgeneralizations Strauss has referred to as "identity spread" in describing other chronic illnesses (Strauss 1975). For dementing illnesses, Gubrium and Lynott (1987) find that once someone has been diagnosed, people see impairment everywhere. People become disease "types" or categories and experience a "loss of self" (Charmaz 1983) greater than the self-deterioration associated with the dementing illness. This treatment may increase anxiety, frustration, and "agitation" among people with dementia, which in turn may increase the demands on staff.

Conceptualizing and treating older people with dementia as children in the "regression" associated with "disease progression" offers some predictability for an unpredictable illness. There is greater certainty in facing the future tasks of caregiving within the biomedical model of dementia and the medical model of caregiving. One of the paradoxical tasks of dementia care, then, is to enable caregivers to cope with the stress of their work without contributing to the distress of their clients.

References

Brody, Elaine M., M.M. Kleban, M.P. Lawton, and H.A. Silverman. 1971. "Excess Disabilities of Mentally Impaired Aged: Impact of Individualized Treatment." *The Gerontologist* 11: 124-33.

Brown, Phil. 1987. "Diagnostic Conflict and Contradiction in Psychiatry." *Journal of Health and Social Behavior* 28: 37-50.

———. 1990. "The Name Game: Toward a Sociology of Diagnosis." *Journal of Mind and Behavior* 11: 385-406.

Chappell, Neena L. 1978. "Senility: Problems in Communication." In *Shaping Identity in Canadian Society*, edited by J. Haas and W. Shaffir. Englewood Cliffs, N.J.: Prentice-Hall.

Charmaz, Kathy. 1983. "Loss of Self: A Fundamental Form of Suffering for the Chronically Ill." *Sociology of Health and Illness* 5: 168-95.

Conrad, Peter, and Joseph W. Schneider. 1980. *Deviance and Medicalization: From Badness to Sickness*. St. Louis: C.W. Mosby.

Folstein, M., S. Folstein, and P. McHugh. 1975. "Mini Mental State: A Practical Method for Grading the Cognitive State of Patients for the Clinician." *Journal of Psychiatric Research* 12: 189-98.

Gubrium, Jaber F. 1975. *Living and Dying at Murray Manor*. New York: St. Martin's Press.

———. 1987. "Structuring and Destructuring the Course of Illness: The Alzheimer's Disease Experience." *Sociology of Health and Illness* 9: 1-24.

Gubrium, Jaber F. 1987. "Measurement and the Interpretation of Burden in the Alzheimer's Disease Experience." *Journal of Aging Studies* 1: 265-85.

Kanner, Allen D., James C. Coyne, Catherine Schaefer, and Richard S. Lazarus. 1981. "Comparison of Two Modes of Stress Management: Daily Hassles and Uplifts Versus Major Life Events." *Journal of Behavioral Medicine* 4: 381-406.

Kielhofner, G. 1983. "Teaching Retarded Adults: Paradoxical Effects of a Pedagogical Enterprise." *Urban Life* 12: 307-26.

Kiyak, H. Asuman, and Eva F. Kahana. 1983. "Predictors of Job Commitment and Turnover among Staff Working with the Aged." Paper presented to the Gerontological Society annual meeting, November.

Lyman, Karen A. 1988. "Infantilization of Elders: Day Care for Alzheimer's Disease Victims." In *Research in the Sociology of Health Care*, vol. 7, edited by Dorothy Wertz, 71-103. Greenwich, Conn.: JAI Press.

Mace, Nancy L. 1987. "Characteristics of Persons with Dementia." In *Losing a Million Minds: Confronting the Tragedy of Alzheimer's Disease and Other Dementias*. U.S. Government Office of Technology Assessment, OTA-BA-323, 59-83. Washington, D.C.: Government Printing Office.

Maslach, Christina. 1982. *Burnout: The Cost of Caring*. Englewood Cliffs, N.J.: Prentice-Hall.

Maslach, Christina and Susan Jackson. 1986. *Maslach Burnout Inventor Manual*. Consulting Psychologists Press. Palo Alto, CA.

Pynoos, Jon, and Candace A. Stacey. 1986. "Specialized Facilities for Senile Dementia Patients." In *The Dementias: Policy and Management*, edited by M.L.M. Gilhooly, S.H. Zarit, and J.E. Birren, 111-30. Englewood Cliffs, N.J.: Prentice-Hall.

Smithers, J.A. 1977. "Institutional Dimensions of Senility." *Urban Life* 6: 251-76.

Strauss, Anselm. 1975. *Chronic Illness and the Quality of Life*. St. Louis: C.V. Mosby.

Further Reading

Jaber Gubrium. 1986. *Oldtimers and Alzheimer's: The Descriptive Organization of Senility*. Greenwich: JAI Press.

S. Kaufman. 1994. "Old Age, Disease, and the Discourse on Risk: Geriatric Assessment in U.S. Health Care." *Medical Anthropology Quarterly* 8(4): 430-447.

Charles Lidz, Lynn Fischer, and Robert Arnold. 1992. *The Erosion of Autonomy in Long-term Care*. New York: Oxford University Press.

Janice Smithers. 1977. "Institutional Dimensions of Senility." *Urban Life* 6: 251-76.

Discussion Questions

1. How do you evaluate Lyman's argument about possible causes of client behavior?

2. What measures should staff members take to preserve client dignity and control? Specify how a medical model would affect their efforts.

3. How are care, control, and staff stress linked in Lyman's depiction of Alzheimer's care?

From *Day In, Day Out With Alzheimer's: Stress in Caregiving Relationships.* Pp. 62-85. Copyright © 1993 by Temple University Press. Reprinted by permission. ✦

18

Narratives of Aging and Social Problems in Medical Encounters With Older Persons

Howard Waitzkin
Theron Britt
Constance Williams

Getting a physician to listen attentively to your health concerns can be difficult. Some research reveals that demographic differences between physicians and their patients can make it difficult for physicians to understand patient perspectives. Higher social status and medical knowledge base distinguish physicians from many of their patients. Oftentimes, practitioners are younger than their patients. In this selection, Howard Waitzkin and his colleagues examine problems of communication that arise in routine medical encounters between physicians and older patients.

Social as well as medical difficulties accompany age. Widowhood, the loss of a home, concern about mobility and declining ability affect older persons' perceptions of health and general well-being. The discourse of medical encounters shows that the health of older persons is embedded in medical and personal concerns characteristic of aging. Here we get a look at how physicians interact with older persons— the questions they ask, and the social issues they avoid. In spite of the emotional—and po-

tentially medical—distress life circumstances may create for older patients, Waitzkin and his coauthors discover that physicians seldom address the personal concerns of their older patients. These concerns profile life incidents characteristic of older populations and reveal complex issues relevant to health care. As you read this selection, think about the link Waitzkin presents between the life worlds of the elderly and common diagnoses. Look carefully at how physicians frequently ignore or marginalize the social problems older persons raise during the course of medical encounters in this account. The way physicians ignore their older patients' social problems not only affects their clinical relationship but also suggests how physicians negotiate medical encounters and care more generally.

... When older people talk with doctors, their conversations often touch on social problems. Bereavement, financial insecurity, isolation, dependency, inadequate housing, lack of transportation, and similar issues cause difficulties for the elderly. In some cases, patients or doctors raise these issues directly. Alternatively, such problems may surface indirectly, in passing, or marginally, as doctors and patients focus on technical concerns.

The appearance of social problems within medical encounters poses a challenge for researchers and practitioners. Certain geriatric programs use multidisciplinary teams, including social workers, to help resolve problems that derive from the social context of medicine; to some extent, these interventions can improve conditions that seniors face. Meanwhile, many older people continue to consult practitioners who feel that the social context is not relevant to the medical task or that their ability to grapple with contextual problems is limited ...

The present study asks how older patients and doctors deal with social problems in the discourse of routine medical encounters. ...

Encounters With Older Patients

... By interpreting these encounters, we do not intend to criticize the particular doctors or patients involved but rather to reveal patterns of discourse that emerge under the constraints of modern medical practice. This encounter, as well as others we have studied, inevitably raises the question of change. That is, how might the structure and process of medical discourse be modified to improve on the conditions revealed here? While this question is not an easy one to answer, we also speculate in the concluding section on this study's implications for change, and present some preliminary criteria that can guide physicians and patients in discussions about contextual issues.

Loss of Home, Community, and Autonomy

Summary: An elderly woman visits her doctor for follow-up of her heart disease. During the encounter she expresses concerns about decreased vision, her ability to continue driving, lack of stamina and strength, weight loss and diet, and financial problems. She discusses her recent move to a new home and her relationships with family and friends. Her physician assures her that her health is improving; he recommends that she continue her current medical regimen and that she see an eye doctor.

From the questionnaires that the patient and doctor completed after their interaction, some pertinent information is available: The patient is an 80-year-old, White high school graduate. She is Protestant, Scottish American, and widowed, with five living children whose ages range from 45 to 59 years; she describes her occupation as "homemaker." Her doctor is a 44-year-old White male, who is a general internist. The doctor has known the patient for about one year, and believes that her primary diagnoses are atherosclerotic heart disease and prior congestive heart failure. The encounter takes place in a suburban private practice near Boston.

Social support and the loss of home and community. Although the patient values her independence, she also tries to maintain a social support network, which she describes without prompting in an incomplete narrative. Allusions to a support network usually arise within this medical encounter as marginal features, which the patient mentions in passing, and which the doctor does not pursue in depth. Among her social contacts, R—,

a friend, appears the most central. The patient tries to see R— regularly for lunch and other get-togethers. Socializing with R— brings her pleasure, advice, and support. For instance, when she describes her current nutritional status and medications, she says:

> P: And I'm trying hard to eat a banana once in a while, trying to eat some tomatoes, and
> D: uh
> P: I ate a R— took me to lunch and I had an elegant lobster salad sandwich.

As a source of advice, R— has raised a question about vitamin A as a factor in the patient's visual symptoms. The patient also mentions that R— has helped her to move and to buy clothing.

Family members figure less prominently as sources of support, and also create some rather burdensome obligations. Most of the family members have moved to other geographical areas. The patient keeps in touch by telephone and mail, especially for birthdays, but she finds herself unable to do as much as she might like, partly because of the number of people involved:

> P: Well I should—now I've got birthday cards to buy. I've got seven or eight birthdays this week—month. Instead of that, I'm just gonna write 'em and wish them a happy birthday. Just a little note, my grandchildren.
> D: Mm Hmm.
> P: But I'm not gonna bother. I just can't do it all, Dr.—.
> D: Well.
> P: I called my daughter, her birthday was just, today's the third.
> D: Yeah.
> P: My daughter's birthday in Princeton was the uh first, and I called her up and talked with her. Don't know what time it'll cost me, but then, my telephone is my only indiscretion.

At no other time in the encounter does the patient refer to her own family, nor does the doctor ask. The patient does her best to maintain contact, even though she does not mention anything that she receives in the way of day-to-day support.

Compounding these problems of social support and incipient isolation, the patient recently has moved from a home that she occupied for 59 years. The reasons for giving up her home remain unclear, but they seem to involve a combination of financial factors and difficulties in maintaining it. She first mentions the move quickly, but then shifts to a visit with R—and her shopping accomplishments:

P: And of course I'd been awful busy changing addresses, 'n-
D: Yeah.
P: And today, I've been to lunch with R—. And I've done all my week's shopping. And here I am.

During silent periods in the physical examination of the heart and lungs, the patient spontaneously narrates more details about the loss of possessions and relationships with previous neighbors, along with satisfaction about certain conveniences of her new living situation. Further, as the patient speaks, the doctor asks clarifying questions about the move, and gives several of his usual pleasant fillers, before he cuts off this discussion by helping the patient from the examination table:

P: Yeah. . . . . ((moving around noises)) Well, I sold a lot of my stuff.
D: Yeah, how did the moving go, as long as (word)
P: And y'know take forty-ni- fifty-nine year's accumulation. Boy, and I've got cartons in my closet it'll take me till doomsday to, ouch.
D: Gotcha.
P: But I've been kept out of mischief by doing it. But I've got a lot to do, I sold my rugs 'cause they wouldn't fit where I am. I just got a piece of plain cloth at home.
D: Mm hmm.
P: Sometimes I think I'm foolish at 81. I don't know how long I'll live. Isn't much point in putting money into stuff, and then, why not enjoy a little bit of life?
D: Mm hmm, (words).
P: And I've got to have draperies made.

D: Now, then, you're (words).
P: But that'll come. I'm not worrying. I got an awfully cute place. It's very very comfortable. All electric kitchen. It's got a better bathroom than I ever had in my life.
D: Great. . . .Met any of your neighbors there yet?
P: Oh, I met two or three.
D: Mm hmm.
P: And my, some of my neighbors from Belmont here, there's Mrs. F—and her two sisters are up to see me, spent the afternoon with me day before yesterday. And all my neighbors um holler down the hall (words) . . . years ago. They're comin', so they say. So, I'm hopin' they will. I hated to move, cause I loved, um I liked my neighbors very much.
D: Now, we'll let you down. You watch your step.
P: You're not gonna let me, uh, unrobed, disrobed today.
D: Don't have to, I think.
P: Well!
D: Your heart sounds good.
P: It does?
D: Yep.

After the doctor mentions briefly that the patient's heart "sounds good," he and the patient go on to other topics. The doctor's cutoff and a return to technical assessment of cardiac function . . . have the effect of marginalizing a contextual problem that involves loss of home and community. From the patient's perspective, the move holds several meanings.

First, in the realm of inanimate objects, her new living situation, an apartment contains several physical features that she views as more convenient, or at least "cute." On the other hand, she apparently has sold many of her possessions, which carry the memories of 59 years in the same house. Further, she feels the need to decorate her new home, but doubts the wisdom of investing financial resources in such items as rugs and draperies at her advanced age.

Aside from physical objects, the patient confronts a loss of community. In response to the doctor's question about meeting new neighbors, the patient says that she has met "two or three." Yet she "hated" to move, because of the affection that she held for her prior neighbors. Describing her attachment, she first mentions that she "loved" them, and then modulates her feelings by saying that she "liked them very much." Whatever the pain that this loss has created, the full impact remains unexplored, as the doctor cuts off the line of discussion by terminating the physical exam and returning to a technical comment about her heart.

Throughout these passages, the doctor supportively listens. He offers no specific suggestions to help the patient in these arenas, nor does he guide the dialogue toward deeper exploration of her feelings. Despite his supportive demeanor, the doctor here functions within the traditional constraints of the medical role. When tension mounts with the patient's mourning a much-loved community, the doctor returns to the realm of medical technique.

Mobility, autonomy, and visual capacity. From the start of the encounter, the patient complains about her vision and its impact on autonomous function in daily life. Although her cardiac symptoms have improved, she still feels "rocky," by which she refers to her visual symptoms:

P: But I:: feel kind of rocky.
D: You are (word).
P: My eyes are bothering me. I can see perfectly, read signs, but R— [friend] said she wondered if I was eating right, and if I, a little vitamin A or something would, ah, when I go back, turn back from a bright lights, it looks dark to me, although I can see.

The patient attaches importance to eyesight as a critical aid for mobility and autonomy. At age 80, she still drives a car and wants to continue. She emphasizes the link between vision and transportation immediately after the doctor refers her to an ophthalmologist. When the patient introduces the topic of driving, the doctor banters with her about safety and speed:

P: I drove my car yesterday, down Arlington Heights
D: Oh, dear, Eighty miles an hour again.
P: No, I didn't. I went thirty.
D: Thirty.
P: Yeah, down Mass Avenue.
D: Well, that's the first time in years you've ever slowed down to thirty.
P: Nope
D: Hm hmm.
P: Yeah. Ha haa.

The doctor's joking demeanor initially diminishes the urgency of the patient's concerns linking mobility and visual symptoms; here the patient reassures the doctor that she has reduced her speed in line with community standards.

A negotiation that follows expresses several themes, which objectify and reify the complex social conditions facing this older person by converting them to a concrete professional decision about physical capacity to use a car. First, the patient depends on her car for many functional necessities and social contacts. She indicates these concerns later:

P: It's all right for me to drive a little bit if I feel like it?
D: I guess we're not gonna stop you.
P: Well, no, that isn't the question. It's whether you feel my-
D: I think it's all right, yes.
P: Like going (words) shopping center on Baker Street.
P: (word) driving, I went to a funeral (words)
D: Yeah. Well, I don't if you use your judgment that way, sure.

The patient requests the doctor's approval for continuing to drive. His response proves less than enthusiastic, as he uses the royal "we" to note that he will not invoke his legal responsibility, as a doctor and agent of social control, to prohibit driving when physical incapacity predictably might interfere with safety. As the patient begins to reply that the doctor's stopping her "isn't the question," she begins to clarify the question, but the doctor interrupts. After the doctor gives tentative approval, the patient alludes to the importance of using the car to go shopping and also for social responsibilities like a recent funeral. Her car thus becomes her means to buy the necessities required for independent living, as well as a way to fulfill social obligations— among which the funerals of friends and relatives figure prominently at her age.

The mobility that the patient's car provides then becomes part of a story about functional capacity that the patient spontaneously narrates. As she lives alone long after her husband has died and her children have departed, autonomy in activities of daily living has become an increasing struggle. For instance, she expresses pleasure in her ability to do housework, to cook, and to feed herself:

P: Now I'll tell you what I did yesterday. Uhm. I did all my own work, and I've been, been doing a fair amount of vegetable cooking, getting better meals for myself.
D: Mm hmm.
P: I managed to get a whole tomato down this week.
D: There you are.
P: And a whole banana. Ha! Kidding. Well, . . ah, I took the car out, then I came home, and I said, "Well I've got (word)." so I ironed.

Later she alludes to gratification in buying groceries on her own:

P: Still I'm getting better, I can, I can move around pretty well. I went ramblin', picked a (word), oh I have two, three weeks ago, all my groceries myself.

While the patient uses a humorous and ironic tone, she takes such accomplishments seriously. The doctor punctuates the narrative with brief conversational fillers ("Mm hmm," "There you are," and so forth), which convey tolerance and support for the patient's efforts to preserve autonomous function.

Financial insecurity. Worries about money come up at several points in the encounter. As already noted, economic considerations are constraining her decisions about decorating her new home. Further, desire to maintain mobility and autonomy by driving a car also creates financial stress:

P: So, uh, I sha'n't do anything about buying something for myself until I get my bills paid. So, and I suppose I was awfully foolish to put my car on the road this year.

Driving thus increases financial pressures while helping her to maintain autonomy.

The costs of medical care also have become a burden. Noting that her insurance coverage remains incomplete, the patient describes a hospital bill that has affected her ability to make needed purchases, for instance, of clothes:

P: So I told R—, I said I'll go and get a dress at a time. I got a nice bill from— Hospital yesterday. Two hundred and forty-one dollars. ((sniff))
D: How about Medicare?
P: I've got, you see I didn't have Medicare D [sic], Doctor. A—didn't think we needed it. And I was so, well, negligent I should have had it. But I am registered for it the first of July.

Like many seniors, she regrets that she had underestimated the need for insurance.

Consistently, the patient initiates consideration of financial problems. While the doctor seldom interrupts the contextual narrative, his style remains nondirective. The patient's financial difficulties thus remain unengaged and ultimately marginal elements of the discourse.

The body's deterioration. The patient knows her age and its implications. She wonders about the wisdom of decorating her new home when the duration of her ability to enjoy it may be not very long. Further, after mentioning her difficulty in keeping up with birthdays in her family, she assumes a pessimistic tone:

P: I don't care, I never go to the movies, and I very seldom watch movies on television even. So, . . . uh (word) oh, if I could only (word) with my own self
D: ((cough))
P: and go like I used to. But what can you expect when I'm, when I'm, when you're almost, when you're gonna, going toward 81?

A scenario of deterioration also appears in a discussion about weight loss and its impact on the patient's wardrobe:

> P: So I ironed. I had three dresses, which I'll never wear because they're about that wide and I'm about that wide. If you want to see something, come here, look at me.
> D: Uh huh.
> P: Look, look at that.
> D: Well, you've lost a little weight, huh?
> P: A little? I've lost about 20 pounds.

After the doctor questions about her diet and performs a brief physical exam, the patient alludes to her continuing attempts to sew clothing for herself.

> P: Oh, the dress, good Lord, I've made my clothes for years. And I'm heart broken because I had a couple of nice summer dresses that I made myself, and, they're miles too big.

In short, the patient is experiencing distress about changes in her body and her image of it. As her body shrinks, she no longer is able to clothe it as she once could. The loss of such clothes that she has sewn for herself then bends with the effects of her other losses. The technical meaning of weight loss remains ambiguous, as the patient never questions the doctor explicitly about it, nor does he offer an explanation. For instance, a possible association between cancer and weight loss remains absent from the conversation. Further, while she has experienced a series of losses and verbalizes a few depressed emotions, the patient does not mention the word "depression"; likewise, the doctor neither asks about depression nor lists it as a possible diagnosis.

Throughout the encounter, death waits in the background. When the patient obliquely refers to the end of her life, the discourse does not encourage exploration of her feelings or plans about dying. In all this, an ideology of stoicism is maintained, as the patient stoically observes her own bodily deterioration (cf. Zola 1991), and as the doctor listens supportively while she describes her attempts to transcend the sadnesses of physical aging.

Context, ideology, and structure. The socioemotional context of aging predominates in this encounter. Typically, the patient initiates such topics; the doctor listens and enunciates brief verbal fillers that convey interest and support. Technical content gives way in most instances to extensive conversation about the experiences of aging. Patient and doctor engage in warm and mutually respectful dialogue, as they both confront troubling issues that presumably remain beyond medicine's reach.

Several ideological assumptions become apparent. Coping with the vicissitudes of aging remains a matter of individual responsibility. This ideological orientation emphasizing individual responsibility is consistent with a dominant ideological pattern in United States society (Sennett and Cobb 1972). Preserving her functional capacity to carry out activities that are typical of women's social role—homemaking, shopping, cooking, feeding, sewing, and so forth—remains a high priority. In the face of physical deterioration and impending death, the dialogue objectifies and reifies the totality of the patient's contextual difficulties, even as it reinforces her stoical attempts to cope.

This encounter shows structural elements that appear beneath the surface details of patient-doctor communication, shown schematically in Figure 18-1. Contextual issues affecting the patient include social isolation; loss of home, possessions, family, and community; limited resources to preserve independent function; financial insecurity; and physical deterioration associated with the process of dying (A). Because of these contextual difficulties, the patient experiences loneliness, frustration, and anxiety, in addition to the physical troubles of heart disease, visual symptoms, and weight loss (B). In a visit with her doctor (C), she expresses concerns about contextual problems at great length. The doctor listens supportively, allowing the patient to describe her situation in detail (D). There is no intervention to improve any of the contextual difficulties that the patient presents. Nevertheless, tensions in the discourse arise that reflect a disjuncture between medicine's technical voice and the contextual issues that most trouble the patient. Facing these ten-

Figure 18-1
Schematic, Structural Elements of a Medical Encounter Involving Loss of Home,
Community, and Autonomy

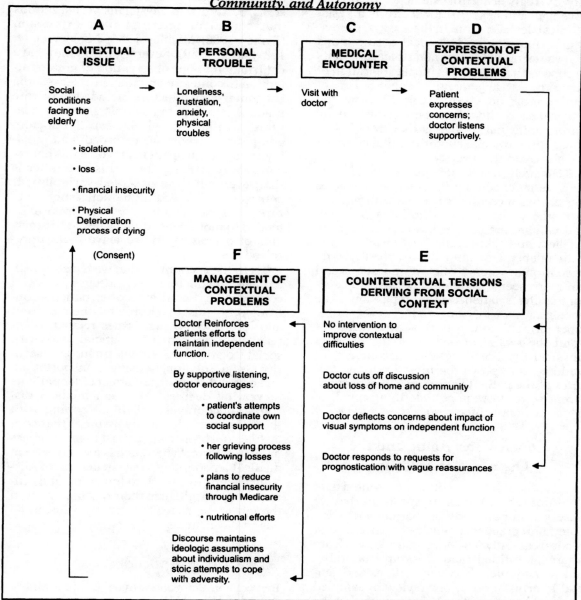

sions, the doctor cuts off a discussion about loss of home and community, and deflects concerns about the impact of visual symptoms on independent function by referring the patient to another specialist (E). To manage the patient's contextual problems, the doctor reinforces her efforts to maintain independent function, although a theme of social control arises about her uncertain ability to drive safely. Through supportive listening, he also encourages her efforts to coordinate a social support network, her grieving process following the loss of a home and community, her plan to reduce financial insecurity by registering for Medicare insurance coverage, and her nutritional efforts to resist physical deterioration. In these ways, the discourse maintains ideological assumptions that value individualism and stoical attempts to cope with adversity. Critical exploration of alternative arrangements to enhance her social support does not occur (F). After the medical encounter, the patient returns to the same contextual problems that trouble her, consenting to social conditions that confront the elderly in this society.

That such structural features should characterize an encounter like this one becomes rather disconcerting, since the communication otherwise seems so admirable. At an advanced age, the patient has retained a keen intellect and takes initiative to lead her life with independence and dignity. She shows no hesitation in voicing whatever questions and emotions seem pertinent. Likewise, the doctor manifests patience and compassion, as he encourages a wide-ranging discussion of socioemotional concerns that extend far beyond the technical details of the patient's physical disorders. Yet the discourse does nothing to improve the most troubling features of the patient's situation. To expect differently would require redefining much of what medicine aims to do. . . .

Conclusions: Aging and the Discourse of Medicine

. . . Although the encounter presented here does not reflect the entire spectrum that we observed in our study or that clinicians encounter in practice, it illustrates patterns that recur frequently. The encounter derives from a large, stratified random sample of audiotaped encounters between patients and general internists. From our review of sampled tapes and transcripts, we also believe that the encounter presented here captures some of the variability in discourse involving doctors and older patients.

Specifically, [the encounter] contains a substantial amount of material concerning the patient's "lifeworld" concerns. . . [In the] encounter, the doctors give the patient more

latitude than one might expect from prior studies, which generally have found very limited discourse concerning lifeworld concerns, partly due to physicians' verbal actions that cut off or interrupt their expression (Fisher 1986; Mishler 1984; Mishler et al. 1989; Todd 1989). Several factors may have contributed to our observation of greater attention to contextual matters in at least some encounters; such factors include the private practice setting of our sample, the prior relationships that existed between the doctors and patients whom we recorded, and possibly the age of the patients involved. What remains very striking about this encounter is that, even with the observed variability, it consistently showed a characteristic structure and sequencing, which eventually tended to move contextual issues to the margins of discourse and to leave them unresolved.

. . . In the encounters that we have studied, patients and doctors rarely discuss the social context in any detail, even when patients confront problems that threaten their current and future well-being. Issues related to bereavement, retirement, financial insecurity, social isolation, retirement, financial insecurity, social isolation, housing, transportation, and other life transitions affect older patients to varying degrees. Although medical discourse encourages individual coping with these problems, it usually assumes that contextual constraints will persist in more or less unaltered form. When such issues do arise in medical encounters, the structure of discourse tends to cut off, to interrupt, and ultimately to marginalize their discussion, even though these issues may create substantial day-to-day distress. . . .

Appendix

Transcription Conventions (modified from Mishler 1984 and West 1984)

1. Speaker D is doctor, P is patient. Speaker is noted at the first line of an utterance and at overlap points.

2. Turn/Utterance Location Each new turn—that is, the beginnings of utterances by speakers in a sequence—generally starts at the beginning of a line in the transcript. Gaps and overlaps are indicated by appropriate markers.

3. Overlap [If a speaker begins to talk while the other is still talking, the point of beginning overlap is marked by a bracket [between the lines.

4. Silence. . . . . Silences within speaker utterances and between speakers are marked by a series of dots; each dot represents one second.

   Long pauses are denoted by number of seconds in parentheses. These silences are assigned to the previous speaker if they occur between speakers; that is, they are given the meaning of a post-utterance pause.

5. Unclarity (cold)/(. . .) Where a word(s) is heard but remains unclear, it is included in parentheses; if there are speaking sounds that are unintelligible, this is noted as dots within parentheses.

6. Speech Features ?/. Punctuation marks are used when intonation clearly marks the utterance as a question or as the end of a sentence. : If a word is stretched, this is marked by a colon as . in "Wel:l". - If a speaker breaks off in the middle of a word or phrase, this is marked by a hyphen,-, as in "haven't felt like-". ((softly)) ((change in tone of voice)) Double parentheses enclose descriptions, not transcribed utterances. .hh, hh, eh-heh, .engh-henh These are breathing and laughing indicators. A period followed by "hh's" marks an inhalation. The "hh's" alone stand for exhalation. The "eh-heh" and ".engh-henh" are laughter syllables (inhaled when preceded by a period). ___(Italics) or CAPS Underline or capital letters are used if there is a marked increase in loudness and/or emphasis.

7. Names —(blanks) To protect confidentiality, blanks substitute for proper names.

8. Deletion in Excerpt* * * (asterisks) Within excerpts from transcripts, three asterisks signify a passage from the original transcript that has been deleted from the excerpt.

References

Mishler, Elliot G. 1984. *The Discourse of Medicine: Dialectics of Medical Interviews.* Norwood, NJ: Ablex.

Mishler, Elliot G., Jack A. Clark. Joseph Ingelfinger, and Michael P. Simon. 1989. "The Language of Attentive Patient Care: A Comparison of Two Medical Interviews." *Journal of General Internal Medicine* 4:325-35.

Sennett, Richard and Jonathan Cobb. 1972. *The Hidden Injuries of Class.* New York: Vintage.

Zola, Irving Kenneth. 1991. "Bringing Our Bodies and Ourselves Back In: Reflections on a Past, Present, and Future 'Medical Sociology.' " *Journal of Health and Social Behavior* 32:1-16.

Further Reading

Jay Katz. 1984. *The Silent World of Doctor and Patient.* New York: The Free Press.

Candace West. 1984. *Routine Complications: Troubles with Talk Between Doctors and Patients.* Indiana: Indiana University Press.

Irving Zola. 1991. "Bringing Our Bodies and Ourselves Back in: Reflections on a Past, Present, and Future 'Medical Sociology'." *Journal of Health and Social Behavior* 32: 1-16.

Discussion Questions

1. Think about your last visit to a physician or other sort of health care provider. Were there issues that you felt your provider ignored? What sorts of issues were they? Medical? Social? Emotional?

2. To what degree do you believe physicians have a responsibility to attend to the social experiences of their patients?

3. What kind of impact do you believe physician nonresponse to social problems has on the overall health of patients?

19

Prevalence and Sources of Patients' Unmet Expectations for Care

Richard L. Kravitz
Edward J. Callahan
Debora A. Paterniti
Deirdre Antonius
Marcia Dunham
Charles E. Lewis

What sorts of things do you expect when you go to your physician for care? In this selection, Kravitz and his coauthors query patients about reports of dissatisfaction following a physician office visit. When patients visit their health care provider, they often have questions they want their physician to address: lack of clarity about the kind and course of treatment, mysterious side effects, family history, explanations and directions from past practitioners, the advice of family and friends. All of these crowd patients' minds, making it hard for patients to see an office visit as "usual business." As the costs of health care increase, policymakers and health care administrators search out ways to keep expenses down. Budget cuts mean the disappearance of high-priced tests and specialty referrals. Often, budgetary decreases reduce physicians' time with patients. As you read about types of patient expectations, consider what health care cutbacks

mean for satisfaction and unfulfilled expectations for care.

Patients' expectations for medical care are of increasing interest to clinicians, policymakers, and researchers. For clinicians, understanding and attempting to meet these expectations is an inherent responsibility[1] and may lead to increased patient satisfaction.[2] For policymakers, patients' expectations warrant attention because of their potential influence on health care utilization[3] and because fulfillment of expectations is one measure of the quality of health care systems[1,4]. For researchers, patients' expectations can serve as both independent and dependent variables in studies of health care utilization, costs, quality, and satisfaction. Thus, further understanding of patients' expectations could improve the clinical process of care, health care delivery systems, and health services research.

Although several studies[5] have highlighted the importance of patients' expectations, none has directly addressed the question of what influences the development and expression of these expectations. Obtaining a more thorough understanding of this process is important for two reasons. First, it may sensitize physicians to patients' concerns and facilitate more effective communication and clinical care; second, it could lead to strategies for helping patients form more consistently reasonable expectations in this era of limited medical resources.

We sought to identify influences on the development of patients' expectations by interviewing patients whose expectations about an office visit were unmet. In doing this, we focused on three questions. First, what is the prevalence of patient-reported omissions of care after visits to internists? Second, what factors influence the development of patients' expectations and patients' perceptions of omission to articulate perceived omissions of care?

After describing the methods by which our data were collected and analyzed, we present the characteristics of the patients who were interviewed and the prevalence of unfulfilled expectations reported by these patients. We then discuss the various sources of patients' expectations. Finally, we discuss the implications of our findings for clinical effectiveness and health policy.

Methods

Sampling of Practices and Patients

Our study was done in three general internal-medicine practices in a mid-sized city in northern California. Two practices were branch offices of a large group-model health maintenance organization. Within these two practices, all patients were members of the health maintenance organization and received care on a capitated basis; the 10 physicians and three nurse practitioners were each paid a salary. The third practice consisted of 8 general internists (2 of whom had additional subspecialty training) and one nurse practitioner, all of whom worked in a single private office and received a combination of salary and productivity bonuses. Patients in this practice were insured under various prepaid and fee-for-service plans. All three practices attempted to schedule patients with their own regular practitioners when possible.

We selected these practices to represent the dominant models of health care in northern California, an area heavily penetrated by managed care. Because managed care providers may have financial incentives to restrict medical care, managed care settings are potential sites of conflict between patients' expectations and the ability of clinicians to meet those expectations.

During 36 half-day sessions (12 sessions per practice) scheduled between October and December 1994, trained research assistants approached patients in waiting rooms and encouraged them to complete a brief form that was designed to identify and thus exclude patients presenting for routine checkups. (In preliminary research, we had found that such patients were relatively unlikely to have unmet expectations.) The form asked two questions: 1) Do you have a new or worsening problem that you wish to discuss with the doctor today (yes or no)? and 2) How concerned are you that you might have a serious disease or condition that has not yet been diagnosed (not-at-all to extremely)? Of the 1221 patients who completed the form, 804 had a new or worsening problem or were at least moderately concerned about an undiagnosed condition and thus were eligible for further study. Of the 804 eligible patients, 688 (86%) agreed to participate in the study and completed a post-visit questionnaire that asked about demographic characteristics, recent health care utilization, health status, satisfaction with the visit, and perceived omissions of care.

The core of the written survey was eight questions about perceived omissions of care. Patients were given the following instructions:

> When people go to the doctor, they usually bring some thoughts about how he or she can be of the most help. Sometimes, however, the doctor may not be able or willing to do exactly what the patient wants. . . . These questions are about things you felt were necessary for the doctor to do today but which (for whatever reason) didn't happen. . . .

These instructions were followed by questions about sets of possible omissions involving physician preparation for the visit; history taking; physical examination; laboratory testing or diagnostic imaging; prescription of medication; referral to specialists; information, counseling, or personal help; and "anything else you felt was necessary or might be necessary for the doctor to do today but which didn't happen." The wording of the instructions reflected semantic concerns reviewed elsewhere[5] and was intended to convey a broad definition of "patients' expectations," emphasizing expectations as things that patients value. Of the 688 respondents, 125 (18%) reported one or more omissions and 108 (86%) consented in writing to participate in a telephone interview within several days of the visit.

Telephone Interviews

Within 1 to 7 days of the visit, one investigator conducted telephone interviews with 90 of the 108 patients who had reported one or more omissions on their questionnaire and who had provided their home telephone numbers as part of the consent process. The interviewer identified himself as a "researcher from UC Davis" but not as a physician (he did say that he was a physician if specifically asked). The interviewing approach was modeled on the critical incident technique[6], which focuses on patients' accounts of events that have actually happened rather than on generalizations or opinions[7]. In this case, the critical incident was the perceived omission of care. Thus, the opening question was, "You mentioned on your questionnaire that you were hoping that the doctor would [perform a particular intervention], but that didn't happen. Can you tell me more about that?" Patient interviews averaged 15 minutes in length.

Data Transformation

Of the 90 interviews, 88 were successfully tape recorded and transcribed. To locate key themes related to the genesis of patients' expectations for care, we used an iterative process, which began with a careful reading by three investigators of approximately 20 randomly selected transcripts. In a series of meetings, the research team developed by consensus a preliminary coding scheme. Codes were developed inductively, consistent with the grounded theory approach used in sociology.[8,9] We focused on the sources and the process of development of patient's expectations. Examples of codes and their definitions are shown in Table 19-1.

In the second stage of the analysis, the lead investigator applied the coding scheme to 50% of the transcripts ($n = 44$) by using a qualitative research tool, the Ethnograph[10]. A health psychologist independently coded 20% of these transcripts. The κ coefficient for inter-rater reliability at the coded-segment level was 0.39, indicating moderate agreement beyond chance. The lead investigator then coded the remaining transcripts, and the study team as a whole reviewed the results and reached a consensus on major concepts and themes.

Results

Patient Characteristics

The patients who completed the post-visit survey ($n = 688$) had a mean age of 51 years and a mean education level of 14.2 years; 63%

Table 19-1
Selected Coding Categories Used To Examine Patients' Expectations for Care

Coding Category	Definition	Example
Symptom Severity	Severity or intensity of symptom or problem, focus of concern on current symptoms	"My main complaint was the horrible headache I had."
Symptom seriousness	Perceived seriousness of symptoms: focus of concern on future implications of symptoms	"I just want to make sure it's not pneumonia"
Vulnerability: family history	Perceived vulnerability due to a family history of illness	"I just thought it might have been a preventive measure to go ahead and give me a mammogram . . . I have had a history of breast cancer in my family."
Personal experience	Expectations derived from past personal experience with a disease, problem, or symptom similar to the one being experienced	"The first [surgery] I had in Illinois was totally successful. Of course I was 10 years younger."
Specialized knowledge: self	Expectations derived from the patient's own education or training in a health-related field	"In my veterinary clinic we always draw a CBC* on the animals when they have a fever."
Media	Expectations derived from books, periodicals, and electronic media	"The last time I saw him I asked if he would please prescribe some estrogen for me because I read an article about it . . ."

* CBC = complete blood count.

were female and 83% were white. Six percent were visiting a physician for an initial, comprehensive evaluation; 49% were making follow-up visits with their own physicians; 38% were being seen on an urgent basis by someone other than their own physicians; and 7% were making other types of visits.

In terms of sex, education level, and the percentage of patients who were making follow-up visits to their own physicians, the group of patients who reported at least one omission of care ($n = 125$) was similar to the group of patients who reported no omissions of care. However, patients with unmet expectations were younger (mean age, 47 years compared with 52 years; $P = 0.001$). The likelihood of reporting one or more omissions was lowest among the 188 patients aged 65 years and older (11% reported one or more omissions), highest for the 127 patients younger than 35 years of age (23% reported one or more omission), and intermediate for the 365 middle-aged patients (20% reported one or more omissions) ($P = 0.007$). Patients who reported at least one omission were less likely than patients who did not report an omission to provide an "excellent" rating for the visit overall (35% compared with 75%; $P = 0.001$).

Prevalence of Unmet Expectations

A total of 125 patients (18.2%) reported at least one unfulfilled expectation within eight broad categories of care (Table 19-2). The prevalence of specific perceived omissions ranged from 2.8% (for failure to provide needed information, counseling, or personal help) to 5.5% (for omission of a component of the physical examination) (Table 19-2). Among patients who reported at least one perceived omission, the mean number of perceived omissions ± SD was 1.9 ± 1.17.

Sources of Expectations

In the telephone interviews, patients identified four major sources of their unmet expectations: somatic symptoms, perceived vulnerability to illness, previous experience, and transmitted knowledge; 95 percent of patients cited at least one of these sources, and 73 percent cited two or more.

Somatic Symptoms. Somatic symptoms influenced the expectations of 74% of the interviewed patients, who described their symptoms in terms of four dimensions: intensity of symptoms, functional impairment, duration of symptoms, and perceived seriousness of symptoms (Table 19-3). Patients often linked salient symptom dimensions to specific goals of care-seeking. For example, patients who had severe or disabling symptoms frequently sought empathy or relief, whereas those with frightening symptoms sought reassurance that they did not have a serious disorder.

Table 19-2
Prevalence of Perceived Omissions of Care

Omission Category	Example	Patients, n (%)[*]	
Physician preparation for the visit	Failing to review chart before patient's arrival	29	(4.3)
History taking	Not asking about specific medical or lifestyle factors	33	(4.9)
Physical examination	Not doing cardiac auscultation	37	(5.5)
Laboratory testing	Omitting cholesterol level measurement or magnetic resonance imagining	35	(5.2)
Prescription of medication	Not prescribing analgesics	24	(3.6)
Referral to specialists	Not recommending a neurosurgical consultation	33	(5.0)
Information and counseling	Not answering questions about prognosis	19	(2.8)
Other		31	(4.7)
Total reporting one or more omissions		125	(18.2)

[*]$n = 688$.

Forty-two percent of patients commented on the intensity or severity of their symptoms. As justification for patients' expectations, symptoms often spoke for themselves ("There is a red hot poker that is drilled through my leg and it's real painful at times.") Other patients explicitly contrasted the severity of their symptoms with the clinician's apparent nonchalance. Distress about symptoms was compounded by concern that the physician was not taking the problem seriously: "Yes, it's my entire body. My extremities, connective tissue, everything is sore and painful. . . It warranted more than, well, let's just talk about it in 2 weeks."

About one sixth of patients emphasized the functional consequences of their symptoms (Table 19-3). These patients focused on resuming short-term responsibilities ("I'm having a really big problem with my back right now and I'm missing work and would like to go ahead and get a refill on my Flexeril") or achieving long-term goals, such as finishing school or having a baby. Implicit in these comments was the belief that the physician had underappreciated the extent of the patient's distress.

Almost half of the patients focused on "how long" instead of "how much" (Table 19-3). Prolonged symptoms not only taxed patients' ability to cope ("My leg is not getting better. . . . I can't stand it"); they also raised questions about therapy ("If something doesn't work, why keep using it?"). These patients viewed refractory symptoms as a signal that the clinician was off track.

More than one third of patients expressed concern about the implications of their symptoms (Table 19-3). The prospect of serious disease triggered anxieties that were not assuaged by attempts to relieve symptoms; these attempts were often dismissed as blind empiricism. "I want to know," said one patient, "Is this exactly what is wrong with me, or is there something else? before I start taking medication that might mask what really is the problem." In this case, the physician misread the patient's primary goal, which was not relief from hand cramps but reassurance that a serious disease was not lurking behind them.

Perceived Vulnerability to Illness. The degree to which patients attended to sensations, interpreted them as abnormal, and developed concerns about them was related to each patient's unique vulnerabilities. Forty-four patients (50%) mentioned at least one specific vulnerability related to one of five factors: aging, a previously diagnosed condition, a family history of illness, personal lifestyle factors, and the utterances of medical office staff (Table 19-3).

Patients' recognition that they were growing older affected their responses to specific symptoms (". . . at my age I'm just kind of getting worried [about my backache]") as well as their perceived susceptibility to illness in general (". . . I'm in my mid-life and I'm thinking a little bit about my age and health. . . . I thought maybe I should have some kind of . . . heart test and a cholesterol test, blood test, urinalysis"). Age-related concerns were reported by 5% of interviewed patients younger than 35 years of age, 15% of

Table 19-3
Sources of Patients' Expectations

Source	Patients, %[*]
Somatic symptoms	74
Intensity of symptoms	42
Functional impairment	14
Durations of symptoms	49
Perceived seriousness of symptoms	35
Perceived vulnerability to illness	50
Related to age	12
Related to a previously diagnosed condition	26
Related to a family history of illness	9
Related to personal lifestyle	9
Derived from remarks of medical office staff	9
Previous experience	42
With similar symptoms or illness	40
Acquired while caring for others	8
Transmitted knowledge	54
Personal education or training in health care field	7
Friends or relatives trained in health care fields	10
Statements by lay friends or relatives	8
Pronouncements of other clinicians	42
The media	7

*n = 88.

those 35 to 64 years of age, and 14% of those older than 65 years of age. Thus, attaining a particular chronological age was neither necessary nor sufficient for the development of age-related expectations.

About one fourth of study participants had a previously diagnosed medical condition that appeared to influence current expectations by magnifying perceived vulnerability to illness (Table 19-3). Symptomatic and asymptomatic patients reacted differently. Having had a medical problem in the past could cast a morbid shadow over otherwise minor symptoms, as it did for one patient with a sty who was unhappy when he was advised to use warm compresses rather than to see an ophthalmologist ("I have extremely poor eyes. . . . Therefore I am always concerned if I have a problem with my eyes. . .").

However, previous or underlying illnesses influenced expectations even among persons who currently felt well. As one 67-year-old patient told us, "So I feel like, having a heart condition where I take two drugs for it, that he automatically should listen to the heart and lungs when I go in. I don't feel like I should have to ask." As a "heart patient," this patient expected that her special medical vulnerabilities would be recognized and acted on by her physician.

For about 9% of patients, personal vulnerability was derived from a family history of illness, often heart disease or cancer (Table 19-3). For these patients, diseases that had killed their relatives colored even the most routine medical encounter. One young woman made such concerns explicit: "I went in for some concerns about ovaries. . . . I was having some lower abdominal pain which was obviously not appendix, and my mother, grandmother, and great-grandmother all died of cancer. I brought it up and nothing was really said about it." Here the patient reflects on family history and feels vulnerable, the physician overlooks or down plays the connection, and the patient feels slighted or endangered.

Even when patients were not concerned about genetic predispositions to disease, recalling the difficult experiences of family members could inspire specific demands for care. As one 46-year old man put it, "Walking pneumonia killed my father, and I know the best way to tell if you have pneumonia is with a chest x-ray, so that is why I'm going back to get this to make sure I haven't caught it."

Another 9% of patients felt vulnerable because of their own health habits (Table 19-3). These patients recognized the threat inherent in ongoing substance abuse or stress, and their concerns were often grounded in epidemiologic reality. However, some patients, such as a 38-year-old man who was experiencing work-related stress and wanted the physician "to take a look at my eyes [to make sure] I wasn't having a stroke" seemed to overestimate their absolute risk.

Expectations sometimes came from odd quarters: "I called and gave them my symptoms on the phone [and] they . . . told me you have to come in because of our meningitis scare. I guess your mind starts to work overtime then." Nurses, technicians, and medical clerical personnel could wield considerable influence. Casual asides led patients to downgrade their perceived health, leading to changed expectations for care.

Previous Experience. For 42% of interviewed patients, unmet expectations for care were shaped by past experiences with similar symptoms or illnesses or by experiences acquired while caring for others (Table 19-3).

Direct personal experience influenced expectations for both diagnosis and therapy. Reasoning by analogy, patients interpreted their current symptoms in light of the past. They also used past experiences to develop definitions of an appropriate diagnostic process. As one woman told us, "Well, I think . . . if you're as tired as I am and everything, that a basic blood test wouldn't hurt. . . . That's how they found out [the last time I was sick]—my blood [platelet] count was down to 5000 on the night they put me in the hospital for my spleen. It was just a simple blood test." We do not know enough about the case to judge whether a blood count might have been diagnostically helpful at this visit, but the patient's commitment to this strategy, derived from her own experience, seems plain enough.

Patients also acquired experience while accompanying relatives or friends to the physician. For example, a 68-year-old man said: "The doctor [my wife] was going to before would do . . . a thorough run-up of tests. All that ceased when we went to [the current health maintenance organization]."

Transmitted Knowledge. A final category of influences on the development of patients' expectations included knowledge transmitted from sources other than personal experience. A total of 54% of patients reported having expectations that had been acquired through personal education and training; through conversations with friends, relatives, and physicians and other health care professionals; or through instruments of popular culture (Table 19-3).

Approximately 16% of our largely middle-class study sample had had formal training in the health professions or were closely related to health care professionals. These patients used their specialized medical knowledge to anticipate or influence their physicians' plans for diagnosis and therapy ("I work in veterinary medicine and we would have routinely done a blood count"). They also tended to react harshly to perceived medical omissions ("I'm an RN, and when someone presents with these symptoms I think I would be inclined to at least examine them.") To these medically sophisticated persons, failed expectations were not merely a source of disappointment but hinted at medical incompetence.

Similarly, patients whose close friends or family members were health care professionals drew on the expertise—real or perceived—of others. Friends, family, and acquaintances were important sources of medical information when they had specialized medical training (" . . . my mother who is a nurse said that it sounded like an infection because of all the other things that were going on") and even when they didn't (" . . . my girlfriend recommended [that I see] a dermatologist since she had seen one herself who she liked a lot"). Patients did not generally disclose their sources of information to the clinician. Only when providers appreciated the influence of informal counselors could they address patients' expectations directly.

Patients also drew on the authority of health care professionals other than the physicians they were currently seeing. More than 40% of patients reported on the salience of pronouncements, admonitions, and asides delivered by previously encountered physicians and nurses (Table 19-3). When the advice of trusted health professionals (often a physician the patient had seen in the past) was challenged, patients became suspicious. One elderly woman stated, "Dr. X thought it was very important once a year that I have that test where they put the dye and you ride the treadmill and then you go into nuclear medicine. . . . [But now] suddenly I don't need it. Now was it because they wanted the money from the insurance or was it because I really did need it? You know, which was it?"

To our surprise, references to the media were relatively uncommon (7%; Table 19-3). Those patients who did mention the media tended to discount its influence. As one patient pointed out, however, the media's influence may be so pervasive that it is often difficult to identify it as a separate factor ("I didn't necessarily read [about needing regular blood tests] in the paper but just because of cholesterol; we live in a high fat society"). In this statement, the patient articulates how preventive health ideology has become part of the social canon, a media-dependent process.

Discussion

Our study both documents the prevalence of patient's unmet expectations for care in office practice and elucidates the multifactorial ontogenesis of those expectations. The complexity of the process by which patients develop expectations may lessen the allure of "demand management," an increasingly popular concept that seeks to discourage health care utilization by helping patients make rational decisions about medical services[12,13]. However, rationality has its limits. Approaches that do not consider patients' underlying vulnerabilities and past experiences will merely encourage patients to express their symptoms in more urgent terms[14]. A more realistic goal would be to support clinicians' efforts to understand patients' expectations and, when necessary, initiate negotiations around them.

Our data allow us to construct a preliminary model of how patients' expectations develop in the context of symptom-driven clinical encounters (Figure 19-1). Each patient comes to the physician's office with a unique set of perceived vulnerabilities, past experiences, and stores of knowledge. These antecedents influence the interpretation of symptoms and lead to the formulation of a response that is expected for the practitioner. The practitioner's actual response is then evaluated in light of the patient's expectations.

For many patients, three symptom dimensions (duration of and lack of alleviation of symptoms, functional impairment, and perceived seriousness of symptoms) were especially salient. Inattention to these dimensions may or may not have affected the ability of physicians to reach a correct biomedical diagnosis, but it surely restricted their ability to impart a sense of concern and understanding. Our data highlight the previously recognized gap between the clinician's focus on objective disease and the patient's subjective experience of illness[15]. A rich and multifaceted understanding of patients' interpretations of symptoms, perceptions of vulnerability, and ways of knowing can enable clinicians to meet patients "where they are" and can lead to more productive clinical negotiation[16].

We found that for at least half of the patients interviewed in our study, symptoms and acquired knowledge were filtered through a mesh of perceived vulnerabilities related to age, previously diagnosed conditions, family history, lifestyle, or the casual utterances of health care professionals or medical office staff. Patients who considered themselves to be at risk for specific diseases tended to have broader expectations about history taking, physical examination, diagnostic testing, and therapy. Because patients often do not voice such concerns unless asked about them, physicians may find themselves arguing with patients about a particular clinical strategy (such as whether antibiotics should be used to treat an upper respiratory tract infection) when the fundamental difference turns on risk assessment—for example, the physician may see a "cold," but the patient thinks of Uncle Charlie, whose fatal case of pneumonia started with the sniffles. Our results argue for the medical relevance of the social and family history. Clinicians hoping to understand their patients' expectations should inquire about a family history of serious illness, anniversaries of significant life events, and previous diagnoses and their meaning to the patient.

Patients' increasing expectations for the application of expensive medical technologies have been cited as an important contributor to increased health care costs[17]. Physicians may feel uncomfortable when patients request costly interventions of equivocal benefit. Yet our data suggest that one of the most powerful influences on patients' expectations is physicians themselves. Physicians can promote inappropriate expectations by prescribing marginally beneficial tests and therapies, couching clinical beliefs as medically authoritative dicta, and giving in to inappropriate patient requests without discussion. In contrast, they may be able to interrupt the development of unrealistic expectations by reducing unjustified practice variation, learning about and sharing with patients some of medicine's inherent uncertainties, and engaging patients as partners in a clinical negotiation[16,18].

Figure 19-1

A preliminary model of how patients develop and report expectations. Perceived vulnerability, past experience, and transmitted knowledge influence expectations both by affecting the interpretation of symptoms and by establishing an implicit standard of care. The behavior of health care practitioners is then evaluated in light of these expectations.

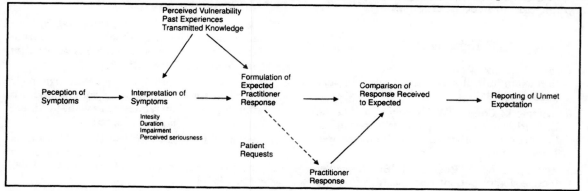

Several patients in our study reported that they received conflicting information from their health care providers. The amount of contradictory advice that patients receive is likely to increase as managed care (and societal mobility) continues to disrupt long-term patient-physician relationships[4]. Policies that encourage continuity of care might not only improve patient satisfaction[19] but also reduce unfulfilled expectations and the clinical conflict that they can cause.

Our data and conclusions should be evaluated in light of our study's limitations. The study was done in three practices (two health care systems) in one geographic region. The sample of patients interviewed was large by qualitative standards, but it comprised only 88 patients. Moreover, we intentionally excluded patients who were presenting for routine check-ups. This strategy probably increased the proportion of patients who had unmet expectations for diagnosis and treatment but eliminated many whose expectations may have centered on prevention.

In summary, we have identified some of the major sources of patients' expectations within three highly managed general internal medicine practices in northern California. By stripping away some of the mystique surrounding patients' expectations, we hope our study will enable physicians to refine their history-taking skills and priorities, to be sensitive to patients' expectations even when these are not made explicit, and to reduce needless clinical conflict. Further study is needed to confirm our findings in other settings, help clinicians elicit patients' expectations efficiently, and evaluate strategies for reshaping expectations when they are unreasonable and in need of change.

References

1. Cleary, P. D., and McNeil, B. J. "Patient satisfaction as an indicator of quality care." *Inquiry.* 1988; 25:25-36.

2. Kravitz, R. L., Cope, D. W., Bhrany, V., and Leake, B. "Internal medicine patients' expectations for care during office visits." *J Gen Intern Med.* 1994; 9:75-81.

3. Speedling, E. J., and Rose, D. N. "Building an effective doctor-patient relationship: from patient satisfaction to patient participation." *Soc Sci Med.* 1985; 21:115-20.

4. Safran, D. G., Tarlov, A. R., and Rogers, W. H. "Primary care performance in fee-for-service and prepaid health care systems." Results from the Medical Outcomes Study. *JAMA* 1994; 271:1579-86.

5. Kravitz, R. L. "Patients' expectations for medical care: an expanded formulation based on review of the literature." *Medical Care Research and Review.* 1996; 53:3-27.

6. Flanagan, J. C. "The critical incident technique." *Psychol Bull.* 1954; 51:327-58.

7. Bradley, C. P. "Uncomfortable prescribing decisions: a critical incident study." *BMJ.* 1992; 304:294-6

8. Glaser, B., and Strauss, A. *The Discovery of Grounded Theory.* New York: Aldine; 1967.

9. Strauss, A., and Corbin, J. *Basis of Qualitative Research: Grounded Theory Procedures and Techniques.* Newbury Park: Sage; 1990.

10. Seidel, J., Friese, S., and Leonard, D. C. *The Ethnograph, v. 4.0: A User's Guide.* Amherst, MA: Qualis Research Associates; 1995.

11. Brody, D. S., Miller, S. M., Lerman, C. E., Smith, D. G., Lazaro, C. G., and Blum, M. J.. "The relationship between patients' satisfaction with their physicians and perceptions about interventions they desired and received." *Med Care.* 1989; 27:1027-35.

12. Vickery, D. M., and Lynch, W. D. "Demand management: enabling patients to use medical care appropriately." *J Occup Environ Med.* 1996; 37:551-7.

13. Partridge, P. "Demand management moving to forefront." *Health Care Strateg Manage.* 1996; 14:14-6.

14. Barsky, A. J., and Borus, J. F. "Somatization and medicalization in the era of managed care." *JAMA.* 1995; 274:1931-4.

15. Kleinman, A., Eisenberg, L., and Good, B. "Culture, illness, and care: clinical lessons from anthropologic and cross-cultural research." *Ann Intern Med.* 1978; 88: 251-8.

16. Lazare, A., Eisenthal, S., and Wasserman, L. "The customer approach to patienthood. Attending to patient requests in a walk-in clinic." *Arch Gen Psychiatry.* 1975; 553-8.

17. Woolf, S. H., and Kamerow, D. B. "Testing for uncommon conditions. The heroic search for positive test results." *Arch Intern Med.* 1990; 150:2451-8.

18. Sox, H. C., and Nease, R. F. "When doctor and patient disagree" [Editorial]. *J Gen Intern Med.* 1993; 8:580-1.

19. Hjortdahl, P., and Laerum, E. "Continuity of care in general practice: effect on patient satisfaction." *BMJ.* 1992; 304:1287-90.

Further Reading

Elliot Mishler. 1990. "The Struggle Between the Voice of Medicine and the Voice of the Life World." *The Sociology of Health and Illness: Critical Perspectives*, edited by P. Conrad and R. Kern, New York: St. Martin's Press. Pp. 295-307.

Terry Mizrahi. 1986. *Getting Rid of Patients: Contradictions in the Socialization of Physicians*. New Brunswick: Rutgers University Press.

Howard Waitzkin. 1991. *The Politics of Medical Encounters*. New Haven: Yale University Press.

Discussion Questions

1. Do you see a connection between what Waitzkin and his coauthors say about discourse and what Kravitz and his coauthors claim about patients' unmet expectations for care?

2. Is it realistic to want physicians or systems of health care to meet the kinds of demands for care reported in this selection? Why or why not?

3. What do unfulfilled expectations mean for a patient's likelihood of compliance with a physician's orders for treatment?

From *Annals of Internal Medicine*, Vol. 125. Pp. 730-737.

Understanding Caretaking: Practitioner Socialization

20

'If It's Not Charted, It Didn't Happen'

Timothy Diamond

Timothy Diamond reports the troubles and triumphs of work and life in a nursing home from his own perspectives as nurse's assistant and sociologist. Diamond shows that the "dirty work" of medicine and health care—aspects of a patient's everyday life, like eating, bathing, walking, and toileting—determine the work routine for nursing assistants. Activities of daily living become specific tasks requiring accomplishment by the shift's end. Assistants learn by doing, sometimes the hard way, how to manage time constraints, unexpected patient troubles and emotional tensions. Diamond shows that the experience of being an assistant is not revealed in hospital charts but in the everyday lives and interactions between nursing assistants and their patients. Pay attention to the kinds of work that Diamond and the other assistants do during the course of the day.

Staff members learn to note task completion by charting. Charting, however, reveals little that assistants learn about patients, about likes and dislikes, easy days and hard ones. Chart records disclose nothing about the kind of job that needs to be done. Most work accomplished by nursing assistants is "invisible work"—work that cannot be charted. Diamond shows us the undocumented work of nursing assistants. Watch how he uncovers webs of hidden relationships between patients and nursing assistants. Complex webs of interaction go uncaptured in the rigid and limited structure of the chart that organizes the work day for the nursing assistant and the patient.

'Don't Worry, You'll Learn'

. . . Mornings began with waking residents. For most nursing assistants it seemed that a certain way of greeting each person developed, not always successfully, but always bearing some relation to the person in bed. Juanita Carmona typified the approach. "You've got to watch that Sagan," she warned. "He's a rough one."

"And what about Mrs. O'Brien?" I asked her.

"Oh, just ignore her, she'll go on griping about having to get up whether you' re there or not." These grumblings about wanting to stay in bed were more subdued than disruptive or violent. While they did make for some conflict during those early morning hours, there was no real debate about whether or not the complainant could stay in bed. It was not as though a right was being claimed.

Waking some was complicated, because it involved immediately cleaning up messes made in the bed during the night. One early lesson in the rigors of the work revolved around such an incident. I approached Monica Stewart, who announced with caution, "I'm afraid I've made a mess today."

"Oh, no problem, Monica, it happens to the best of us," was my naive response. But as I folded back her sheets, now confronted with the real work of "getting them out of that," Monica could see me get weak and pale. "Um . . . I'll be right back." I sputtered, rushing off first to the toilet, then to Mrs. Johnson, a co-worker and veteran of ten years. "Mrs. Johnson, ah . . . I don't feel too good today, and Monica has made a terrific mess. Could you help me?"

"Sure," came her reassuring response.

"Good morning, Monica," Mrs. Johnson began with an uplifting chuckle. "C'mon, let's get you up and rolling!" Without hesitation, continuing her talking, she folded the blankets to the bottom of the bed and with her right hand rolled Monica over on her left side, deftly wrapping the soiled bottom sheet toward the center of the bed, then turned to me with, "Here, hand me that Kleenex box. Quick! you got to be quick about this!" and turned to Monica, talking and cleaning, "Okay, up once, okay, now over," and lifted her lower half completely with just one arm, folded the clean parts of the old bottom sheet under her to help finish the cleaning, unwrapped a new bottom sheet and another for protection and slid them down the side of the bed where Monica was not lying, simultaneously turning to me, "Now that washcloth and towel, quick! You've got to have these right at your side before you start," and to Monica, "There you go," rolling her over onto the new bottom sheets and folding a new top sheet and blankets over her. I gasped in amazement. Mrs. Johnson had executed the entire operation, turning it into one continuous fluid motion, in little more than two minutes.

"Don't worry," she said, scurrying out the door, "you'll learn."

I did not learn, even after months, in any way that matched the orchestration, agility, timing, strength, speed, compassion, or rapport that Mrs. Johnson demonstrated in her expertise of "getting them out of that."

Little by little, however, I did pick up on the skills of the next task on the agenda, feeding someone. As with cleaning, the actual work of feeding had not been described in class or in the text, nor was there any code or guide in the charts other than a box to check as to whether the patient ate or refused to eat.

"You feed Alice today," came an early instruction. Alice McGraw sat confused, still groggy from sleep, mouth tightly closed. Somehow the food had to get into it to stimulate her taste buds. Mrs. Carmona advised, "Try doing just like we do everything else with Alice. Try a song." "Okay. Ahem. Alice! Hello? When Irish eyes are smiling, all the world is bright and gay." Eventually, recognition dawned, and with some egg held long enough under her nose to smell and see, she opened her mouth a crack.

Learning how to become someone else's tastebuds, how to vary portions and kinds of food and drink, was a complicated puzzle, the more so for being slightly different for every person. "Keep looking in their eyes, especially the ones who don't talk," Mrs. Bonderoid had taught us in school. After many frightening chokings, and many refusals, these skills slowly began to develop. Some residents, unable to perform all the complex tasks of eating, needed assistance. Feeding someone began by selecting a portion of food, or more likely drink, since thirst was frequently intense. Then the food: a piece of the scrambled egg to begin, how much or little depending on the person, then offering it, waiting for it to be chewed and swallowed, then some milk, and more waiting, then toast, dipped in the milk for easier chewing, a pause to avoid regurgitation or a choke, and another piece enhanced by the single pad of jam, then coffee. With some it could be a pleasant exchange, feeding someone and watching them smile.

But there was always pressure when several people needed special help. It was considered a bad day when it fell to a nursing assistant to have to help more than two or three, because it was intrinsically a very slow process. "C'mon, will yah, Ellen, eat the damn food, and let's go!" I urged under my breath, while residents urged back, "C'mon, will yah, I'm hungry, let's go!" Buried underneath this pressured moment was the delicate, sometimes frightening process of feeding a frail, sick person. It often seemed one of the most refined nursing skills of the day as I watched a seasoned nursing assistant sensitive to the slow pace of an old person's eating, knowing how to vary portions and tastes, how to reinforce nonverbally while feeding—a refined and complicated skill, but unnamed and suppressed when forced into a forty-minute task.

Because the rush was on to finish by 8:40 when the kitchen worker arrived to pick up the trays, the work involved juggling: feeding one person, handing a drink to second, grabbing a third to sit her back down, dodging the nurse and her cart as they moved along dispensing the morning medications. By 8:20, with feeding not half done, the requests began. "Toilet, take me to the toilet." "Is someone free? I need to go." "Got any second helpings?" "Nurse! nurse!". . .

At first it seemed odd that all of this had to be done by 8:40 A.M. But by 8:45 the reason was clear: there was a lot of work on the schedule. After breakfast one nursing assistant was assigned to beds, one to showers, two to day room coverage and toileting. Some residents made their own beds, but many did not. Changing and making forty beds seemed at first a simple enough, menial task that anyone could do. After a while such a perspective seemed simplistic, a view that could be maintained only by someone who did not do the work. It is simple enough for someone with a lower back strong enough for three straight hours of constant bending at the body's center and a blood pressure low enough to avoid dizziness at each quick rise. Dorothy Tomason was convinced that over the years this constant up-and-down motion contributed to her high blood pressure. Vera Norris associated it with chronic back pain. . . .

While Vera agreed with Dorothy on the health hazards of this task, she preferred it to the alternative. "I get weak doing beds, sure, but I'd still rather do them than showers."

Each person who lived in the home had to take a shower every third day. Showers were going on continually through the morning and afternoon hours. Vera's reason for not liking to give showers was straightforward: "I can't stand the screams."

Sometimes the screaming was about water temperature, which dropped as the day went along. "You get in here and try it," Marjorie McCabe protested. "You know testing the water with your hand isn't the same as

being here." A few of the more frail were frightened just by the shower itself. For many, with brittle bones and highly sensitive body thermometers, it was an effort just to stand or sit underneath it, and for the nursing assistants it was a challenge to provide adequate support and force, while managing to stay out of the shower.

"You all right in there, Hazel?" I inquired of Mrs. Morris.

"Yeah," she yelled, thus freeing me to get a towel and check on Harriet Bowler in the next stall. Within thirty seconds Hazel fell to the floor. Luckily, she had fallen first against the wall out of dizziness, and only slowly drifted downward. After that, maintaining those delicate balances took on new meaning as an integral part of the work. It took a constant anticipatory vigilance to keep ahead of potential accidents.[1]

In the charts, boxes were marked after each shower. There was no space to note the work of nervous monitoring or residents' fears, not to mention their screams. Hazel Morris. Shower. Check. If it wasn't charted, it didn't happen, but much more happened than got charted. What happened to the work that wasn't charted? It seemed as if much of it was being made invisible. The chart makers needed to have certain information. I began to wonder whether, in order to accomplish their objectives, they also needed to leave certain information out.

In the late morning one day after I had worked for about two months, I was assigned to clean and change linen for Bill Hackett. Bill had spent his life as a bartender. In his late sixties he got liver disease, and he did not have long to survive. At first it was frightening and embarrassing for me to be with him, and no doubt he felt the same, as I bumbled along trying to clean him, get accustomed to the smells, avoid sickness, and feign a smile. Most days I tried to bear in mind the advice of registered nurse Mary Collins. "There's one good way to get beyond your feelings of embarrassment. Think of theirs." Over time, as we got to know each other, the encounter became easier. Bill held on to the humor that must have made him an excellent bartender, and he came out with great quips about nursing home life. It was something of a turning point in learning this work when one day I left Bill's room and realized that while cleaning him I had not even noticed the assault on my senses that had so dominated the encounter when he was a stranger.

By 11:45 A.M. it was time to serve lunch. . . .

It was one of the pleasures of the work to help a blind person with a meal. Nursing Supervisor Marian Moran summarized it, "If you don't do it right, sometimes they just don't eat." Still, it was easy to overstep boundaries. To get to know Peter Prince, who was also visually impaired, was to realize that he resented many offers of service, especially relating to food. He had just finished telling me to get out of his way when Robbie from the next table asked him, "Hey, Prince, what did you get for dessert, cookies or peaches?"

"I don't know," said Mr. Prince, his fingers creeping around his tray. "I haven't found them yet."

In Here They Get Their Feelings Hurt Awfully Easy

. . . Dressing someone was another skill that took some practice to coordinate, especially with people who could not help much. Ellen McMahon, for example, had almost no power of movement, so lifting her took some strength. Yet at almost a hundred years old, her bones were eggshell brittle; one false move while coaxing her fingers and arms through the sleeve of a blouse or sweater could mean a broken bone. To lift her in and out of the wheelchair took holding her bobbing head and her limp legs while trying to secure her pencil-thin arms at her sides. These tasks required both strength and delicacy and knowing how to distinguish which among her almost inaudible utterances were deep breaths and which were muted grunts of pain.

Her roommate, Edna Barrett, showed that the act of dressing involved some emotional delicacy as well. Edna was in the public aid phase of her nursing home life when we met, but the fine wool and cotton clothes in her closet suggested that in her earlier days she had been a woman of some wealth. It was not easy to lift her spirits. When approached for the afternoon face washes she responded glumly, "Who cares?" and "What does it matter?" So one day I decided to help her dress up in one of her finer suits, with a necklace and bracelet. "There, you look good, Edna," I said. Smiling, she followed me into the day room. Then to the nurses' station. Then into someone else's room. Then down the hall. Much of Edna's time in the home she wanted to follow someone around, but now following had taken on a different dimension. She was engaged in being dressed up, and she wanted to continue sharing the occasion. The problem was that she stayed about two feet behind me for almost an hour. I could neither get the work done nor persuade her to sit down or go back to her room. Eventually, I had to sit her down and tie her up. That hurt her feelings.

In this work it was difficult to learn when to hold back, how not to offer too much. LPN Pearl DeLorio, a veteran of several years' work, understood the dilemma. "It's tough," she said, "You never know when you're going to hurt their feelings. In here they get their feelings hurt awfully easy."

Anna Ervin got her feelings hurt regularly in the course of one of the nursing assistants fulfilling her assigned job. At some point between 1:00 and 2:00 p.m. Bessie Miranda approached Anna to persuade her to go to the bathroom. On Anna's chart, which Bessie held in her hand during these encounters, it was recorded that her bowel activity was irregular, and Bessie was carrying out orders designed to correct the problem. The idea was that if Anna could be encouraged to go at a regular time each day her intermittent difficulties with constipation and incontinence could be avoided. The regimen was called bowel and bladder training. Anna disliked the training, as did Bessie, as was obvious from their loud yelling.

Bessie coaxed, "Did you go yet, Anna? C'mon, let's go. I don't want to fight with you today."

Anna screamed, "Get away from me! I was an LPN myself, you know. I don't need you telling me when to go to the bathroom. Besides, I tried earlier. What do you expect, miracles? Get away from me!"

Bessie could not get away, not without failing at her assigned task. "C'mon, Anna, it's time, let's go," she insisted, while pulling her along. The argument raged daily as Anna was escorted to the bathroom, usually under duress.

By 2:00 p.m. interpersonal crashes were subdued. It was the peak period for visitors. Nursing assistants' instructions for this period were succinct. They were based on maintaining a good appearance to the outsiders, with special reference to physicians or Board of Health inspectors who might happen to drop in. The assistant head nurse told us, "When you are in the day room never stay in one place. Keep moving. You never know when they'll pop in for an inspection. If somebody comes in, grab a chart or fold some sheets, or take some blood pressures. Look busy." Looking busy was hardly difficult: there were beds that needed making, more showers, orienting a new arrival, being interrupted by an emotional crisis, helping the registered nurse change a catheter or bandage, cleaning tables, washing faces, sorting clothes. . . .

Nursing assistants went about trying to organize their day as best they could. It took continual mental work to balance the tasks from above with the contingencies of the moment. Schedules were completed, if sometimes late: beds got made, showers given, vitals and weights taken, diapers changed. Yet if these activities were all that happened, all that the work consisted of, the contours of the day would have been very different from what they actually were in the everyday world.[2]

The official tasks were difficult, sometimes unpleasant, and took some skill. But there was also a host of unspoken, unnamed demands before, during, and after the tasks that presented problems, both physical and emotional. . . .

As the afternoons went along, moving around meant passing in front of a row of people sitting in their chairs, sometimes coming upon someone who had slid down or fallen over and needed repositioning. In such a circumstance, the fact that there were still six more beds and two more showers before shift change had little bearing on the immediate need. Often at this time of day the pace of the staff and their duties came into conflict with the pace of the people who lived there. "C'mon, c'mon, will you, I haven't got all day" was a legitimate plea of a nursing assistant trying to tend to her eighteen or twenty people. That plea contrasted with the slow pace of the people who lived there, who kept asking, "What did you say? I can't hear you" or "Please walk slower. I can't keep up with you" or who, in answer to a question like "How are you today?" Doris responded "Oh . . . fine . . . and . . . you. . . ?"—by which time we were halfway down the hall.

Nursing also meant trying to learn each person's peculiar mental and physical problems. This skill was not static; it evolved as personal relations developed. . . .

When nursing assistants described their work, they often referred to gaining experience or skills in terms of getting to know people. In getting to know someone, the knowledge of anticipating their needs and desires took shape. Being able to sense in advance who needed water, moisturizing lotion, or a change of clothing took experience in the work and knowing the people. . . .

'Don't Ever Tell These People You Know How They Feel'

By the start of the 3:00 to 11:00 shift, many of the medical tasks were done for the day, but a lot of person-to-person work lurked ahead. Perhaps the most difficult part of the caretaking work was just keeping up its necessary conversations. When the shift began, nursing assistants left the nurses' station with some objective in mind, perhaps to gather a pile of clean sheets or clothing. The objective was reached only slowly, for to leave the station was to be met with a barrage of conversation from a few of the residents. Some expected a nod of recognition as soon as we came on duty, some a handshake or other touch that meant a greeting, and they were quietly insulted if we walked by without making it. Moving out from behind the nurses' station meant fielding many overtures, sometimes simultaneous: "Hi! What's for dinner?" "Can you fix my belt?" "Have you got a quarter?" "Guess what I did today?" and most of all, the ever-ready "How are you?"— often made in the hope of more than just a one-line response.

. . . Amid the rushing, changing, and charting, there was the never-ending listening to comments and questions that accompanied them. Frequently, the questions were not easy. From Edna Barrett who was slowly dying with cancer, "Am I going to die?" From Elizabeth Stern, "My mind keeps wandering. Am I crazy?" From Sharon Drake, far along the path of poverty, "You know, you have to believe you won't be here forever. Do you think I'll be here for the rest of my life?" Regardless of the prospects, a cool yes to any of these questions did not work well, but neither did a transparent no. It took something in between, including some knowledge of the person asking the question.

"Above all," advised veteran Mrs. Carmona, referring to Robbie, confined to a wheelchair, "don't ever tell these people that you know how they feel. You don't."

In the training manuals and records the tasks appeared as discrete acts, as though they were performed one at a time, but the actual work always involved more than one focus, at least mentally. Arriving at the end of the hall to sort out some clean clothing meant simultaneously listening to the day room several yards away, attentive to its potential incidents. The rule was "coverage"; someone had to be present in the day room to oversee the thirty to forty people sitting in it. With three nursing assistants on the floor, and recurrent emergencies calling us away, it was a rule impossible to follow. Usually, just as soon as we left the day room for an instant, we had to rush back, for someone was likely to have seized the moment of our absence to wriggle partly out of her restraint vest.

"Nurse, nurse!" yelled Bernice Calhoun, who kept a vigilant eye out for such potential catastrophies. "Mary Ryan's out again!" At that instance the clean clothing was dropped for the more urgent demand to rush back to reposition her or another of the eager escapees; that is, reposition and try to negotiate.

"Mary, please stay put this time, will you?"

"Stay put?" Mary Ryan screeched back. "You're all crazy in here. I don't trust anybody in white anymore. Look at my arms!" She pointed to black and blue marks on her arms, the result of continuous struggle with the restraints.

"Just try to relax, please; dinner will be here soon," I said, as if I had any idea what either "relax" or "soon" meant to her.[3] Then it was back to get some changes of clothing and fresh linens, and perhaps to squeeze in one of the showers that had been delayed earlier . . . .

By 4:30 visitors, family members, and volunteers filtered out. It frequently fell to the nursing assistants to encourage this, subtly at first, more strongly as the dinner hour approached, since we had to rearrange the day room into a dining room for the thirty or so residents who did not leave the floor. When the visitors departed they sometimes left an emptiness that could be seen on their relatives' faces. This was especially true of those for whom visits were rare. It was part of the work to be there when the visitors left, to try to fill the vacuum made by their absence. . . .

When the evening meal approached, nursing assistants seized whatever moments were available between 5:00 and 5:30 to attach the bibs, which involved their moving toward people from behind, not always announcing the approach. Marjorie McCabe once let out a shriek when the bib came around her neck. "Didn't anybody ever teach you not to come up to somebody from behind?" she reacted with rage. And Elizabeth Stern scolded when I touched her back once without any prior eye contact. It seemed like a friendly gesture as we waited for the trays to arrive. Instead it was an insult. "Don't ever touch me like that," she insisted indignantly. "It's not natural."

Usually staff members were either moving or standing, while the people who lived there were sitting or lying down. Consequently, even with the best of intentions, it was the staff who became the touchers, those in the chairs the touched. Marjorie and Elizabeth seemed especially sensitive about this asymmetry, as though part of their practice of patienthood was learning how to deal with staff's unsolicited touch and how to avoid their invasions of presumed familiarity.

Dinner trays arrived between 5:15 and 5:30. Another strict regulation from the Board of Health was that plastic hats and gloves had to be worn when food was distributed. "Don't get caught without those gloves and hat," warned Kenny Obaku, a co-worker from Nigeria, "or at least have them close by so you can grab them. If the administrators or head nurse see you without gloves and hat, it's suspension for sure." Meanwhile, the work of serving included encouraging people to eat. These negotiations sometimes meant inventing ways to make food palatable and trying to generate appetite for someone, especially when the materials at hand, the tepid hot dog and chunky mashed potatoes from the steam tables, did not lend themselves to the challenge. . . .

After dinner there were showers and linen changes which had not been finished earlier, and vital signs of all the residents had to be taken.

The crucial significance of the vital signs procedure was brought into bold relief one evening about seven o' clock. Taking blood pressures, temperatures, and pulses was a five-minute task, barring interruptions. Mary Karney's turn came up, and on this particular evening she sat at the edge of her bed, head slumped over, crying—not at all typical of her usually jovial, if cynical, demeanor.

"Mary, what's the trouble?" I probed. No response. Wait. Responses sometimes came very slowly. "Can I check your pulse and blood pressure?" She offered her arm and looked away. Her blood pressure was a bit high, but within a normal range. Pulse, normal, check.

What was charted happened, but was the nursing care over? I waited, fiddling around with some blankets at the foot of the bed, apparently idle, waiting for Mary to speak. It was clearly idle to the charge nurse who was rushing down the hall. Seeing that I had completed the task in Mary's room, she called me out into the hall, beckoning me to get going on the appointed rounds. Looking at her watch, then at me, she said, "Let's get back to work. You've got sixteen more vitals to do." She rushed off to change a dressing, and while Mary continued to sit silently, I moved on to the next room to the prescribed and enforced work of measuring life signs.

The blood pressure cuff, nicknamed the sphygmo (for sphygmomanometer), was an important piece of technology in the homes, continually in use and frequently in demand. While finishing the vital signs one evening, I was alerted by one of the staff: "Bring the sphygmo! Bring the sphygmo, quick!"

Lorraine Sokolof had stumbled on the freshly waxed floor, twisting her ankle and nearly fainting for an instant afterwards. The charge nurse alerted the nursing supervisor downstairs, who called an ambulance. The charge nurse then rushed with the two nursing assistants to Lorraine's aid. "Here, give me that," she instructed, grabbing the blood pressure instrument. As Lorraine regained composure she sat on the floor while the nurse wrapped its slip around her arm. She studied the gauge, then recorded Lorraine's blood pressure. That accomplished, the three members of the staff and three curious and helpful residents waited with her for the ambulance. Eventually the other nursing assistant, Kenny, asked, "Is there anything you would like?"

"Yes," Lorraine answered, "a glass of water."

In certain contexts, when someone nearly faints, the first gesture is to offer a glass of water. At that moment it was an afterthought, after the prescribed emergency measures for an incident had been executed. It was not permitted that any of us, including the charge nurse, deal directly with Lorraine's ankle, as, for example, by wrapping it with an elastic bandage. "We don't wrap without doctor's orders," explained Kenny. The primary health care delivery consisted of measuring and recording Lorraine's vital signs and waiting for the ambulance to arrive. Off she went for X-rays and a hospital stay, at considerable cost, leaving her husband to worry if he'd ever see her again.

. . . Establishing control brought out behavior that came across as cruelty. Some of us, including me, slipped into this mode. As 10:00 p.m. came, it was time for lights out. "C'mon, now, off with the TV."

"Oh, just a little while longer."

"No. You know the rules." If they were not obeyed there was force to be wielded. We had the power to press the rules, even in the face of residents' opposition. I became amazed at my own capacity as an enforcer.

"Turn that off now. Do you hear me, Rose? "

"Yes," she mumbled.

"Do you hear me?" I barked again louder.

"Yes!" she repeated on cue, also louder. I had demanded that yes be repeated just to hear my own power through someone else's acquiescing voice.

"Can I have an extra cookie for snack?" was a common request.

"Let's see, have you had any bad behavior this week?"

"Oh, no, not me."

"All right, then, just one extra cookie." Within such relations of power and powerlessness it became easier to understand how Mary Karney came to derive and deliver her ironic "Thank you, Mommy."

I was fast enough at picking up on the power to lord it over my charges and efficient in deploying the drilled technologies. The learning that came later, and slowly, was how to think, listen, see, feed, touch, change, clean, and talk. These skills were buried deep within the complex of "assist as needed." Within this vast dimension was the knowledge most of the women brought to the job from their skills as mothers, wives, daughters, and other kinds of caregivers. I had none of these skills, as I came to realize daily. It was not a lack of emotions or concern; like the other staff I had these in adequate supply. What came so slowly were the actual skills of performance.[4] It became clear there was a base of skill behind that which was named, stemming from experience in unnamed domains, that was simply presupposed and written into the job.

That is, written out of the job. Just after most residents had gone to bed, and before the night shift arrived, we hustled to finish our charting of the bedmaking, bath schedule, bowel and bladder regimens, restraint and position sheets, weights and vital signs. Then nursing assistants were considered by the authorities to have performed their tasks. But these documentary requirements had little to do with how the night closed, or with much of what had gone on during the day, in terms of human contact. The coming of night meant coaxing brittle bones into night clothes, while negotiating with those who wore them to get into bed, calm down, and

try to sleep. Then it meant slipping out the door and turning off the light as quietly as possible. Soon the shift would be over and we could go home, usually exhausted, not just from the physical labors that were officially specified for the job, but quite as much from executing the invisible skills of caretaking on which they depended. . . .

'You've Got to Practice Hallway Amnesia'

When the night shift got under way, room check was the first designated task to complete. On a good night this meant a passing peek into the rooms. Occasionally it required changing someone's sheets, offering a drink of water, some turning, some noting of danger signals, like heavy wheezing, for the charge nurse. It may also have meant cleaning a body, wiping a nose or mouth to clear away phlegm, patting a perspiring brow, quieting a scream, a fear, a cough, a shiver.

Often it involved work that was more intensely interpersonal. "Oh . . ." moaned Edna Barrett one night when she heard the door open. "Please stay here for a while, will you? I can't sleep. It's awful to be in the dark and not know anyone."

"Ah, I'll be back, Edna, just as soon as I check on the rest of the rooms." Upon my return in half an hour, Edna was still awake. She liked it when one of us could stay long enough for her to fall asleep—past just the closing of her eyes, which she did often during the day and night, past a few minutes of silence, until ultimately her deep sigh and slight snore signified that she was calm.

One evening, Dorothy Tomason and I returned from room check about 12:30 when the charge nurse stopped us at the nursing station. "Diamond, go put some lotion on Charlotte." Deferring to Dorothy's fourteen years on the job, she asked rather than ordered, "Dorothy, do you have time to change Arthur?"

Dorothy responded with an ironic smirk, "Honey, I'm a nurses' aide. I don't *have* time for nothing. I just make time to do what's got to be done." Then she turned to me with an instruction regarding Charlotte. "Don't ever put lotion directly on their skin. Old people are too sensitive for that. Always put it on your hands first and rub it around. Warm it up.". . .

"Oh. . . I got to sit down," moaned Dorothy around 2:00 a.m. most nights, with her hand on her sore lower back. "Pain don't know no time."

"Yeah" said I, "me, too." Her eyes darted at me, expressing doubt. It was my only shift of the day, and Dorothy's second.

"God, how do you get some of these people out of your mind?" I asked her, with Charlotte's moans still echoing in my ears. "Well," she said after a moment's reflection, "you've got to treat everybody a little different. But when you walk out of the room, you've got to leave them there and start moving on to somebody else. You've got to practice hallway amnesia."

We sat tidying up some charts. As I glanced over Mary Karney's vital signs, I remembered the incident when she was crying on the bed and I was told to keep moving. Here were the records of her life signs; they made it clear that formally the nursing assistant's job had nothing to do with talking with Mary. It had, in fact, been more efficient and productive not to do so, the faster to collect the measurements. In an early lecture in the school we were told "Nurses do the paperwork now, your job is to do the primary care." It turned out that often it was our job as well to walk away from primary care. To stay to give Mary Karney an emotional outlet for her trouble was supplanted by the act of taking vitals and moving on. Who was the giver and who the taker got confusing as I kept taking Mary's vitals. Tasks produced numbers that, rather than folded in as part of human relations, were extracted out as though they stood apart; then they dictated the form that interaction took between staff and residents.

Documentation reflected the physical life of the people who lived there and, in turn, generated a conception of nursing work as physical. Staff continually cursed at being overwhelmed with paperwork. Kenny once waved his hand at the whole row of binders containing these records. "Oh, they're just a formality," he said. They were a formality with a force—made of forms, and forming

the contours of doing the prescribed work and in certifying that it had been done.

Sometimes they formed the way we spoke. A new nursing assistant once approached a charge nurse who had been at work at this home for two years. Resident Frances Wasserman, who lost her purse, had now been at the home for two months and was crying out loudly in her room. "Is there anything I can do for her?" asked the nursing assistant.

"Oh," said the nurse, her mind immersed in the medications checklist, "don't worry about it, it's nothing physical, just emotional." Here in the night it was easy to see how readily such a comment could be voiced, for we were all thinking in physical terms: "Did I get the right vital signs? Is there enough linen? Is the place clean? Are we looking busy?" These were the issues monitored by the authorities and thus crucial to keeping our jobs.

Thinking was also shaped in terms derived from disease categories. Among Frances Wasserman's diagnoses was Alzheimer's disease. One time she was babbling and crying and moaning. "Oh," said the same charge nurse, "that's the way Alzheimer's people are." Frances's actions became explained as a manifestation of her disease, as though they were devoid of any personal, emotional, or situational content, and flowed purely as a consequence of knots in her brain. What would have explained her crying had this category not been readily available? Might her lost purse have come into focus? Or her son, who was going too near the deep water? Whether or not these might have had a place in a different context, they were considered irrelevant in this intellectual climate, permeated as it was by concepts of physical life and mental disease. . . .

By 4:00 a.m. lights were on in many of the rooms. The nursing assistants had thirsts to relieve, conversations to carry on, pain to acknowledge if not alleviate, nightmares to banish, sleep to coax back. "Go see what Henry wants, will you?" asked Dorothy around 5:00 a.m. one morning. He had awakened with his recurrent chant, "I'm gonna die, I'm gonna die."

"No, no, Henry, you're not! Please try to calm down," one of us appealed, while offering a cool cloth, or a hand, and a presence until he was quiet. After this it was back to the charts, where none of that happened. It was just another physically and emotionally draining moment of nonwork. . . .

Shortly after 6:00 a.m. it was time to begin preparing people for the day to begin. En route down the hallway I began to anticipate two of the forthcoming encounters. One was surely going to be a struggle, while the second hardly unpleasant at all. Yet both involved almost the same physical activity of cleaning and dressing someone. Erma Douglas's advice from the clinical training came to mind. Her prompt response when I approached her with trepidation about cleaning George was "Just go in there and pretend he's your father." By calling on this trick of fictive kin, she was telling me to put the exchange into some kind of personal context, even if I had to pretend one. In the early mornings I headed toward Mary Ryan and Alice McGraw. With Mary, unceasingly bitter and enraged, it was going to be difficult. With Alice the encounter would be partly in a fantasy world as she sang lullabies to people who were not really there. Erma's other lore began to make more sense as well. "After a while when you get to know these folks, it's like your baby" she said with a smile. "You'll find out whose shit stinks and whose don't." Erma's advice, besides being graphic and funny, was usually framed in a narrative of relations. Relationships, good and bad alike, were not something distinct from the work but integral to how it got accomplished.

But what Erma was telling me to do to get the work done, the charting process was prescribing *not* to do. Just as Erma's instruction was to put the tasks into a social relation to carry them off, the chart demanded that whatever happened as a human encounter be eliminated from the recording of the event. Recording the work in the charts came to be no more than jotting down numbers and check marks, transforming it out of social contexts into a narrative of tasks. Just as patient emerges into a social status in the meeting of sickness and institution, so the job emerged as a set of menial, physical tasks in the meeting of the actual work and the documentary products of it: the menial risks were

only a part of a larger human context in their actual execution, but they became simply menial and mechanical as recorded.

After rolling back the curtains to let the light into Sharon Drake and Mary Reynold's room, there was work to do, and much of it involved talk. "I'm dizzy when I first get up, you know," Mary grumbled, "so don't rush me."

"Yeah, I'm dizzy, too. Sorry, no Bloody Marys today. We're out of Tabasco."

"Sagan, rise and shine," as I tried to rouse him from sedated sleep. He awoke kicking, screaming, and cursing—always a rough one, as Mrs. Carmona had warned. We went along, waking, actively listening, filtering, and guessing who needed the most attention. We learned to cheer and to be cheered by Jack Sagan's two roommates. "How are you this morning, Juan?"

"Useless in here, thank you. I just hope my kids don't get a taste of this."

"Oh, c'mon, it's not so bad. The sun is shining. Get ready for breakfast, you'll feel better."

The third man, Art Jacobs, cheered the staff with his early morning renditions of "You Are My Sunshine." Even waking somebody was often more than just a mechanical task; there had to be some personal exchange to carry it off.

Like the residents who had to learn to live within that institutional order, nursing assistants had to learn to work within the people's specific visions of reality. Many were senile and spoke in their own obscure idioms that became understandable only after a time. Every day Jack Phillipson got up and put on his coat and tie, ready to go to work as he had for forty years. We called on nursing assistant Mimi Girard, who knew best how to reason with him. "No, Jack, no work today, breakfast first," she coaxed, "then a shower, okay?"

He paused, trying to figure this out, then asked, "Is the car in the garage?"

"Yes, Jack," she assured him, "the car is safe and sound." Somewhat settled, he walked to the day room. Getting him there was more than "assist residents to day room," as listed in the job manual, and coaxing him to take off his coat and tie to take a shower was more than "give shower." To carry it off took knowing each other and an exchange based on familiarity within partnerships of caretaking.

In time I concluded that supervisors and other passing authorities often did not know the work. Even if they knew the skills, they did not know the relationships within which they were accomplished. "My Frankie" was distinctly not someone else's Frankie. Aileen Crawford's "I'm gonna miss that old goat" was about someone she had tended for two years. Feeding Helen Donahue's memories of her daughter or Sharon Drake's of her restaurant developed only with time.

Yet in the narrative of the charts a clear line was drawn between giver and receiver, and what was given was measured. The social and emotional work was distilled into measures of productivity, and a responsive job was made over into a prescribed set of tasks. The process erased work such as waiting for someone to make an endlessly slow walk down the hall or knowing how to touch someone in the right spots and not to touch someone else in the wrong ones, just as it erased work that was not named or even noticed until left undone, like making the sheets clean enough to be called dirty. No terms connected with caring, relations, or emotions found their way here to muddy up the smooth, carefully calculated records of care. The job was organizationally produced as menial and mechanical, industrially streamlined to complement the making of patients.

As those nights ended and as we waited for the next shift to relieve us and start a new day, the sign over the nurses' station reminded us that if it's not charted, it didn't happen. Still, even if not charted, a lot had happened. The nights and days moved along, aided by the intricate skills, including the mother's wit, that caregiving involved. Erma Douglas's position had now become a little clearer from the time when she stood across that bed explaining the complexity of her work with just five words: "This is what I do."

Notes

1. Regarding the skills of monitoring and anticipating needs, I draw from Alison Griffith and Dorothy E. Smith, "Mother's Work and School," paper delivered at the conference on "Women in the Invisible Economy," Simone de Beauvoir Institute, Concordia University, 1985; also Mary E. Hawkinson, "Women's Studies Office Workers." *Sojourner* 13 (1986): 4-8.

2. The schedule of tasks that eliminates the mental and emotional aspects of the work exemplifies "the organization of power in texts and the relations of ruling mediated by texts." Smith, *The Everyday World as Problematic*, 212.

3. On the passage of time in medical settings, see David R. Maines, "Time and Biography in Diabetic Experience," *Mid-American Review of Sociology* 8 (1983): 103-17; Evitar Zarubel, *Patterns of Time in Hospital Life* (Chicago: University of Chicago Press, 1979).

4. On caretaking as a complex set of skills as well as emotions, see Hilary Graham, "Caring: A Labor of Love," in *A Labour of Love*, ed. Finch and Groves, chap. 1; and Clare Ungerson, "Why Do Women Care?" in *A Labour of Love*, chap. 2. See also Emily K. Abel and Margaret K. Nelson, "Circles of Care: An Introductory Essay," in *Circles of Care*, ed. Abel and Nelson, chap. 1; and Berenice Fisher and Joan Tronto, "Toward a Feminist Theory of Caring," chap. 2.

Further Reading

Renee Rose Shield. 1990. *Uneasy Endings: Daily Life in an American Nursing Home*. Ithaca: Cornell University Press.

V. Tellis-Nayak and Mary Tellis-Nayak. 1989. "Quality of Care and the Burden of Two Cultures: When the World of the Nurse's Aides Enters the World of the Nursing Home." *The Gerontologist* 29(3): 307-313.

Carolyn Weiner and Jeanie Kayser-Jones. 1990. "The Uneasy Fate of Nursing Home Residents: An Organizational-Interactional Perspective." *Sociology of Health and Illness* 12: 84-104.

Discussion Questions

1. What kinds of work make up the "invisible work" of a nursing assistant? What does it mean to define this work as "invisible"?

2. Explain how patient familiarity helps nursing assistants cope with some of the emotionally difficult aspects of their work.

3. What webs of relationships are important in getting through the work day? How are these similar to and different from the relationships between residents characterized by William Yoels and Jeffrey Clair?

21

Mr. Kilwauski

Frederic Hafferty

During their early years in training, medical
students learn to interview patients. From
these interviews, students learn something
about how and why a patient's health deteriorates. Students learn about patients through a
complex set of questions meant to investigate
previous medical history, significant life relationships, and social dilemmas. In previous
selections, Waitzkin et al. and Kravitz et al. illustrate the significance of the social problems
in patients's lives. Instructors intend students
to understand the social problems that affect
patients' lives, and therefore, their health. For
students, this is not an easy task.

   In an interview with an elderly patient, Mr.
Kilwauski, an unlikely turn of events allows us
to examine the ways students learn to cope
with death. Frederic Hafferty talks with students and instructors about the sudden death
of Mr. Kilwauski. Listen to what their accounts
reveal about how students acquire the rigid
roles of medical professionals. In this selection, we see how who medical students learn
to become affects how they learn to treat their
patients. We witness part of the transformation
of students from lay person to professional.
Students' feelings about Mr. Kilwauski's death
transform over a short period of time. Guilt becomes irritation. Fear becomes anger. Empathy becomes blame. These responses echo victim-blaming in the larger culture. Think about
how these changes in students' emotions reveal perspectives toward patients and ideas
about caring.

   . . . In the case of Mr. Kilwauski, dying and
death were merged in a more time-proximate
and realistic fashion, becoming graphically
juxtaposed. More important . . . the death of
Mr. Kilwauski was an unscheduled event. Mr.
Kilwauski was not supposed to die, at least

not during a class on interviewing skills. It is
precisely the unscheduled nature of this incident that allows us to view, from yet another
vantage point, how medicine attempts to
structure meanings around the process of dying, the event of death, and the object . . . in
question. Similarly, the unanticipated nature
of Mr. Kilwauski's death provides us with a
relatively uncensored view of how the culture
of medicine defines its practitioners . . . as
emotional beings. Faced with traumatized
students, and confronted by student charges
of neglect and responsibility, the faculty
found themselves embroiled in a crisis that
demanded immediate and forceful action.
Thus, the death of Mr. Kilwauski allows us to
examine how a medical-school faculty and
administration sought to restore order and
meaning in the face of chaos and unrest, and
ultimately how medicine seeks to construct a
distinctly "medical" reality of death and dying.

   The dying and death of Mr. Kilwauski will
also provide us with a brief . . . visit to how
these physicians-to-be view the social worth
and social significance of the elderly. . . . As
we will see, the fact that Mr. Kilwauski was
in his eighties was quickly adopted by students as a rationale for many of their subsequent redefinitions of his death.

The Setting

On November 13, Mr. Kilwauski and seven
other nursing home residents traveled to City
Medical School to take part in a first-year
course on human behavior and psychiatry.
The course had several goals. Students were
expected to develop an awareness of some of
the issues physicians face in working with
different types of patients . . . as well as to
gain an understanding of basic interviewing
techniques.

   The class was divided into small groups of
about twelve students each. Each group was
led by two preceptors. The interviewing exercises were structured so that one of the group
leaders would initially assume the interviewing responsibilities, with students being
given the opportunity to ask their own questions approximately halfway through each
session. Students were also expected to turn
in a written evaluation of each subject inter-

viewed. On this November day, half of the students at City were to interview an elderly nursing home resident and the other half another type of "patient." In the following weeks, each group of students would rotate through a variety of patient types. For the students in Group 7, Mr. Kilwauski was the first patient they would formally interview in medical school. . . .

When Mr. Kilwauski entered the room, students saw a man of 81 who, according to them, "looked a lot younger" and who was dressed "very neatly—dress shirt, tie, sweater, suit, and everything." As the interview began, the students found Mr. Kilwauski "pleasant," "cheerful," "engaging," "a charming old man." The first part of the interview was conducted by the associate instructor, a psychiatric social worker, who touched on a wide variety of topics, including Mr. Kilwauski's nursing home . . . his life experiences, his present state of health . . . his family, and his attitudes about death. . . .

Looking back on this session, the students and proctors recalled three aspects of Mr. Kilwauski's verbal and physical behavior. First, they noted that Mr. Kilwauski preferred to speak in generalities; in the words of one student, "He presented a philosophy of life and world events." According to the instructor: "He came with something to say, that he wanted to say, and he enjoyed the opportunity. He went ahead and said what he came to say in spite of what I was asking him. He turned my questions around to give himself an opportunity to tell the students what he wanted to tell them about life from the point of view of an eightyish-year-old man—which was very charming." One of the students echoed this view:

The meaning of this whole interview for that guy was different from the meaning that we had. The meaning for that guy is: "Here is my chance to tell these people about life and I know something about life because I have experienced it all these years, and my personal life isn't so important because I want to be a teacher. And I'm going to teach these people something, and any individual life is not so important in terms of teaching them in the philosophical way [I am] trying to do." So the fact that he didn't want to talk about

his personal life was not so much because he was defensive about it but simply because it was a small thing compared to the macroscopic world kind of events that he came to talk about.

Second, all the students and both instructors mentioned Mr. Kilwauski's reluctance to answer questions about his personal life, particularly about his wife, who had been institutionalized in another state for the past twenty years; his relationship with his sons, which students gathered was not close; and his contact with his grandchildren, which occurred, in Mr. Kilwauski's words, "about as often as can be expected."

They [the proctors] said, "This is the class; they'll be asking some questions." And he said, "What kind of questions will they be? How much will I have to answer? I can't tell you everything about my life. There are some things I just won't discuss."

The initial thing that I picked up was that when the caseworker said to him, "We're going to ask you some questions," he said, "What kind of questions?" and she said, "Well, we'll just have to see how it goes along." Right away I noted on my notes that there seemed to be some question on his part as to what was going to be asked of him.

I honestly don't think he knew we'd be asking personal questions. I actually don't think he knew what he was getting into.

The third aspect of Mr. Kilwauski's behavior recalled by all parties was that early in the interview he began to cough and that the cough grew more frequent and intense as the session proceeded.

At the beginning he coughed maybe once the first five minutes, a few times the next five minutes. Then he started coughing more, but I didn't pay any attention to it. People cough; all old people cough. I was used to seeing that in old people.

He was coughing once in a while, and I know I was thinking maybe we should get him water. And it turned out afterwards a lot of other people were thinking the same thing. But I thought, "If he wants water, he'll ask for it. The psychiatrist is there. He can bring the water. He's a doctor."

Of course, now it all looks significant in retrospect. But at the time, we didn't think anything about it.

About the time the questioning was being turned over to the students, Mr. Kilwauski's respiratory problems rapidly grew more serious. Coughing more frequently and with greater intensity, he paused for a moment, jokingly remarked that he was the only person wearing a tie, and then removed it. At this point, two of the students began to question Mr. Kilwauski. The first student asked why he did not move closer to his wife, or vice versa. Following Mr. Kilwauski's answer, the second student asked what turned out to be the last question of the session. As this student recalled: "I asked him the last question, which ironically was something like, 'Here you are, you're eighty-eight [eighty-one] years old, and you've lived your life, and I'm just beginning mine essentially. Can you tell me anything? Can you give me anything you think would be of any assistance to me?' He didn't answer. He couldn't. He just died."

As this question was being asked, Mr. Kilwauski began to cough violently, rose to his feet, and moved toward the student "as if he didn't hear my question." Mr. Kilwauski then moved past the student into a corner of the room and began to cough up phlegm spasmodically into a wastepaper basket. At this point, the group leader asked Mr. Kilwauski if he wanted some water or would like to lie down. Mr. Kilwauski, still coughing, did not answer. The group leader and a student then assisted Mr. Kilwauski out of the room and into the corridor, where, unbeknownst to the students and instructor who remained in the room, Mr. Kilwauski collapsed. Additional help was summoned, and after approximately twenty minutes of unsuccessful resuscitation efforts by two physicians, Mr. Kilwauski was pronounced dead in the hallway. . . .

Following the associate instructor's directive, the students began to discuss the interview, mentioning Mr. Kilwauski's pattern of shifting to generalities and his "avoidance" of questions about his wife and family. No reference was made to his state of health or what might be happening to him now that he had left the room. Meanwhile, Mr. Kilwauski lay outside in the hall, dying. About ten minutes after this discussion began, the group leader entered the room and told the class that Mr. Kilwauski had suffered a heart attack, and that two physicians experienced in emergency work were "covering the case." On his next visit, a few minutes later, he informed the class that Mr. Kilwauski's condition had stabilized, but that even if he recovered he would be a very sick man with a strong likelihood of brain damage and related pathologies due to a lack of oxygen in his system. On his final trip back into the room, the group leader told the class, "It's all over, they pulled the sheet over his head." He did not specifically use the words death, died, or dead. Finally, somewhere in this series of messages was the information that Mr. Kilwauski had been carrying nitroglycerin pills.

The first overt indications of student anxiety and guilt began to surface with the news that Mr. Kilwauski had suffered a heart attack. Following a collective "Oh, wow!" the heretofore academically based discussion shifted to a series of anxious questions and opinions about whether Mr. Kilwauski had been pushed too hard during the interview, whether his pulmonary distress was indicative of an impending or full-blown heart attack, and whether or not the interview should have been stopped.

When [the group leader] came back, and until we found out he had died, even after we found out he had died, from the time that he told us he had suffered a heart attack until the session ended, most of the discussion was on—Had we been too hard on him? Had we pushed him too far? Was the content of the interview too difficult for him? Should we have realized sooner that he was under stress?— basically trying to ascertain if we could have done something to prevent this, done something to cause his attack—a lot of intellectualization, hypothesizing or whatever.

For most students, the message "cardiac arrest" came as a complete surprise. All students recalled that this was the first time they realized that he was seriously ill, but still none reported entertaining the notion that he was dying.

At first, I wasn't affected. It seemed like a very unreal situation. He was sick and wasn't doing too well. But when the psychiatrist came back in and said he was in cardiac arrest, I really didn't know what he meant. Like, what do you mean cardiac arrest? How do you know he's in cardiac arrest? I didn't say anything, and it really didn't dawn on me that it really was cardiac arrest until later.

It was a big shock, but I really didn't think he was going to die. It didn't really seriously occur to me that he was going to die before that [the last message]. I've never been that close to a person who died before.

I'd like to think that we all just didn't want to believe. I like to think that I didn't want to believe that the man was really sick and I didn't want to admit to myself that he was really going to die.

With the increasing seriousness of each message, the conversational level became more strained. "Most people started to get very worried. There were a lot of silences—people making quiet comments to each other. A lot of people didn't feel like talking about it very much."

The final message that Mr. Kilwauski had died brought all conversation to a halt. Following a shocked moment, students began to scramble for explanatory rationales. Most began to retrace the interview, raising questions of cause and culpability. A few withdrew into silence, occasionally punctuated by outbursts of anger toward those who were speaking. Almost immediately, the class's attention focused on the one student who had witnessed the death. He had anticipated that he would be asked how he felt when he returned to the room, and he dreaded that moment. It was the group leader who asked the question. In the student's words:

I said that it really surprised me that it bothered me so much, that I thought I was one of those guys that could handle anything, and I couldn't handle this. I told them, "I don't know how you people are going to take it, but I'm very

shocked". . . . Everyone's going to go through it sooner or later, and I guess I'm going through it now. . . . I don't know how someone is supposed to react. I'm just reacting. . . . It's a strange feeling to talk to someone that's alive and then realize that they're no longer there, and no longer existing. And it's also a shock [because you have the feeling that] . . . "You can't do this to me. I'm not ready for it yet." If this had taken place in an emergency ward, something you would have expected . . . I didn't expect this man to die. I sort of felt he had no right to because I wasn't ready for it. It was a tremendous shock.

The student who had asked Mr. Kilwauski the second-to-last question pressed the group leader about why Mr. Kilwauski had not stopped the interview and why he had refused to take his nitroglycerin pill. In interviews with me, two other students joined in this attempt to assign some measure of blame to Mr. Kilwauski himself. . . . A fourth student attempted to draw an analogy between what was happening in the room and a recent neurology exam, and succeeded only in arousing anger in the group. A fifth student, directing her comments to no one in particular, verbalized guilt for not having acknowledged and responded to Mr. Kilwauski's coughing.

I sort of withdrew from the group. I *really* felt badly about the old man. I really got to liking him while he was talking. I really enjoyed listening to him talk, respected him the way he continued to carry on after all he had been through. And here he was, he had just passed away, and some tears started forming in my eyes. I didn't make any effort to try and hold back. I really felt touched. I was turned off with the whole interviewing business after that. I was shocked, really shocked, that this had happened and the way some of the people were responding to it.

That was the part that upset me the most, after he died. I was completely upset with both [the two instructors] and everybody else for participating in a discussion. People were saying, "Boy, I'm upset!" and yet they were intellectualizing about what we could have done, what we shouldn't have done—like Whose fault was it? Could we have prevented it? . . . First of all, I couldn't see how you could say you're upset and talk about it at the same point. This was the first time. At least it was for me. What I was thinking about, basically, I'm saying to myself, "Two minutes ago this guy was sitting in front of me and he was alive, and now he's lying out there and he's dead.". . . .

I never encountered something like that. I can't believe this just happened. And what bothered me most was that afterwards, people were complaining that the interview had been pushed and that there were certain topics forced upon him that had caused him stress. People who argued against the intellectualizing after we learned he had a heart attack and had died—these were the same people who had done all the discussing, all the intellectualizing and prophesying.

Not every student in the group reported feeling emotionally shaken. Two students characterized their initial reaction as "surprise" and reported that they had "adjusted" almost immediately, without feelings of guilt or questions of responsibility.

My chain of thought changed, but only in that I knew now he was dead. . . . That here I was talking to him ten minutes ago, he was a thinking organism, and now he's nothing; that thinking organism no longer exists. . . . I worked it out in my head immediately, and that was it. It's a silly thing to linger over. . . . I just accepted the situation. . . . I was just sitting there thinking, "How awful." No, that's not what I was thinking. I was just sort of thinking to myself, "Yes, his chest *was* really heaving up and down." I said to myself, "I *did* see that his lips were blue." So, I just sort of was a little pleased with myself that I saw that something was wrong.

It didn't upset me that much. . . . It was something we were going to confront sooner or later and the thing was just to go through it. You don't become personally attached with the dead person.

The group leader, in a somewhat disjointed fashion, recalled his efforts to keep the class going:

I don't think I reacted to it [the death] emotionally at all. I don't think so. In fact,

at that hour, the technical problem had to be handled. I didn't feel anything until that night. . . . I think during the action, I was really concerned with keeping the class going and keeping it intact as a group. . . I don't think I had the intention of saying anything. I wanted to see what their reactions were and handle the problems with it because I remember thinking that night that I really should explain things about the physiology, what actually must have occurred. I know I couldn't have explained it that day.

Student recollections of what the group leader said during this time were more specific and accusatory:

He kept on going back to saying that we shouldn't feel guilty because it was the man's own fault—that he had been told he was coming, and he did have his nitroglycerin pills. And we shouldn't feel bad, and "You're all going to be professionals; with all of the hassles that are going to happen to you, you've got to learn how to deal with death." He was going on like that.

What [he] was trying to get at was, these things happen. When you get onto the wards, these things happen, and the thing you have to try and do is not become too emotional. Otherwise, it's going to interfere with your daily routine work in the hospital. So the thing [that the psychiatrist was saying] was not to dwell so much on the old man who died—not to let the whole thing get into us so much that we wouldn't be able to talk intelligently about death.

The preceptors in the group took it all as an educational experience. They made it into an exercise for us, and I thought this was extremely inappropriate, and many other people thought so also.

The social worker and psychiatrist wanted to sit down and talk about it as a learning experience and something you're going to have to get used to, even given the fact that most people you're going to see in a cardiac arrest in emergency medicine you're not going to know ahead of time . . . And nobody was really ready to do that. I thought it was a little amusing to expect people to bounce back from an experience like that, that they expected us to talk about it.

He said that there was no reason to feel uncomfortable about it. This would have happened under any circumstance, that this was not extraordinary. You tell him how you feel and he says, "Well, you shouldn't feel that way." It doesn't tell you why you shouldn't feel that way. That's no answer, to say he would have died anyway, that it could happen anywhere. That's no answer.

Amid all the discussion, rationales, and definitions of the situation, two or three students abruptly and emotionally left the room, thereby terminating the class.

Picking Up The Pieces: The Institution Responds

Two days later, at the close of a lecture in another class, the psychiatrist who had overall responsibility for the human behavior course addressed the entire first-year class on the matter of Mr. Kilwauski's death. Several students walked out of the room, labeling the event a "waste of time," but most of the class, including all of the students in Group 7, stayed. The course leader announced that he had a three-point agenda. First, he said he felt it was incumbent upon him, as course leader, to formally report to the whole class that a man had died during one of the interview sessions. Second, he wanted to provide the students with "the facts of the case" and thus "dispel or counteract" any "unfounded rumors" that might be circulating. Third, he wanted to open the floor to any questions, complaints, or comments the students wished to make.

The students in Group 7 initially felt supportive of the course leader and his position. Several sympathized with his "plight" and, in hind-sight, even acknowledged that he "certainly had to do something." They saw the information provided by the course leader . . . as relevant to gain a better picture of what had happened. The comment that Mr. Kilwauski's sons had felt their father's death was a "good" death, however, was received with disbelief and the feeling that the course leader was trying to "patronize" them: "[He] mentioned that he spoke to his sons and they weren't uptight about it. Again it was the message, 'They're not upset about it and they're his sons, so don't you get uptight.' But we were there, they weren't, and I had already put together that he wasn't getting along too tight with his sons. So why should they care?"

By this time, the students in Group 7 were feeling more agitated and alienated.

It was sort of a whitewash. Most of the people that I've talked to thought that he didn't really say anything, that he was up there placating people . . . What he did say was that this guy had a good death as most deaths go. He went quickly. He was doing something he enjoyed right beforehand. That he didn't have to suffer any prolonged incapacitations, and things like that. He didn't really say anything of substance after that, but there were a lot of comments from the class. Some negative feelings. I know I spoke up about the whole attitude of the preceptors in the discussions that went on afterwards.

Q: Did he reply to you?

A: No, he'd say something, but it didn't have anything to do with the question, and he didn't answer other people's questions. It was mostly just to calm everyone down and not to raise any more controversy . . . his whole attitude was, it was something that happens, you're going to have to deal with it, and it's upsetting, but you shouldn't be too upset about it.

Other students in Group 7 echoed these feelings.

At one point he said that he had talked with last year's class about how they would like to die and they said at an old age and very quickly. I thought that was irrelevant. He said that the people in the nursing home weren't nearly as upset as you seem to be, which sort of indicates that we were really taking it too seriously. The same old message, "After all he was an old man; he was going to die anyway, and he died very quickly." I kind of resented that because, well, I don't think it's fair. For a man who's alive, he's just as much alive to himself as [the course leader] is at his young age . . . you're just as much alive in your eighties as when you're forty, or ten, or anything. When I get old I would hate it because people would say, "Well, she's not worth much. She's been around for eighty years." That's a really wrong attitude.

[The course leader] is a pain in the ass. The thing was, he was really, really treating it as a learning exercise and it really offended me. Perhaps it shouldn't. If somebody can die and I can use his cadaver as a learning exercise in anatomy, there's no reason why I shouldn't use his death as a learning experience in psychiatry. But I didn't like it. I really didn't.

The students in Group 7 experienced antagonism and anger not only toward the course leader but also toward several of their classmates.

I kind of had the feeling that this was a mistake to do this kind of thing because the people who were involved were the people who were there, and the other people didn't really give a shit. They weren't there. They didn't know. They didn't care. For them it was an incident that happened over there and they'd rather have it over there. Some people who weren't in the group came in and rapped and intellectualized it. They put it rather harshly in that this was a learning experience and the whole bit about how we were supposed to get something out of class. They were coming off with a "Get what you can out of it and store it for later use." That kind of thing—real heavy stuff that didn't ring too well with me. I didn't like it. What I did catch was really negative. They weren't there so it was easy for them to come off like that.

People were saying how this is the first of a series of deaths you're going to be seeing and you'd better get used to it now, folks, because after all, you're going to have to become really callous by the time you leave. That whole attitude is really bad because it's teaching you that you're expected to get used to it. . . . Why should you have to get used to it? Obviously, you shouldn't be shocked when a patient dies, if you know a patient is going to die. . . . But I don't understand why you have to be taught that you're not supposed to get upset or that you have to learn to deal with things. Why can't you just be left alone? . . .

Issues

There is no question that Mr. Kilwauski's unexpected death triggered massive guilt and anxiety for the students in Group 7. The news that he had died established a radically new definition of the situation. The students had previously viewed themselves as simply "talking to a nice old man." In this context, they considered Mr. Kilwauski's cough essentially meaningless and their own subsequent analysis of his "defensive" behavior an appropriate class exercise. Following the news of Mr. Kilwauski's death, however, these events took on new meaning. Students now saw themselves . . . as having "peppered a dying man with quesions." What had been a "class discussion" was recast as a group of people who sat around "coolly" while Mr. Kilwauski was out in the hall "fighting for his life." Mr. Kilwauski himself was transformed from a "somewhat private person" into someone whose "denial" had "quite possibly contributed to his own death." Had Mr. Kilwauski left the room as he did but returned to the nursing home with nothing more than a bad cold, the group's discussion of his defense mechanisms would most probably have continued uneventfully and without further reflection. But this is not what transpired. Mr. Kilwauski did die and the situation was transformed from something routine into something extraordinary.

Let us not, however, lose sight of the fact that Mr. Kilwauski did not leave the room in apparent good health. He did not leave under his own power. Yet an observer who witnessed only the first ten minutes or so of the group discussion following Mr. Kilwauski's exit from the room would have received no indication that anything out of the ordinary had occurred during the interview. In short, we might ask at this point, why was it necessary for Mr. Kilwauski to die in order for students to recognize that something was wrong with his health? Why were the visual cues of illness given such a low level of salience that his incapacitating cough was defined as normal, insignificant, or even meaningless? Most students chose to center their explanations around the themes of avoidance and denial. One student offered a structural interpretation: "We ignored the man's signs of distress because that wasn't on the agenda. He wasn't supposed to be having a heart attack. He was supposed to be letting us observe the interview."

Assigning Blame

What of the questions students raised about their own responsibility for Mr. Kilwauski's death? According to one student: "It's a hard thing to escape, the two situations, us asking him questions and his condition worsening. They did parallel each other, and whether or not there was a cause and effect we don't know, and we'll never know, but obviously it was a source of guilt feelings."

By the following week and second interviewing class, all but four of the twelve students in Group 7 were convinced that the interview itself was not too highly pressured and that the timing of Mr. Kilwauski's heart attack was basically a coincidence. The students no longer felt, as they had on the day Mr. Kilwauski died, that the class had "bombarded" him with questions. The death had become both decontextualized and depersonalized. Most of the students had accepted that neither they nor the interview situation was responsible for Mr. Kilwauski's death.

> There is no basis for feeling guilty because this could have happened that day as he was sitting in the old-age home. If something like that [the questions] could bother him to that extent, he must have been on the brink already. I think it was just a bad coincidence . . . what happened was he had a heart attack and his lungs filled up with fluid as a result. That's why he was coughing so much . . . We didn't ask him right away about his family and his kids [the questions being asked at the time Mr. Kilwauski's stress became most evident], which meant that he was having these symptoms before anyone asked him [about that].

Within a week, students' outpourings of emotions and self-accusations were replaced by phrases such as "he would have died anyway" and "that was his day." These were the messages they had heard not only from the class preceptors and the course leader, but also most frequently from their own classmates.

. . . The unequivocal messages of "no responsibility" which rapidly surfaced and then gained almost universal acceptance, although possibly accurate, reflected a cultural response more than a complete representation of diagnostic and etiologic possibilities.

Blaming the Victim

One of the most interesting reactions to Mr. Kilwauski's death was the contention that he himself might be the most culpable actor in this entire chain of events. The strategy of blaming the victim, although not unknown in medicine, has been documented most frequently in situations where patients were seen as occupying some socially undesirable status—for example, drug addicts, prostitutes, criminals injured in the course of some crime, alcoholics (Sudnow 1967). Mr. Kilwauski, on the other hand, fit none of these categories. He was articulate, sober, and of apparently good moral character. If he did possess a social flaw, it was his status as an elderly person. The fact remains, however, that this articulate and well-dressed person was eventually considered by some students to be culpable because he "lied" about his condition during his interview. Although several students insisted that "he must have known what was happening" and that "he misled us about his medical condition," the study interviews clearly established that Mr. Kilwauski was not asked about his medical history or his use of medications at any point during the interview. The only remotely connected question asked was the general, "How are you feeling today?" but there was no indication that Mr. Kilwauski interpreted this question as anything other than a general conversational gambit and social greeting. Even if he did interpret it as a medical probe, the depth of detail called for was still ambiguous. As noted by one student: "When we asked him about his health, he said he was fine and he was all right, but at eighty-one it could be that . . . walking around with a bottle of nitro is a definition of fine and all right for eighty-one."

By the end of the week, only four students continued to express concern about the social conditions surrounding Mr. Kilwauski's death. . . .

He came here in a kind of pathetic way . . . he thought he was going to get to talk about his life, and he just ended up being analyzed and picked apart. He came thinking he was going to get to make speeches about what it was like to be old. Instead, he was being asked questions about his wife . . . about his kids and his relationships. I don't think that put stress on him—that it caused the heart attack. I just thought it was pathetic to die. You know, people were saying "Isn't it wonderful he died so rapidly?" But I think it's pathetic to die in such a situation. It's not that the interview is such a personalized situation where people care about you. You're being used. You're being used for a bunch of medical students. Your life is being put on display, and he died in that situation. Yeah, it wasn't very dignified. . . . I told the class something like that, something to the effect of, "My God, if this was my grandmother, if I had seen her coughing, I would have offered her a glass of water, asked, 'Is something the matter? Do you want to stop?'" I wouldn't have continued the interview at all.

The issue raised here is not whether Mr. Kilwauski's death was a "good" or "bad" death or whether the proctors or students should have been more clinically astute. Rather, it is an issue of role rigidity and why neither students nor proctors responded to an old man's distress. Clinical culpability aside, the fact remains that Mr. Kilwauski was not treated with the same consideration the students and proctors would have expected to receive had the roles been reversed. Unfortunately, Mr. Kilwauski was anchored in his role as a learning tool, and remained so right up until the time of his death. Within this medical setting, Mr. Kilwauski lost the social attentiveness that might have been routinely extended to others in a more neutral social setting. It was not Mr. Kilwauski "the nice old man" who died in that hallway, it was Mr. Kilwauski the interview subject or Mr. Kilwauski the learning tool. Similarly, the man who "lied," "covered up," and "caused

his own death" was not Mr. Kilwauski the subject, but Mr. Kilwauski the object. Of all of the changing definitions of the situation witnessed during this episode, it was this transformation of Mr. Kilwauski's self that set the stage for all that was to follow.

Generating a Medical Definition of Responsibility

The unexpected and unscheduled nature of Mr. Kilwauski's death, coupled with the emotional nature of the students' reactions, forced faculty into an unplanned and unrehearsed attempt to provide students with more "appropriate" ways of perceiving the symbols associated with dying and death.

The messages students encountered emphasized their lack of responsibility for cause, an attribution of cause to the other party, a denial of responsibility for situational conditions, and a "good death" definition that concentrated largely on the physiological aspects of dying. Students were also told that other people, particularly those closer to Mr. Kilwauski . . . were less upset than the students were. Within this pool of normative messages, the actions of the course director stand out most clearly. Speaking one week after Mr. Kilwauski's death—and thus, in contrast to the session leaders, safely distanced from the immediacy of the event itself—this individual had both the time and the opportunity to organize a presentation. He was also faced with a relatively unemotional audience. . . .

Overall, the data strongly indicate that in the immediate situation . . . there was little, if anything, the proctors could have said that the students would not have criticized as inappropriate. Virtually everything said in the room was characterized by another as involving "intellectualization" or "avoidance of the real issues." According to one: "There was a helluva lot of discussion going on. I was there. I was watching this, and I don't understand how anyone could say they weren't intellectualizing. Maybe they want to give it another label. There was a lot of discussion going on, if not intellectualizing."

On the other hand, it seems clear that had his death occurred at a time and place in which medical definitions of death, dying, and emotional competence were paramount, little guilt would have been assigned, and few, if any, charges of incompetence or responsibility would have been leveled. Instead, what emerges from the data presented thus far is a picture of students caught in a situation in which common, everyday, lay norms of reaction were defined as inappropriate, but new norms defining a new set of medically appropriate behaviors and feelings were not yet fully operational. . . .

The Big Picture

Most of the Group 7 interview questions focused on establishing the particulars of Mr. Kilwauski's death and the subsequent events. One additional question, however, asked students if there were any "big messages," lessons to be learned, or long-range perspectives that they had developed as a consequence of all that had happened.[1] For the two students who professed that Mr. Kilwauski's death had little impact on them, the answer was "no." For them, Mr. Kilwauski's death was an unfortunate coincidence, nothing more. For three other students, Mr. Kilwauski's death demonstrated weakened links in their emotional armor; they concluded that the feelings they experienced were counterproductive to their development as physicians.

Well, I guess part of what it taught me, and I guess it didn't teach me very well because I still do this constantly, was to stop seeing your father and your boyfriend and the rest of the world as your patient, and yourself of course. I mean, to some extent, but don't get quite that involved. I don't think this means being callous. I think it just means adopting a more self-protective reserve.

You just can't jump right in with issues of your fault, my fault. It was just the type of situation where we couldn't do anything about it and maybe in the future we'll know not to get so hysterical, not to lay blame on anybody till all the facts are in, to be aware of people being stressful [stressed] and hold yourself back and not contribute to it. I guess the big thing is that the second time, the next time, maybe out of insensitivity, it will be a lot easier to handle.

With this situation, there's nothing I can take out of it. It's like a scar. It just heals and it stays there and it doesn't bother you any more, and you just shrug it off.

Interestingly, the more effusive responses came from the students who were identified . . . as those who had been the most overtly emotional following the death of Mr. Kilwauski. There was no central theme to these observations, except that they were all worth sharing. One said, "One thing was that I was glad that it was upsetting me, and I said this to [a classmate], 'Look, at least we haven't become so insensitive, we haven't become totally numbed, things can still get to us, we can be thankful for this,' even though it's hard to say that I'm thankful for this incident." A second student highlighted a theme of altruistic detachment:

From seeing that man, I came to realize that . . . there are going to be other people my age that I'm going to have to help instead of helping myself. That was about the one major thing I got out of it—that I'm going to have to help other people. I'm going to have to be concerned with how other people feel and think rather than what's going on with me. . . . And I became very serious at that point about medicine.

A third also spoke of detachment and its relationship to compassion:

The one thing I hoped I would pick up was some kind of compassion about death, about someone dying. You hear all sorts of stories about doctors being fairly impersonal about death and dying. And obviously it is much easier to do if you don't know the person. . . . What I hoped for was a kind of feeling that this is a person, as a whole, and not someone that was going to jump into my daily routine for me to look at. Some kind of a more personal attitude toward the patient and even one who is in very bad shape and even, in all probability will die, despite anything that I or anybody else could do for him. So that is what I hope I would take away from my experience. That's justifying it to myself somewhat, I suppose. I can't say it was a good experience to go through. It obviously is not a good experience when anybody dies. I hope I can look at it in the right way.

And then there was the student who spoke first about denial and the indignity of death:

> You never really believe anybody is going to die until they're really dead. There was a period of time when we knew he was very sick but you don't really realize that you have a denial mechanism going on in you. That you don't really believe they're dead until they're just completely gone, and that's a scary thing. The other thing is just the indignity of death. There's the guy gasping for air. It was pathetic to watch it. Even though the person is old, it's very scary, it's very real . . .

and then closed with an observation that in its own way touches upon the core of the relationship of medicine, death, and the emotional socialization of medical students:

> I don't know if it's anything you can ever really learn to deal with. I tend to be skeptical about the whole situation of coping with death. I don't know what it really means. If it just means going on living and ignoring it, that's one way of dealing with it, but I'm not really sure. But I guess ultimately that's what you do, you say, 'Oh, yes, I'm going to die, too,' and then you just forget about it.

In an era that cries out for "humanistic" physicians and sensitizing course materials, I find this student's conclusion pessimistic—and haunting.

Notes

1. As previously noted, the framing of Mr. Kilwauski's death as a "learning opportunity" was one of the principal messages delivered

by faculty to the students at City. My interview question was intended not to reaffirm that perspective (although it might have), but only to tap what the content of any such "lessons" might be.

References

Sudnow, David. 1967. *Passing On: The Social Organization of Dying.* Englewood Cliffs, N.J.: Prentice-Hall.

Further Reading

Allen C. Smith and Sherryl Kleinman. 1989. "Managing Emotions in Medical School: Students' Contacts with the Living and the Dead." *Social Psychology Quarterly* 52: 56-69.

Deborah Leiderman and Jean-Anne Grisso. 1985. "The Gomer Phenomenon." *Journal of Health and Social Behavior* 26: 222-32.

Harold Lief and Renee Fox. 1963. "Training for 'Detached Concern' in Medical Students." *The Psychological Basis of Medical Practice*, edited by H. Lief, V. Lief, and N. Lief. New York: Harper and Row, pp. 12-35.

Discussion Questions

1. What does Hafferty mean when he claims students' abilities to cope with the death of Mr. Kilwauski resulted from "role rigidity"?

2. Outline the process of "assigning blame" to death in the case of Mr. Kilwauski.

3. Using the example of Mr. Kilwauski's death, explain how patients become the *objects* of medical work.

Section 4

Professional and Organizational Constraints

Transformations in American health care affected both institutional structures and health care practices (Starr 1982). Physicians working for hospitals and other health care organizations now experience more constraints than physicians have in private practice. Most American health care organizations, like most businesses, attempt to provide health care at minimal organizational cost. Cost cutting involves enlisting physician assistance to limit expenditures on care and means organizational restructuring. Physician participation in reducing organizational costs of care have been encouraged by payment incentives and "gag" clauses about care alternatives that physicians might discuss with patients. Personnel substitutions mean more patient treatment comes from nurse-practitioners and physicians' assistants rather than physicians. These changes reflect institutional constraints on health care practices and professions. The transformations also draw attention to professional boundaries of medical practice; they highlight turf wars to protect domains of medical practice. In the previous section, we saw examples of constraints on individual patients and providers. In this section, we explore those constraints further by examining professional

relationships and organizational demands that constitute contemporary health care.

Changes in the structure of health care impact practitioners and available therapies and, consequently affect patients. Adjustments to structure and costs of care also affect medical professionals. Challenges to professional boundaries and structural changes impact physicians in particular. As organizations downsize and try to control expenditures, physicians' occupational responsibilities increasingly fall to other health care professionals. Mark Mesler notes that clinical pharmacists take greater responsibility than physicians for educating and counseling patients about compliance with drug regimens. Pharmacists now do the work of physicians in discussing drug therapies and medications with patients. This change alters task definition and specialized knowledge for both professions. Task definition and specialized knowledge are properties that have traditionally distinguished occupational territories (Freidson 1970). Auxiliary and alternative care providers now threaten physicians' exclusive rights to care and to cure. New groups of health care professionals—like acupuncturists, clinical pharmacists, and chiropractors—dilute the authority of physicians, as once auxiliary health

219

professionals take a more directive role in patient education and care.

Emergent work responsibilities in auxiliary professions present unique occupational problems. Daniel Chambliss discusses how troubles of occupational territory plague nurses as they move into positions of greater professional power as medical practitioners. Nurses' traditional training as subservient to physicians (Reverby 1987) contradicts what happens in contemporary work. Although nurses remain legally accountable to medical authority they must take immediate responsibility for important moral decisions (Stein 1967). Chambliss illuminates the extraordinary ethical decisions nurses make as part of their everyday work. Yet, institutional routines and struggles over professional territories with physicians and other health care providers blur complex dimensions of nurses' work that include intensely moral decisions. Lacking clearly designated roles, nurses often overlook the moral significance of their work.

Michelle Harrison discusses the freedom and conflict generated by ideological changes in medicine, medical work, and care resulting from women's presence in medicine. Her personal account highlights the influence of feminist ideology and women in medicine on patient awareness and caretaking directions. Still, new ideologies, whether patient or practitioner-based, must contend with the structure of current systems. Barbara Katz Rothman discusses the influence of women-centered birthing practices of nurse-midwives and standard hospital definitions of birth. Differing technological values and philosophies of care distinguish home birth-midwives from hospital nurse-midwives. As we see in Rothman's account, technologies mean different things to midwives who find themselves in the home and in the hospital. Struggle over the place of technology and the normal standards set by technological design circumscribe forms of work and of birthing. Both groups of practitioners define themselves as midwives, yet their practices, the structure and location of care, and the responsibilities they can assume are determined by medical and legal designations of birth and birthing processes. The medical work of midwives is characterized by constraints of institutions and professions.

Organizational ideologies influence the structure of work and of professions. Hospice organizations share a philosophy about moral decisions in death and dying that contrasts with standard hospital ethos of care (Mor 1987). Invisible work and high emotional tension make it hard for workers to reconcile their own experiences of tension with the ideology of "good death." Judith Levy and Audrey Gordon discover that moral notions of death with dignity circumscribe an ethic of work at great cost to staff and volunteers of hospice organizations. The "death with dignity" work ethic creates high rates of burnout for hospice employees.

The hospice movement provides an example of institutional barriers to translating ideology to direct experience for staff and volunteers. Ideologies about organizational involvement in workers' health blends the private lives of workers with the public realm of work. Movements to transform workers' health may benefit individuals and organizations. But worker health movements also make the worker a product of organizational transformation. Healthy employees cost less for organizations to maintain in terms of lost productivity and health care needs. Peter Conrad addresses the phenomenon of work-site promotion campaigns and worker wellness. He points to the fact that organizational transformations may come at tremendous costs to individuals (Conrad and Walsh 1992; Nelkin and Tancredi 1989).

As you read through the selections in this section, consider the boundaries that frame professional patterns of work and define health care organizations. Changing professional boundaries means that territories of responsibility for care are contested. The transformation of professional and organizational parameters signals a new dawn for health care, a new set of responsibilities and burdens for individuals who seek and who provide care. The transformation also suggests increased reliance on alternative therapies and possibilities for healing in the future.

References

Peter Conrad and Diana C. Walsh. 1992. "The New Corporate Health Ethic: Lifestyle and the Social Control of Work." *International Journal of Health Services* 22(1):89-111.

Elliot Freidson. 1970. *Professional Dominance*. Chicago: Aldine.

Vincent Mor. 1987. *Hospital Care Systems: Structure, Process, Costs, and Outcome*. New York: Springer.

Dorothy Nelkin and L. Tancredi. 1989. *Dangerous Diagnostics: The Social Power of Biological Information*. New York: Basic Books.

Susan Reverby. 1987. *Ordered to Care: The Dilemma of American Nursing*. New York: Cambridge University Press.

Paul Starr. 1982. *The Social Transformation of American Medicine*. New York: Basic Books.

Leonard Stein. 1967. "The Doctor-Nurse Game." *Archives of General Psychiatry* 16:699-703. ◆

Defining Domains of Practice

22

My Past

Michelle Harrison

In this brief account, Michelle Harrison points out changes that have arisen as women enter the medical profession and as feminist ideology influences some patients and practitioners. Controversies over home births shaped the practice of obstetric and family medicine. These controversies determined the experiences of some groups of women. Harrison struggles with what these changes mean for her patients and for her treatment perspective as a physician. As you read this selection, look for some of the dilemmas—personal and professional—that Harrison confronts.

. . . "Family medicine" was a new specialty, which under its "grandfather clause" allowed physicians in practice who took the requisite continuing medical-education courses to pass an examination for board certification without having to take a family medicine residency. Determined to obtain this specialty certification, I took courses, studied and passed the examination. I began teaching at a local medical school and at a residency program where I both supervised residents and saw patients myself. Because my salary came out of teaching money, I was able to enjoy spending enough time with patients (i.e., I was not compelled to be cost-effective through the practice). The teaching

scared me at first and I was unsure of myself, but I came to enjoy my work both with the students and with the patients.

Life was fairly peaceful. Heather's day-care-center hours were similar to those of my work. Often we had mornings at home together; I would take her on my bike to the center, and then I worked for the afternoon. I became more involved in the women's health movement and there found a group of women who were responsive to my feminism, my feelings about motherhood, and even my medical knowledge. Being a physician has often isolated me from the people to whom I have felt closest. For the first time, both my feminism and my work became a unified part of my life.

Years before, when I was still a resident in psychiatry, I had attended home births, but when I tried to tell my friends at work about what I was doing, I was usually warned that I could lose my license. It upset me that women were having babies in a field unattended, so I did it anyway. My first home birth, in a trailer in Maryland, was also the first time I had ever been alone with a woman throughout her labor. It took hours. There were no nurses, no shifts, no system to shield me from how long having a baby really takes. I remember opening my obstetrics book, examining the curve of labor charted on the page and feeling reassured, for the hours of the woman's labor were no longer than the hours of the curve. It only seemed longer because I wasn't used to being with the woman all that time.

When I moved to South Carolina, I didn't think about home births. There, I was taking care of a population which had just turned away from the granny midwives. Women wanted to give birth in the hospital. They wanted anesthesia, not natural childbirth. They did not breast-feed, even if that meant taking the baby home to an inadequate diet.

Our society was teaching them that almost anything was better than "old-fashioned" breast-feeding, and these mothers were committed to providing "the best" for their babies. Breast-feeding didn't regain acceptance in that community until after I had my child and was seen nursing her.

In the midst of New Jersey affluence, though, women were having babies at home without anyone in attendance, so I was again forced to confront my fears of becoming involved. After sitting on the fence for a few months, I knew that if I really believed a woman had the right to choose, I should be helping her do it safely. Little of my life remained unaffected by my decision to attend births, although there were not many actual hours involved. For example, it was necessary to give up emergency-room work, when someone's life might be endangered by my inability to be present. A woman delivering at home must have her doctor or midwife there or she is without trained help. There aren't other nurses or doctors passing in the hall who can step in and help. Always on call, I carried a beeper wherever I went. At night my sleep took on a vigilance that was a part of my work, including dreams that warned me when there was a difficult birth ahead.

Heather came with me to some of the births; her official job was to kiss the baby after it was born. Sometimes she waited in another room; at other times she was actually present for the birth. Within the growing home-birth movement, enough children have attended home births that at a national childbirth conference I once did a workshop for children who had been present either in their role as siblings or as the children of those of us who had attended women at home. Children see birth differently from adults. They say, "You see, as the baby starts to come out, it turns its head and then it twists the rest of its body so there is room," and while the children talk they demonstrate to one another how the baby makes its way out. They describe the baby as an active participant both in the timing of birth and in the process of being born. "Babies like to come

out when it's dark because it's more like inside the mother."

The births were a source of great pleasure for me, but also of fear. With each one that went well, I wondered how I could have been so worried. When things didn't go well, I agonized over what I should have done differently.

Although my official duties at the medical school were to teach family medicine, I also lectured on women's health care, and especially the rights of women to give birth as they choose. Appointed to the New Jersey State Medical Society Committee on Maternal and Infant Welfare, I sat with heads of OB departments throughout the state discussing such issues as midwife privileges. I accepted my function as a bridge between orthodox medicine and a community which trusted little of what medicine had to offer.

In spite of my good intentions, though, I was still suspect in the lay community because I was a physician. Originally I had planned to attend home births to support the midwives, but as it turned out, I found myself much more alone than I had anticipated. The fear surrounding home birth had affected midwives as well as physicians.

"Home birth is child abuse" was the statement coming from the American College of Obstetrics and Gynecology (ACOG). Throughout the country, doctors attending home births were being threatened with loss of both hospital privileges and malpractice insurance. Residents attending home births either had been expelled from their training programs or were being threatened with expulsion. Legislation to limit midwife privileges was being introduced in many states. Midwives were being charged with murder if a baby died after a home birth.

Eventually, however, some competent and dedicated midwives and I began to work together and to give one another support in the face of increasing pressure to refuse our services to women. At about this time it became clear that I, especially because of the growing publicity about my work, would not be able to go on attending home births and still work within teaching institutions.

I was a family physician, not an obstetrician. If a woman I was taking care of developed any complications I had to turn her over to others who, although more trained in the technological aspects of medical care, rarely shared my political or moral views or those of the women I treated. I wanted to do more obstetrics in the hospital as well as at home. Sometimes at the medical school, counseling students about their future, I found myself wishing I were younger and had the chance to get more training.

The development of part-time residency positions around the country began to render my hopes more attainable. Up to now I'd been stopped from going on with my training because I knew that a full-time program was more than I could manage as a single parent. Another reason I was reluctant to take more training was that I didn't believe it was possible to give the kind of care I wanted to give in a hospital. Every time I walked into a hospital, I changed, without wanting to. I became cooler, more removed, less human, more antiseptic. Patients changed too, in ways that made them turn over their destinies to professionals like me.

The birthing of a young woman named Anna gave me the sense that I *could* work in a hospital and still be myself. Anna was only eighteen when I attended her birth, and her husband seemed about the same age. When Adrienne, a nurse who worked with me, and I first arrived at the house, Kurt confessed that they hadn't practiced the childbirth exercises and he seemed frightened because he didn't know what to do. Relieved that he was not expected to "coach" his wife, he was able to be there solely as support. There is something absurd about expecting a young male, who will never experience childbirth, to be able, after six lessons, to "coach" a woman through labor and childbirth.

The young couple were living with Kurt's parents, who, along with other relatives, hovered outside the bedroom, anxiously awaiting all news. Anna labored for many hours, but then for some time she made no progress. She was a small woman with what seemed to be a large baby. A decision was made to move her to the hospital, with everyone in agreement and seemingly quite relieved.

We went to a nearby hospital where, although I did not have privileges, I did have an informal agreement that I would stay with Anna. I took her in and remained with her while she labored many more hours. The obstetrician, Anna and I agreed to postpone x-rays, since within the safety of the hospital we could just watch to see what happened. Our nurse Adrienne worked in this hospital at night on obstetrics, so she was able to assist in relations between the nursing staff and me. We didn't have privacy, because there were several nurses curious about what we were doing, but Anna didn't mind their presence.

Most important, though, was my decision not to leave the room for any reason at all. I did not take calls and there was no communication between the obstetrician and myself that did not include Anna. No conversation outside the room aligned me with the staff separate from the patient. I stayed locked in her room as if we had been at her home.

Anna was pushing and having a hard time. She tried several positions—on her knees, then standing and pushing. She stood at the side of the bed, with Kurt beside her applying pressure to her back when she wanted him to, while I stood in front of her so she could lean on me. She was leaning and breathing. We were all breathing with her. As she leaned forward, I placed my hands under her thighs to give her more support so she could bend her knees and put some of her weight on my hands. And then suddenly I realized that her feet were no longer touching the floor and that the full weight of her body was resting on my hands, in my arms. I held her that way while she pushed her baby.

The rest of the birth was as beautiful. She delivered her baby up on the bed finally, with Kurt sitting cross-legged behind her and holding her, with Adrienne listening intermittently to the unborn baby's heartbeat, with me doing perineal massage to ease the passage out, with the obstetrician and the nurses watching and learning.

Reassured by this experience that I could sustain myself against institutional intimidation, I felt able to seek more training within a hospital. Strengthened by Anna's birthing, I felt I could become an obstetrician and that my hands and arms could still hold women in labor.

Further Reading

Margaret Campbell. 1973. *Why Would a Girl Go into Medicine?* Old Westbury: The Feminist Press.

Judith Lorber. 1984. *Women Physicians: Careers, Status, and Power.* New York: Tavistock.

William J. Sweeney. 1973. *Woman's Doctor: A Year in the Life of an Obstetrician-Gynecologist.* New York: Morrow.

Discussion Questions

1. What kinds of dilemmas and tensions did Harrison notice in her transition into family medicine?

2. What general issues will a new specialty area present to any profession?

3. Explain how some controversies over home births as discussed by Michelle Harrison might help to shape the practice of medicine. How did they shape her own views of medicine and family?

23

Radicalization: Going Through Changes

Barbara Katz Rothman

In this selection, Barbara Katz Rothman expands on boundary tensions between practitioners adhering to standard medical models of birth and those subscribing to alternative definitions. Visiting the domains of hospital and home, Katz Rothman queries midwives on their work and guiding perspectives in these two worlds of care. Hospital nurse midwives, under the medical model of care, adhere to rigid timetables when monitoring the birth process. Deviations from medically prescribed schedules are constituted as medically defined abnormalities in the birth process. Hospital midwives learn to deal with deviations through instrumentation and medical procedures. Home birth midwives view birthing differently. Note the differences in the hospital and the home birthing models. Think about the philosophies of caring and medical work that make the home birthing model different from the traditional medical model of hospital nurse midwives.

Katz Rothman discovers that adherence to a medical model of birthing accounts for the bulk of differences between hospital and home birth perspectives. Using the comparison between hospital and home births offered by Katz Rothman, consider some of the ways in which technology affects birth and definitions of treatment.

A British-trained midwife, after working in an American hospital, reflected on the transition from home to hospital births:

I knew I was being turned about . . . she was getting dehydrated and instead of getting her something to drink, I put up an IV, thinking this was good management, you know, thinking that this was a great thing. And the next thing I take her blood pressure and it's up, really sky-high . . . So she now has two IV solutions . . . Then of course the contractions stopped, right, and we put up an IV on the other hand. So we now have the monitor attached to the lady, one arm has two IV bottles and the other has one. The woman was in agony, you know, when I could've just given her apple juice, walked her around, and talked to her. And that was the first time I really realized what was happening.

An American-trained midwife talked about the transition from hospital to home births:

Over there the maternity floor is on the eighth floor, and I heard this poor woman from where she had come in on the sub-basement admitting unit, all the way up on the elevator, in such distress, and my thought was, my word, these Spanish people really have a frightful concept of labor. She was noisy and out of control, it was just nightmarish, and I felt, "I hope I don't have to take care of too many Puerto Rican women in my career." Well, the first home birth I went out on was a Puerto Rican family, and I almost dropped my teeth, because there was the mother, when we arrived, very close to pushing, and she was lying peacefully propped up on her bed with her cousin speaking soft Spanish in her ear. She was eating a banana between contractions. I was sort of an observer, and the senior student actually received the baby, and assisted the midwife. But it was like watching a silent movie. I came away and I thought, what are we doing to people in hospitals to put them into this frantic stress I had observed?

Giving birth at home changes things. It reshapes the experience of birthing women and their families. It lessens the monopoly that hospitals have had on childbirth in this country. And it deeply affects the nurse-midwives.

For a nurse-midwife with standard hospital-based training, doing home births is a radicalizing experience. It makes her think hard about her work and its meaning. In this new setting she has to question many of the taken-for-granted assumptions of the medical setting and the medical model. And she finds herself constructing a new model, a new way of explaining what she sees. This is the process of *reconceptualization*, taking something you've confronted maybe a hundred times, and suddenly seeing it anew, seeing it as something else entirely. . . .

For the nurse-midwife making the transition from hospital to home births, many anomalies will present themselves. The nausea that she was taught was part of labor may not be there. She may begin to see that in the hospital this discomfort was caused by not letting the woman eat or drink anything during labor. The amount of time something takes, such as expelling the placenta, may begin to look, in this new setting, very different from the way it did in the hospital delivery room. At first she will try to apply the medical model in the new setting, attempting to utilize the knowledge gained in the hospital to what she is seeing in the home. That won't always work for her. When she is faced with an anomaly in the medical model that she cannot ignore or "normalize," she has a radicalizing experience: she rejects at least part of the medical model. She may share that experience with other nurse-midwives, and many such stories are told. Hearing the resolutions achieved by others supports and furthers her own radicalization. Certain themes develop in these stories; one common theme is that of women controlling their own labors and births by an act of will.

Autonomy and Control

The majority of the nurse-midwives I interviewed had their original training and experience in hospitals. Training in nurse-midwifery does differ from training in obstetrics, yet both are hospital based. In the hospital it is the obstetrician's version of reality that has legitimacy. There may be, as suggested earlier, some inherent contradictions in the role of the nurse-midwife, but once midwifery moved into the hospital as nurse-midwifery, the medical ideas and beliefs surrounding labor and delivery prevailed. One midwife described the medicalization of midwifery, as she experienced it in her own home births, eighteen and sixteen years earlier. She was attended in the first birth by midwifery colleagues who had been trained doing home births. She described the reactions of her hospital-trained colleagues to her second home birth:

> Well, when the second birth was due two years later, the nurse-midwives who were going to be the main call group were those who had graduated from [hospital] and they were the first ones really to come through the large medical-program. And I displayed my wares again, the same homespun equipment, and they were politely acknowledging what I had, and then one said, "Well, where do you plan to have the oxygen tank?" and "Where will you get intravenous?" and "Suppose you need some anesthesia," and on and on, and *it was a completely different concept* . . . there had been such a change in just two years.

The idea that obstetric paraphernalia are absolutely essential indicates a shift in the center of action from the mother, who is, after all, giving birth, to the attendant, who is the manipulator of the equipment. That is, if one *needs* an IV in order to give birth, then the person who attaches the IV is necessary. When the attendants and their equipment are perceived as necessary, then manipulating the equipment appears to bring about the birth.

. . . Anything that appears to shift control back to the mother becomes a challenge to the medical model. In other words, it becomes an anomaly. The prepared-childbirth movement has come close to doing just this, notably by defining the mother's conscious and active pushing efforts as bringing the baby down the birth canal. But that movement has stopped just at the point of presenting a real challenge, by assigning the directions for these expulsive efforts to the doctor. Women can push, but they need to be told when, to be "given permission."[1] ("You can push now, Marion.") The mother is instructed not to push until she's told it's all right, and conversely, must push when she is told to, whatever her own urges are telling her. Her work and her efforts are thus viewed as *helping the doctor* to deliver the baby. Control of the situation remains with the doctor.

. . . The stories that are told by the nurse-midwives I interviewed and observed are about a different kind of control, a more conscious and positive control. The most common stories are about going into labor, or into active labor. As one of the nurse-midwives herself pointed out, "It's an area you can't document that well—it's more or less anecdotal." She then told me about a woman she had attended who had begun labor on a Sunday, "petered out," then came to the birth center in labor on Tuesday. Once again she began to "slow down to nothing." They talked, and she learned that the couple's son had been sick for four days. The husband called home, and came back to report that the child was okay and eating. Labor picked up and the baby was born in a couple of hours.

In the medical model, labor does not stop and start. A stopped labor is either "false labor," and therefore never really started, or, if it is labor, then slowing down is seen as a symptom of a pathological condition that requires treatment. When the nurse-midwife told me this story of a stopped labor, she said that she had seen such things (labor stopping and starting) but not "understood" the phenomenon until she heard Ina May . . . describing how she had dealt with a similar situation. Ina May had asked a woman whose labor was stopping what was worrying her. Once the problem was resolved she "felt free" to go on in her labor. In this instance, the nurse-midwife was very aware of turning from the medical model to the alternative view of women laboring when they are comfortable doing so.

Other nurse-midwives told similar stories, including one who described her own labor as slowing down at four centimeters (early labor) until her two-year-old was brought to her. After seeing that the child was being taken care of and happy, she quickly went on to full dilatation. Some nurse-midwives also pointed out that women who were not really comfortable with a home or birth-center birth, but felt safer in a hospital, would not make progress in labor until they were hospitalized. "One way a woman can cope with not wanting to deliver in a certain place is by not doing it, so that labor process can stop." And from another nurse-midwife, "There has to be a willingness to let it happen." A birth-center nurse-midwife who had been at the center since its first days said that they used to have more women who "failed to progress," who slowed down to a halt for no apparent reason. But as the midwives themselves got more comfortable working outside of the hospital, the mothers too became more comfortable in the new setting; the rate of halted labors, failure to progress, fell off sharply. Now, she said, when a labor slows down they can usually find a specific reason, such as the baby's being turned in an awkward position or, very rarely, being too large for the mother's pelvis. When that happens, the mother will transfer to the hospital for medical assistance—a forceps delivery, or a cesarean section if necessary. But the slowing down for no physical reason, the woman's just stopping her labor because she doesn't want to be there, has mostly disappeared. When labor slows to a halt in the hospital, it is either diagnosed by the medical staff as "false labor" or treated, usually with drugs, as a pathologic condition.

It is not only entering labor and its active phase that the nurse-midwives are now seeing as being under the mother's control. One nurse-midwife described a situation in which she came to see the third stage of labor, the expulsion of the placenta, as requiring the mother's attention and effort. The mother had given birth, and after the first brief flurry of excitement, still holding the baby, she began to make phone calls. She called her family, her friends. The nurse-midwife stood by, growing more and more anxious as time passed and the placenta did not. She finally asked the woman to give the baby to someone else and get off the phone, that there was still work to be done. The mother complied, and within a few minutes her contractions started and she expelled the placenta. This too is the kind of situation that will not be seen in the hospital. Not only is the possibility of social distractions much more severely limited, but, more significant, the obstetrician sees his job as removing the baby and the placenta, and he proceeds directly from one to the other. If the woman wants to celebrate, acknowledge, or share her motherhood, that has to wait until the surgical procedure has been completed. It is still standard procedure in most hospitals simply to hold the baby up in front of the mother for a moment before passing it on to the pediatric staff. A woman's initial extrauterine contact with her baby may be delayed for hours, sometimes as much as a day, even for normal births. Other social contact, with the possible exception of her husband, must wait until she has returned from the recovery room. In the hospital, the birth is, first and foremost, a surgical procedure.

One story I was told by several nurse-midwives on different occasions referred always, to the best of my knowledge, to the same birth. A nurse-midwife found herself at a birth without an assistant and running into trouble. The baby needed suctioning and assistance, and the mother was bleeding too heavily. Instead of smiling at the mother and saying it would all be okay, she told the mother, "The baby needs help and you're bleeding too much. I'll take care of the baby. You try and stop bleeding." And the mother did. Very clearly this would never have occurred in a hospital, where the bleeding would have been medically treated.

Thus, a radicalizing experience for one midwife is shared and so moves that midwife and her peers toward an alternative ideology. What's more, it also opens the door for more such experiences, as midwives try to reproduce these phenomena in their own work. It becomes common practice, for example, to try to find out what might be bothering a woman whose labor is slowing down, or to ask for the mother's conscious assistance in expelling the placenta or in controlling her bleeding.

Seeing the mother as having *more* control is part of the story. The other side is that the birth attendant at home may be seen as having *less* control than in the hospital. For example, one of the contributions many nurse-midwives feel that a good midwife can make to a birth is, ideally, getting the baby out "over an intact perineum," or at least with very minimal damage to the mother, and avoiding the surgical incision (episiotomy) that has

become routine in American obstetrics. On a delivery table the woman is so positioned that the birth attendant has complete access to her perineum and the forthcoming baby. But since the use of stirrups makes tearing likely,[2] "control" is exercised by the attendant performing an episiotomy. In a home birth, or any nondelivery-table birth, the woman will usually position herself so that the midwife can have "good head control," can support her perineum and use oils, massage, or a variety of techniques to control the damage done to it. One nurse-midwife described to me a home birth in which the mother was squatting and the nurse-midwife felt that she could not control the perineum:

> I don't know how much control we really do have . . . She ripped a little bit, but not any more you have "quote" control over—so, y'know, I don't really think I contributed anything more in any other situation where I think I have control.

Without the institutional supports that encourage the practitioner to think (s)he is in control, control may come to be seen as an illusion; and the soundness of the medical model, so firmly based on the practitioner's *doing* the birth, is shaken for the nurse-midwife. Eventually she may move away from the medical model completely. One nurse-midwife who was fully involved in home birth and had essentially completed the transition expressed her view of control in labor:

> Every woman gives birth to her own baby, and no midwife delivers any baby. Every contraction and every push, the woman controls.

Timetables

Timetables are basic to the medical management of birth. They provide a way of structuring and a justification for controlling what is happening. By setting up ideas of what "on time" means—whether for due dates or length of a particular stage of labor—medicine also sets up the occasions for medical intervention to bring women back on schedule. There are timetables for each stage and phase of the pregnancy-birth process.

Pregnancy

To be pregnant implies something other than simply containing a conceptus, the product of conception. Approximately 30 percent of all conceptions are lost with the menstrual period, so that many women are "pregnant" for a few days without knowing it at all. That is in fact the principle behind one of the forms of birth control, the intrauterine device. The IUD is generally believed not to interfere with the majority of sperm-egg unions, but to prevent the fertilized ovum from implanting in the uterus. If pregnancy meant containing a conceptus, then the answer to the question "Have you ever been pregnant?" might be "Yes, probably thirty or more times," for a woman using an IUD for "contraception."

A woman who is menstruating considers that menstrual period as a sign of her non-pregnant state. Yet if two weeks later she conceives, a physician will date her pregnancy from the first day of her last menstrual period. The very date on which she knows she is not pregnant becomes, retroactively, the first day of pregnancy. It is not usually possible to become "officially pregnant" the sixth week, the earliest time to get a positive result on the standardly available pregnancy tests. Furthermore, the pregnancy is always approximately two weeks older than the fetus whose existence presumably determines the pregnancy. A full-term pregnancy is forty weeks, a full-term fetus, thirty-eight. This professional definition is not particularly well suited to the needs or perceptions of women themselves. For example, the seven to twelve weeks considered optimal for an early abortion include those first six weeks, two of which are prior to conception.

In pregnancy the medical profession not only validates the woman's claim to pregnancy; it creates its own unique version of that condition. This in turn legitimizes the profession's control over "diagnosis." A woman may "suspect" early pregnancy, but medical evaluation is needed for verification. Even the "at-home" pregnancy tests instruct the woman to have medical verification of the test results.

When women construct pregnancy timetables, they refer to a variety of different "checkpoints": conception, missed period, "showing," "feeling life," or quickening are the starting points that are important, rather than the "LMP," last menstrual period. The medical definition of pregnancy as dating from the last menstrual period is now widely accepted, even within the home-birth movement. Midwives and nurse-midwives may be more trusting of a woman's reports of known conception times, however, and will not automatically disregard the woman's reports, as doctors will.[3] But quickening, once considered by early midwives to be crucial, is largely rejected in favor of more "objective" measures. Quickening is subjective: it is when the woman *feels* life.

Decision Making and Timetables

In the medical model a full-term pregnancy is forty weeks. There is a two-week allowance made on either side for "normal" births. Any baby born earlier than thirty-eight weeks is "premature"; after forty-two weeks, "postmature." The nurse-midwives accept this definition of prematurity. If a woman goes into labor much before the beginning of the thirty-eighth week the nurse-midwives will send her to the hospital, where the premature fetus can get medical services. (This is not to imply that the nurse-midwives are in agreement with the medical *management*, only that they share the same set of definitions.) The nurse-midwives I interviewed had few clients go into labor prematurely. Undoubtedly selection plays a part—the "screening" process—as may, too, the better nutrition. Postmaturity, however, has become something of an issue.

The medical treatment for postmaturity is to induce labor, either by rupturing the membranes or by administering hormones to start labor contractions, or both. Both of these practices are viewed as "interventionist" or "risky" by midwives. Physicians appear to be relatively comfortable with inducing labor purely for convenience, even without any "medical justification."[4] Induction for postmaturity is certainly not something that appears to bother doctors, and is a standard procedure.

Induced labors are very much more difficult for the mother and the baby. Contractions are longer, more frequent, and more intense. The contractions close down the baby's oxygen supply. The mother may require medication to cope with the more difficult labor, thus further compromising the baby. In addition, once the induction is attempted, doctors will go on to delivery shortly thereafter, by cesarean section if necessary. The nurse-midwives' clients do not want to face hospitalization and induction and are therefore motivated to negotiate for time and to find "safe" and "natural" techniques for starting labor. Nipple stimulation causes uterine contractions, and some nurse-midwives suggest that to women who are going past term. Sexual intercourse in a comfortable position or masturbation are also suggested to stimulate labor, as castor oil and enemas may also be.

The problem of postmaturity seems to come up relatively often, leading some lay midwives and home-birth advocates to suggest a reevaluation of the length of pregnancy. They point out that the medical determination of the length of gestation is based on observations of women under medical care. Many of these women have been systematically malnourished by medically ordered weight-gain limitations. Teenage women in particular are known to have a high level of premature births, and are also known to be particularly malnourished in pregnancy because of the needs of their own growing bodies as well as their poor eating habits. The argument offered is that very well nourished women are capable of maintaining a pregnancy longer than are poorly or borderline nourished women. Thus, the phenomenon of so many women going past term can now be viewed as an indication of even better health, instead of as the pathological condition of "postmaturity."

Going Into Labor

The traditional medical model of labor is best represented by "Friedman's curve," a "graphicostatistical analysis" of labor, introduced by Emanuel A. Friedman in seven separate articles between 1954 and 1959 in the major American obstetrical journal.[5] "Graphicostatistical analysis" is a pompous name for a relatively simple idea. Friedman observed labors and computed the average length of time they took. He broke labor into separate "phases," and found the average length of each phase. He did this separately for primiparas (first births) and for multiparas (women with previous births). He computed the averages, and the statistical limits—a measure of the amount of variation. Take the example of height. If we computed heights for women, we would measure many women, get an average, and also be able to say how likely it was for someone to be much taller or much shorter than average. A woman of over six feet is a statistical abnormality. What Friedman did was to make a connection between *statistical* normality and *physiological* normality. He uses the language of statistics, with its specific technical meanings, and jumps to conclusions about physiology:

> It is clear that cases where the phase-durations fall outside of these [statistical] limits are probably abnormal in some way. . . . We can see now how, with very little effort, we have been able to define average labor and to describe with proper degrees of certainty the limits of normal.[6]

Once the false and misleading connection is made between statistical abnormality and physiological abnormality, the door is opened for medical treatment. Thus, *statistically abnormal labors are medically treated.* The medical treatments are the same as those for induction of labor: rupture of membranes, the administration of hormones and cesarean section. Using this logic, we would say that a woman of six feet one inch was not only unusually tall, but that we should treat her medically for her "height condition." For many years medicine held very closely to these "limits of normal" for labor; many doctors are still being trained with the idea that all labors should follow the statistical norm.

How does this work in practice? The first phase of labor Friedman identified was the *latent* phase. This he said began with the onset of regular uterine contractions and lasted to the beginning of the *active* phase, when cervical dilation is most rapid. But how can one know when contractions are "regular"? There is no way to examine a particular contraction and identify it as "regular." It can only be determined retroactively, after contractions have been *regularly* occurring for a while. This brings us to the confusion over "false labor." The only difference between "false labor" and "true labor" is in what happens next: true labor pains produce a demonstrable degree of effacement (thinning of the cervix) and some dilatation of the cervix, whereas the effect of false labor pains on the cervix is minimal.[7] The difference is then one of degree: how *much* effacement and dilatation, and how *quickly?*

The concept of "false labor" serves as a buffer for the medical model of "true labor." Labors that display an unusually long "latent phase" or labors that simply stop can be diagnosed as "false labors." Doctors can continue to believe that labor does not start, even after they have seen it, because they can retroactively diagnose the labor as "false." Friedman pointed out that the latent phase may occasionally be longer than the time limits, yet the active phase be completely normal. He explained these "unusual cases" by saying that part of the latent phase must really have been "false labor." That way his tables of what is statistically normal still work out. These are of course techniques that are used to prevent anomalies from being seen, to "normalize" the events one observes so that they conform to the medical model.

In the midwifery model, strict time limits are abandoned: each labor is held to be unique. Statistical norms may be interesting, but they are not of value for the management of any given labor. When the nurse-midwives have a woman at home or in the birth center, there is a very strong incentive to keep her out of the hospital, both for the client's benefit and the midwife's. Arbitrary time limits are "negotiated" and the midwife looks only for *progress*, some continual change in the direction of birthing. ("I am comfortable as long as I find there's progress." "We look for progress.") Yet a more medically oriented nurse-midwife expressed her ambivalence about the two models: "They don't have to look like

a Friedman graph walking around, but I think they should make some kind of reasonable progress." She was unable to define "reasonable" progress, but the emphasis was on "reasonable" to distinguish it from "unreasonable" waiting.

A more midwifery-oriented nurse-midwife expressed her concern in terms of the laboring woman's subjective experience:

> There is no absolute limit—it would depend on what part of the labor was the longest and how was she handling that— was she tired? Could she handle that?

Another nurse-midwife described her technique for dealing with long labors:

> Even though she was slow, she kept moving. I have learned to discriminate now, and if it's long I let them do it at home on their own and I try to listen carefully, and when I get there it's towards the end of labor. This girl was going all Saturday and all Sunday, so that's forty-eight hours worth of labor. It wasn't forceful labor, but she was uncomfortable for two days. So if I'd gone and stayed there the first time, I'd have been there a whole long time; then, when you get there you have to do something.

"Doing something" is the cornerstone of medical management. Every labor that takes "too long" and cannot be stimulated by hormones or by breaking the membranes will go on to the next level of medical intervention, the cesarean section. Breaking the membranes is an induction technique that is particularly interesting in this regard. The sac in which the baby and the amniotic fluid are enclosed is easily ruptured once the cervix is partially opened. Sometimes that happens by itself early on in labor, and "the waters breaking" may even be the first sign of labor. But once broken, the membranes are no longer a barrier between the baby and the outside world. Physicians believe that if too many hours pass after the membranes have been ruptured, naturally or artificially, a cesarean section is necessary in order to prevent infection. For women who are exposed to the disease-causing microorganisms in the hospital, especially through repeated vaginal examinations to check for dilatation, infection is a genuine risk. Yet because in the hospital medical personnel always proceed from one intervention to the next, there is no place for feedback: that is, one does not get to see what happens when a woman does stay in the first stage for a long time, without her membranes being ruptured. Instead there are three times as many cesarean sections for "first-stage arrest" among women laboring in the hospital, compared to those who planned a home birth.[8]

While one might think that women laboring in a hospital would have longer labors because of the stress of the hospital situation compared to that of home births, the opposite is true. Hospital labors are shorter than home-birth labors, and, it would appear, are getting shorter all the time.

Length of labor is not a basic, unchanging biological fact, but is subject to social and medical control. The fourteenth edition of *Williams Obstetrics*, in the early 1970s, was still reporting data gathered in 1948 for length of labor. Presumably the authors believed that length of labor is physiologically determined and saw no need to get more current data. But there are big differences between what *Williams* reports as length of labor in 1948, and what Mehl's study of 1,046 matched planned home and hospital births found, and what the 1980 edition of *Williams* reports.[9]

Mehl found that the average length of the first stage of labor, from onset to complete dilatation, for first births was 14.5 hours for home-birth women and 10.4 hours for hospital women. In 1948 the average length of the first stage for first births was 12.5 hours. For multiparas (women having second and later births), Mehl found that first-stage home births take 7.7 hours, and hospital births, 6.6 hours. *Williams* 1948 data reported 7.3 hours. It seems that 1948 hospital births were comparable to present-day home births, and hospital births now are shorter than in 1948, suggesting an increase in "interventionist obstetrics," as home-birth advocates claim. The most current *Williams* reports even shorter labors than Mehl found: 8 hours for first births and only 5 hours for later births. These data are summed up in Table 23-1.

Table 23-1
Length of First Stage of Labor, in Hours

Birth	Home 1970s	Williams Hospital 1948	Hospital 1970s	Williams Hospital 1980
First	4.5	12.5	10.4	8
Subsequent	7.7/8.5*	7.3**	66/5.9*	5**

*2nd birth
**2nd and all subsequent births

Second Stage: Delivery

The medical literature defines the second stage of labor, the delivery, as the period from complete dilatation of the cervix to the birth of the fetus. According to *Williams*, in 1948 this second stage took an average of 80 minutes for first births, and an average of 30 minutes for all subsequent births. As with the first stage, contemporary home births are comparable to the 1948 hospital births: for first births delivery averaged 94.7 minutes, and for second and third births, 48.7-21.7 minutes. Contemporary medical procedures shorten second stage in the hospital to 63.9 minutes for first births and 19-15.9 minutes for second and third births. And in 1980 *Williams* states that the average is 50 minutes for first births and 20 minutes for subsequent births.

Table 23-2
Length of Second Stage of Labor, in minutes

Birth	Home 1970s	Williams Hospital 1948	Hospital 1970s	Williams Hospital 1980
First	94.7	80	63.9	50
Subsequent	48.7/21.7*	30**	19/15.9*	20**

*2nd births/3rd births
**2nd and all subsequent births

The modern medical management of labor and delivery is geared to hastening the process along. In delivery, this is done most obviously by the use of forceps and fundal pressure (pressing on the top of the uterus) to pull a fetus, rather than waiting for it to be born. Friedman presented averages for the second stage of 54 minutes for first births and

18 minutes for all subsequent births. His "limits of normal" were two and a half hours for first births, and 48 minutes for subsequent births. Contemporary hospitals usually hold even stricter limits of normal, and allow only two hours for first births and one hour for later births at maximum. Time limits vary somewhat within American hospitals, but one will not get to see a three-hour, and certainly not a six-hour, second stage in most hospital training or practice. "Prolonged" second stage will be medically managed so as to effect immediate delivery. In Mehl's study, low or outlet forceps, used when the scalp is visible, were fifty-four times more common; and mid-forceps (used when the head is engaged but not yet visible), twenty-one times more common for prolonged second stage and/or protracted descent in the hospital than in home births. This does not include the *elective* use of forceps (without "medical indication"), a procedure that was used in none of the home births and 10 percent of the hospital births (4 percent low forceps and 6 percent mid-forceps). Note that any birth which began at home but was hospitalized for any reason, including protracted descent or prolonged second stage, was included in home-birth statistics.

Midwives and their clients are even more highly motivated to avoid hospitalization for prolonged second stage than for prolonged first stage. There is a sense of having come too far—through the most difficult and trying stage of labor—to switch to a hospital. Once the mother is fully dilated she is so close to birth that one hesitates to start moving her, knowing she could end up birthing on the way to the hospital. The mother is usually not in pain during second stage, and very anxious not to be moved.

In a standard hospital birth, the mother is moved to a delivery table at or near the end of cervical dilatation. She is strapped into leg stirrups and heavily draped. The physician is scrubbed and gowned. The anesthetist is at the ready. It is difficult to imagine the scene continuing for three, four, or more hours. The position of the mother alone makes such a thing impossible. In a home birth the mother is usually feeling much better as dilation is completed. Her birth attendant has been with her for hours. There may be less of a sense of urgency and immediacy about getting the birth done. There is also the emphasis on the individual and unique nature of each labor, so that each must be judged and managed on its own terms. "Progress" again becomes the most important criterion.

> Second stage, I think, could be longer than the conventional two hours some hospitals think, or one hour even, and that would depend on the pattern of the labor.
>
> If there was some definite progress, however slow, whether the baby was posterior or anterior, size of baby, if it all was going well, baby's heartbeat reflecting no stress whatsoever, I think you could be in stage two well over three hours, maybe four.

That nurse-midwife went on to give an example of a six-hour second stage with no complications.

In the medical model second stage begins with complete cervical dilation. Cervical dilatation is an "objective" measure, determined by the birth attendant rather than the mother. That means that the birth attendant defines second stage and so controls the time of formal entry into second stage. One of the ways nurse-midwives quickly learn to "buy time" for their clients is in when and how they measure cervical dilation:

> If she's honestly fully dilated I do count it as second stage. If she has a rim of cervix left I don't, or any cervix at all, the slightest minuscule cervix left, I don't count it, because I don't think it's fair. A lot of what I do is to look good on paper.

"Looking good on paper" is a serious concern. Nurse-midwives expressed their concern about leaving themselves out on a legal limb if they do, for example, allow second stage to go for more than the one- or two-hour hospital limit, and then want to hospitalize the woman. One told of allowing a woman to be in second stage for three hours, and then hospitalizing her for lack of progress. The mother, in her confusion and exhaustion, told the hospital staff she had been in second stage for five hours. The nurse-midwife risks losing her backup at that hospital.

Nurse-midwives talked about the problems of writing down on the woman's chart the start of second stage:

—If I'm doing it for my own use, I start counting when the woman begins to push in a directed manner, really bearing down. I have to lie sometimes. I mean, I'm prepared to lie if we ever have to go to the hospital, because there might be an hour or so between full dilatation and when she begins pushing and I don't see—as long as the heart tones are fine and there is some progress being made—but like I don't think in this city—you'd be very careful to take them to the hospital after five hours of pushing. They would go crazy.

—All my second stages I write down under two hours: by hospital standards two hours is the upper limit of normal but I don't have two-hour second stages, except that one girl that I happened to examine. If I had not examined her, I probably would not have had more than an hour and a half written down because it was only an hour and a half that she was voluntarily pushing herself.

Not looking for what you do not want to find is a technique used by many of the nurse-midwives. They are careful about not examining a woman if she might be fully dilated, for fear of starting up the clock they work under:

I try to hold off on checking if she doesn't have the urge to push, but if she has the urge to push, I have to go in and check.

Some nurse-midwives have taken this a step further, and redefined second stage itself. Rather than saying it starts with full dilatation—the "objective," medical measure—they measure second stage by the subjective measure of the woman's urge to push. Most women begin to feel a definite urge to push and begin bearing down at just about the time of full dilatation. But not all women have this experience. For some, labor contractions cease after full dilatation. These are the "second-stage arrests," which medicine treats by the use of forceps or cesarean section. Some nurse-midwives now think "second-stage arrest" may just be a naturally occurring rest period at the end of labor, instead of a problem requiring medical intervention. Some women, they claim, have a rest period after becoming fully dilated but *before they begin* second stage. In the medical model, once labor starts, it cannot stop and start again and still be "normal." If it stops, that calls for medical intervention. But a nurse-midwife can call the "hour or so between full dilatation and when she starts pushing" as *not* second stage. This is more than just buying time for clients: this is developing an alternative set of definitions, changing the way she sees the birth process.

Midwives who did not know each other, who did not work together, came to this same conclusion:

—My second-stage measurement is when they show signs of being in second stage. That'd be the pushing or the rectum bulging or stuff like that. . . . I usually have short second stages [laughter]. Y'know, if you let nature do it, there's not a hassle.

—I would not, and this is really a fine point, encourage a mother to start pushing just because she feels fully dilated to me. I think I tend to wait till the mother gets a natural urge to push. . . . The baby's been in there for nine months.

It may be that buying time is the first concern. In looking for ways to avoid starting the time clock, nurse-midwives first realize that they can simply not examine. It makes sense not to look for what you don't want to find. They then have the experience of "not looking" for an hour, and seeing the mother stir herself out of a rest and begin to have a strong urge to push. The first few times, that hour is an anxiety-provoking experience. Most of the nurse-midwives were able to tell anecdotes of "the first time I let—go for—time," and of their own nervousness. The experience of breaking the timetable norms and having a successful outcome is a radicalizing experience. They then talk not only about techniques for buying time and looking good on paper, but about a whole new version of the event. This opportunity for feedback simply does not exist in the hospital. In its tight control of the situation, medicine prevents anomalies from arising. A woman who has an "arrested" second stage will not be permitted to simply nap, and therefore the diagnosis remains unchallenged. Forceps and/or hormonal stimulants effect the delivery. The resultant birth injuries are perceived as inevitable, as if without the forceps the baby would never have gotten out alive.

Third Stage: Afterbirth

Third stage is the period between the delivery of the baby and the expulsion of the placenta. In hospitals the third stage is expedited as quickly as possible, and takes five minutes or less. A combination of fundal massage and pressure and gentle traction on the cord are used routinely. *Williams Obstetrics* says that if the placenta has not separated within three to five minutes of the birth of the baby, manual removal of the placenta should probably be carried out.[10] In Mehl's data, the average length of third stage for home births was twenty minutes.

For the nurse-midwives the third stage sometimes presented problems. It occasionally happens that the placenta does not simply slip out, even in the somewhat longer time period they may have learned to accept. Their usual techniques—suckling, squatting, walking—may not show immediate results:

—I don't feel so bad if there's no bleeding. Difficult if it doesn't come, and it's even trickier when there's no hemorrhage, because if there's hemorrhage then there's a definite action you can take, but when it's retained and it isn't coming it's a real question—is it just a bell-shaped curve? and that kind of thing. . . . In the hospital if it isn't coming right away you just go in and pull it out.

—I talked with my grandmother. She's still alive, she's ninety, she did plenty of deliveries, and she says that if the placenta doesn't come out you just let the mother walk around for a day and have her breast-feed and it'll fall out. And I believe her. Here I would have an hour because I am concerned about what appears on the chart.

Like the ninety-year-old grandmother, a very midwifery-oriented nurse-midwife with a great deal of home-birth experience said:

If there was no bleeding, and she was doing fine, I think several hours, you know, or more, could elapse. No problem.

Why the Rush? Institutional Demands and the Birth Process

There are stated medical reasons for rushing the second and third stages of labor. A prolonged third stage is believed to cause excessive bleeding. The second stage is rushed to spare the baby and the mother because birth is seen as traumatic for both. Even in 1980, *Williams* still refers to using the baby's head as a "battering ram." The clean, controlled, medically wielded forceps are trusted more than the mother's body and her efforts. There is another factor as well. *Williams* states:

The vast majority of forceps operations performed in this country are elective low-forceps. One reason is that all methods of drug-induced analgesia and especially conduction analgesia and anesthesia often interfere with the woman's voluntary expulsive efforts, in which circumstances low-forceps delivery becomes the most reasonable procedure.[11]

Williams goes on to affirm that this does not constitute an indictment of the procedures for analgesia, but merely requires the proper use of forceps. The lithotomy position also contributes to the need for forceps because the baby must be pushed upwards. This is the phenomenon that home-birth and midwifery advocates refer to as the "snowballing effect" of obstetrical intervention:

Like a snowball rolling downhill, as one unphysiologic practice is employed, for one reason or another, another frequently becomes necessary to counteract some of the disadvantages, large or small, inherent in the previous procedures.[12]

Besides the medical reasons given, there are also institutional demands for speeding up birth. In Rosengren and DeVault's study of time and space in an obstetric hospital, the authors discussed the importance of timing and tempo in the hospital management of birth.[13] Tempo relates to the number of deliveries taking place in a given period of time.

Physiological tempo will be kept at a pace appropriate to functional tempo, the needs of the institution. If there were too many births, the anesthetist slowed them down—an unphysiologic and dangerous but time efficient practice. An unusually prolonged delivery will also upset the tempo; there is even competition among obstetrical residents to maintain optimal tempos. A resident said:

Our [the residents'] average length of delivery is about 50 minutes, and the Pros' [the private doctors'] is about 40 minutes.[14]

That presumably includes delivery of baby and placenta, and possibly episiotomy repair as well. . . . Once the baby is quickly and efficiently removed, the staff will certainly not wait twenty minutes or more for the spontaneous expulsion of the placenta. One could watch innumerable hospital births and never learn that the placenta can emerge spontaneously.

In the home and to a lesser extent in birth-center births the motivations for maintaining institutional tempo are not present. Each birth is a unique event, and birth attendants do not move from one laboring woman to the next. Births do not have to be meshed with each other to form an overriding hospital schedule. Functioning without these demands, nurse-midwives are presented with situations that are anomalous to the medical model, such as labor stopping and starting, second stage not following immediately on first, or a woman taking four hours to push out a baby with no problems. Without obstetrical interventions, things that were defined as "pathologies" may be seen to right themselves, and so the very idea of what is pathological and what is normal is challenged.

Hospitals so routinize the various obstetrical interventions that alternatives are unthinkable. A woman attached to an IV and a fetal monitor cannot very well be told to go out for a walk or to a movie if her contractions are slow and not forceful. A woman strapped to a delivery table cannot take a nap if she does not feel ready to push. She cannot even get up and move around to find a better position in which to push. The entire situation reinforces the medical model. Once a laboring woman is hospitalized, she will have a medically constructed birth.

In a home birth, and possibly to a lesser extent in a birth-center birth, the routine and perceived consensus are taken away. In a woman's home a birth is, whatever else it may be, a unique life event. Each nurse-midwife stressed the individuality of each out-of-hospital birth, that each birth was a part of each mother and family. They described tight-knit extended-kin situations, devoutly religious births, partylike births, intimate and sexual births—an infinite variety. The variety of social contexts seems to overshadow the baby-out-of-vagina sameness. Medical "management" has to occur within the birth as a personal life event. The mother as *patient* must coexist with or take second place to the mother as *mother*, or wife, daughter, sister.

Stripped of institutional supports, the nurse-midwives perceive the functions of timetables. They are a way of managing women in labor, a way of controlling the situation in a medically appropriate manner.

Notes

1. See, for example, Arthur Colman and Libby Colman, *Pregnancy: The Psychological Experience* (New York: Herder and Herder, 1971).
2. Doris Haire, *The Cultural Warping of Childbirth.* (Seattle: International Childbirth Education Association, 1972).
3. See Rita Seiden Miller, "The Social Construction and Reconstruction of Physiological Events: Acquiring the Pregnant Identity," in Denzin, ed. *Studies in Symbolic Interaction* (JAI Press, 1977).
4. Ronald R. Rindfuss, "Convenience and the Occurrence of Births: Induction of Labor in the United States and Canada" (Paper presented to the Seventy-second Annual Meeting of the American Sociological Association, 1977).
5. For an overview of Friedman's work, see Emanuel Friedman, "Graphic Analysis of Labor," *Bulletin of the American College of Nurse-Midwifery* (1959): 94-105.
6. Ibid., p. 97.
7. Louis M. Hellman and Jack A. Pritchard, eds., *Williams Obstetrics*, 14th ed. (New York: Appleton-Century-Crofts, 1971).
8. Lewis Mehl, "Research on Childbirth Alternatives: What Can It Tell Us about Hospital Practice?" in David Stewart and Lee Stewart, eds.,

21st Century Obstetrics Now! (Chapel Hill: NAPSAC, 1977).

9. Mehl, "Childbirth Alternatives"; Hellman and Pritchard, eds., *Williams Obstetrics*; and Jack A. Pritchard and Paul C. McDonald, eds., *Williams Obstetrics*, 16th ed. (New York: Appleton-Century-Crofts, 1980).

10. Ibid., p. 425.

11. Pritchard and McDonald, eds., *Williams Obstetrics*.

12. Ibid., p. 1044.

13. William R. Rosengren and Spencer DeVault, "The Sociology of Time and Space in an Obsetrical Hospital," in Eliot Freidson, ed., *The Hospital in Modern Society* (New York: Free Press, 1963).

14. Ibid., p. 282.

Further Reading

Emily Martin. 1992. *The Woman in the Body: A Cultural Analysis of Reproduction.* Boston: Beacon Press.

Sue Fisher. 1986. *In the Patient's Best Interest: Women and the Politics of Medical Decisions.* New Brunswick: Rutgers University Press.

Rose Weitz and Deborah Sullivan. 1986. "The Politics of Childbirth: The Re-emergence of Midwifery in Arizona." *Social Problems* 33: 163-175.

Discussion Questions

1. Describe the different philosophies and models of care that guide the practice of hospital nurses and home birth midwives. How do these philosophies determine models of care? What influence do they have on the birth process?

2. What is the relationship between each model of birthing and technology?

3. Which model of birthing do you think is the best strategy? Why? Under what circumstances might the alternative prove a better strategy?

24

Boundary Encroachment and Task Delegation: Clinical Pharmacists on the Medical Team

Mark A. Mesler

In this selection, Mark Mesler identifies a restructuring of medical practice and the emergence of a new profession: clinical pharmacy. Consider the kinds of conflicts that arise in the (re)definition of a profession. In his discussion, Mesler emphasizes problems in introducing a new professional into medicine. Definitions of work roles change. Statuses are threatened. Boundaries are blurred. As the position of clinical pharmacy emerges, we see tensions within the profession of medicine. The new role of pharmacists threatens territorial domains of work and professional expertise. Historically, pharmacists worked at the peripheries of medical teams, providing drug therapies and prescriptions for use. Technological change helps fuel increasing numbers of clinical pharmacists on hospital teams. Note what happens as pharmacists begin a more active and patient-oriented role in disseminating information about drug therapies and prescriptions. The participation of clinical pharmacists on a medical team provides us a vivid example of negotiated territories of medical work. As you read this piece, think about the issues that might obscure the boundaries of medical work.

Introduction

The research presented here is concerned with changes in the world of medicine, specifically with pharmacists' attempts to expand their role boundaries as members of the medical team. Especially since World War II, changes in the nature of health care in the U.S. (and many other countries) led to the making of several new medical roles and fostered the remaking of many traditional ones (Bullough 1966; Bullough and Bullough 1964; Freidson 1970; Kronus 1976; Starr 1982). About twenty years ago these changes led pharmacists to redefine their role to be more patient-oriented, to take increased responsibility for medication therapy, and the term 'clinical' pharmacy gained increased prominence to express the nature of these expanded boundaries (Tyler 1968). This more active, clinical role has been seen by some, pharmacists and outside observers alike, to be one of the most promising strategies for 'reprofessionalising' pharmacy's status (e.g., Apple 1981; Birenbaum 1982). As is generally the case with such changes, pharmacy's extended role boundaries have the potential to affect incumbents of other roles with whom they interact, particularly physicians and nurses. . . .

I argue that the bipolar perceptions of pharmacy's clinical role are not so much contradictory as they are incomplete; they do not do justice to the interactive processes or role expansion and boundary construction taking place. To provide a context for this argument, presented first is a brief historical background on pharmacy and the methods and settings of the data collection. A discussion of role boundaries and the medical team is broken down into three interdependent elements: the first section, role expansion, involves a comparison of the more traditional with the expanded, clinical pharmacy role; the next section is on boundary conflicts and resolutions, where pharmacy's expanded clinical boundaries affect other members of the medical team and, in the third section, the boundaries perceived by relevant participants on the medical team are discussed. In concluding, a few observations are made regarding pharmacy's 'clinical' role, and the sociological perception of occupational role boundaries in general.

Historical Background

At one time the role boundaries between pharmacists and physicians were rather ambiguous. In the original division of labour, pharmacists were not only the distributors but the compounders of medications, and the esoteric knowledge required to perform their role granted them a relatively professional status in society and medicine. Around the turn of the twentieth century, however, the role of the pharmacist began to undergo significant change (Kronus 1976; Starr 1982).

For example, as early as the 1920s the synthesis of potent medications became standardised and manufactured on a large scale. Beginning in the 1950s with the development of, and demand for, various 'miracle' drugs (e.g. antibiotics, tranquillisers, psychotropics), pharmacy's major production functions were gradually taken away by manufacturers making high quality, inexpensive, mass-produced dosage forms of many medications (Kramer et al. 1979; Tyler 1968). As drugs became the treatment of choice in varied medical contexts (Lennard et al. 1971), the resulting proliferation brought with it an increased educational requirement for pharmacy. Together with their loss of function as compounders, pharmacists became boxed into a role of over-educated distributors; the pharmacists in this research described their traditional role as being 'counters and pourers' or 'lickers and stickers', who merely filled and passed on doctors' prescriptions. By the 1960s even this role was becoming threatened by those receiving a minimum of technical training; pharmacy 'techs' were taking over many of the rote distribution functions (Tyler 1968).

It is difficult to determine exactly when the notion of clinical pharmacy began; the word appeared in the literature in the 1920s and the idea was debated off and on for the rest of the century(Frank 1974; Smith and Swintosky 1983). However, several factors occurred in the 1960s that played a major part in its current status. The sequence of events discussed and the growing number of pharmacy technicians motivated pharmacists to explore alternatives to their traditional role. Beginning in the late 1950s and early 60s, with drugs playing an increasingly important part in our society's health care, the federal government took an active interest in coordinating and disseminating available drug information. A number of organisations, including the American Society of Hospital Pharmacists (ASHP), took part in providing this information (Martin 1971). Also in the early 1960s the first research reports on medication errors and adverse drug reactions in hospital patients were being published. As a function of these factors, the pharmacy literature during the latter 1960s reflects the emergence of three related responses: the unit dose drug distribution system, hospital-based drug information centres, and the ideology of clinical pharmacy (Ray 1979; Smith 1969, 1971).

Methods and Settings

Although the research presented here is focused on the role of the clinical pharmacist, much of the data were collected under the auspices of a university research project funded to study student socialization into that role. My part was that of lone field researcher to a three-person team headed by two professors, one in the department of sociology, the other in the department of pharmacy.

One of the biggest advantages I had in joining an established project was access to the field settings. Although I learned that entree in a setting is much more a process than an event, access to the setting and negotiating with the 'gatekeepers' at all levels (see Broadhead and Rist 1976) was already taken care of by the time I entered the scene. Nonetheless, passing through these otherwise closed doors as an outsider posed its own set of unique problems.

Although my role had been formally prescribed as a pharmacy student, this proved to be only a place on stage, so to speak, an assigned character in an improvisational scene.

While dressing like the pharmacists and pharmacy students (in a shirt, tie and white labcoat) granted me general acceptance in the hospital setting, I was an outsider to the established life, the department of pharmacy, and the cohort of students I was observing. This inherent problem of participant observation was resolved in my circumstances by a process very much analogous to that discovered in the research. I attempted to negotiate my role through the development of rapport; I varied my emphasis on participation and observation by running errands (e.g., carrying messages), taking part in hospital activities (e.g., participating in patient exams), and sharing thoughts when it seemed appropriate. By letting the participants in the setting get to know me and lying back in my observational stance, I was able to gain acceptance as a nonthreatening other.

Entree had been gained at two different teaching hospitals (both affiliated with the same university) where pharmacy students were being socialised into clinical practice. I conducted the major part of the research on two full working days during two spring semesters of the 1981 and 1982 academic years. After successfully renegotiating my own entree, I carried out additional observations and interviews during the summer months of the latter year, and conducted my final interviews following a significant proportion of the analysis some two years later. My interviews were generally tape recorded, semiformal, guided conversations. In total I conducted interviews with 14 pharmacists, 16 physicians, two clinical librarians, two head nurses, three pharmacy administrators, and the Associate Dean for Clinical Affairs in the university school of pharmacy.

I carried out the first semester's observations at Suburban hospital, an approximately twenty-five-year-old, 200-bed university-operated facility located in a fairly affluent suburban neighbourhood. There were eight bachelor-degreed clinical pharmacists at Suburban who worked with a unit dose distribution system. In this system pharmacists were not only responsible for preparing and properly dosing all individual patient medications, but they could also personally distribute the medications to each care unit and carry out the more clinical functions of their role (described below). Clinically, these pharmacists had specialised their services to the extent that, while usually covering two or three floors per day, each pharmacist was primarily responsible for a particular floor or care unit. In this way, there were pharmacists who had concentrated their expertise in one of four areas: general medicine, paediatrics, cardiac care, or psychiatric care.

The second research setting was Urban Hospital. It was some one hundred years older, considerably larger (approximately 900 beds), and located in the heart of a city whose population well exceeded 100,000. Urban was the city's oldest and most prestigious hospital, providing the widest scope of available medical services. At Urban there were six pharmacists providing specialised clinical services in one of the following areas: general medicine, paediatrics, surgery, infectious disease, cancer treatment and total parenteral nutrition (TPN—for those patients who require total sustenance without eating). In addition to these basic distinctions, the clinical pharmacists at Urban were also unusual in their field; most had attained a Pharm. D. (Doctor of Pharmacy) degree, and they were totally divorced from distributive functions.[1]

Role Expansion

Prior to the changes which begin in the 1960s and 70s, hospital pharmacists generally practised with a ward stock drug distribution system, often dispensing in virtual anonymity from the basement of the hospital. In a ward stock-type system pharmacists were responsible for keeping the appropriate supply of medicines in each care unit from which nurses administered according to physicians' orders. On the whole, where such systems existed, the nursing staff had responsibility for proper selection, dosing and identification of medication errors. The ward stock system fostered only the more traditional, dispensing tasks of pharmacy; what the pharmacists in this research referred to is product-oriented tasks. At the time this research was being conducted, a transition from ward stock to unit dose distribution seemed to be taking place in hospitals throughout the U.S., but was as yet incomplete. The unit dose system (described below) was considered to provide a safer method of drug distribution and was being advocated by many pharmacy leaders as a facilitator of the more patient-oriented, clinical role; it was placing pharmacists in a better position for interacting with members of the medical team and practising their clinical tasks (Borgsdorf et al. 1973; Hood 1977).

This distinction between 'traditional' and 'clinical' pharmacy has itself produced some factionalism within the field (e.g. Carroll and Gagnon 1984; Zelnio et al. 1984). As such, clinical pharmacy could be considered a 'segment' within pharmacy which has become a professionalising social movement[2] and, as Bucher (1962: 40) noted, one of the problems of segmentation is '. . . opposition to older entrenched groups . . .'. That is, pharmacists have been negotiating their expanded boundaries not only interprofessionally but intraprofessionally. At least in part as a result of this segmentation, a lack of consensus has developed among pharmacists regarding the clinical concept and its application (see Smith and Swintosky 1983; Wardwell 1974). With this in mind, the initial focus of the present research involved the pharmacy participants' understanding of the clinical role.

Among the first questions asked of both the clinical pharmacy students and the clinical pharmacists was, 'What is it about your expanded role that makes it clinical; what activities make pharmacy a clinical practice?' Their responses were then compared to the tasks outlined in two contemporary articles on the subject, one from pharmacy (Smith 1982), the other from sociology (Ritchey and Raney 1981). By collapsing and/or expanding categories, all sources more or less corresponded, the ideology had been internalised at both settings, so that the ideal clinical role would include the following tasks: 1) Pharmacists provide *drug information* to allied personnel in various forms, through spontaneous interaction, complex questions necessitating referral, or requests for formal consultation requiring elaborate literature review and write-up. 2) *Drug monitoring*, surveillance of patient medications, is performed to detect and correct inappropriate dosage levels, potential for adverse reactions, and drug/drug or drug/illness interactions.[3] 3) In conjunction with medication monitoring, pharmacists employ other data (e.g., patients' diagnoses and treatment plans found in the charts) to *evaluate* the effectiveness of *drug therapy* and make recommendations accordingly. 4) Pharmacists accompany physicians on *patient care rounds* and provide various pharmacy services (e.g., drug information/education) while keeping abreast of patient conditions and progress. 5) Pharmacists collect medication histories and *counsel patients* on the use of, and possible reactions to, their medications. 6) Allied personnel, particularly physicians and nurses, are provided information and education on *pharmacokitietics* (the biomedical action of drugs in the body), and how to properly dose and monitor drug levels for optimum therapeutic value. (This also plays a role in pharmacists' monitoring function.) 7) Pharmacists provide formal and informal *clinical education* (regarding medications) to other medical personnel as well as, in some cases, to advanced pharmacy students. 8) Pharmacists conduct different types of *research* on the various aspects of drug utilization, from the simple (e.g., drug case studies) to the more complex (e.g., bone marrow absorption rates).

The clinical pharmacists at both hospitals had come to a similar understanding of what the clinical ideology entailed. However, the boundary encroachment literature suggested that few of these tasks were being performed. The research focus thus turned to a comparison of the ideal with the realities of practice. This entailed an understanding of pharmacists' work life in these hospitals and the contextual influences which enabled and/or constrained clinical practice.

At Suburban Hospital, pharmacists practised their clinical tasks in conjunction with the unit dose drug distribution system: medication orders were picked up from each care unit by a pharmacist, checked against the Medication Administration Record (MAR) for each patient, and delivered to the pharmacy to be filled. A unit dose cart for that unit was then filled with each patient's individualised medications and wheeled to the unit floor for double-checking by the pharmacist. In this way, each patient's medications were systematically monitored for correspondence with physicians' orders and for potential dosage or drug/drug interaction problems (through the MAR). Since the pharmacists were brought to the unit floor, their opportunities to perform other clinical tasks were also enhanced; they would, for example, monitor patient charts for drug/illness interactions and evaluate the effectiveness of medications for physicians' therapeutic goals, coordinate laboratory tests, counsel patients about their medications, and interact with other members of the medical team.

At Urban Hospital distribution of medication was handled by a separate component of the pharmacy department through a ward stock system, and the graduate-educated pharmacists were freed from those more traditional tasks specifically to perform clinical ones. This level of clinical practice has generally been associated with graduate education, the teaching of pharmacy students or both. The combination of these factors (freedom from distribution, advanced degrees and teaching) made clinical practice at Urban an ideal example of clinical pharmacy specialization. For these pharmacists the day generally started by making rounds with the physicians in their particular care unit. If it was a matter of deciding between several groups of physicians, each covering different groups of patients (as it usually was), the pharmacists generally made rounds in their ICU where patients required the most attention (and usually the most or most powerful medications). The rest of the day was anything but routine; it usually consisted of doing what needed doing most: e.g., following up on other patients that were being monitored through the charts, completing formal consultations or drug information requests from physicians, counselling with patients face to face, coordinating with the laboratory for test results, working on their own research in their offices, or completing paperwork required by the administration.

Because of the differences in the way pharmacy was practised in these two settings, both hospitals had established some clinical priorities that their systems fostered. For ex-

ample, Suburban's pharmacists emphasised monitoring (new orders against the MAR, double-checking filled cassettes) and providing drug information (to those with whom the pharmacists interacted on the floor) as a function of unit dose distribution; they had less time for going on rounds, counselling patients or calculating pharmacokinetics. The clinical specialists at Urban had more time for going on rounds, counselling patients and pharmacokinetics, but without any responsibility for distribution these pharmacists had little opportunity to monitor all patient medications. While the true ideal would allow for all clinical tasks to be performed fully and equally in all settings, and this was not the case, both were practising some degree of all tasks promoted by the clinical ideology, and were attempting to take responsibility for the management of drug therapeutics. Moving beyond the more traditional tasks of distribution thus required acceptance of these expanded role boundaries by the other members of the medical team.

Boundary Conflicts and Resolutions

The medical team in these settings represented an approach to treatment more than an organised arrangement of medical staff. Depending upon the patient's status (e.g., heart disease, kidney dysfunction, physical trauma or a combination of problems), different members of the medical staff became involved in treatment. That is, various medical personnel had carved out a piece of territory for which they claimed some degree of expertise and, thus, management of therapy. A variety of medical personnel were frequently heard from: laboratory technicians, radiologists (MDs), radiographers (technicians), orthopaedic surgeons, physical therapists, social workers, dieticians and occupational therapists. However, all of these occupational roles were called into action only with specific patients, when their particular expertise was required. The expanded, clinical role for pharmacy did not appear to threaten, nor was it threatened by any of these team members.

The 'core' of the medical team, constant and visible in virtually all care areas, were physicians and nurses. Where the clinical pharmacy role was being applied in these settings, the pharmacists were attempting to become the newest members of this visible core, taking responsibility for all patients' medication therapy. As such, they found themselves in the position of establishing role boundaries with these more institutionalised members (see also Wardwell 1974).

Following the implementation of the clinical ideology in the two research settings, about the late 1960s and early 1970s, pharmacy had been assigned some of the responsibilities that used to belong to nursing. For example, at Suburban unit dose distribution had taken away the responsibility of retrieving, measuring, and distributing medications out of ward stock. In both settings preparing intravenous (IV) solutions was no longer totally the responsibility of nursing; IVs were prepared by pharmacists under the more controlled conditions of the hospital pharmacy, and administered under pharmacy supervision. Such transfer of 'territory' was more a product of technological change than a traditional exercise of power. As noted, the cognitive and technological resources of the pharmacy were being advocated and perceived as more appropriate for these tasks, and the nurses in these hospitals did not eagerly guard them.

The area which held the most potential for boundary conflicts with nursing involved pharmacists' contact with patients, whether on rounds or for counselling. The patient is the axis around which nurses' role boundaries have been constructed. As one nurse put it, 'Nurses are trained to have the patient as their product, their central focus, their primary concern.' While the clinical pharmacists did interact with patients, more as a part of clinical specialization than unit dose distribution, a greater percentage of the clinical pharmacists' time at both hospitals was spent as a patient advocate: keeping abreast of patients' status through making rounds, reading charts, or monitoring the MARs. was an outgrowth of pharmacy's responsibility for medication therapy. Consequently, pharmacy's expanded tasks did not overlap considerably with nursing's. With the pharmacists attempting to be the drug 'experts' on the

medical team, and the physician's role involving the writing of patients' drug orders, pharmacists' boundary conflicts with physicians appeared to be of greater significance.

Finding and correcting medication problems was a daily occurrence for these pharmacists. While this could be perceived as a resource for the exercise of power, documentation of physicians' medical errors being used as leverage toward acceptance of pharmacy's expanded role, even if this were desired by some pharmacists the concept of error in medicine is rarely black and white. As Bosk (1979: 27) discovered in his observation of surgeons, medical error is an 'essentially contestable' matter: 'By this I mean that the grounds for fixing the label "error" to any section are always arguable.'

This was particularly so for the clinical pharmacists because their assessment of 'error' was so often tied to a physician's diagnosis. Unless the mistake was clear (as in a misplaced decimal point in dosing),[4] the appropriateness of a treatment depended to a great extent upon the physician's diagnosis and treatment goals. Pharmacists' reliance upon physicians' judgments was readily acknowledged. A ten-year veteran of clinical pharmacy at Urban exemplified this well in his description of pharmacists' monitoring function:

> You're looking at the drug regimens that the people are on, hoping that the therapeutic goals have been defined, where they have not been defined, trying to firm them up as to why we are using this drug, how long we are going to use it, what do we expect to see, what parameters do we expect to see change.

Even when the pharmacists felt a particular therapy to be inappropriate, such an assessment did not often rest solely upon their judgment. This pharmacist continued by saying,

> It's a matter of degree. You know, how much attention does something need: getting into this optimum/suboptimum versus appropriate/inappropriate. . . . Sometimes we are very strong in our approach. . . . Other times, what may be important to you may not be important to the physician.

Further, pharmacists bring knowledge of medicinal chemistry and drug research to the medical team as quality control agents, but physicians tend to value their own clinical experience more than scientific sources of information (Avorn et al. 1982, Bosk 1979). Thus, pharmacists were able to quote the literature on a drug's usage, but physicians tended to follow the lessons of personal experience if that differed. An attending psychiatrist had this to say of their differences in judging therapy:

> Are there many inappropriate orders which they can recognise? Yes. Are there some inappropriate orders they cannot recognise? Yes. Are there some orders which are appropriate which they could deem inappropriate? Yes. . . . There may be times when they are not familiar with, or have not used a drug in a certain way. Where I have used it in that certain way, and I can feel comfortable in giving it.

One of the more experienced pharmacists acknowledged the difference and the value of clinical experience. He said, 'Just because the books or papers say this is what's going to happen doesn't mean that's what's going to happen. The more you work in this, the more you realize that.'

In these settings potential conflicts were sometimes resolved in physicians' favor because of their power to define appropriate therapy, often based on their personal experience. Thus, as Broadhead and Facchinetti (1985: 432; emphasis original) have noted, 'Because errors, mistakes and refinements in drug treatment are contestable matters, *the importance and impact of clinical pharmacy is also contestable.*' It is, in great part, for this reason that the pharmacists in these settings were working diligently to gain acceptance on the medical team, to make the work of the team easier and improve patient care. As professionalising subordinates, these pharmacists were deploying the resources at their disposal to influence the activities of both nurses and physicians in this regard.

These pharmacists were aligning themselves with nurses not just structurally, as ancillary members of the medical team, but deliberately, using the expanded boundaries of their role to address the immense responsibilities, and thus the complex needs, of nursing. As the Director of pharmacy at Suburban put it, 'Nurses get hammered from all sides; pharmacists help take some of their responsibility.' For example, shifting responsibility for drug dosing and IV therapy to the pharmacy had relieved some of nursing's burden, yet these pharmacists deployed their resources further by devising new forms that helped nurses take blood samples, and teaching them aspects of drugs that benefited their role. Also, as mentioned earlier, pharmacy's responsibility for medication therapy often required consultation with patients. This provided for autonomous use of their drug expertise, but these pharmacists granted nurses the courtesy of asking before entering a patient's room, and pharmacy students were instructed to do likewise. Although some conflictual interactions between pharmacists and nurses were observed, they were not patterned around role boundaries, and the vast majority of interactions were of a cooperative nature.

Similarly, available resources were being employed with physicians. For example, an integral aspect of pharmacy's expanded role boundaries involved the information recorded in the patient's chart, a legal document. A Patient Oriented Medical Record (POMR) system had been established at both hospitals that allowed all members of the patient's medical team to enter their contributions in the progress notes of the chart. Since much of clinical pharmacy practice entailed finding potential problems with medication orders, and recording even this therapeutic input might raise the spectre of liability for physicians, such pharmacy input had become a matter of consultation with the physician involved (see also Davis 1976).[5]

As a general rule, however, pharmacists perceived potential medication problems either while monitoring patient medications or making rounds with the medical team, and communication took place outside the patients' charts. If a question arose during monitoring, the ideal practice (time permitting) would be to research the potential problem by reviewing the patient's chart or reading up on the research in the problem area. In any case, if questions still remained then the physician would have to be sought out and approached, when he or she was alone, face to face if possible. One of the younger pharmacists indicated his apprehension when describing his approach. He said that he would go to the intern who was 'in charge' of the patient first (despite the fact that interns didn't write medication orders), then work his way up the echelon to the resident and attending physician if the intern couldn't get the problem fixed. His agitated mannerisms and tone of voice when relating this approach conveyed what a tenuous situation it became for him to go beyond the intern. Even the more venerable pharmacists admitted that they did indeed 'pick their spots' when approaching physicians; as one put it,

> Sometimes you pick the person to speak to depending on your relationship with them, and what kind of person you perceive them to be, or what kind of person you've been told they are. Some physicians, frankly, are more open to outside input.

All the pharmacists related that factors such as physicians' age, status, clinical experience, type of practice, personality and medical socialisation influenced their acceptance of pharmacy input (see also, Avorn et al. 1982; Bosk 1979; Kane and Kane 1969; Ritchey and Raney 1981).

When approaching physicians about their orders, the pharmacists generally couched questions in terms of clarifying understanding. The Director of pharmacy at Suburban put it this way,

> I always preface, or attempt to preface questioning (physicians) on an educational basis—'What were you thinking of when you wrote this order; what was your goal?'—and then when they tell me their goal, I'll say, 'Well this probably won't get you there for this reason' or 'I understand your goal; this makes sense.'

As would be expected, this approach was most common among the pharmacists at Suburban, where monitoring was an ongoing function of distribution, independent of the team.

When pharmacists perceived potential problems while making rounds with the team, their approach often took a different form. First of all, there was often no time to research the question before expressing it. If pharmacists doubted the legitimacy of their question, and the potential consequences were not severe, the question was held and it was researched following rounds. Then the approach resembled that just discussed. More often, however, the question was at least a legitimate one and the pharmacist had to raise it, tactfully, before the entire team. This approach was best exemplified by the pharmacists at Urban. Field notes taken during morning rounds reflect these pharmacists' approach:

> Most of this pharmacist's input to questions asked had to do with the kinetics of the drugs involved, particularly coverage attained over time and, subsequently, when the doses should be scheduled. I also heard this female pharmacist talk about absorption rates and half-life information in conjunction. On the last patient she had her own input on drug treatment. She said, 'Tell you what we're going to do. . .', indicating her level of comfort within the medical team; however, she paused to change her phrasing to 'why don't we. . .', indicating her awareness of leaving the doctor in charge. She went on to explain the peak and trough levels of the drug when these should be drawn. As she explained, the resident wrote these as orders in the chart.

Most of the boundary conflicts between pharmacists and physicians took place and were resolved at this level of daily interaction. These pharmacists generally deployed their drug knowledge and communication skills in subtle ways to influence patients' therapy. However, there were stories of more conflictual interactions earlier in pharmacists' negotiations. For example, a few times a pharmacist had approached the prescribing physician about therapy that was perceived as potentially dangerous, and the physician had neither convinced the pharmacist of the therapeutic rationale nor changed the order. When the pharmacist felt that the problem was only potentially dangerous, documentation of this interaction in the patient's chart sufficed to clear the pharmacist of responsibility for the consequences. When the problem was considered sufficiently serious, however, some pharmacists went to the physician's superior to get the order changed, or simply refused to dispense the medication. Deployment of these resources required some fairly objective criteria for concern on the part of the pharmacist as well as the support of the pharmacy department. Therefore, as the Director of Pharmacy at Suburban said, 'You can count on your hand the number of times that's happened.' Most of the boundary conflicts occurred less contentiously, and by the time this research was drawing to a close, pharmacists' place on the medical team seemed fairly clear to all concerned.

The Boundaries Constructed

Concluding research interviews focused on the perception of role boundaries among clinical pharmacists, nurses and the physicians who were most likely to resist 'clinical' pharmacy input: those in higher risk specialisations, with higher status and/or who were accustomed to the higher autonomy model of medical practice. All conveyed a fairly stable understanding of their boundaries. Pharmacists were responsible for appropriate medication therapy, nurses for patient care; physicians remained in charge of the total patient, from diagnosis, through treatment goals and prognosis, to ultimate responsibility for the outcome.

Nurses perceived pharmacists as helpful allies, as this response from a head nurse at Suburban reflects:

> They're always accessible and provide us with good information. . . . Also, the pharmacy has taken over some of the old nursing responsibilities. . . . They're expanding the department to help.

A head nurse at Urban added,

> Well, before they came I would have said there was no need for a pharmacist full-time on the unit. Now that they're here, I don't know how we did without them. . . . Before the pharmacists came we probably hurt a lot of people.

An attending physician for Suburban's pulmonary ICU reflected the perceived boundary for physicians this way:

> You can't let somebody hurt anybody else. So (the pharmacists) are not going to do something that they think is categorically wrong. But because it's a teaching institution, and because they may be wrong in the question they're raising, I think that after they make sure the situation is going to fail in a safe fashion, they need to contact the physician who's responsible for the patient.

One of the more experienced pharmacists expressed their perception:

> A lot of the pharmacists writing in the literature now are too aggressive about being on the floor and in the charts. These are the subtle kinds of things that doctors pick up on, those pharmacists that feel they know more than the doctors. Some make diagnostic recommendations; even if they're right, it's beyond their role. I feel that this causes a combative situation. We have to be very careful.

The general sentiment regarding clinical pharmacy's role within these boundaries was expressed well by the Director of the surgical ICU at Urban:

> It's a matter of how much information one person can maintain at their fingertips and use appropriately and intelligently without the minimum of morbidity. The fact is that physicians are no longer able to know everything there is to know about medications, and the ones we use in there are frequently potentially dangerous medications. I mean not only the direct effects of, but the interactions of the medications as well as simple dosages, you know. And no longer is any dosage really simple, but you deal now with levels, kinetics and pharmacokinetics. So, the role of the clinical pharmacist in that is, I think, extremely important.

Discussion and Conclusion

As part of a larger professionalising social movement, the pharmacists in two northeastern teaching hospitals were attempting to make an expanded 'clinical' role that was beyond the expectations and involved the evolution, of other roles on the medical team, particularly those of nurses and physicians. These clinical pharmacists were deploying professional and interpersonal resources to influence the activities of the medical team and make a difference in the way patients were treated in these settings. Moreover, the extended boundaries of their clinical role had been accepted so that both nurses and doctors had generally come to welcome the expertise in medication therapy they provided. . . .

The pharmacists in the present research had responded to technological changes in health care, expanding their task boundaries to include responsibility for patients' medication therapy. They attended patient care rounds, monitored and evaluated patients' medications (including pharmacokinetic assessments), counselled patients, and provided drug information to other members of the medical team. Often their expertise was unsolicited, provided autonomously, but either behind the scenes, so to speak, or in such a manner that nurses and physicians were left 'in charge.' Further, many nurses and physicians had become aware of the need for such assistance from pharmacy and were relinquishing (some even gladly) the burden of keeping pace with drug technology. There was, in essence, a slow process of encroachment and delegation taking place.

. . . In this case, unlike most sports, becoming a new member of the 'team' does not mean that someone else had to leave. This is not to say that occupational structures and role boundaries do not exist, or that role players do not attempt to maintain them. Rather, role boundaries are both constructed and maintained through social interactions in their contexts. In the contexts reported here, pharmacists deployed the resources at their disposal to influence the activities of physicians and nurses to make a difference in the way patients were treated and gain acceptance as new members of the medical team. . . .

Notes

1. Both research settings must also be recognised in this regard: most hospitals are not teaching hospitals with clinical pharmacy preceptors, let

alone this many practitioners. Further, their northeastern urban location places them within a professional milieu for pharmacy which strongly emphasises clinical practice.

2. Although clinical pharmacy can be considered a social movement, the 'segment' which branched off from traditional pharmacy is distinguished from those originally discussed by Bucher and Strauss (1961) and Bucher (1962) in that 'clinical' pharmacy is not a specialty practice within the 'profession' so much as it is a practice orientation which is advocated for all pharmacists. It is discussed as a segment here as it was originally, and still is, an orientation not necessarily advocated by all pharmacists.

3. Drug/drug interaction problems refer to the potentially harmful effects some drugs produce when used in combination and/or without carefully monitoring dosages. A common drug/illness interaction problem concerns the proper functioning of the patient's kidneys and their subsequent ability to clear the medications properly from the body.

4. Mistakes such as misplaced decimal point in dosing, although potentially lethal in consequence, are what Bosk (1979) would call 'technical' errors, the kind everyone makes and are medically excusable (at least when corrected).

5. The recording of pharmacy input in the patient's chart has also been an issue of documentation for pharmacy, in trying to establish their clinical functions as cost effective. In an economic climate of cost constraints, hospital administrations ask all departments to document the cost effectiveness of their personnel. By not recording their therapeutic input in the patient's chart, clinically oriented pharmacists have struggled to find alternative means of documentation (see Broadhead and Facchinetti (1985), and Mesler (1989) for a discussion of these problems for clinical pharmacy; and see Burkle et al.; Chrymko and Conrad (1982); Saklad et al. (1984), and Smith (1982) for examples of pharmacy's attempts to resolve them).

References

Apple, W. S. (1981) Introspection and challenge anticipating pharmacy's future, *American Pharmacy*. NS21, 30–8.

Avorn, J., M. Chen, and R. Hartley. (1982) Scientific versus commercial sources of influence on the prescribing behavior of physicians, *American Journal of Medicine*. 73. 4–8.

Birenbaum, A. (1982) Reprofessionalizition in pharmacy, *Social Science and Medicine*. 16, 871–8.

Borgsdorf, L. R., D. C. McLeod, W. E. Smith Jr., and D. S. Tatro. (1973) Implementing clinical pharmacy services—an AJHP roundtable discussion, *American Journal of Hospital Pharmacy.* 30, 672–82.

Bosk, C. L. (1979) *Forgive and Remember: Managing Medical Failure* Chicago: University of Chicago Press.

Broadhead, R. S. and N. Facchinetti. (1985) Drug iatrogenesis and clinical pharmacy: The mutual fate of a social problem and a professional movement, *Social Problems.* 32, 425–36.

Broadhead, R. S. and R. C. Rist. (1976) Gatekeepers and the social control of social research, *Social Problems.* 23, 325–6.

Bucher, R. (1962) Pathology: A study of social movements within a profession, *Social Problems.* 10, 40–51.

Bucher, R. and A. Strauss. (1961) Professions in process, *American Journal of Sociology.* 66, 325–34.

Bullough, V. L. (1966) *The Development of Medicine as a Profession* New York: Hafner Publishing Co.

Bullough, B. and V. L. Bullough. (1964) *The Emergence of Modern Nursing* New York: The Macmillan Co.

Burkle, W. S., R. L. Lucarotti, and G. R. Matzke. (1982) Documenting influence of clinical pharmacists, *American Journal of Hospital Pharmacy.* 39, 481–2.

Carroll, N. V. and J. P. Gagnon. (1984) Pharmacists' perceptions of consumer demand for patient-oriented pharmacy services, *Drug Intelligence and Clinical Pharmacy.* 18, 640-4.

Chrymko, M. M. and W. F. Conrad. (1982) Effect of removing clinical pharmacy input, *American Journal of Hospital Pharmacy.* 39, 641.

Davis, N. M. (1976) A question: Should pharmacists make permanent entries on patients' charts? *Hospital Pharmacy.* 11, 336–50.

Frank, D. E. (1974) The importance of an historical perspective, *Drug Intelligence and Clinical Pharmacy.* 8, 55.

Freidson, E. (1970) *Professional Dominance* New York: Atherton.

Hood, J. C. (1977) The role of clinical pharmacists in an industrial setting. In Walker, C. A. and J. R. Fox (eds.) *Practical Clinical Pharmacy* New York: Stratton Intercontinental Medical Book Company.

Kane, R. L. and R. W. Kane. (1969) Physicians' attitudes of omnipotence in a university hospital, *Journal of Medical Education.* 44, 684–90.

Kramer, A. H., M. C. McCarvey, P. H. Holmes, R. Zwirb, P. K. Pitch, and D. F. Lean. (1979) *Drug Product Selection: Staff Report to the Federal Trade Commission* Washington: Bureau of Consumer Protection.

Kronus, C. L. (1976) The evolution of occupational power: An historical study of task boundaries between physicians and pharmacists, *Sociology of Work and Occupations.* 3, 3–37.

Lennard, H. L., et al. (1971) *Mystification and Drug Misuse* San Francisco: Jossey-Bass.

Martin, E. W. (1971) Drug information resources. In Martin, E.W. (ed.) *Dispensing of Medication* Easton, PA: Mack Pub. Co.

Mesler, M. A. (1989) Negotiated order and the clinical pharmacist: The ongoing process of structure, *Symbolic Interaction.* 12, 139–57.

Ray, M. P. (1979) Administrative direction for clinical pharmacy, *American Journal of Hospital Pharmacy.* 36, 308.

Ritchey, F. J. and M. R. Raney. (1981) Medical role-task boundary maintenance Physicians' opinions on clinical pharmacy, *Medical Care.* 19, 90–103.

Saklad, S.R., L. Ereshefsky, M.W. Jann, and M.L. Crismon. (1984) Clinical Pharmacists' impact on prescribing in an acute adult psychiatric facility, *Drug Intelligence and Clinical Pharmacy.* 18, 632–4.

Smith, H. A. and J. V. Swintosky. (1983) The origin, goals, and development of a clinical pharmacy emphasis in pharmacy education and practice, *American Journal of Pharmaceutical Education.* 47, 204–10.

Smith, W. E. (1969) Drugs, the patient and the hospital, *Drug Intelligence aid Clinical Pharmacy.* 3, 244–7.

Smith, W. E. (1971) Hospital pharmacy. In Martin, E.W. (ed.) *Dispensing of Medication* Easton, PA: Mack Publishing Co.

Smith, W. E. (1982) A conceptual model for evaluating a pharmacist's clinical practice in the hospital setting, *Drug Intelligence and Clinical Pharmacy.* 16, 400–3.

Starr, P. (1982) *The Social Transformation of American Medicine* New York: Basic Books.

Tyler, V. E. (1968) Clinical pharmacy: The need and an evaluation of the concept, *American Journal of Pharmaceutical Education.* 32, 764–71.

Wardwell, W. I. (1974) Clinical pharmacy in cross-professional perspective. In Wertheimer, A.I. and Smith, M. (eds.) *Pharmacy Practice: Social and Behavioral Aspects* Baltimore: University Park Press.

Zelnio, R. N., A. A. Nelson, and C. E. Beno. (1984) Clinical pharmaceutical services in retail-practice: I. Pharmacists' willingness and abilities to provide services, *Drug Intelligence and Clinical Pharmacy* 18, 917–22. Reprinted from *Sociology of Health & Illness Vol. 13 No. 3 1991 ISSN 0141-9889.*

Further Reading

Arnold Birenbaum. 1982. "Reprofessionalization in Pharmacy." *Social Science and Medicine* 16: 871-878.

Eliot Freidson. 1970. *Professional Dominance*. Chicago: Aldine.

Ferris J. Ritchey and Marilyn R. Raney. 1981. "Medical Role-Task Boundary Maintenance: Physicians' Opinions on Clinical Pharmacy." *Medical Care* 19: 90-103.

Leonard Stein. 1990. "The Doctor-Nurse Game Revisited." *The New England Journal of Medicine* 322: 546-49.

Discussion Questions

1. Describe how boundary encroachment might threaten traditional models of medical work.

2. Explain how differing views of medical professionals and philosophies of treatment help circumscribe work boundaries.

3. Extend Mesler's analysis to midwives, chiropractors, acupuncturists, and other health practitioners. What might Mesler's argument mean for changes in the organization of health care tasks for professionals? For restructuring treatment alternatives for patients?

4. What would be the future for pharmacy if it did not move in the direction Mesler describes?

25

What It Means to Be a Nurse

Daniel F. Chambliss

Ethical and moral decision making are part of the medical world. These dilemmas plague medical work. In this selection, Chambliss finds moral judgments embedded in the contradictory missions of nurses—to be "in charge" and simultaneously "under control." Sick and dying patients. Treatment decisions. Paperwork. Rush orders from physicians. Yet, for nurses, nothing is extraordinary. Consider the kinds of ambiguities that challenge medical professionals, especially nurses. Note that these dilemmas are not often easily resolved.

Organizational ethos and hospital schedules determine how nurses should perform work tasks. Notice how decision making is embedded in and becomes part of the ordinary work day. Ethos and schedules determine who the nurse is. See if you can uncover the taken for granted back drop that blurs ethical decisions and moral dilemmas into the work routine. Chambliss argues nursing ethics to be the ethics of the powerless, of the organizational "doers." Think about Mark Mesler's discussion of the territory of clinical pharmacy as you read about nurses' troubles with duties and boundaries.

So what . . . does it mean to be a nurse?
. . . For the nurse, the hospital is a normal place, and with routinization even traumatic events that occur there appear normal. What once was a frightful emergency to the novice has become, more and more, just the "same ol' same ol'." The nurse now casually handles naked bodies, measures output of stool, suctions fluid from patients' lungs, passes knives to surgeons, and, just as routinely, cares for the dying. None of this, once she has made the "leap" into a routine, disrupts her daily life or causes her any special concern.

This attitude radically separates nurses and other health workers from the rest of us, and the separation is *morally* relevant, a distance between what nurses and laypersons see as "the right way to behave." Patients are regularly subjected to events no one outside the hospital would willingly undergo. Invasive procedures, humiliating exams, and radical surgery are considered not only acceptable but even in a sense good; the staff rarely gives them a passing thought. Not only is there a shift in what is thought good and what is thought bad; some very serious matters are not much thought about at all. Routinization means that once-crucial issues have been set aside: "These," it declares, "need not concern us."

Of course, routinization of hospital life is not peculiar to nursing. Physicians undergo a similar process, becoming bored with routine physical exams, hurrying through colonoscopies, pelvic exams, and assorted consultations; so too, in varying degrees and in their own activities, orderlies, blood technicians, and respiratory therapists find their work taking on the rhythm of everyday life. Occupational therapists may work every day with children who have cerebral palsy, surgeons quickly get used to removing gall bladders, aides get used to wiping bottoms, and hospital secretaries learn to comfort crying relatives and guide wandering geriatric patients back to their rooms. In all of the health care professions, repeated encounters with messiness, confusion, and tragedy dull the senses a bit, professional jargon softens the hard edges, and jokes become genuinely funny. All hospital workers experience routinization; nursing is not special in this.

But some things *are* special about nursing. The nurse is a particular kind of hospital worker, one with at least three difficult and sometimes contradictory missions. The hospital nurse is expected, and typically expects herself, to be simultaneously (1) a caring individual, (2) a professional, and (3) a relatively subordinate member of the organization. Nurses will argue, even among themselves, just what these directives require, or even that they should exist. (Many nurses will say, for instance, that they should not be subordinates.) Regardless, these three principles tell us who nurses really are and what they really do.

The inherent conflict of these demands makes nursing a prototype case for a dilemma of many workers in an organizational society: I want to do good, but the boss won't let me. The directives conflict: be caring and yet professional, be subordinate and yet responsible, be diffusely accountable for a patient's total well-being and yet oriented to the hospital as an economic employer. Perhaps no other occupation suffers so great a conflict between the practical requirements of the job—and nursing is, rhetoric aside, still fundamentally a job, a paid assignment—and the explicitly moral goals of the profession. Perhaps these are dilemmas of all the "caring" professions (teaching, social work, nursing). Or perhaps they somehow typify predominantly female professions. With more women entering the labor force, with the caring professions growing, and with an increasing proportion of all Americans working under the control of large organizations, increasing numbers of Americans may face conflicts such as those faced by nurses.

In this selection, these three requirements of the nurse's role will be examined—the directives of caring, being a professional, and being a subordinate. Then the difficult theoretical issue of nursing as a "female" profession will be considered. Finally, I will suggest why nursing ethics should matter to the rest of us. In nursing, I think, we can see how morally concerned but subordinate people in organizations handle moral problems in their work.

Nurses Care for Patients

"Care" is the key term in nursing's definition of itself, and crucially defines what nurses believe is their task. . . . Care, some nurses say, distinguishes nursing from medicine: "Nurses care, doctors cure;" and while physicians may dispute the connotations of that slogan, few would completely deny its message. . . .

As nurses use the term, "care" seems to include four meanings: face-to-face working with patients, dealing with the patient as a whole person, the comparatively open-ended nature of the nurse's duties, and the personal commitment of the nurse to her work. All of these are included in what nurses mean by "caring." To a moderate degree, "caring" describes what nurses actually *do*; to a great degree, it describes what nurses believe they *should* do.

1. *Nursing care is a hands-on*, face-to-face encounter with a patient. Unlike in medicine, in nursing there can be no quick review of lab reports, a scribbling of orders, and then a fast exit down the hall. Nurses carry out the scribbled orders, deliver the medications, pass the food trays, monitor the IV's and the ventilators. Nurses give baths, catheterize patients, turn patients who cannot move themselves, clean bedsores, change soiled sheets, and constantly watch patients, writing notes on their patients' progress or deterioration. Close patient contact, with all five senses, is nursing's specialty. "I could never be a nurse," says one unit clerk. "I couldn't stand all those smells." Nurses are constantly talking with, listening to, and touching their patients in intimate ways; the prototypical, universal dirty work of nursing is "wiping bottoms." One nurse explains why in her unit nurses no longer wear the classic white uniform:

> It wouldn't stay white very long: there's red blood, feces of various colors, green bile, yellowish mucous, vomit, projectile defecations. [Field Notes]

Physicians visit floors to perform major procedures (inserting tubes into the chest, bronchoscopies); but most of what is done to patients is said and done by bedside nurses.

The nurse works primarily in a contained space, on one floor or unit; if the patients are very sick, she stays in one or two rooms. She is geographically contained and sharply focused, on this room, this patient, perhaps even this small patch of skin where the veins are "blown" and the intravenous line won't go in. She remains close to this small space, or on the same hallway, for a full shift, at least eight hours and in intensive care areas twelve hours; often she is there for two or even three shifts in a row. With the chronic shortage of nurses she frequently stays and works overtime. I have known a sizable number of nurses, in different hospitals, who worked double and triple shifts—up to twenty-four straight hours—on both floors and in ICUs. One such nurse enjoys double shifts because "I don't have to rush [to finish paperwork] . . . if it isn't done in the first shift, I'll get it done in the evening." So nurses have close contact with their patients over time, hour by hour if not minute by minute, for an extended period of time—"around the clock," they say, and sometimes this is precisely true. This close contact, over time, in a confined space, can give nurses the sense that they know better than anyone else what is happening with their patients; and they may resent any other view:

Doctor, commenting on geriatric patient: "She looks better today."

Nurse: "You haven't had to fuck with her all morning."

Doctor (pause, then tentatively): "She looks better than when she came in." [Field Notes]

No doubt, the "continuity of care" by nurses can be exaggerated by nurses themselves. In fact, with rotating nursing schedules, shifting assignments, the short turnaround time of many nursing tasks, and the constant turnover of nursing personnel, it is not clear that nurses provide continuity at all. Few nurses are actually on the scene "around the clock," and only occasionally is one nurse responsible for the total care of a particular patient. Nevertheless, the geographical restriction of a nurse to one area does enhance her knowledge of the condition of those patients, even when she isn't personally caring for them.

To care for patients, then, first means that one works directly, spatially and temporally, with sick people.

2. *Care means that the patient should be treated not merely as a biological organism* or the site of some disease entity, but as a human being with a life beyond the hospital and a meaning beyond the medical world. Nurses certainly handle the physiological treatment of disease, but they also spend time teaching patients (on dialysis units, e.g., this may be

their major task), answering the family's questions, listening to the patient's worries, calling for social service consultations, helping fill out insurance forms, or even, to use a fairly common example, helping an old person find a pair of glasses lost somewhere in the sheets or under the bed. In caring for AIDS patients, nurses often manage negotiations between families and lovers, or among relatives and friends, when families often don't know the true diagnosis. In all these ways, nurses seem focused on the personal experience of illness:

[N]ursing appears to be directed to more immediate and experiential goals than medicine: a compassionate response to suffering is more closely identified with nursing than with medicine. Nurses also more often express an interest in disease prevention and health maintenance than physicians. Nurses are less wedded to the physiological theories and diagnostic modes of medical practice. And nursing has a more global and unified science approach to health care.[1]

"Care," then, includes a broad range of the patient's concerns, not just the physical disease itself.

3. *The nurse's duties are open-ended.* Perhaps because of the nurse's sheer physical availability, her job often expands to fill the gaps left by physicians, orderlies, or even families. Some duties are prescribed, but many are not. "To care" for a nurse comes to mean that the nurse will handle problems that arise, whether or not they are part of her official tasks. This occurs for practical reasons. "The nurse," in the words of Anselm Strauss," comes and stays while others come and go. . . . *The role of nurse is profoundly affected by her obligation to represent continuity of time and place.*"[2] Being on the scene, around the clock, means that nurses are there to integrate the different aspects of hospital work: "Since there's no general agreement about what a nurse is, there are no obvious limits to the job."[3]

Thus the nurse takes on more and more tasks, cleaning up the physical and social messes left by others. When doctors don't explain a diagnosis to the patient, when a unit clerk isn't there to answer the phone, when housekeeping has left a sink unwashed or a floor unmopped, when administration hasn't provided the staff to cover the unit, when chaplains aren't around to listen to a family, when the transportation aide hasn't shown up to take a patient to X-ray—then, often, nurses take over and do these jobs themselves, probably grumbling in the process but realizing that it must be done and that nurses will have to live with the results if they don't:

> Everybody else says: "What do you do as a nurse?" And I say, "I do everything that nobody else wants to do." [Interview]

Nurses might say they do this work *because* they "care;" but here there is no distinction between doing and caring. To care is to *do* the leftover work, to take that responsibility, whether ordered to or not.[4]

4. *Caring requires a personal commitment of the nurse to her work.* It requires a commitment of the nurse herself, as a person, to her work. There is an intertwining of professional skills and personal involvement; in a sense, the involvement is the work, in a way not true of more technical occupations. Nurses would say that some excellent surgeons are horrible human beings; but perhaps it is not theoretically possible to be simultaneously an excellent nurse and a despicable person.[5] The job itself seems to call for decency.

In practice, nursing often elicits a deep personal involvement. In the best cases, nurses give and receive with their patients, first giving of themselves and then receiving, in turn, an unusual intimacy and personal satisfaction from helping another person in his or her most difficult time. Patients can be more open with nurses than with their own families, for a variety of reasons: to spare loved ones the truth of suffering, to maintain the dignity of one's body with a spouse, or to protect children from the reality of their mother's imminent death. The caring professional hears of these things without falling apart, so patients often tell nurses what they wouldn't tell anyone else.

> It's the nurse who's there when the patient is upset and crying, especially on those long, dark nights. It's also the nurse who develops a day-to-day rapport with the patient. Patients can feel comfortable sharing their physical and emotional pain. There is a lot of intimacy involved; it's the same intimacy found with anyone who is terminal. For some reason, people who are dying tend to lessen their barriers. It's a sad phenomenon that we wait until that time to establish those relationships. But it's a privilege for nurses to work in this area [with AIDS patients and dying patients generally], because in no other type of work are you invited into another's soul.[6]

So the first imperative of nursing is to give care—direct, person-to-person, relatively open-ended care. When nurses tell of their best moments in nursing, they tell of giving such care—not of their technical expertise, or their ability to follow complicated orders without bungling, but of care. This is what nurses define as the meaningful heart of nursing.

Obviously "caring" is also an ideological term, an idealized way of talking about nursing. It is openly used as a weapon in nurses' conflicts with physicians, to distinguish what nurses do ("care") from what doctors do ("cure"), and to assert the nurse's moral superiority. The more challenging "care" is, the greater the moral prestige of the nurse. So when nurses say they "care," this is more than an empirical description of duties: it is a defense of their own importance. . . .

Nurses Are Professionals

So nurses care—but others care as well. Parents care for their children, lovers for their beloved, children for their pets. For nurses, though, caring is a *job*, an economically rewarded task. And it is a certain *kind* of job, one with high demands for education and responsibility and a claim to a special status, commonly called "professional." The first imperative of nursing is to care; the second imperative of nursing is to behave like a *professional*.

Being a professional means (1) doing a job (2) that requires special competence and (3) that deserves special status.

1. *Most basically, a profession is a job*— and a good one at that. The most accurate generalization about nurses is not that they care for patients; it is that they are *paid* to care for

patients. For many, ideology aside, this is the primary motivation. Nurses typically have little trouble finding work in America, or almost anywhere in the world. It is easy to move in and out of the nursing workforce, taking time out for raising a family, pursuing other careers, or just taking vacations. The unemployment rate for nurses in the United States is typically close to zero, and nurses' salaries rose significantly during the 1980s in the United States, so that by 1990 their typical starting income was close to $30,000. . . .

Since nursing is a job, the nurse is frequently required to deal with unpleasant colleagues, uncooperative patients, frustrating bureaucracies, and the routine difficulties of paid work. Even when nurses hate their patients or disapprove of their identities (casualties of gang wars, drug dealers shot in a deal gone bad), or feel that patients are to blame for their own predicament (smokers with emphysema, or alcoholics with gastrointestinal bleeding), they claim to care for them fully. In a sense, I believe, nurses' talk about disliking certain patients reinforces the pride of professionalism. Whoever the patients are, the nurse still goes to work, delivers meal trays, fills out forms, listens to supervisors, delivers medications, and cleans up messes. She can't just walk away, as a volunteer could, or care only for loved ones, as a mother could. Professionalism, then, first means performing the job.

2. Second, *professionalism requires special competence.* Nursing work is often neither simple nor easy; it can be intellectually, emotionally, and physically demanding. So sheer competence is a value, perhaps the central value in nursing.[7] Some people just can't do the work, aren't organized or responsible enough, lack the manual dexterity to insert IV's or give injections, or don't understand the necessary physiology. Nurses can quickly differentiate the good nurses from the bad based on their ability to do the job, finish the assigned tasks, and not make the disastrous mistakes that can so easily happen. They know which nurses can be trusted and which ones can't:

> "If my baby comes in here," said one pregnant neonatal nurse to her colleague, "swear to me that you'll take care of him.

I don't want R——[another nurse] taking care of my kid." [Field Notes]

Professional competence is most challenged in those emergencies when routines break down. Normally, the professional cares for her clients in the form of a "detached concern"[8]— holding her personal feelings in check while remaining open to the feelings of the patient. A special effort is required for a nurse to keep this "professional" detachment when a critically ill patient, after coming close to recovery, suddenly codes and dies.

> Right after the code had started, Madge, laughing nervously as the team worked on Mrs. B——, said to me, "Oh, God, I'd just written her assessment" [saying she was improving].

> After Mrs. B.'s code was over, and they'd declared her dead, Madge (who had nursed her for the past week) immediately sat at the rolling desk outside the room and wrote notes for at least 1/2 hour, very persistently, almost through tears—her face was flushed—when people said anything to her, she answered only vaguely, kept her head down writing. [Field Notes]

"Being professional" here may mean, as it often does, going into a bathroom to cry, then cleaning up and coming back out to continue working for the rest of the shift, trying to act as if nothing happened. "Competence" includes technical expertise as well as the personal fortitude to maintain that expertise under pressure.

3. *A professional deserves special status.* A professional, nurses feel, deserves respect. Nurses typically feel that they deserve more respect than they receive, from their colleagues (especially physicians) and from laypersons. They are paid for their work, but good pay is not sufficient.

> No amount of money is worth what you have to do and what you have to put up with. That's it: what you have to put up with . . . patients throwing full urinals at you, slapping you, biting, fighting, swearing. [Interview]

As professionals, nurses feel they deserve an improved status and better treatment: polite treatment by doctors, the listening ear of administrators, the respect of outsiders who too often treat nurses like maids or waitresses.

In trying to be professionals, nurses strive to differentiate themselves in the public eye from other occupations. A nurse, they emphasize, is *not* a maid, *not* a waitress, *not* a servant.[9] Nurses commonly mention these "antiroles" in talking about their work, to distinguish nursing from those jobs, even if the tasks themselves may sometimes be similar: answering patient call bells, changing sheets, emptying bedpans, helping patients dress or turn over. Nurses do some things maids do. How then does one change sheets "professionally?" The public, they feel, doesn't understand:

> It bothers me, the chronic stupid image of the nurse, the hand-maid-to-the-doctor thing. I don't take well to people who kiddingly say, "You just empty bedpans all day long." The public has no idea what nursing really is all about. They can see you giving baths, carrying bedpans, taking blood pressures, temperatures, whatever. And they think that's all nurses do. [Interview]

A major part of nursing's effort to improve its status has come in changing the educational requirements for becoming an R.N. Initially, such requirements were more vocational than academic. From the late nineteenth century until the middle of the twentieth, most nurses were trained by hospitals, often the Catholic Hospitals run by religious orders of nuns, and after three years they were awarded a diploma. These nursing students worked as poorly paid apprentices and received, in turn, the skills to go out and practice on their own. The training was rigorous, often notoriously so, and very applied. The nurses received training, the hospitals had cheap labor.[10]

But since the 1960s, many of the hospital schools have closed down, replaced by academic university or community-college programs. With this change, the tone of nursing has changed.

> Nursing is no longer the calling it once was, says P.W.; the influence of nuns, so pervasive when she was younger, is now fading, being replaced by the university-trained academic model of nursing. [Interview]

The collegiate nurse has come, perhaps unfairly, to represent the ascendance of education, of science, of classroom training, and of the increased social status of higher education. By comparison, the older, hospital-trained nurse represents more traditional values, the more ready subservience to doctors, the hands-on experience, the "school of hard knocks." As can easily be imagined, this split in the profession, and in what counts as "real" nurse's education, makes a truly unified effort to improve nurses' status difficult. In addition, social class divisions in nursing between the typically middle-class B.S.N. nurses and the more working-class A.A. or diploma nurses are themselves the basis of much contention.[11] Even nurses' caps, which once symbolized a nurse's status, are now considered by most to be outdated and symbolic of lesser prestige; nurses are abandoning the traditional white uniform dress in favor of scrub suits or even civilian clothes.[12]

Many younger nurses see such changes as good; they mark the path to professionalism. Their formal education is longer, their occupational class is higher, their pay is greater, and their expectations for respect and individual initiative have increased. Professionalism is an ideal, but one which, especially through increased education, can improve their social standing.

Nurses Are Subordinates

Finally, nurses are subordinates in the hospital hierarchy. Not surprisingly, nurses see this feature of nursing less positively than the injunctions toward care and professionalism. Nurses want to care, and they want to be professionals. They don't always want to be subordinates but without doubt they are, and for the most part they accept this as part of their role. The old hospital-based nursing schools actively reinforce this: "under the dominance of male doctors and administrators, schools of nursing grew; and they were not noted for their development of independent, thoughtful nurses. Students entered nursing schools already expecting that women would defer to men, and, therefore, that nurses would defer to doctors."[13] Nurses' daily work is guided by others: by administrators, some of whom come from nursing; by head nurses who assign them patients; and by physicians, whose detailed orders structure their medical tasks. Nurses arrive at work at an ordered time, on an ordered shift, on specified days. They report at rounds when scheduled, read reports according to custom, answer beepers, fill out charts, and deliver medications as ordered. It is nurses who prepare the patients before procedures, and who clean up afterward, changing the sheets, mopping blood, counting sponges, and calming the patients. . . .

Nurses aren't always directly under the orders of others, of course. In ICUs, nurses frequently make quick decisions on their own, when no physician is available; in dialysis units, it is nurses who teach patients how to dialyze themselves, who write the manuals for patients to use at home, who decide how long dialysis will continue, and who evaluate the patient's tolerance of the side effects. The nurse's subordination, then, is situational: it is almost total in the operating room, where the entire staff is under the command of a surgeon; in long-term nursing home care, by contrast, nurses are in charge. Nurses often supervise other workers, such as aides, orderlies, and therapists of various sorts. And as nurses climb the status hierarchy, other workers fill the lower positions and are subject to the abuse nurses themselves have long known:

A nurse made a passing comment to L—, a respiratory therapist (and an older, black woman), about how she, the nurse, would have to do some procedure; as a therapist, L. wasn't supposed to do it. Over the next ten minutes, L. kept saying when spoken to, "Don't talk to me, I'm just a therapist," or "You don't want to ask me anything, I'm just a therapist," or "You asking me? A *therapist???*" etc. [Field Notes]

If there is a single dominant theme in nurses' complaints about their work, it is the lack of respect they feel, from laypersons, from coworkers, and especially from physicians. It is nearly universally felt and resented. "The docs never listen to us," they say, "you don't get any recognition from doctors";

doctors don't read the nurse's notes in the patients' chart, don't ask her what she has seen or what she thinks, they don't take her seriously. The daily evidence for this is truly pervasive; I was genuinely surprised at how common the obvious disrespect is. One day I was talking with several staff nurses in a conference room when a young male physician—probably an intern—walked in and asked what a drug was for. Immediately, the assistant head nurse explained quickly and in detail. "Oh yeah," said the doctor, "that's right," and walked out. The nurses began to laugh, and one said to the advisor, "You get an A." And doctors also often ignore nurses' opinions:

Attending not present today, so the Fellow took charge of doc's round in the ICU. In discussing one patient, a resident asked the nurse taking care of this patient if she had anything to add. Before the N finished her first sentence, the Fellow was looking away, visibly uninterested; by the second sentence he had started talking with the other intern. [Field Notes]

Sometimes such ignoring of the nurse's view can have serious consequences:

At Tuesday's conference on Geriatric floor, with residents, attending, social workers, etc., all present, Asst. HN said repeatedly, "You should look at Mr. F.'s foot, it will be a big problem," etc. She didn't seem to make an impression on the docs.

They did nothing about it. Saturday morning, the residents called an emergency surgery consultation because the foot was badly necrosed. Surgeon looked, said had to amputate above the ankle, maybe even above the knee, to check the sepsis. The Asst. Head Nurse, who had warned them on Tuesday, was standing off to one side during this discussion, was visibly exasperated. [Field Notes]

Even medical students put down nurses in small ways.

In psychiatry unit: during nursing rounds, one nurse reads aloud, written on chart, as doctor's order: "Make sure patient voids [urinates]."

"Who wrote that?"

"Doctor R.'s little med. student." A good laugh about this, as if the nurse would overlook something so obvious. Getting no respect from docs—even future docs—is a source of aggravation and sometimes laughs. [Field Notes]

Here, then, may begin a cycle: doctors don't trust nurses; nurses, not trusted even when they are correct, slack off. The mutual lack of respect shows in various ways. Some nurses complain that doctors doing research projects try to recruit nurses as unpaid research assistants—"You're charting this anyway, can't you just keep another copy of it for my data, too?"—and then become angry if the nurse misses six hours of this charting and the data are lost. Generally, nurses' time is considered less valuable, her work less pressing, her opinions less worthy of consideration.

Outside the door of a middle-aged woman patient, with a steady stream of visitors going in, two nurses and the resident are arguing about acidosis and ventilator settings and what Respiratory Therapy should be doing to suction the patient, all in very technical jargon, decreasing this and increasing that. The nurse who takes care of this patient is very angry, with a constant forced smile she puts on in these situations, and repeating, "I don't really want to discuss it anymore," and "It's obvious what we should do. Just sedate her, that's all you need to do." But the resident isn't sure at all, and the nurses are at the end of their rope. [The patient died within days.] [Field Notes]

There are, then, pervasive problems in nurses' work relationships with doctors.[14] In part, the difficulty results from different views of what the nurse's task actually is. To doctors, the nurses are there to carry out physician's orders.[15] Indeed, doctors (and many nurses) regard nursing as a sort of "lesser" medicine, with the subordination of nursing dictated by the shorter period of training.

Dr. M., explaining why he should make the DNR decisions—and why the nurses should not—explains that the difference between him and the nurses is "years of training—I have 6 or 10, depending on how you count, and they have 2 or 4—I just understand things better." [Interview]

Dr. M. here assumes that nursing is essentially the same as medicine but with less training. He assumes that nurses share medicine's basic theory of disease (a physiological disturbance with psychological ramifications) and share medicine's ideas of the goals of treatment. For many physicians, laypersons, and even nurses, nursing is basically second-tier medicine, and nursing education consists of watered-down physiology courses, using textbooks written by physicians, teaching nurses how to be "the doctor's helper."

In recent years, this position is formulated in a description of nurses as "physician extenders," a cost-effective substitute in areas where there aren't enough physicians—a kind of "Hamburger Helper"[16] who does the same work for less money. So the nursing viewpoint is not merely subordinated; indeed, it is often invisible as a distinct approach. . . .

Many, if not most, staff nurses accept the assumption that medicine is superior and that nursing is simply a lesser form of medicine. They try to enhance their own prestige by a kind of "drift to medicine": by going into the more "medical" areas of nursing, like emergency work, or ICUs; by appropriating the scientific and pathophysiological model of disease; and by getting into the "medical macho" of high technology, invasive procedures, and massive pharmacological inventions, all the while setting aside the lower status "dirty work" of nursing. Although nursing as a profession tries to distance itself from medicine, establishing its own expertise, the typical nurse takes respect where she finds it, from her close association with doctors.[17]

To some extent, nurses' subordination lessened, or at least changed its character, during the period of my research from the late 1970s to the early 1990s. Nurses now more often will openly confront physicians rather than practice subterfuge; they have more ready support from independent nursing schools; perhaps because of the women's movement, nurses are somewhat more likely to expect to be treated with respect, if not really as equals. Still, despite some movement in these directions nurses remain fundamentally unequal to doctors in their power and status. They are clearly subordinates, much more than their professional leaders or even staff nurses would like to believe. They do important work, and many of them do it with deep personal commitment and a high degree of skill. Yet their subordinate position, more than professionalism and perhaps even more than "caring," is a crucial component of most hospital nursing.

Here we see the dilemma of the nurse's role. On the one hand, she would like to raise her status by both differentiating her work from medicine ("we care, doctors cure") and by claiming to be a professional. On the other hand, by being a necessary member of the medical team she can borrow some of the prestige of medicine. The three components of the nurse's role—caring, professionalism, subordination—all represent in some degree what nurses empirically do and how they interpret what they do. In some ways they are conflicting requirements, fortified by conflicting parties: nursing schools with their admonition to professionalism, administrators with their efforts at controlling nurses, journals with their calls to "care." In some ways, managing these conflicts is inherent in the job of being a nurse. . . .

Nursing is a female occupation, not essentially but empirically. That fact, along with the other particulars we've discussed of the nurse's role, shapes the nurse's view of moral issues in the hospital.

The Nurse's Role: Implications for Ethics

. . . We have already seen that nurses treat their work in the hospital routinely and experience the hospital as a relatively normal place. Nurses understand their work as falling under the sometimes conflicting imperatives of caring for patients, behaving as professionals, and working as subordinates in the hospital organization. These imperatives are simultaneously *prescriptive*—saying what nurses should do—and somewhat *descrip-tive*—that is, actually reflecting what nurses in fact do. Nursing is basically a female occupation, with low visibility of its work and moderate prestige accorded to it. All of these components of the nursing role are suffused with moral implications: they carry moral judgments about who the nurse is and how she should do her work.

That role has implications for the ethics of nurses and for the rest of us. The nurse's position is not so unusual. Many Americans work in the "helping professions," broadly defined, and many more would characterize their work as serving others. While most do not consider themselves professionals, they do take their work seriously. And a growing number of workers are female. The ethical challenges of nurses may suggest the ethical challenges of any caring but subordinate person working in a large organization today. In trying to understand the ethics of nursing, then, we can begin to understand the ethical problems of the rest of us as well.

For this new variant of ethical analysis, several steps are required:

1. *Rediscovering the unappreciated.* Probably the most frequent question I am asked about my research is "Why are you studying nurses?" or even "Why do you care about nurses?" Most people don't care about nurses and, not surprisingly, don't understand the significance of their work. Much of nursing is invisible—to doctors, to patients, and to the layperson. What is noticed—baths, turning patients, routine monitoring—is seen as unimportant, except by patients: "A patient complains about not getting a box of tissues. That may seem unimportant. Yet if the person is lying there with his nose running and he can't get up, that box of tissues becomes monumental."[18] Naturally enough, nurses resent this lack of appreciation; a popular recent book on nursing, by a pair of nurses, is titled, with quotation marks and all, *"Just a Nurse."*[19]

Even when doing recognizably important work, as in the ICUs or operating rooms, nurses are regarded as skilled helpers to the doctors, adjuncts to the people doing the "real" work. It's easy, when watching surgery, to be drawn to the action, to the surgeon who is cutting, and away from the nurses arrayed around that center, or walking in the background. On rounds, physicians do the talking while nurses stand by holding charts or quietly attending to some task. With physicians holding the dramatic center stage of medical work, nurses become stagehands, secondary figures. The physician's work is valued; nurses' work is valued only as it mimics the physicians: "The most valued forms of competence currently tend to reflect scientific and technological interests—what people consider intellectually difficult, exciting, and challenging—rather than what is most directly related to patient good or to public health."[20] To rediscover their own work and see what they do—to put them, for a moment at least, at the center of their own world—is a first step to understanding who nurses are.

The recovery of unappreciated work is especially relevant when analyzing women's work. As Miller puts it, "All of these things, the things women are allowed to do, are in a significant way removed from the life of one's time. Women's place is outside the ongoing action. To nurse the old, the sick, and the disabled is taking care of those who are temporarily or permanently retired; raising children is an involvement with those who are not yet in the main action. Women even take care of those who are in the main action during the hours of the day when they are out of action—that is, they provide care and comfort to the tired man when he comes home at night. Women's other role, the biological production of the next generation, is deemed essential, but also positions them effectively outside the action of their own generation. This is one of the circumstances that women refer to when they say they feel they have lost touch with 'the real world'.[21] But perhaps theirs is the real world, and it is the observers who have lost touch.

2. *Finding the appropriate ethics for nursing.* Nursing ethics is hardly a recognized field of inquiry, even for academics. Books on nursing ethics typically borrow the principles of medical ethics and apply them to nursing situations, with little recognition that the nurse's situation is profoundly different from that of the doctor. Doctors often make critical decisions with little outside help. The prototype medical ethics scenario involves a dramatic case, choices of heroic intervention, a situation of crisis: and now the doctor must choose. Medical ethics is thus characterized by dilemmas in which the lone individual must decide the right thing to do. Philosophical medical ethics largely assumes this freedom of the practitioner to choose; the ethical problem lies in deciding what choice is morally right. But in nursing, the problems are frequently those over which nurses have no control; they are not dilemmas, in the sense of an individual's quandary, at all, and the language of "ethical dilemmas" hardly works for a profession whose work is so determined by choices of other, more powerful, actors. For doctors, the dilemma may be, "Do we save this baby?" For nurses, the problem is, "How can I care for this baby who is needlessly suffering?" The doctor often *decides;* the nurse more often then *does.*

Since nursing ethics is usually written as a variant of medical ethics, medical hegemony in health care is perpetuated; the distinctive voice of nursing is lost; and the distinctive moral situation of the nurse is lost.

3. *A distinctive ethical analysis is required.* If we are truly to recognize the position of the nurse and see that nursing is not merely a branch of medicine, then a different sort of ethical analysis is required. Medical ethics deals with dilemmas faced by relatively powerful people, but nursing ethics needs to consider the distress suffered by much less powerful people—in this case, the nurses. While trying to do good, nurses are embedded in an organization, responsible for some people and ordered by others. Nurses are enjoined to care for the patient, to be concerned with the patient as a person, and to be professionally responsible. At the same time, devoutly prolife nurses may be asked to help with abortions, to let deformed infants die, to disconnect ventilators from terminal cancer patients. In each of these cases, they may feel the decision is morally wrong. Nurses often must carry out policies they deplore, orders they believe wrong, and treatments they believe cruel. They have little time to consider a range of options, little power to change current routines, and almost no freedom to leave the situation.

Nursing ethics, then, is the ethics of powerless people; the ethics of witnesses, not decision makers; the ethics of implementers, not choosers; the ethics of those whose work goes unnoticed. Perhaps, too, as its practitioners are predominantly women, it is the ethics of more personal relationships: "In particular, it is well known that many women—perhaps most women—do not approach moral problems as problems of principle, reasoning, and judgment."[23] Nursing ethics is the ethics of most of us: not in charge; carrying out the commands of others; trying, within imposed limits, to do the job. There is no special virtue in this. Much of the nursing literature suffers from an exaggerated idealism, and many nurses will in effect say, "I would do things differently if I were in charge." But they aren't in charge, and if they were, experience shows us, they probably would do things the way the people in charge do. Simply being a nurse does not guarantee righteousness. As Zussman says, "[T]hey are more concerned than physicians with comfort and emotional adjustments to illness, less concerned with cure. But this perspective does not make nurses angels of mercy."[24]

In summary, we have seen that nursing has a distinctive moral core—a set of directives that nurses accept as their own, even when they feel short of those standards. The distinctive role of nursing entails a combination of care, professionalism, and a subordinate position, and the style of the profession is obviously female. In many ways, the ethics of nursing points to a broader ethics of organizational life. In understanding nursing, we may better understand the moral position of other organizational subordinates. . . .

Notes

1. Andrew Jameton, *Nursing Practice: The Ethical Issues*, p. 256.(Englewood Cliffs, NJ: Prentice-Hall, 1984.)

2. Anselm Strauss, "The Structure and Ideology of American Nursing: An Interpretation," in Fred Davis, *The Nursing Profession: Five Sociological Essays*, pp. 117, 120. (New York: John Wiley and Sons, 1966.)

3. Peggy Anderson, *Nurse*, p. 31. (New York: Berkeley Books, 1978.)

4. For further elaboration, see Hughes, *Men and Their Work*, p. 74. (Westport, CT: Greenwood Press [1958] 1981.)

5. "The one-caring, in caring, is present in her acts of caring. Even in physical absence, acts at a distance bear the signs of presence: engrossment in the other, regard, desire for the other's well being." Nel Noddings, *Caring: A Feminine Approach to Ethics and Moral Education* (Berkeley: University of California Press, 1984), p. 19.

6. Janet Kraegel and Mary Kachoyeanos, *"Just a Nurse"* (New York: Dell Publishing, 1989), p. 16.

7. Jameton, *Nursing Practice*, chap. 6.

8. Robert K. Merton, *Sociological Ambivalence and Other Essays* (New York: Free Press, 1976); the concept is discussed in a number of places in the text.

9. I once made the mistake, in a lecture to a nurses' association, of comparing nurses' work to that of these other stereotypically female occupations. The audience didn't actually jeer, but they were visibly displeased by the comparison.

10. Jo Ann Ashley, *Hospitals, Paternalism, and the Role of the Nurse* (New York: Teacher's College Press, 1977). See also Barbara Melosh, *The Physician's Hand: Work Culture and Conflict in American Nursing* (Philadelphia: Temple University Press, 1982); and Reverby, *Ordered to Care*.

11. "[C]lass divisions within the nursing culture made a feminist politics difficult to achieve," Reverby, *Ordered to Care: The Dilemma of American Nursing, 1850-1945* p. 6. (Cambridge University Press, 1987.)

12. The shift in number of registered nurses coming from diploma programs versus associate and baccalaureate (college-based) programs is dramatic: "More than 90 percent of the nurses [practicing in 1984] who graduated before 1960 were graduates of diploma schools. . . . During the period 1980 to 1984, only 17 percent of all registered nurse graduates were graduated from a diploma program." *American Nurses' Association: Facts about Nursing 86-87*, p. 21. (Kansas City, MO: American Nurses' Association, 1987.)

13. Martin Benjamin and Joy Curtis, *Ethics in Nursing*, p. 79. (New York: Oxford University Press, 1981.)

14. The classic article on how the nurse "plays the game" is C. K. Hofling et al., "An Experimental Study in Nurse-Physician Relationships,"

Journal of Nervous and Mental Disorders 143 (1966), pp. 171-180.

15. Diana Crane, *The Sanctity of Social Life: Physician's Treatment of Critically Ill Patients*. (New Brunswick: Transaction Books, 1977.) Anderson, *Nurse*, pp. 246-248.

16. I borrow the characterization from Gretchen Aumann, R.N.

17. Perhaps to the long-term detriment of nursing's effort to independent status. See W. Glasen, in Davis, *The Nursing Profession*, p. 27.

18. Anderson, *Nurse*, p.106

19. Kraegel and Kachoyeanos, "*Just a Nurse.*"

20. Jameton, *Nursing Practice*, p. 85.

21. Jean Baker Miller, *Toward a New Psychology of Women, 2nd Edition* p. 75. (Boston: Beacon Press, 1986.)

22. Noddings, *Caring*, p. 28.

23. Robert Zussman, *Intensive Care*, pp. 71-72. (Chicago: University of Chicago Press, 1992.)

Further Reading

Fred Davis (ed.). 1966. *The Nursing Profession*. New York: John Wiley.

Virginia L. Olesen and Elvi W. Whittaker. 1968. *The Silent Dialogue*. San Francisco: Jossey-Bass.

Susan Reverby. 1987. *Ordered to Care: The Dilemma of American Nursing, 1850-1945*. Cambridge: Cambridge University Press.

Robert Zussman. 1992. *Intensive Care: Medical Ethics and the Medical Profession*. Chicago: Chicago University Press.

Discussion Questions

1. What does it mean for a nurse to be a professional and a subordinate simultaneously?

2. Explain how ethical and moral dilemmas become encoded in the work routine of hospital nurses. Why do nurses' ethical and moral decisions go unnoticed?

3. In what ways might Mesler's analysis of medical boundaries apply to the nurses Chambliss describes? How do boundary tensions obfuscate the job of the nurse?

4. What does Chambliss mean when he argues that nursing ethics is the ethics of the powerless? What is the greatest ethical danger for nurses?

Organizational Definitions of Health and Wellness

26

Wellness in the Work Place: Potentials and Pitfalls of Work-site Health Promotion

Peter Conrad

Peter Conrad raises some intriguing questions about health promotion in the work place. As you read through this selection, consider these questions in light of Michael Goldstein's and Deborah Lupton's arguments from Section One. Most agree that health and fitness are not only honorable but necessary for employee wellness. Many employers, employees, and medical experts view worksite programs as universally beneficial. Still, controversy over whether these programs reduce health risks continues. What drives worksite promotion campaigns?

Examining a range of worksite programs, Conrad discusses the benefits and pitfalls of wellness in the workplace. Employees enjoy the improvement that these movements bring to

the workplace and to their general sense of self. But organizational health promotion alters individual perceptions of self. It reforms perceptions of what individual health means and what it should be. Conrad points out that large-scale benefits of organizational health promotion may come at great cost to the individual. See whether or not you agree. Then contemplate the parallels between health promotion campaigns in the workplace and public health movements more generally.

In the past decade worksite health promotion or "wellness" emerged as a manifestation of the growing national interest in disease prevention and health promotion. For many companies it has become an active part of their corporate health care policies. This article examines the potentials and pitfalls of worksite health promotion.

Worksite health promotion is "a combination of educational, organizational and environmental activities designed to support behavior conducive to the health of employees and their families" (Parkinson et al. 1982, 13). In effect, worksite health promotion consists of health education, screening, and/or intervention designed to change employees' behavior in order to achieve better health and reduce the associated health risks.

These programs range from single interventions (such as hypertension screening) to comprehensive health and fitness programs. An increasing number of companies are introducing more comprehensive worksite wellness programs that may include hypertension screening, aerobic exercise and fitness, nutrition and weight control, stress management, smoking cessation, healthy back care, cancer-risk screening and reduction, drug and alcohol abuse prevention, accident prevention, self-care and health information. Many programs use some type of health-risk appraisal (HRA) to determine employees' health risks and to help them develop a regimen to reduce their risks and improve their health.

Worksite health promotion has captured the imagination of many health educators and corporate policy makers. Workers spend more than 30 percent of their waking hours at the work site, making it an attractive place for health education and promotion. Corporate people are attracted by the broad claims made for worksite health promotion (see O'Donnell 1984). For example:

> Benefits of worksite health promotion have included improvements in productivity, such as decreased absenteeism, increased employee morale, improved ability to perform and the development of high quality staff, reduction in benefit costs, such as decreases in health, life and workers compensation insurance; reduction in human resource development costs, such as decreased turnover and greater employee satisfaction; and improved image for the corporation (Rosen 1984, 1).

If these benefits are valid, probably no company would want to be without a wellness program.

Many major corporations have already developed worksite health promotion programs, including Lockheed, Johnson and Johnson, Campbell Soup, Kimberly-Clark, Blue Cross-Blue Shield of Indiana, Tenneco, AT&T, IBM, Metropolitan Life, CIGNA Insurance, Control Data, Pepsico, and the Ford Motor Company. Nearly all the programs have upbeat names like "Live for Life," "Healthsteps," "Lifestyle," "Total Life Concept," and "Staywell."

The programs' specific characteristics vary in terms of whether they are on- or off-site, company or vendor run, on or off company time, inclusive (all employees eligible) or exclusive, at some or no cost to employees, emphasize health or fitness, year-round classes or periodic modules, have special facilities, and are available to employees only or families as well. All programs are volun-

tary, although some companies use incentives (from T-shirts to cash) to encourage participation. In general, employees participate on their own time (before and after work or during lunchtime). The typical program is on-site, with modest facilities (e.g., shower and exercise room), operating off company time, at a minimal cost to participants and managed by a part-time or full-time health and fitness director.

The number of worksite wellness programs is growing; studies report 21.1 percent (Fielding and Breslow 1983), 23 percent (Davis et al. 1984), 29 percent (Reza-Forouzesh and Ratzker 1984-1985), and 37.6 percent (Business Roundtable Task Force on Health 1985) of surveyed companies had some type of health-promotion program. It is difficult to interpret these figures. Not only are there serious definitional problems as to what counts as a program, but many may yet be only pilot programs and not available to all employees and at all corporate sites. Estimated employee participation rates range from 20 to 40 percent for on-site to 10 to 20 percent for off-site programs (Fielding 1984), but accurate data are very scarce (Conrad 1987a).

Worksite health promotion as a widespread corporate phenomenon only began to emerge in the 1970s and has developed largely outside of the medical care system with little participation by physicians. The dominant stated rationale for worksite health promotion has been containing health care costs by improving employee health. Business and industry pays a large portion (estimated at over 30 percent) of the American national health care bill, and its health insurance costs have been increasing rapidly. By the late 1970s corporate health costs were rising as much as 20 to 30 percent a year (Stein 1985, 14). This has become a corporate concern. In an effort to reduce these costs, corporations have redesigned benefit plans to include more employee "cost-sharing," less coverage of ambulatory surgery, mandated second opinions, increased health care options and alternative delivery plans (e.g., health maintenance organizations and preferred provider organizations), as well as worksite health promotion programs. Although wellness programs are only a piece of a multipronged cost-containment strategy, they may be especially important as a symbolic exchange for employer cost shifting and reductions in other health benefits. They are moderate in cost and very popular with employees.

Corporations are restructuring their benefit packages to shift more cost responsibility to employees in the form of deductibles, cost sharing, and the like. A national survey of over a thousand businesses found that 52 percent of companies provided free coverage to their employees in 1980; by 1984 only 39 percent did so. In 1980 only 5 percent had deductibles over $100; four years later 40 percent had such deductibles (Allegrante and Sloan 1986).

Cost containment may be the most commonly stated goal of wellness programs, but it is not the only one. Reducing absenteeism, improving employee morale, and increasing productivity are also important corporate rationales for worksite health promotion (Herzlinger and Calkins 1986, 74; Davis et al. 1984, 542). "Hidden" absenteeism can be very costly, especially when skilled labor is involved (Clement and Gibbs 1983). Improved morale is expected to reduce turnover, increase company loyalty, and improve workforce productivity (Bellingham, Johnson, and McCauley 1985). The morale-loyalty-absenteeism-productivity issue may be as important as health costs in the development of worksite wellness. The competitive international economic situation in the 1980s makes the productivity of American workers a critical issue for corporations.

Despite the broad claims for worksite health promotion, the scientific data available to evaluate them are very limited. While more scientific data could better enable us to assess the claims of the promoters of worksite wellness, it is not necessarily helpful for addressing some of the difficult social and health policy issues raised by worksite health promotion. To examine these more policy-oriented dimensions, it is useful to distinguish between potentials and pitfalls—potentials roughly aligning with the claims made for worksite programs, the pitfalls with less-discussed sociopolitical implications. These distinctions are for analytic purposes and are somewhat arbitrary; there may be downsides to potentials as well as upsides to pitfalls. This framework, however, provides us with a vehicle for examining worksite health promotion that includes yet goes beyond the dominant corporate/medical concerns of reducing individual health risks and containing costs.

Potentials

The Worksite Locale

More people are in the "public" (i.e., non-home or farm) work force today than ever before—estimated to be 85 million in the United States. Roughly one-third of workers' waking hours are spent in the work place. Work sites are potentially the single most accessible and efficient site for reaching adults for health education. From an employee's perspective, on-site wellness programs may be convenient and inexpensive, thus increasing the opportunities for participation in health promotion. The work site has potentially indigenous social support for difficult undertakings such as quitting smoking, exercising regularly, or losing weight. Worksite programs may raise the level of discourse and concern about health matters, when employees begin to "talk health" with each other. And since corporations pay such a large share of health costs, there is a built-in incentive for corporations to promote health and healthier workers.

One of the most underdeveloped potentials of the work site is possible modification of the "corporate culture." When the term "corporate culture" is used by the health promotion advocates, they generally mean improved health changes in the organizational culture and physical environment. Some also include changing company norms or the creation of the healthy organization (Bellingham 1985), often meaning making healthy behavior a desirable value among employees and management. Such goals, however noble, are vague and difficult to assess. In practice, changing the corporate culture has meant introducing more concrete interventions like company smoking policies (Walsh 1984), "healthy" choices and caloric labeling in cafeterias and vending machines, fruit instead of donuts in meetings, and developing on-site fitness facilities. Very rarely, however, have proposed wellness interventions in the corporate culture included alterations in work organization, such as stressful management styles or the content of boring work, or even shop floor noise.

Health Enhancement

Screening and intervention for risk factors are the most common vehicles for enhancing employee health. Medical screening includes tests for potential physiological problems; interventions are preventive or treatment measures for the putative problem. Medical screening at the work site, including chest X-rays, sophisticated serological (blood) testing, blood pressure and health risk appraisals (HRAs), can identify latent health problems at a presymptomatic stage. To achieve an improvement in health, however, worksite screening must also include appropriate behavioral intervention, medical referral, and backup when necessary. Thus far, hypertension screening has produced scientific evidence supporting positive worksite results (Foote and Erfurt 1983).

The scientific evidence available to support specific worksite interventions is also, as yet, limited. Examining the extant literature on specific interventions, Fielding (1982) found good evidence for the health effectiveness of worksite hypertension control and smoke-cessation programs. He concluded that the data on physical fitness and weight reduction were not yet available. Hallet (1986), on the other hand, argued that well-controlled studies of work-place smoking intervention are not yet available. The evidence for physical fitness is still contentious (e.g., Paffenbarger et al. 1984; Solomon 1984) although the health effects of 30 minutes of vigorous exercise three times a week are probably positive, at least for cardiovascular health. There are reports of using work-place competitions (Brownell et al. 1984) or incentives (Forster et al. 1985) for increasing weight reduction, but the studies are short term and lack follow-up.

In the past few years large research projects to study the effects of worksite health promotion were initiated at AT&T (Spilman et al. 1986), Johnson and Johnson (Blair et al. 1986a) and Blue Cross-Blue Shield of Indiana (Reed et al. 1985). Most of the results currently available are from pilot programs or one or two years of worksite health promotion activity (except the Blue Cross-Blue Shield of Indiana study, which is a five-year evaluation). In general, these studies show health improvements in terms of exercise (Blair et al. 1986a), reduced blood pressure and cholesterol (Spilman et al. 1986), although the findings are not entirely consistent. The 5-year Blue Cross-Blue Shield of Indiana study also found that interventions led to a significant reduction in serum cholesterol and high blood pressure and a lesser reduction in cigarette smoking (Reed et al. 1985). These reductions in risk factors are positive signs of health enhancement, but the studies are too short term to measure actual effect on disease. Limited scientific evidence aside, the interventions are at worst benign, since few appear harmful (save infrequent exercise-related injuries) and likely health effects seem between mildly and moderately positive.

Cost Containment

The effect of worksite health promotion on health costs, while highly touted, is difficult to measure and has engendered little rigorous research. Most companies do not keep records of their health claims in a fashion that is easy for researchers to assess. Since most research in this area tends to be short-term, and cost-containment benefits may be long-term (say five to ten years), the long time frame makes rigorous research on this topic unattractive to corporations and expensive for investigators. Finally, it is difficult to ascertain which, if any, worksite wellness interventions effected any changes in corporate health costs. Many studies of health promotion "project" potential cost savings from reductions in risk, which while unsatisfactory for scientific evaluation often satisfy the corporate sponsors.

There are a few studies of cost benefits that report promising findings. A national survey of 1,500 of the largest United States employers conducted by Health Research Institute found that health care costs for employers with wellness programs in place for 4 years was $1,311 per employee compared to $1,868 for companies without such programs (*Blue Cross-Blue Shield Consumer Exchange* 1986, 3). Such cross-sectional surveys, however, do not adequately control for confounding variables (e.g., different employee populations or benefit plans) that certainly affect health costs. Blue Cross-Blue Shield of California initiated a single intervention—a self-care program—through 22 California employers, that reduced outpatient visits, especially among households with first dollar coverage (Lorig et al. 1985, 1044). The authors don't calculate the estimated cost savings, but since the cost of the intervention was small, the cost-savings potential is high.

The most compelling cost-containment data to date come from the Blue Cross-Blue Shield of Indiana (Reed et al. 1985; Gibbs et al. 1985) and Johnson and Johnson (Bly, Jones, and Richardson 1986) studies. The Blue Cross-Blue Shield study tracked and compared claims data for participants and nonparticipants (N = 2,400) in a comprehensive wellness program for 5 years. They found that although participants submitted more claims than nonparticipants (i.e., had a higher utilization), the average payment per participant was *lower* throughout the course of the study. When payments were adjusted in 1982 dollars, the mean annual health cost of participants was $227.38 compared to $286.73 for nonparticipants. For 5 years, the average "savings" per employee was $143.60 compared to the program cost of $98.60 per person, giving a savings to cost ratio of 1.45. A possible selection bias in terms of who is attracted to the program could have affected the results. Overall, the 5-year cost of the program was $867,000, with a saving of $1,450,000 in paid claims and an additional $180,000 saved in absence due to illness. The savings is estimated to be 8 to 10 percent of total claims (Mulvaney et al. 1985).

The Johnson and Johnson study compares health care costs and utilization of employees over a 5-year period at work sites with or without a health-promotion program (Bly, Jones, and Richardson 1986). Adjusting for differences among the sites, the investigators found that the mean annual per capita inpatient cost increased $42 and $43 at the two sites with the wellness program as opposed to $76 at the sites without one. Health-promotion sites also had lower increase in hospital days and admissions, although there were no significant differences in outpatient or other health costs. The investigators calculate a cost savings of $980,316 for the study period. What is interesting is that this study was based on *all* employees at a work site. The suggestion here is that a worksite wellness program may produce a cost-containing effect on the entire cohort, not just on participants. The "Live for Life" program is an exemplary and unique program in terms of Johnson and Johnson's corporate investment in wellness; the effect of health promotion on an entire employee cohort needs to be replicated in other worksite settings.

Without further prospective studies, cost containment remains a promising but unproven benefit of worksite health promotion. Changes in health status—which are more easily measurable—do not automatically translate into health cost savings. It is often difficult to quantify health effect and subsequent cost savings. High employee turnover, discovery of new conditions, and other factors may affect actual cost benefits. On the other hand, the usual calculations do not take into account the cost of replacing key employees due to sickness or death. As Clement and Gibbs (1983, 51-52) note, the cost savings may be affected by characteristics of the company:

> For example, more benefits would be achieved by firms with highly compensated, high-risk employees, where turnover is low, recruitment and training costs are high, benefit provisions are generous and employees are likely to participate.

If corporations are serious about using health promotion to contain health costs, programs may need to be reconceptualized and expanded beyond their current scope. An important reality is that roughly *two-thirds* of corporate health costs are paid for spouses and dependents, who are not part of most worksite wellness programs, and that a large portion of health costs is expended for psychiatric care, which may only most indirectly be affected by wellness programs.

Cost containment is an overriding concern for some managers and program evaluators, especially in terms of "cost-benefit ratios." It may be that the current corporate political climate demands such bottom-line rhetoric for the implementation of worksite health promotion, but very few programs have been closed down due to lack of cost effectiveness.

Improving Morale and Productivity

The effects of worksite health promotion on morale and productivity are more difficult to measure than health effects. Participating in wellness activities, especially exercise classes, has several potentially morale-enhancing by-products. Current evidence is only anecdotal, but is generally in a consistent direction. First, there is the "fun" element. In the course of a year's observations at one corporate wellness program, I regularly observed banter, joking, and camaraderie among participants during program activities. There is a sense of people working together to improve their health. Programs that are open to all employees may create a leveling effect; often employees from varying company levels participate in the same classes and corporate hierarchical distinctions make little difference in sweatsuits and gym shorts. As one participant told me, "We all sweat together, including some of the higher ups." But rigorous studies on the effect of the programs on job satisfaction are not yet available.

Despite a legion of claims, virtually no one has even attempted to measure increased productivity as a result of worksite health promotion. Although changes in productivity are difficult to assess, there are two productivity-related effects about which we have some information. Several studies have found a reduction in absenteeism among wellness program participants (Reed et al. 1985; Baun, Bernacki, and Tsai 1986; Blair et al. 1986b). It is generally believed that a reduction in absenteeism can lead to an increase in overall productivity. Second, several observers have noted that participants often say they "feel" more energetic and productive

from participating regularly in the program, especially in terms of exercising (Spilman et al. 1986, 289; Conrad 1987b). This kind of "subjective positivity" that results from wellness participation may be related to improved morale and productivity, although we are not likely to obtain "hard" measures.

The symbolic effects of offering a worksite wellness program should not be underestimated. Worksite health-promotion programs are often among the most visible and popular employee benefits. The mere existence of a program may be interpreted by employees as tangible evidence that the company cares about the health of its workers, and as contributing to company loyalty and morale. Programs are also a plus in recruiting new employees in a competitive marketplace.

Individual Empowerment

Worksite health promotion presents a positive orientation toward health. Its orientation is promotive and preventative rather than restorative and rehabilitative and provides a general strategy aimed at *all* potential beneficiaries, not only those with problems ("deviants," or troubled or sick employees). This makes participation in wellness nonstigmatizing; in fact, the opposite is possible—participants may be seen as self-actualizing and exemplary.

The ideology of health promotion suggests that people are responsible for their health, that they are or ought to be able to do something about it. This may convey a sense of agency to people's relation with health, by seeing it as something over which individuals can have some personal control. Positive experience with these kinds of activities can be empowering and imbue employees with a sense that they are able to effect changes in their lives.

Pitfalls

In their enthusiasm for the positive potentials of worksite health promotion, the promoters and purveyors of wellness programs usually neglect to consider the subtler, more problematic issues surrounding worksite health promotion. I want to examine some of the limitations and potential unintended consequences of promoting health in the work place.

The Limitations of Prevention

Many wellness activities, such as smoking cessation, hypertension control, and cholesterol reduction, are more accurately seen as prevention of disease than promotion of health. Disease prevention may be useful, but these interventions are not specific to the mission of health promotion (i.e., enhancing positive health).

Research within the lifestyle or "risk factor" paradigm has unearthed convincing evidence that a variety of life "habits" are detrimental to our health (e.g., Breslow 1978; U.S. Department of Health, Education, and Welfare 1979), but it is not always clear that this translates directly to health enhancement. Promoters of health promotion have frequently oversold the benefits of intervention (Goodman and Goodman 1986), which are not always well established (Morris 1982), and have ignored such equivocal evidence as the MRFIT study (Multiple Risk Factor Intervention Trial Group 1982). Moreover, just because a behavior or condition is a "risk factor" does not mean automatically that a change (e.g., a reduction) will lead to a corresponding change in health. In addition, clinicians and social scientists do not yet know very well how to change people's habits—witness the mixed results of various smoking-cessation programs or the high failure rate in diet and weight reduction.

In terms of modifying health risks, over what do people actually have control? Surely, there are some behavioral risk factors, but what about the effects of social structure, the environment, heredity, or simple chance? Clearly, the individual is not solely responsible for the development of disease, yet this is precisely what many worksite health-promotion efforts assume (Allegrante and Sloan 1986).

The overwhelming focus of work-site health promotion on individual lifestyle as the unit of intervention muddles the reality of social behavior. The social reality, including class, gender, and race—all known to affect health as well as lifestyle—is collapsed into handy individual risk factors that can be remedied by changing personal habits. This approach takes behavior out of its context and assumes "that personal habits are discrete and independently modifiable, and that individuals can voluntarily choose to alter such behaviors" (Coriel, Levin, and Jaco 1986, 428). At best this is deceptive; at worst it is misguided and useless.

It is often assumed that prevention is more cost effective than treatment and "cure." As Louise Russell (1986) has persuasively shown, for some diseases prevention may actually add to medical costs, especially when interventions are directed to large numbers of people, only a few of whom would have gotten sick without them. She concludes that prevention and health promotion may be beneficial in their own right, but in general should not be seen as a solution for medical expenditures. Ironically, for corporations for whom cost containment is a major goal, there is an additional problem in that if employees are healthier and live longer (by no means yet proven), corporations will have to pay higher retirement benefits. In any case, prevention seems a limited vehicle for medical cost containment. To the extent that controlling health costs is a major rationale, worksite wellness may seem peripheral when the results are limited.

Blurring the Occupational Health Focus

Worksite health promotion's target for intervention is the individual rather than the organization or environment. While the history of health and safety movement is replete with examples of corporate denial of responsibility for workers' health and individual interpretations of fault (e.g., "accident prone worker") (Bale 1986), by the 1970s a strong measure was established to change the work environment to protect individual workers from disease and disability. This was both symbolized and in part realized by the existence of the Occupational Safety and Health Administration (OSHA). But the promulgators of wellness are uninterested in the traditional concerns of occupational health and safety and turn attention from the environment to the individual. One virtually never hears wellness people discussing occupational disease or hazardous working conditions. Whether they view it as someone else's domain or as simply too downbeat for upbeat wellness programs is difficult to know. But this may in part explain why worksite health promotion has been greeted with skepticism by occupational health veterans.

The ideology of worksite wellness includes a limited definition of what constitutes health promotion. For example, it does not include improvement of working conditions. As noted earlier, wellness advocates neglect evaluating the work environment and conceptualize "corporate cultures" in a limited way. In fact, the individual lifestyle focus deflects attention away from seriously examining the effects of corporate cultures or the work environment. Little attention is given to how the work-place organization itself might be made more health enhancing. Perhaps it is feared that organizational changes to improve health may conflict with certain corporate priorities. For example, by focusing on individual stress reduction rather than altering a stressful working environment, worksite health promotion may be helping people "adapt" to unhealthy environments.

The ideology of health promotion is creating a "new health morality," based on individual responsibility for health, by which character and moral worth are judged (Becker 1986, 19). This responsibility inevitably creates new "health deviants" and stigmatizes individuals for certain unhealthy lifestyles. While this process is similar to medicalization (Conrad and Schneider 1980) in that it focuses on definitions and interventions on the individual level and fuses medical and moral concerns, it is better thought of as a type of "healthicization." With medicalization we see medical definitions and treatments for previously social problems (e.g., alcoholism, drug addiction) or natural events (e.g., menopause); with healthicization, behavioral and social definitions and treatments are offered for previously biomedically defined events (e.g., heart disease). Medicalization proposes biomedical causes and interventions; healthicization proposes lifestyle and behavioral causes and interventions. One turns the moral into the medical; the other turns health into the moral.

The worksite wellness focus on individual responsibility can be overstated and leads to a certain kind of moralizing. For example, although personal responsibility is undeniably an issue with cigarette smoking, social factors like class, stress, and advertising also must be implicated. With other cases like high blood pressure, cholesterol, and stress, attribution of responsibility is even more murky. But when individuals are deemed causally responsible for their health, it facilitates their easily slipping into victim-blaming responses (Crawford 1979). Employees who smoke, are overweight, exhibit "Type A" behaviors, have high blood pressure, and so forth are blamed, usually implicitly, for their condition. Not only does this absolve the organization, society, and even medical care from responsibility for the problem, it creates a moral dilemma for the individual. With the existence of a corporate wellness program, employees may be blamed both for the condition and for not doing something about it. This may be especially true for "high risk" individuals who choose not to participate. And even relatively healthy people may feel uneasy for not working harder to raise their health behavior to the new standards. Thus, work-site health promotion may unwittingly contribute to stigmatizing certain lifestyles and creating new forms of personal guilt. In a sense, health promotion is engendering a shift in morality in the workplace and elsewhere; we need to, at least, raise questions about what value structure is being promoted in the name of health and what consequences might obtain from taking the position that one lifestyle is preferable to another. While it is assumed that worksite wellness is in everyone's interest—I've heard it termed a "winwin" situation—it is important to examine what we are jeopardizing as well as what is gained (cf. Gillick 1984).

Enhancing the Relatively Healthy

In several ways worksite wellness focuses its attention on relatively healthy individuals. Were we to consider the major global or national health problems from a public health perspective, workers would not be listed among the most needy of intervention. Research for decades has pointed out that lower social class (Syme and Berkman 1976) and social deprivation (Morris 1982), in general, are among the most important contributors to poor health. Workers in spite of having real health problems are a relatively healthy population. Occupational groups have generally lower rates of morbidity and mortality than the rest of the population. This so-called "healthy worker effect" implies that the labor force selects for healthier individuals who are sufficiently healthy to obtain and hold employment (Sterling and Weinkam 1986). There is, furthermore, some evidence suggesting that unemployment may have a detrimental effect on individual health (Liem 1981). The main target of worksite health promotion is a relatively healthy one.

Even within the worksite context, who is it that comes to wellness programs? Although data are limited, a recent review suggests some self-selection occurs:

> Overall, it appears participants are likely to be nonsmokers, more concerned with health matters, perceive themselves in better health, and be more interested in physical activities, especially aerobic exercise, than nonparticipants. There is also some evidence that participants may use less health services and be somewhat younger than nonparticipants (Conrad 1987a, 319).

In general, the data suggest that participants coming to worksite wellness programs may be healthier than nonparticipants (see also Baun, Bernacki, and Tsai 1986).

Finally, the whole health-promotion concept has a middle-class bias (Minkler 1985). Wellness advocates ignore issues like social deprivation and social class, which may have health effects independent of individual behavior (Slater and Carlton 1985), when advocating stress reduction or health enhancement. The health-promotion message itself may have a differential effect on different social classes. As Morris (1982) points out, in 1960 there was little class difference between smokers; by 1980 there were only 21 percent smokers in class I while there were 57 percent smokers in class V. And what little evidence we have suggests that overwhelmingly the participants in worksite wellness programs are white-collar workers (Conrad 1987a). For

a variety of reasons—including scheduling, time off, and priority setting, blue-collar workers have been less likely to participate (see Pechter 1986). Thus, worksite health-promotion programs may generally be serving the already converted.

Expanding the Boundaries of Corporate Jurisdiction

The boundaries of private and work life are shifting, particularly as to what can legitimately be encompassed under corporate jurisdiction. Worksite programs that screen for drugs, AIDS, or genetic makeup are more obvious manifestations of this, but worksite wellness programs also represent a shift in private corporate boundaries.

Worksite health-promotion programs, with their focus on smoking, exercise, diet, blood pressure, and the like, are entering the domain of what has long been considered private life. Corporations are now increasingly concerned with what employees are doing in off-company time. We have not yet reached a point where corporate paternalism has launched off-site surveillance programs (and this is, of course, highly unlikely), but employers are more concerned about private "habits," even if they do not occur in the work place. These behaviors can be deemed to affect work performance indirectly through a lack of wellness. This raises the question of how far corporations may go when a behavior (e.g., off-hours drug use) or condition (e.g., overweight) does not *directly* affect others or employee job performance. Yet, screening and intervention programs are bringing such concerns into the corporate realm.

With the advent of health insurance, especially when paid for by employers, the boundaries between public and private become less distinct. That is, health-risk behavior potentially becomes a financial burden to others. The interesting question is, however, why are we seeing an increased blurring of boundaries and corporate expansion in the 1980s? The danger of this boundary shift is that it increases the potential for coercion. The current ideology of worksite wellness is one of voluntaryism; programs are open to employees who want to participate. But voluntaryism needs to be seen in context.

> Bureaucracies are not democracies, and any so-called "voluntary" behavior in organizational settings is likely to be open to challenge. Unlike the community setting, the employer has a fairly long-term contractual relationship with most employees, which in many cases is dynamic with the possibility of raises, promotions, as well as overt and covert demotions. This may result in deliberate or inadvertent impressions that participation in a particular active preventive program is normative and expected (Roman 1981, 40).

Employers and their representatives may now coax employees into participation or lifestyle change, but it is also likely that employers will begin to use incentives (such as higher insurance premiums for employees who smoke or are overweight) to increase health promotion. At some point companies could make wellness a condition of employment or promotion. This raises the spectre of new types of job discrimination based on lifestyle and attributed wellness.

In a sense, what we are discussing here is the other side of the "responsible corporation" that cares about the health and well-being of its employees. The crucial question is, are corporations able to represent the individual's authentic interests in work and private life?

Conclusion

Worksite health promotion is largely an American phenomenon. Few similar programs exist in Europe or other advanced industrial nations. Worksite wellness is a response to a particular set of circumstances found in the United States: the American cultural preoccupation with health and wellness; the corporate incentive due to the employer-paid health insurance; and the policy concern with spiraling health costs. Its growth is related to a disenchantment with government as a source of health improvement and a retrenchment in the financing of medical services. Its expansion is fueled by the commercialization of health and fitness

and the marketing of health-promotion and cost-management strategies (cf. Evans 1982). Moreover, worksite wellness aligns well with the fashion in the 1980s for private-sector "corporate" approaches to health policy.

In their enthusiasm, the promoters of worksite health promotion make excessive claims for its efficacy. The worksite wellness movement has gained momentum, although it may still turn out to be a passing fad rather than a lasting innovation. It seems clear that worksite wellness programs have some potential for improving individual employees' health and will perhaps contribute to reduce the rate of rise in costs. The scientific data on program effects, however, are by no means in and to a large extent corporations are operating on faith. The actual results are likely to be more modest than the current claims. How much data are necessary for policy implementation is an open question. For despite the rhetoric of cost containment, corporate concern over health costs may be more of a trigger than a drive toward wellness programs. Concern about morale, loyalty, and productivity—corporate competitiveness in the marketplace—may be of greater import than health.

Rigorous scientific evaluation will enable better evaluation of the potentials of worksite health promotion for improving employee health, reducing costs, and improving morale and productivity. But such data remain largely irrelevant for assessing the more sociopolitical pitfalls of worksite wellness. These can be only adequately evaluated in the context of the social organization of the work place, the relation between employers and employees, and as part of an overall health policy strategy. They cannot be simply counted in terms of reduced employee risk factors or saved corporate health dollars.

Worksite health promotion has the appearance of corporate benevolence. Health is a value like motherhood and apple pie. In modern society, health is deemed a gateway to progress, salvation, and productivity. Despite the pitfalls discussed in this article, worksite health promotion does not appear to be an overt extension of corporate control, at least not in terms of so-called technical or bureaucratic control (Edwards 1979). In fact, on the surface worksite wellness appears as more of a throwback to the largely abandoned policies of "welfare capitalism" (Edwards 1979). Whether worksite health promotion is a valuable health innovation, the harbinger of a new type of worker control, or an insignificant footnote in the history of workers' health remains to be seen.

References

Allegrante, J. P and R. P. Sloan. 1986. "Ethical Dilemmas in Worksite Health Promotion." *Preventive Medicine* 15:313-20.

Bale, A. 1986. *Compensation Crisis.* Ph.D. diss., Brandeis University. (Unpublished.)

Baun, W. B., E. J. Bernacki, and Shan P. Tsai. 1986. "A Preliminary Investigation: Effect of a Corporate Fitness Program on Absenteeism and Health Care Cost." *Journal of Occupational Medicine* 28:18-22.

Becker, M. H. 1986. "The Tyranny of Health Promotion." *Public Health Reviews* 14:15-25.

Bellingham, R. 1985. Keynote address delivered at the 1985 *Wellness in the Workplace* conference, Norfolk, Va., May.

Bellingham, R., D. Johnson, and M. McCauley. 1985. "The AT&T Communications Total Life Concept." *Corporate Commentary* 5(4):1-13.

Blair, S. N., P. V. Piserchia, C. S. Wilbur, and J. H. Crowder. 1986a. "A Public Health Intervention Model for Worksite Health Promotion: Impact on Exercise and Physical Fitness in a Health Promotion Plan after 24 Months." *Journal of the American Medical Association* 255:921-26.

Blair, S. N., M. Smith, T. R. Collingwood, R. Reynolds, M. Prentice, and C. L. Sterling. 1986b. "Health Promotion for Educators: The Impact on Absenteeism." *Preventive Medicine* 15:166-75.

Blue Cross-Blue Shield Consumer Exchange. 1986. "Plan Hopes to Spur Worksite Health Promotion and Wellness Programs." May, p. 3.

Bly, J. L., R. C. Jones, and J. E. Richardson. 1986. "Impact of Worksite Health Promotion on Health Care Costs and Utilization: Evaluation of Johnson and Johnson's Live for Life Program." *Journal of the American Medical Association* 256:3235-40.

Breslow, L. 1978. "Risk Factor Intervention in Health Maintenance." *Science* 200:908-12.

Brownell, K. B., R. Y. Cohen, A. J. Stunkard, and M. R. J. Felix. 1984. "Weight Loss Competitions at the Work Site: Impact on Weight, Morale and Cost-Effectiveness." *American Journal of Public Health* 74:1283-85.

Business Roundtable Task Force on Health. 1985. *Corporate Health Care Cost Management and Private-sector Initiatives.* Indianapolis: Lilly Corporate Center.

Castillo-Salgado, C. 1984. "Assessing Recent Developments and Opportunities in the Promotion of Health in the American Workplace." *Social Science and Medicine* 19:349-58.

Clement J. and D. A. Gibbs. 1983. "Employer Consideration of Health Promotion Programs: Financial Variables. *Journal of Public Health Policy.* 4:45-55.

Conrad, P. 1987a. "Who Comes to Worksite Wellness Programs?" *Journal of Occupational Medicine* 29:317-20.

—— 1987b. "Health and Fitness at Work: A Participant's Perspective." *Social Science and Medicine.*

Conrad, P., and J. W. Schneider. 1980. *Deviance and Medicalization: From Badness to Sickness.* St. Louis: Mosby.

Coriel, J., J. S. Levin, and E. G. Jaco. 1986. "Lifestyle: An Emergent Concept in the Social Sciences." *Culture, Medicine and Psychiatry* 9:423-37.

Crawford, R. 1979. "Individual Responsibility and Health Politics in the 1970s," in S. Reverby and D. Rosner (ed.), *Health Care In America,* 247-68. Philadelphia: Temple University Press.

Cunningham, R. M. 1982. *Wellness at Work.* Chicago: Blue Cross Association.

Davis, M. K., K. Rosenberg, D. C. Iverson, T. M. Vernon, and J. Bauer. 1984. "Worksite Health Promotion In Colorado." *Public Health Reports* 99:538-43.

Edwards, R. 1979. *Contested Terrain: The Transformation of the Workplace in the 20th Century.* New York: Basic Books.

Evans, R. 1982. "A Retrospective on the 'New Perspective'." *Journal of Health Politics, Policy and Law* 7:325-44.

Fielding, J. E. 1982. "Effectiveness of Employee Health Programs." *Journal of Occupational Medicine* 24:907-15.

——1984. "Health Promotion and Disease Prevention at the Worksite." *Annual Review of Public Health* 5:237-65.

Fielding, J. E. and L. Breslow. 1983. "Health Promotion Programs Sponsored by California Employers." *American Journal of Public Health* 73:533-42.

Foote, A., and J. C. Erfurt. 1983. Hypertension Control at the Worksite. *New England Journal of Medicine* 308:809-13.

Forster, J. L., R. W. Jeffrey, S. Sullivan, and M. K. Snell. 1985. "A Worksite Weight Control Program Using Financial Incentives Collected through Payroll Deductions." *Journal of Occupational Medicine* 27:804-8.

Gibbs, J. 0., D. Mulvaney, C. Hanes, and R. W. Reed. 1985. "Worksite Health Promotion: Five-year Trend in Employee Health Care Costs." *Journal of Occupational Medicine* 27:826-30.

Gillick, M. R. 1984. "Health Promotion, Jogging and the Pursuit of Moral Life." *Journal of Health Politics, Policy and Law* 9:369-87.

Goodman, L. E. and M. J. Goodman. 1986. "Prevention: How Misuse of a Concept Undercuts Its Worth." *Hastings Center Report* 16:26-38.

Hallet, R. 1986. "Smoking Intervention in the Workplace: Review and Recommendations." *Preventive Medicine* 15:213-31.

Health Research Institute. 1986. *1985 Health Care Cost Containment Survey—Participant Report* (Summary). Walnut Creek, CA.

Herzlinger, R. E., and D. Calkins. 1986. "How Companies Tackle Health Costs: Part 3." *Harvard Business Review* 63(6).70-80.

Levenstein, C., and M. Moret. 1985. "Health Promotion in the Workplace." *Journal of Public Health Polity* 6:149-51.

Liem, R. 1981. "Economic Change and Unemployment Contexts of Illness," in G. Mishler (ed.), *Social Contexts of Health. Illness and Patient Care*, 55-78. New York: Cambridge University Press.

Lorig, K., R. G. Kraines, B. W. Brown, and N. Richardson. 1985. "A Workplace Health Education Program that Reduces Outpatient Visits." *Medical Care* 23:1044-54.

Minkler, M. 1985. "Health Promotion Research: Are We Asking the Right Questions?" Paper presented at the annual meeting of the American Public Health Association, Washington, November 18.

Morris, J. N. 1982. "Epidemiology and Prevention." *Milbank Memorial Fund Quarterly/Health and Society* 60(l): 1-16.

Multiple Risk Factor Intervention Trial Group. 1982. "Multiple Risk Factor Intervention Trial: Risk Factor Changes and Mortality Results." *Journal of the American Medical Association* 248:1465-77.

Mulvaney, D., R. Reed, J. Gibbs, and C. Henes. 1985. "Blue Cross and Blue Shield of Indiana: Five Year Payoff in Health Promotion." *Corporate Commentary* 5(l):1-6.

Neubauer, D. and R. Pratt. 1981. "The Second Public Health Revolution: A Critical Appraisal." *Journal of Health Politics, Policy and Law* 6:205-28.

O'Donnell, M. P. 1984. "The Corporate Perspective," in M.P. O'Donnell and T.H. Ainsworth (ed.), *Health Promotion in the Work Place*, 10-36. New York: Wiley.

Paffenbarger, R. S., R. J. Hyde, A. L. Wing, and C. H. Steinmetz. 1984. "A Natural History of Athleticism and Cardiovascular Health." *Journal of the American Medical Association* 252:491-95.

Parkinson, R. S., and Associates (eds.). 1982. *Managing Health Promotion in the Workplace*. Palo Alto: Mayfield.

Pechter, K. 1986. "Corporate Fitness and Blue-Collar Fears." *Across the Board* 23(10):14-21.

Reed R. W., D. Mulvaney, R. Bellingham, and K. C. Huber. 1985. *Health Promotion Service: Evaluation Study*. Indianapolis: Blue Cross-Blue Shield of Indiana.

Reza-Forouzesh, M., and L. E. Ratzker. 1984-1985. "Health Promotion and Wellness Programs: An Insight into the Fortune 500." *Health Education* 15(7):18-22.

Roman, P. 1981. *Prevention and Health Promotion Programming in Work Organizations*. DeKalb: Northern Illinois University, Office for Health Promotion.

Rosen, R. H. 1984. "Worksite Health Promotion: Fact or Fantasy." *Corporate Commentary* 5(l):1-8.

Russell, L. B. *Is Prevention Better Than Cure?* 1986. Washington: Brookings Institute.

Slater, C. and B. Carlton. 1985. "Behavior, Lifestyle and Socioeconomic Variables as Determinants of Health Status: Implications for Health Policy Development." *American Journal of Preventative Medicine* 1(5):25-33.

Solomon, H. A. 1984. *The Exercise Myth*. New York: Harcourt Brace Jovanovich.

Spilman, M. A., A. Goetz, J. Schultz, R. Bellingham, and D. Johnson. 1986. "Effects of a Health Promotion Program." *Journal of Occupational Medicine* 28:285-89.

Stein, J. 1985. "Industry's New Bottom Line on Health Care Costs: Is Less Better?" *Hastings Center Report* 15(5):14-18.

Sterling, T. D., and J. J. Weinkam. 1986. "Extent, Persistence and Constancy of the Healthy Worker or Healthy Person Effect by All and Selected Causes of Death." *Journal of Occupational Medicine* 28:348-53.

Syme, L. S., and L. F. Berkman. 1976. "Social Class, Susceptibility and Illness." *American Journal of Epidemiology* 104:1-8.

Walsh, D. C. 1984. "Corporate Smoking Policies: A Review and an Analysis." *Journal of Occupational Medicine* 26:17-22.

U.S. Department of Health, Education, and Welfare. 1979. *Healthy People: The Surgeon General's Report on Health Promotion and Disease Prevention*. Washington.

Further Reading

J. Fielding. 1984. "Health Promotion and Disease Prevention at the Worksite." *Annual Review of Public Health* 5: 237-65.

Carlos Salgado-Castillo. 1984. "Assessing Recent Developments and Opportunities in the Promotion of Health in the American Workplace." *Social Science and Medicine* 19: 349-58.

"Worksite Health Promotion." 26:5. 1988. *Social Science and Medicine*. Special Issue.

Discussion Questions

1. In your opinion, what are the strengths and weaknesses of worksite wellness programs for employees?

2. What does Conrad mean when he claims that worksite wellness serves as an example of the healthicization of individuals? How is this similar to the process of medicalization that you read about in other selections?

3. Can you identify similarities in Michael Goldstein's and Deborah Lupton's arguments about public health and wellness and Conrad's claims about individual wellness in the workplace? What consensus do these authors reach regarding individual responsibility and health?

From *The Milbank Quarterly*, 1987, 65:2. Pp. 255-275.

27

Stress and Burnout in the Social World of Hospice

Judith A. Levy
Audrey K. Gordon

Beginning in the United States in the 1970s, the hospice movement promoted a "good death" philosophy. Throughout their history, hospice organizations have attempted to practice this ideology. A hospice death offers an alternative to the dying experience—institutionally and personally—for patients and health care staff. Tensions in advancing hospice philosophy are as strong today as they were twenty years ago at the inception of the movement.

In this piece, Judith Levy and Audrey Gordon illustrate how the ideals of the hospice movement conflict with the life experiences of hospice staff and volunteers. Hospice workers in this selection tell us about hidden work and emotional stress. These create tension. Stress becomes difficult to reconcile with the "good death" ideology. Staff burn out. The "good death" ideal spurs numerous organizational and personal tensions for health care workers. Think about the specific organizational difficulties that create stress for hospice staff. As you read this selection, consider the perspectives of Karen Lyman and Timothy Diamond regarding chronic care settings and invisible work. Consider the general implications of these works for the workers and patients of chronic care institutions.

Most studies of hospice burnout tend to locate its source within the emotional stress of working with dying persons and their families (Koff 1980; Roche 1981). This research suggests a second source of stress potentially leading to burnout: the ideological expectations of the movement itself. Drawing upon a social world perspective that views society as a set of subworlds, each bound by a universe of shared meaning, we explore how the hospice movement has constructed a world-view of the "good death" and attempts to achieve that goal. Stress and the possibility for burnout arise, we suggest, from staff attempts to fulfill the ideals that this view represents. The discussion ends by suggesting a set of strategies and techniques for reducing the likelihood that stress and burnout related to ideology will occur. . . .

Method

The observations for this study were collected using multiple methods. First, data were drawn from a 12-month field study of hospice activities in a large Midwestern city (Levy 1982). As part of this field research, a snowball sample technique was used to solicit 75 in-depth interviews with individuals who participated in the hospice movement or whose occupational positions intersect with the delivery of hospice services. In addition, 49 hospice program directors located throughout the surrounding state were asked to administer a mail survey to their volunteers. The survey instrument included both forced choice and open-ended questions that requested volunteers to recount their experiences and stresses in working with patients and families. Twenty-seven hospices responded to yield a total of 260 respondents. Response rates of volunteers by hospice varied from a low of 5 percent to a high of 100 percent. The data collected from the three methods were coded and cross-validated. Such triangulation helps to assure the reliability and validity of observations (Denzin, 1970). In all cases, participants were assured that their responses would be kept confidential.

Social Worlds of the Dying

Over the last seventy years, the locus of death in industrial societies has shifted from the home to hospital, nursing home, and other health care facilities (McCuster 1983; McDonnell 1986; Quint 1979). Within these institutions, the patient has access to regularized treatment, high-tech intervention, and skilled nursing care. But as Blauner (1966) observed, hospitals and nursing homes also function as special death worlds where the dying are separated from the mainstream of life, and death can be lonely and painful. Indeed, research has shown that the social world of dying people often becomes restricted as caregivers and significant others avoid interaction (Gubrium 1975a).

Hospice represents an attempt to create a new social world for the dying person where family and friends participate, palliative procedures minimize physical discomfort, and patients are helped to live as fully as possible until they die (Levy 1982). This goal demands a redefinition of such organizational and personal values as to what constitutes an appropriate death, how and where things should get accomplished, and who will take charge.

Like all social worlds (Shibutani 1961), the perimeters of hospice are defined and bound by a shared universe of meaning that structures participation within it. Language is used to construct social reality, and terms like "to live as fully as possible," "death with dignity," "pain-free death," and "death as a final stage of growth," are part of a shared vocabulary of values through which staff describe and orient themselves to their work. These concepts and the values that they represent are reinforced through hospice literature, staff education, case reviews, and everyday hospice practice; as such, they constitute the ideology or structure of beliefs through which decisions are made.

The standards of the "good death" and the expectations of the hospice setting produce necessary guidelines for forging new patterns of death and terminal care. Yet, they can also become a source of strain or disappointment in situations where the ideal is not obtained. When viewed from this perspective, the hospice construction of the good death is, to some extent, also the collective production of ideological stress. As is true for all work situations, effective intervention rests upon understanding the genesis of the problem.

This task begins by examining the good death as a service ideal.

The Social Construction of the Good Death

All social worlds emerge from and are organized around the coordinated efforts of their members (Becker 1976; Unruh 1980). Within the world of medicine, staff activities are directed toward producing medical cure, and such organizational components as a hierarchical division of labor, an ethical system for valuing life, and the technical procedures of medical practice shape the productive process (Finn Paradis 1985). Within medical ideology, death is the final enemy, and dying serves as a visible sign of staff failure.

In contrast, the world of hospice is organized around the social production of the good death (Lofland 1978). This concept refers to one that is pain-free, is attended by significant others, takes place in a home-like setting, is controlled to some degree by patient and family choices, and brings an orderly resolution to the life that is ending. Burger (1980, p. 134) summarizes the ideal hospice death by noting that ". . . the dying patient should be free of physical, mental, social, and spiritual pain in order that he may live as fully as possible, hopefully at home with his family." The good death also is referred to as a "natural death," "appropriate death," and "death with dignity" in hospice literature and practice (Vanderpool 1978).

According to hospice belief, intervention in the dying process is helpful since "dying, like birthing, is a process typically requiring assistance" to run smoothly (Stoddard 1978, p. 7). It is this assistance that produces the good death, implying that, without this service, many deaths would be "bad." Consequently, individuals who undertake hospice work have high expectations for themselves, including their ability to relieve the diverse problems of terminally ill patients and their families (Munley 1984). As one volunteer explains about the mission of her work:

I feel simply that I am a help to the family—some extra support. In some cases, this is the first time the family has had this type of difficulty, they don't know what to do, what is expected of them, how they are "supposed" to act. Sometimes I think that it's part of my role to let them know that whatever they feel, as long as there is love, is fine. At times, I feel that what I am doing is to help the patient and family to become close. (survey, #16)

Where such goals fail, the resulting disappointment and/or disillusionment form the basis for stress (Friel and Tehan 1980). Contrast this account, for example, to the one above.

The wife only heard what she wanted to hear. Everyone thought she knew her husband was dying because she could talk about it. When the time came, she was shocked. She blames the doctor and still holds a great deal of anger toward him. The husband (the patient) curled up in a ball and refused to talk to anyone. He became pretty withdrawn. The 16-year-old son blamed God for his father's death, had violent temper tantrums where he did physical damage to the house, and threatened suicide. (survey, #101)

In the latter case, the volunteer reported feeling a great deal of distress. Put simply, for those who believe in their ability to help construct a phenomenon called the "good, ideal, appropriate, or natural death," deviation from its parameters poses the potential for stress as it implies failure to achieve a goal (Vachon 1983). This outcome can be seen by examining the interactional patterns that surround a hospice death.

Dramaturgical Constructions

Hospice, like all social worlds, is characterized by a dramaturgical order that defines the participation of various social actors and roles that they play. As in all social worlds, maintaining a definition of the situation and a satisfying role performance typically requires the cooperation of more than one participant. Goffman (1959, p. 79) uses the word "team" to refer to "any set of individuals who cooperate in staging a single routine." In hospice, the concept of team is more than a metaphoric convention used by social scientists to understand human interaction. Interdiscipli-

nary teams are the basic core of hospice service delivery. They represent an organized effort to respond to the full range of patient and family needs on a timely and comprehensive basis.

Hospice teams consist of nurses, physicians, pastoral or other counselors, dietitians, social workers, one or more other hospice professional staff (Proffitt 1985). . . . In hospice, the patient plays the central part around which other supportive roles are organized. Patients are encouraged to take charge of their death so that, as they die, death unfolds in a manner consistent with the values and styles with which they have lived (Weisman 1972). Hospice personnel learn they are expected to honor each patient's personal script as part of their special training. Nonetheless, putting this belief into practice can be a source of tension for those individuals who are used to taking charge of problems. Moreover, family or circumstance can pressure staff to override patient preferences.

Such an override took place in one hospice where the caseload included a patient who insisted upon smoking in bed. Perhaps due to the medication he was taking, the patient would fall asleep, drop his cigarette, and set his mattress on fire. Attempts to induce him to restrict his smoking to those times when someone was in the room failed. So did the strategy of keeping a bucket of water near the bedside so that he could douse his cigarette as he fell asleep. Finally, his wife and the volunteer decided to hide his cigarettes and to allow him only to smoke when they were present.

While this decision might be justified on the basis of safety, denying the patient control over his or her final days was considered sufficiently serious to warrant hours of staff discussion. The central issue revolved around specifying those circumstances where the needs of the living take precedence over the dying. This quandary, common throughout hospice, permeates many of the day-to-day decisions staff and volunteers make. It becomes a source of stress or discomfort where answers are not readily discernible.

Although hospice philosophy provides staff with a general guideline for carrying out their work, all people engage in "role creation" (Bucher and Stelling 1969). When a person joins a hospice team, she or he receives training in how to do hospice work and a grounding in its basic philosophical tenets. Yet, even with the same preparation, no two volunteers or staff will deliver precisely the same service. Each, to some extent, will tailor the generalized role to coincide with his or her own values or image of what the work should entail.

Where these tailorings fit within the goals of a particular hospice, little or no problems exist. A rich variation in staff composition makes for more knowledgeable teams and aids the hospice in matching the volunteers' interests to those of the clients. Difficulties emerge, however, where the personal style or work performance of the staff do not match those of the other team members or conflict with organizational objectives. Where the breach is serious, most hospices take steps to remove or severely discourage the offender. With less troubling offenses, the staff person is pulled from direct patient care or kept closely monitored.

Such reprimands arising from organizational policy or style can prove stressful to the person to whom they are directed. Take the case of Kathy, for example. Although she was certified as an RN, her hospice felt that she overstepped her staff role by physically relieving her patient of a bowel impaction. Since her hospice was licensed as a volunteer program, "hands-on" nursing care was not considered a service component. Home health care agencies were used wherever nursing care was required, and Kathy was expected to respect this arrangement. Yet, Kathy found that she "couldn't let the patient suffer just because the home care nurse wasn't there." In another instance, a volunteer left hospice service after she was chastised by volunteers at a support meeting for not attempting the same level of intimate and personal connections with the family as did the other volunteers. Since hospices differ in policy and role expectations, both Kathy's and the volunteer's actions might have passed without incident had they been employed by different programs.

For some individuals, reducing stress may be merely a matter of changing to a different hospice. While hospice groups share a common philosophy about death, like all organizations, each has its own organizational culture. Which values are stressed or how service is delivered differs among hospices. This uniqueness is a product of managerial preferences, organizational history, the composition of the particular executive board, and staff idiosyncrasies. Staff and volunteer work satisfaction depends, in part, upon how closely the dynamics of a particular hospice fit with their own work style and values.

A mismatch in values also creates tension where staff, patient, or family hold different death expectations. Not all participants who take part in a hospice death are committed team players. Sometimes, for example, a hospice is called in over the objections of a family member:

> In one case, the husband assumed his wife wanted hospice. I was assigned to her and it became apparent very quickly that she resented my presence and was probably automatically linking me with "death" in a *very* negative fashion. (Survey, #55)

In other instances, the family members may be at odds and volunteers or staff get pulled into the conflict.

Teamwork also breaks down when nonhospice staff subscribe to those values of medicine that hospice is designed to ameliorate. In such instances, the nonhospice staff may actively engage in behavior that allows their own definitions and priorities to prevail:

> On Thursday when I came to work, I saw a little old woman who was dying of cancer and was very lonely. She needed hospice care so I went to the director and asked, "couldn't we get her into the hospice?" The director approached the woman's doctor and he said definitely not; she wasn't ready yet. He still wanted to give her active care. But a few days later I saw she had gone into a coma, so I slipped in and held her hand. (Interview, #17)

Defying a noncooperative teammate like this recalcitrant physician can cause considerable strain, as can being dependent upon a reluctant medical staff for the resources that a good death entails. As Moser and Krikorian (1982) found, having to rely upon a slow or noncooperative physician to order necessary drugs poses a great source of tension for many hospice workers.

The hospice movement was built upon a dramaturgical belief that lay helpers are as important to hospice care as trained professionals. These egalitarian beliefs were particularly pronounced in the early days of the movement as hospice was first getting started. Many hospices were staffed entirely by volunteers during this formative period. Now the tendency is to recruit staff with professional degrees or formalized management skills. Meanwhile, people from outside the movement increasingly are being hired to fill critical positions. This growing emphasis on professional training has become a source of frustration for personnel who prefer the movement's original lay orientation. In describing her own resignation, for example, one volunteer disclosed another volunteer's dissatisfaction:

> Lynn is going to quit too. I think that they (members of the executive board) want a nurse to direct things. They never were too happy with Lynn wanting to do the patient assessment. They want a professional. She did a good job, but somehow they never trusted her because she didn't have the proper degree. The thing is that volunteers are what hospice is all about—being nonprofessional—and yet here they are replacing her with a more professional person. (Interview, #41)

As a result of such professionalization, those in the movement without formal credentials are likely to experience shrinking opportunity for service or career mobility within hospice organizations. . . .

Spatial Constructions

Social worlds, and the places within them, vary as to "the degree to which they are dramaturgically open or concealed" (Lofland 1975, p. 280). Lyman and Scott (1967) suggest public, home, interactional, and body territories as four types of space where be-

havior is ordered. Focusing solely on the stress that comes from delivering the good death, let us consider each territory as it applies to hospice.

"Public territories are those territories where the individual has freedom of access, but not necessarily of action . . ." (Lyman and Scott 1967, p. 237). Hospitals and nursing homes are public territories in that various categories of people enter and routinely use space within these facilities. Because public territories are open to many individuals and multiple social networks, they tend to discourage participants from claiming sections as their own. The object of a hospice inpatient unit is to obviate this anonymity by creating a "home territory" where patients are encouraged to stake out personal space and where each person's uniqueness is preserved. Such home territories, according to Lyman and Scott (1967, p. 238), are social arenas where people enjoy "a relative freedom of behavior and a sense of intimacy and control over the area."

Creating a home territory within an institution presents a series of problems. For example, stress arises from attempts to maintain consistency of care and philosophy between the home territory of the hospice unit and the public territory of the host facility. Often the everyday routines of institutional business-as-usual overshadow hospice attempts at implementing social service reform.

Control over nonhospice staff (x-ray technicians, phlebotomists, etc.) poses additional problems for creating a home territory within an institution. For example, open communication with the family is part of hospice philosophy but such candidness is not always characteristic of institutional policy. Family members who expect open communication from hospice staff often have difficulty differentiating who is part of the hospice team, and who is not. Thus, where there are complaints about poor communication or unsatisfactory nursing services, the hospice team often bears the brunt of the family's displeasure. From the standpoint of ideological control, inpatient units are less stressful for staff than delivering hospice services to isolated beds scattered throughout the institution (McArdle

1985, pp. 130–132). In the case of hospice accreditation standards the Joint Commission on Accreditation of Hospitals requires that all hospice beds be in the same unit, an intervention that contributes to easier transmission of hospice ideology.

Hospice care delivered in the home presents stress of a different nature. The image of the home as a secure, safe, known place—the very womb of the family—is central to hospice philosophy. In circumstances where it becomes necessary to transfer a patient from the home to a nonhospice setting, wrenching the patient from this symbolic womb, represents a generally disappointing outcome to hospice staff.

The symbolism of the home extends into the belief by some volunteers and staff that families should be loving, close, and supportive of one another. Strain occurs where hospice staff have values and expectations about the meaning of home or family that differ from that of the family or patient. In one instance, for example, the volunteer found that the patient's son misappropriated his mother's savings account for a vacation. Handling this information posed a difficult dilemma for the volunteer. Although she felt that the woman should be told of her son's actions, she perceived that such a disclosure would hurt the woman deeply. Caught between two adverse outcomes, she decided to keep the knowledge to herself.

The hospice team take on hospice work with the expectation that they will participate in the "interactional territories" that surround the death trajectory. Yet, families are themselves semiprivate worlds that have secrets and rituals not easily shared with outsiders. The barriers that protect the family from outside view can also bar the staff from some of the family's central activities. Rejection, even when it is not a conscious decision, can be personally hurtful to the staff who feel left out of the action. One volunteer describes what she considers one of her most difficult cases:

> Occasionally a family gave me the feeling of being an intruder. There were a few families who told nurse and staff when they first came to the unit that they'd let us know when they needed or wanted

someone or help, but to otherwise let them alone. (Survey, #60)

In other instances, overparticipation in family dynamics can engulf volunteers and hospice staff. Where the hospice caregiver is heavily influenced by the ideal of the "caring person," he or she may find it difficult to say no or to establish adequate self-boundaries.

How a family responds to interactional overtures is a product of both need and ability to tolerate the presence of hospice staff in the role of an "intimate stranger" (Gordon and Rooney 1984; Levy 1982). Volunteers perform tasks such as shopping, babysitting, cooking, and respite care. In the course of their duties, hospice staff frequently become privy to intimate family life in a way that threatens the privacy of a closed family system (Kantor and Lehr 1975). For example, one hospice volunteer reports that a patient:

> . . . stated in her first contact that she felt it strange to share one of life's most intimate events, referring to her death, with a stranger. I believe she turned to a sister, which became difficult for me in a sense and yet I felt good. Where there is great division in a family and no one trusts anyone else, the situation makes it difficult to be objective because one begins to feel that everyone is lying. (Survey, #82)

Some families respond to hospice intrusion by closing off interactional territories to the volunteer and professional staff except in those situations where circumstance denies them this luxury. Such cases tend to occur where family or patient cannot afford paid services and therefore must rely upon volunteers regardless of family preference.

The very intimacy of hospice work brings volunteers into close association with the otherwise forbidden "body territories" that comprise what Gubrium (1975b) called "bed and body work." This concept refers to personal service to the body and other caregiving functions in which private body territories and interactional territories intersect. Volunteers as intimate strangers assist with nonmedical "bed and body work," a role usually performed elsewhere by healthcare professionals or family members. Yet, an experienced volunteer stated that ". . . even after 2 years, I still feel uncomfortable trying to assist the patient with the bedpan." In such instances, the protective screen of the home territory his been torn aside as the volunteer encounters the private spaces of the patient. The result is discomfort for both parties.

Sentimental Constructions

All social worlds contain an "intangible but very real patterning of mood and sentiment" (Glaser and Strauss 1965). The sentimental order of hospice takes its cues from the concept of a "death with dignity" where the patient's wishes are respected. The honoring of this sentiment manifests itself as a holistic approach to services in which spiritual care of the patient and family is as important as physical care. Dying is not perceived as failure, as it is in medicine, but as a final stage of growth. Beliefs and attitudes about the nature of life and death, good and evil vis-à-vis the dying process, and certain assumptions about family dynamics shape the organization of hospice work. Meanwhile, narcotics and palliative care measures provide relief from pain so as to insure the person's ability to sustain life in relative comfort.

Establishing trust between the team, the patient, and the family is critical to good hospice service. Yet, building such bonds of confidence are complicated by the circumstances under which the patient and hospice meet. At what stage of the service trajectory a patient enters the program makes a difference:

> It's difficult to serve families of patients who are very near death and you haven't had contact with them. I personally believe that credibility and trust need to be built to adequately serve in such a situation. (Survey, #128)

A patient's or family's personality or past experience is a critical issue. In one case, a patient entered a hospice program after several months in a nursing home where petty theft of patient belongings was a recurring problem. Whenever the patient mislaid something, she would accuse the volunteer of theft until the article was found. The volunteer's pique at being called a thief hindered hospice attempts at building positive sentiment.

Much of volunteer training focuses on laying groundwork for the sentimental order by praising volunteers for those special qualities that allow them to do such difficult work under sometimes trying conditions. Neophytes routinely are told that working with patients will "make you feel good about yourself." Yet, the expectations and possible stress that arise from this practice can be seen in the following account.

In this instance, the volunteer's first major hospice activity involved taking her patient to the doctor. The trip was highly complicated by the patient's infirmity teamed with her somewhat anxious manner. Later, as the volunteer described the experience, she ended the conversation by disclosing, "Funny, I didn't feel the uplift I expected." A more seasoned volunteer hastened to reassure the neophyte that she would feel more rewarded as she knew her patient better. Indeed, the number of volunteers who report feeling uplifted by helping their patients suggests that such a transformation in sentiment is common. Yet, should such an initial letdown continue, the volunteer may begin to doubt his or her calling as a volunteer.

In sum, the sentimental ideology of the good death is deeply mirrored in staff and volunteer behaviors and expectations. Experience that runs counter to these beliefs potentially disturbs the collective sentiment of the hospice program and places stress upon its staff and volunteers. When a death occurs according to expectations everyone is gratified. Where it does not, such moods as doubt, ambivalence, anger, frustration, and reduced self-esteem emerge.

Temporal Constructions

The human lifespan is organized according to a series of culturally-defined life stages. Each stage has its own particular norms and set of expectations. Dying represents the last phase of the human life cycle within this temporal ordering; In hospice, it also signals a final opportunity for the dying person's personal growth and development. A primary goal of hospice services is to help patients and their families to construct a temporal social world where this final stage of growth optimally can occur.

Where successful, growth-work that helps patients to realize their potential can prove quite rewarding. But the work also can be discouraging where patients remain embittered or angry:

> I really didn't like Bob (the patient). I really thought he was unnecessarily cruel to his daughter. You'd think he'd be nicer to her as he came closer to death . . . but he never was. (Interview, #5)

In the case of Bob, staff notes reveal that the volunteer frequently attempted to bring patient and daughter amicably together. Her feelings of frustration, self-recorded in the patient's case records, also attest to the strain of unrealized expectations. Death in this instance could not be construed as a final stage of growth, at least in terms of forging better father-daughter relations.

While death is the common fate of all people, how people die takes on individualized expression including its own temporal ordering. Glaser and Strauss (1968) noted that attempts to fix the actual timing of death is complicated by various permutations of the bio-medically known combined with the uncertain. Such ambiguity makes it difficult for staff, the patient, and family to anticipate future problems or to schedule their own participation in the death. Consequently, the person who dies before an expected time or at an untimely moment creates strain for others. Likewise, the person who takes too long may outlive his or her earthly welcome. This was the case of Brenda, a patient volunteers admitted they sometimes wished would die. These feelings were sparked by Brenda's excessive demands and the burden they posed for her family.

Dying time is limited in that it is measured in months, days, hours, and minutes (Koff 1980). It is sacred time in that its priorities override the profane time and demands of everyday life. Dawson (1981, p. 82), for example, observed that:

> Time is important in hospice care. Opportunity may be once and for all. Need may require long periods of undivided at-

tention from the staff. The development of themes that arise may require a great deal of effort from a great many people.

Such temporal valuations encourage hospice staff and volunteers to view their personal life as less important than meeting the needs of the dying person. For the most part, however, hospices vary in how closely they accept or hold to this tenet.

Where personal and service schedules conflict, knowing which timetable to follow is simpler for those staff for whom the decision rule entails honoring patient priorities. On the other hand, team members who try to balance personal needs against conflicting patient demands are far more likely to report "feeling pulled in two directions." In such instances, they often require team encouragement or support to feel comfortable with their decisions.

Organizations also have their own expectational timetables that compete with those of staff, patients, and families. In hospice, the "six months to live" rule for patient admissions represents an attempt to bring some temporal certainly to case management. Moreover, six-month trajectories also increase the likelihood that patients and families will learn to trust the hospice staff, as this comment suggests:

> Relationships become close if the length of time becomes great. Friendships become close as people learn they can depend on you and they develop confidence. Many people are overwhelmed by the caring of those who come to the home. Contact is made between home visits mostly by phase. (Survey, #82)

While the six-month rule is an official statement of organizational policy, many patients actually enter hospice in the last weeks or days of life. In such instances, building close rapport in the short period before death poses a difficult challenge for staff. As one volunteer reports following initial contact with the family, "The patient expired after about two weeks without me ever getting to meet her."

In general, hospice work ideally is organized around a service trajectory that begins with patient and family acceptance into the program and ends with bereavement and follow-up care. Patients and families, however, do not always envision the same service scheduling as the hospice or even agree among themselves as to when things should happen. Where disagreement occurs, patient/family counter-definitions create potential difficulties for staff. A staff member reported the following example of too early and intense a case-entry:

> I knew that the family didn't need me or want me right away, but X (the director) insisted that I keep on calling. I guess she wanted them to know that we were there and waiting. But I suspect they got tired of having me call. (Interview, #68)

At the other end of the spectrum are those families who are reluctant to relinquish hospice services long after the organizationally defined bereavement period has ended. These cases can drain staff and volunteers who are ready to go on to other patients or interests. Thus, some hospices have written policies on how long volunteers may remain assigned to a family after the death. These regulations provide a mechanism to prevent families from becoming permanently dependent upon hospice services and to keep volunteers from becoming over involved emotionally in a family system.

The Social Construction of Intervention

While it has been used in multiple ways, the term "burnout" typically refers to the progressive loss of idealism, energy, and purpose experienced by people in the helping profession as a result of their work conditions (Edelwich and Brodsky 1980, p. 14). Throughout the analysis, we have shown how collective ideals of hospice become a source of stress and pose the possibility for burnout. . . .

The concept of the good death, when applied to actual practices implicitly promises more than hospice staff routinely can deliver. Stress occurs where deviations from the ideal are perceived as failure by either hospice staff or the families they serve.

One intervention strategy involves helping staff to develop realistic expectations. This includes identifying those elements within hospice ideology and organizational culture that contribute to a distorted view of what occurs. In terms of the sentimental order, for example, the tendency exists in hospice training to emphasize the high motivations and ideals of hospice staff. The staff person who later becomes bored or discouraged may later feel too ashamed to admit to emotions that contradict the feelings ascribed to others or those which they anticipated. Young, well-educated staff appear particularly vulnerable. (Masterson-Allen, Laliberte, and Monteiro 1985; Mor and Laliberte 1984). Staff members need to know that it is organizationally acceptable *not* to feel uplifted by the work. They also need the reassurance of being entitled to their own opinions and values where these run counter to hospice, patient, or family expectations. Part of the work role of the support group can be directed toward helping staff mediate these contradictions.

Another tendency of hospice training is to skim over the drawbacks to hospice services to avoid frightening the neophyte. The more technical or potentially problematic aspects of care typically are reserved for the final sessions. While such temporal tactics of gradual disclosure does allow time to adjust to fears, hospice training must be careful to provide a comprehensive and realistic overview to hospice by the time training has ended.

Hospice policy dictates seven-day-a-week, 24-hour availability of the team to meet patient and family needs. In fulfilling this ideal, hospice organizations must be careful that staff members and volunteers do not fall into the trap of thinking that they personally must be available at all times and under all circumstances. This is where many of the dramaturgical dilemmas of hospice emerge as staff and volunteers attempt to carry out their roles and responsibilities. Hospice regulations should specify carefully when and where caregiving will be done and by whom. Provisions for meeting emergencies, competing priorities, and possible work overload need to be formally addressed and periodically updated. Specific periods of time off to participate in other timetables and social worlds need to be enforced. To avoid stress buildup, volunteers must be paced in their case-load according to their personalities and the difficulties of the situation they encounter. Those volunteer groups that devise specific strategies for maximizing members' time tend to cut down on staff attrition (Moore 1963).

Hospice caregiving takes place in multiple settings and under a variety of conditions. The home territories of the patient and family may be sentimentally or socioeconomically different from those of the hospice team. Meanwhile, the spatial territories of the hospital or nursing facility frequents that compete with those governing how hospice is practiced.

Stress can be reduced by formulating clear guidelines that specify hospice intraorganizational relationships including the interactions that surround issues such as case management, reimbursement, and home care. Intraorganizational tension also can be reduced by contracting only those outside service providers who are willing to complete hospice training in palliative care, narcotic regimen, and hospice philosophy. Also, both nonhospice staff and hospice personnel who feel caught between ideological beliefs or upset by a particular family circumstance may need help to cope with this conflict. Special attention to discussing family systems as a component of staff and volunteer training has particular merit. Periodic inservice education further enhances the ability of volunteers and staff to handle difficult family problems. Intervention in family dynamics should include the information necessary to understand what is occurring while also providing social support to accept those factors that cannot be changed.

A final intervention may lie in substituting the concept of the *better* death for the good death as a service ideal. In each case *better* would be relative to the situation in which the patient/family initially finds itself. Success would be measured by volunteers' and staffs' ability to make a positive difference in contrast to unrealistic attempts to bring about an ideal state. The concept of the better death along with an open discussion of avoiding ideological pressure would become an essential component of volunteer and staff training. Then hospice ideology, as a framework for constructing new social worlds for the dying, would offer a service goal that is both feasible and rewarding

also producing less stressful outcomes for volunteers and staff.

References

Becker, H. S. (1976). "Art worlds and social types." *American Behavioral Scientist, 19.* 703–719.

Blauner, R. (1966). "Bureaucratization of modern death control." *Psychiatry, 29.* 383–387.

Bucher, R. and J. Stelling. (1969). "Characteristics of professional organizations." *Journal of Health and Social Behavior, 10.* 3–15.

Burger, S. (1980). "The approaches to patient care: Hospice, nursing homes and hospitals," in M. Hamilton and H. Reed (eds.), *A hospice handbook: A new way to care for dying.* (pp. 131–144). Grand Rapids: William B. Eerdmans.

Dawson, P. (1981)."Meeting the psychosocial needs of the patient," in J. M. Zimmerman (ed.), *Hospice: Complete care for the terminally ill* (pp. 79–96). Baltimore: Urban and Schwarzenberg.

Denzin, N. (1970). *The research act: A theoretical introduction to sociological methods.* Chicago: Aldine.

Edelwich, J. and A. Brodsky. (1980). *Burn-out.* New York: Human Sciences Press.

Finn Paradis, L. (1985). "The development of hospice in America" in L. Finn Paradis (ed.), *Hospice handbook: A guide for managers and planners* (pp. 3–24). Rockville, MD: Aspen Systems Corporation.

Friel, M. and C. B. Tehan. (1980). "Counteracting burnout for the hospice caregiver." *Cancer Nursing, 3.* 285–293.

Glaser, B. G. and A. L. Strauss. (1965). *Awareness of dying.* Chicago: Aldine.

———. (1968). *Time for dying.* Chicago: Aldine.

Goffman, E. (1959). *The presentation of self in everyday life.* Garden City: Doubleday Anchor Books.

Gordon, A. and A. Rooney. (1984). "Hospice and the family: A systems approach to assessment." *American Journal of Hospice Care, 1.* 31–33.

Gubrium, J. F. (1975a). "Death worlds in a nursing home." *Urban Life, 4.* 317–338.

Gubrium, J. F. (1975b). *Living and dying at Murray Manor.* New York: St. Martin's Press.

Kantor, D. and W. Lehr. (1975). *Inside the family.* New York: Harper Colophon Books.

Koff, T. H. (1980). *Hospice: A caring community.* Cambridge: Winthrop.

Levy, J. A. (1982). *The hospice movement: Creating new social worlds for the dying.* Unpublished doctoral dissertation, Northwestern University, Evanston, IL.

Lofland, J. (1975). "Open and concealed dramaturgic strategies: The case of the state execution." *Urban Life*, 4. 272–295.

Lofland, L. (1978). *The craft of dying*. Beverly Hills: Sage.

Lyman, S. M. and M. B. Scott. (1967). "Territoriality: A neglected sociological dimension." *Social Problems*. 15. 236–249.

Masterson-Allen, A., V. Mor, L. Laliberte, and L. Monteiro. (1985). "Staff burnout in a hospice setting." *The Hospice Journal*. 1. 1–15.

McArdle, K. (1985). "Management of the hospital inpatient unit," in L. Finn Paradis (ed.), *Hospice handbook: A guide for managers and planners* (pp. 127–146). Rockville, MD: Aspen Systems Corporations.

McCuster, J. (1983). "Where cancer patients die: An epidemiologic study." *Public Health Reports, 98*(2). 170–176.

McDonnell, A. (1986). *Quality hospice care*. Owings Mills, MD: National Health Publishing.

Moore, W. (1963). *Man, time and society*. New York: Wiley & Sons.

Mor, V. and L. Laliberte. (1984). "Burnout among hospice staff." *Health and Social Work*. 9. 274–283.

Moser, D. H. and D. A. Krikorian. (1982). "Satisfaction and stress incidents reported by hospice nurses: A pilot study." *Nursing Leadership*. 5. 9–16.

Munley, A. (1984). *The hospice alternative*. New York: Basic Books.

Proffitt, L. (1985). "Management of the hospice home care program," in L. Finn Paradis (ed.), *Hospice handbook: A guide for managers and planners* (pp. 173–190). Rockville, MD: Aspen Systems Corporation.

Quint, B. J. (1979). "Dying in an institution," in H. Wass (ed.), *Dying* (pp. 137–268). New York: McGraw Hill.

Roche, K. (1981). "Self selection, education and evaluation," in J. M. Zimmerman (ed.), *Hospice: Complete care for the terminally ill* (pp.113–123). Baltimore-Munich: Urban and Schwarzenberg.

Shibutani, T. (1961). *Society and personality*. Englewood Cliffs, NJ: Prentice Hall.

Stoddard, S. (1978). *The hospice movement*. New York: Stein and Day.

Unruh, D. (1980). "The nature of social worlds." *Pacific Sociological Review*. 23. 271–296.

Vachon, M. S. (1983). "Staff stress in care of the terminally ill," in C. A. Corr and D. M. Corr (eds.), *Hospice care: Principles and practice* (pp. 237–245). New York: Springer.

Vanderpool, H. Y. (1978). "The ethics of terminal care." *Journal of the American Medical Association*. 850. 239.

Weisman, A. D. (1972). *On dying and denying*. New York: Behavioral Publications.

Weisman, A. D. (1981). "Understanding the cancer patient: The syndrome of caregiver's plight." *Psychiatry,* 44. 161–168.

Wilson, D. C. and D. J. English. (1980, July). *An assessment of the existing staffing patterns and personnel required in a hospice to deliver interdisciplinary patient care and the problems related to delivering humanistic care to hospice* (DHEW Contract No. HRA 232-79-0082). Hyattsville, MD: Bureau of Health Professions, Health Resources Administration.

Yancik, R. (1984a). "Coping with hospice work stress." *Journal of Psychosocial Oncology, 2*(2). 19–35.

Yancik, R. (1984b). "Source of stress for hospice staff." *Journal of Psychosocial Oncology, 2*(1). 21–31.

Yasko, J. M. (1983). "Variables which predict burnout experienced by oncology nurse specialists." *Cancer Nursing,* 6. 109–116.

Further Reading

Joan Kron. 1976. "Designing a Better Place to Die: Structural Characteristics of the Hospice." *New York Magazine* March: 43–49.

Anne Munley. 1983. *The Hospice Alternative: A New Context for Death and Dying*. New York: Basic Books.

Rockwell Schulz, James R. Greenley, and Roger Brown. 1995. "Organization, Management, and Client Effects on Staff Burnout." *Journal of Health and Social Behavior* 36(4): 333–345.

Genevieve Strahan. 1993. "Overview of Home Health and Hospice Care Patients." *Advance Data* 235: 1–12.

Discussion Questions

1. How might you define a "good death" as an alternative to modern day death and dying experiences?

2. In what ways do Karen Lyman's and Timothy Diamond's accounts support Levy and Gordon's arguments about worker "burnout"? How might Lyman's and Diamond's perspectives conflict with Levy and Gordon's conclusions?

3. Consider some organizational changes that might be effective in minimizing staff and volunteer "burnout." How might these changes be enacted?

Section 5

Social and Cultural Structures of Care

When we think about health and illness, we need to consider the populations and social groups affected by disease and the kinds of diseases that affect them. We should also consider those groups who remain healthy. Social epidemiology emphasizes these issues precisely. Sociologists, health services researchers, clinicians, and scientists are the people who do epidemiological research. Social epidemiologists investigate the links between aspects of social life—gender, race, class, age, or occupation, for example—and the distribution and spread of illness and health. Their data generally take numeric form, and unlike most of what you have read in previous sections, their analyses of those data are usually quantitative and are presented in tables, charts, and graphs. These data become important in identifying trends in disease, defining social and clinical problems, designing interventions, and formulating health policy.

Our understanding of disease and its spread has grown significantly with advanced methodologies in quantitative analysis, more developed technologies for recognizing and describing disease, and expanded acceptability in topics of epidemiological investigation.

Historically, epidemiologists studied epidemics, diseases that caused a large number of people in a given area to become sick or to die in a time period that seemed unreason-able for the number, area, or prognosis. Contemporary epidemiologists focus on a wider range of problems since many of the agents that caused early epidemics have all but been eradicated by housing, sewage, and water systems, and by scientific achievements in "cell theory" and "germ theory" leading to simple preventive measures and vaccinations.

Modern epidemiologists also study morbidity and mortality trends in epidemics. Morbidity is sickness or illness; mortality, death. But modern epidemiologists also examine rates of health and illness related to accidents, occupational hazards, violence (*JAMA* 1995), and other injuries. Hence, the field of epidemiology has expanded from its traditional focus on epidemic diseases, such as the black plague and the spread of cholera, to rates of accidents and illness related to teen tobacco and drug use (Altman et al. 1996; APHA 1997), firearm injuries, and environmental disasters (MacKay 1993). Epidemiologists are interested in describing the prevalence and incidence of the phenomena they study. Prevalence is an epidemiological measure that suggests the total occurrence of a particular illness, disease, or health related behavior at a given point in time. In epidemiology, this measure is often contrasted with disease incidence, a measure that reflects the occurrence of a particular illness, disease, or health related behavior over a specifically defined period of time.

Yet, as the focus of epidemiology has changed, so have methods of data collection. Early studies of the relationship between illness and social factors often involved a method of data collection known as "shoe leather epidemiology." This method required epidemiologists to go door-to-door or to sites where disease was spread and to interview those who had the illness or who may have come in contact with someone who did. Many recent epidemiological studies use large computerized databases that are collected from hospitals and clinics, government institutions, and medical research sites, like the Centers for Disease Control, to study trends in illness and health in a population. Although the use of computerized data bases has been a very effective way to examine disease patterns in a population, researchers from the Centers for Disease Control who first began to examine the spread of AIDS used the early technique of shoe leather epidemiology, finding interview data which suggested sexual transmission as a common mode of contracting the human immune deficiency virus that leads to AIDS (Brandt 1987).

The selections in this section examine the spread of disease due to social factors in various populations. They indicate a range of definitions of illness and health and point to how social factors—gender, race, class, age, occupation, and history—affect the distribution of health and illness in individuals and populations in the United States.

A nation's health is best represented by its life expectancy and by its rates of infant mortality. While the United States has some of the most advanced systems of medical technology and training in the world, David Himmelstein and Steffie Woolhandler show that it does not have the best health outcome measures for infant mortality compared with other countries. Health outcome measures enumerate the effects of particular social and clinical variables on health. For example, social variables that contribute to or cause health outcomes of infant mortality might include parents' socio-economic status; clinical variables might be low laboratory test scores indicating physiologic dysfunction. Sociologists David Williams and Chiquita Collins argue, however, that factors related to poor health outcomes, like social class, make infant mortality a social problem rather than a problem of medicine and health. Pay attention to their discussion about the construction of "race" as a variable in analyzing health and illness, and critically consider other cause and effect models related to health outcomes reported in scientific and popular literatures.

Marsha Lillie-Blanton and her colleagues argue that long standing social inequalities account for health differences between minority and nonminority women in the United States. These authors contextualize health as the result of the environments and life experiences of women. As a result, they examine how factors like self-perceived health, environmental and occupational circumstances, and access to health services contribute to different health and illness outcomes for minority and nonminority women. Lois Verbrugge looks at health differentials between men and women. Like Williams and Collins, she challenges biological characteristics as determining the gendered gap in morbidity and mortality. Gaps in morbidity and mortality can be accounted for, in part, by an individual's social support system. Although sociological research has resulted in conflicting findings regarding the impact of social support, health services researchers Howard Gordon and Gary Rosenthal show that social support, indicated by patients' marital status, is an important determinant of hospitalized patients' health outcomes, including in-hospital death. Each of the selections in this section underscores the significance of social over biological structures for understanding health outcomes.

Over time, the incidence of disease, illness, and health related behaviors change. Some of these changes are marked by advancements in medical technologies; others, by improved access to health care and illness preventive measures. Still other changes are marked by practitioner definitions of problems and the health seeking behaviors of patients as consumers.

Emily Martin notes the significance of metaphors for characterizing women's bodies—how the image of a woman's body as a factory implies ideal functioning and how anything outside this standard can be labeled as dysfunction or disease. Compare the effects of these metaphors with definitions of bodies shaped by the rise of cosmetic surgery in the United States, where malformed bodies are thought to benefit from medical intervention (Sullivan 1993). Kathy Davis documents changing conceptions of bodies resulting from the marketing of reconstructive surgery as a business. But cosmetic reconstructive surgery has not been the only medical enterprise to become a market commodity. Gary Albrecht documents how rehabilitation products and services are marketed to attract consumers and to create profit. Marketing strategies are built into how health care is managed in the U.S. today. In turn, management priorities overshadow medical needs. Thus, these strategies determine parameters of business and also critically affect the organization of care.

As we examine issues of health care and attend to meaningful social and cultural structures, we see that disease incidence and prevalence, complex causal explanations, historical forces, and cultural definitions present daunting problems for health policy makers and national health care systems. Vicente Navarro emphasizes how vested interests and social class relations determine the organization of health services and the distribution of health and illness outcomes in the United States. He shows that class systems of dominance over care financing and institutional administration eliminate options for the organization of health services.

Other national health care systems, like the Canadian system, provide alternative examples for the structure and provision of care. Yet sentiment in the United States about the structure of Canadian health care has not been favorable. Many believe that single-payer government regulated care will limit access to innovative practices. The selection by David Himmelstein and Steffie Woolhandler addresses this concern by showing that access to cancer treatment and transplantation does not differ significantly in Canada

and the United States. Looking at structure more specifically, John Iglehart explores the organization of health care in Japanese society—the obligations of corporate business toward employees and the role of national health insurance for those who are under-insured or unemployed. This selection, along with a personal account of a Japanese patient's hospital experience described in the selection by Hiroko Akiyama, allows us conceive of experiences of health care unlike those in the United States. As you read about differences in accessibility and resource distribution resulting from different systems of care in the United States, Canada, and Japan, think about the philosophies of society, patient, and care that define the organization of health services.

Eastern philosophies have had increasing appeal in the West as people face the uncertainty of chronic and lengthy terminal illness. Alexandra Dundas Todd's account states the significance of patient-centered conceptions in the treatment of disease. Her account depicts how eastern philosophies of healing can alter the illness experience and draw attention to deficits in western conceptions of disease, patient, and the healing process.

What lessons do we learn about health, illness, and possibilities for healing when we investigate the structures that characterize the distribution of health and illness? Consider alternative directions for the provision of care with critical attention to the physical, social, organizational, and philosophical structures that shape individual and national experiences of health and illness as you read the subsequent selections.

References

David Altman, Douglas Levine, Remy Coeytaux, John Slade, and Robert Jaffe. 1996. "Tobacco Promotion and Susceptibility to Tobacco Use Among Adolescents Aged 12-17 Years in a Nationally Representative Sample." *American Journal of Public Health* 86(11): 1590-1593.

American Public Health Association. September 1997. *The Nation's Health.*

Allan Brandt 1987. *No Magic Bullet: A Social History of Venereal Disease in the U.S. Since 1880.* New York: Oxford.

Journal of the American Medical Association. 1995. 273(2), Special Issue on Violence.

Judith MacKay. 1993. *The State of Health Atlas.* New York: Simon and Schuster.

Deborah Sullivan. 1993. "Cosmetic Surgery: Market Dynamics and Medicalization." *Research in the Sociology of Health Care* 10: 97-115.

Further Reading

The Nation's Health. Official Newsletter of the American Public Health Association.

U.S. Department of Health Services. *Morbidity and Mortality Review.* Massachusetts Medical Society. ✦

The Social and Cultural Shaping of Medical Care

28

Medical Metaphors of Women's Bodies: Menstruation and Menopause

Emily Martin

A *metaphor substitutes one thing for another. Comparing two dissimilar things asks us to take a fresh look at them. Writers use metaphor to reveal deeper meaning, a hidden truth. A well-chosen metaphor startles us with its sharp image, clarity, and, perhaps, emotional intensity. Many metaphors are obvious and simply provide a novel view of a familiar phenomena. For example, seeing the body as a business focuses our attention on defining losses and gains, balancing accounts, managing the parts, and concentrating on efficient functioning.*

Other metaphors may be taken for granted and viewed as some kind of truth. Think about the implications of metaphors in medical care of the nurse as "handmaiden," cancer "victim," and "fighting" disease. Such metaphors may be applied as if concrete reality, rather than as a way of portraying it. Menstruation as a patho-

logical condition invites identifying women as temporarily "sick." Menopause as a reproductive breakdown reaffirms the Detroit model of aging as deterioration, deficiency, disconnection, and decay—losses and deficits. Loss of production then equals loss of function. Martin shows how medical metaphors portray beliefs about similarities and differences between male and female bodies, borrow imagery and social issues from the cultural and historical epoch in which they are invoked, and reinforce women's position in society. See if you can find which metaphors speak to each of these views.

Metaphors in Descriptions of Female Reproduction

. . . In overall descriptions of female reproduction, the dominant image is that of a signaling system. Lein, in a textbook designed for junior colleges, spells it out in detail:

> Hormones are chemical signals to which distant tissues or organs are able to respond. Whereas the nervous system has characteristics in common with a telephone network, the endocrine glands perform in a manner somewhat analogous to radio transmission. A radio transmitter may blanket an entire region with its signal, but a response occurs only if a radio receiver is turned on and tuned to the proper frequency . . . the radio receiver in biological systems is a tissue whose cells possess active receptor sites for a particular hormone or hormones.[1]

The signal-response metaphor is found almost universally in current texts for premedical and medical students (emphasis in the following quotes is added):

The hypothalamus *receives signals* from almost all possible sources in the nervous system.[2]

The endometrium *responds directly* to stimulation or withdrawal of estrogen and progesterone. In turn, regulation of the secretion of these steroids involves a well-integrated, highly structured series of activities by the hypothalamus and the anterior lobe of the pituitary. Although the ovaries do not function autonomously, they *influence*, through *feedback* mechanisms, the level of performance *programmed* by the hypothalamic-pituitary axis.[3]

As a result of strong stimulation of FSH, a number of follicles *respond* with growth.[4]

And the same idea is found, more obviously, in popular health books:

Each month from menarch on, [the hypothalamus] acts as elegant interpreter of the body's rhythms, *transmitting messages* to the pituitary gland that set the menstrual cycle in motion.[5]

Each month, *in response to a message* from the pituitary gland, one of the unripe egg cells develops inside a tiny microscopic ring of cells, which gradually increases to form a little balloon or cyst called the Graafian follicle.[6]

Although most accounts stress signals or stimuli traveling in a "loop" from hypothalamus to pituitary to ovary and back again, carrying positive or negative feedback, one element in the loop, the hypothalamus, a part of the brain, is often seen as predominant. . . . The female brain-hormone-ovary system is usually described not as a feedback loop like a thermostat system, but as a hierarchy, in which the "directions" or "orders" of one element dominate (emphasis in the following quotes from medical texts is added):

Both positive and negative feedback control must be invoked, together with *superimposition* of control by the CNS through neurotransmitters released into the hypophyseal portal circulation.[7]

Almost all secretion by the pituitary is *controlled* by either hormonal or nervous signals from the hypothalamus.[8]

The hypothalamus is a collecting center for information concerned with the internal well-being of the body, and in turn much of this information is used *to control* secretions of the many globally important pituitary hormones.[9]

As Lein puts it into ordinary language, "The cerebrum, that part of the brain that provides awareness and mood, can play a significant role in the control of the menstrual cycle. . . . It seems evident that these higher regions of the brain exert their influence by modifying the actions of the hypothalamus. So even though the hypothalamus is a kind of master gland dominating the anterior pituitary, and through it the ovaries also, it does not act with complete independence or without influence from outside itself . . . there are also pathways of control from the higher centers of the brain."[10]

So this is a communication system organized hierarchically, not a committee reaching decisions by mutual influence.[11] The hierarchical nature of the organization is reflected in some popular literature meant to explain the nature of menstruation simply: "From first menstrual cycle to menopause, the hypothalamus acts as the conductor of a highly trained orchestra. Once its baton signals the downbeat to the pituitary, the hypothalamus-pituitary-ovarian axis is united in purpose and begins to play its symphonic message, preparing a woman's body for conception and child-bearing." Carrying the metaphor further, the follicles vie with each other for the role of producing the egg like violinists trying for the position of concertmaster; a burst of estrogen is emitted from the follicle like a "clap of tympani."[12]

The basic images chosen here—an information-transmitting, system with a hierarchical structure—have an obvious relation to the dominant form of organization in our society.[13] What I want to show is how this set of metaphors, once chosen as the basis for the description of physiological events, has profound implications for the way in which a change in the basic organization of the system will be perceived. In terms of female reproduction, this basic change is of course menopause. Many criticisms have been made of the medical propensity to see menopause as a pathological state.[14] I would like to suggest that the tenacity of this view comes not only from the negative stereotypes associated with aging women in our society, but as a logical outgrowth of seeing the body as a hierarchical information-processing system in the first place. (Another part of the reason menopause is seen so negatively is related to metaphors of production, which we discuss later in this chapter.)

What is the language in which menopause is described? In menopause, according to a college text, the ovaries become "unresponsive" to stimulation from the gonadotropins, to which they used to respond. As a result the ovaries "regress." On the other end of the cycle, the hypothalamus has gotten estrogen "addiction" from all those years of menstruating. As a result of the "withdrawal" of estrogen at menopause, the hypothalamus begins to give "inappropriate orders."[15] In a more popular account, "the pituitary gland during the change of life becomes disturbed when the ovaries fail to respond to its secretions, which tends to affect its control over other glands. This results in a temporary imbalance existing among all the endocrine glands of the body, which could very well lead to disturbances that may involve a person's nervous system."[16]

In both medical texts and popular books, what is being described is the breakdown of a system of authority. The cause of ovarian "decline" is the "decreasing ability of the aging ovaries to respond to pituitary gonadotropins."[17] At every point in this system, functions "fail" and falter. Follicles "fail to muster the strength" to reach ovulation.[18] As functions fall, so do the members of the system decline: "breasts and genital organs gradually atrophy,"[19] "wither,"[20] and become "senile."[21] Diminished, atrophied relics of the former vigorous, functioning selves, the "senile ovaries" are an example of the vivid imagery brought to this process. A text whose detailed illustrations make it a primary resource for medical students despite its early date describes the ovaries this way:

> The *senile ovary* is a shrunken and puckered organ, containing few if any follicles, and made up for the most part of old corpora albincantia and corpora atretica,

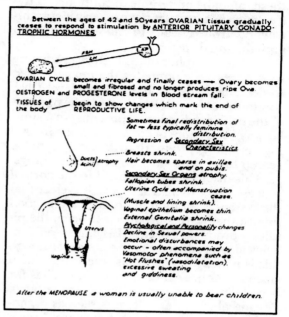

Figure 28-1
Menopause

Between the ages of 42 and 50years OVARIAN tissue gradually ceases to respond to stimulation by ANTERIOR PITUITARY GONADO-TROPHIC HORMONES.

OVARIAN CYCLE becomes irregular and finally ceases ⟶ Ovary becomes small and fibrosed and no longer produces ripe Ova.
OESTROGEN and PROGESTERONE levels in Blood stream fall.

TISSUES of the body — begin to show changes which mark the end of REPRODUCTIVE LIFE.

Sometimes final redistribution of fat ⟶ less typically feminine distribution.
Regression of Secondary Sex Characteristics.
Breasts shrink.
Hair becomes sparse in axillae and on pubis.
Secondary Sex Organs atrophy.
Fallopian tubes shrink.
Uterine Cycle and Menstruation cease.
(Muscle and lining shrink).
Vaginal epithelium becomes thin.
External Genitalia shrink.
Psychological and Personality changes
Decline in Sexual powers.
Emotional disturbances may occur - often accompanied by Vasomotor phenomena such as "Hot Flushes" (vasodilatation).
excessive sweating and giddiness.

Ducts] Atrophy
Acini]
Uterus
Vagina.

After the MENOPAUSE a woman is usually unable to bear children.

the bleached and functionless remainders of corpora lutia and follicles embedded in a dense connective tissue stroma.[22]

The illustration in Figure 28-1 summarizes the whole picture: ovaries cease to respond and fail to produce. Everywhere else there is regression, decline, atrophy, shrinkage, and disturbance.

The key to the problem connoted by these descriptions is functionlessness. Susan Sontag has written of our obsessive fear of cancer, a disease that we see as entailing a nightmare of excessive growth and rampant production. These images frighten us in part because in our stage of advanced capitalism, they are close to a reality we find difficult to see clearly: broken-down hierarchy and organization members who no longer play their designated parts represent nightmare images for us. . . . One woman I talked to said her doctor gave her two choices for treatment of her menopause: she could take estrogen and get cancer or she could not take it and have her bones dissolve. Like this woman, our imagery of the body as a hierarchical organization gives us no good choice when the basis of the organization seems to us to have changed drastically. We are left with breakdown, decay, and atrophy. Bad as they are, these might be preferable to continued activity, which because it is not properly hierarchically controlled, leads to chaos, unmanaged growth, and disaster.

... The metaphor of the factory producing substances ... dominates the imagery used to describe cells. At the cellular level DNA communicates with RNA, all for the purpose of the cell's production of proteins. In a similar way, the system of communication involving female reproduction is thought to be geared toward production of various things. ... This discussion is confined to the normal process of the menstrual cycle. It is clear that the system is thought to produce many good things: the ovaries produce estrogen, the pituitary produces FSH and LH, and so on. Follicles also produce eggs in a sense, although this is usually described as "maturing" them since the entire set of eggs a woman has for her lifetime is known to be present at birth. Beyond all this the system is seen as organized for a single preeminent purpose: "transport" of the egg along journey from the ovary to purpose: the uterus[23] and preparation of an appropriate place for the egg to grow if it is fertilized. In a chapter titled "Prepregnancy Reproductive Functions of the Female, and the Female Hormones," Guyton puts it all together: "Female reproductive functions can be divided into two major phases: first, preparation of the female body for conception and gestation, and second, the period of gestation itself."[24] This view may seem commonsensical and entirely justified by the evolutionary development of the species, with its need for reproduction to ensure survival.

Yet I suggest that assuming this view of the purpose for the process slants our description and understanding of the female cycle unnecessarily. Let us look at how medical textbooks describe menstruation. They see the action of progesterone and estrogen on the lining of the uterus as "ideally suited to provide a hospitable environment for implantation and survival of the embryo"[25] or as intended to lead to "the monthly renewal of the tissue that will cradle [the ovum]."[26] As Guyton summarizes, "The whole purpose of all these endometrial changes is to produce a

highly secretory endometrium containing large amounts of stored nutrients that can provide appropriate conditions for implantation of a fertilized ovum during the latter half of the monthly cycle."[27] Given this teleological interpretation of the purpose of the increased amount of endometrial tissue, it should be no surprise that when a fertilized egg does not implant, these texts describe the next event in very negative terms. The fall in blood progesterone and estrogen "deprives" the "highly developed endometrial lining of its hormonal support," "constriction" of blood vessels leads to a "diminished" supply of oxygen and nutrients, and finally "disintegration starts, the entire lining begins to slough, and the menstrual flow begins." Blood vessels in the endometrium "hemorrhage" and the menstrual flow "consists of this blood mixed with endometrial debris."[28] The "loss" of hormonal stimulation causes "necrosis" (death of tissue).[29]

The construction of these events in terms of a purpose that has failed is beautifully captured in a standard text for medical students (a text otherwise noteworthy for its extremely objective, factual descriptions) in which a discussion of the events covered in the last paragraph (sloughing, hemorrhaging) ends with the statement "When fertilization fails to occur, the endometrium is shed, and a new cycle starts. This is why it used to be taught that 'menstruation is the uterus crying for lack of a baby.'"[30]

I am arguing that just as seeing menopause as a kind of failure of the authority structure in the body contributes to our negative view of it, so does seeing menstruation as failed production contribute to our negative view of it. We have seen how Sontag describes our horror of production gone out of control. But another kind of horror for us is *lack* of production: the disused factory, the failed business, the idle machine. In his analysis of industrial civilization, Winner terms the stopping and breakdown of technological systems in modern society "apraxia" and describes it as "the ultimate horror, a condition to be avoided at all costs."[31] This horror of idle workers or machines seems to have been present even at earlier stages of industrialization. A nineteenth-century inventor, Thomas

Ewbank, elaborated his view that the whole world "was designed for a Factory."[32] "It is only as a Factory, a *General Factory*, that the whole materials and influences of the play."[33] In this great workshop, humans' role is to produce: "God employs no idlers—creates none."[34]

> Like artificial motors, we are created for the work we can do—for the useful and productive ideas we can stamp upon matter. Engines running daily without doing any work resemble men who live without labor; both are spendthrifts dissipating means that would be productive if given to others.[35]

Menstruation not only carries with it the connotation of a productive system that has failed to produce, it also carries the idea of production gone awry, making products of no use, not to specification, unsalable, wasted, scrap. However disgusting it may be, menstrual blood will come out. Production gone awry is also an image that fills us with dismay and horror. Amid the glorification of machinery common in the nineteenth century were also fears of what machines could do if they went out of control. Capturing this fear, one satirist wrote of a steam-operated shaving machine that "sliced the noses off too many customers."[36] This image is close to the one Melville created in "The Bell-Tower," in which an inventor, who can be seen as an allegory of America, is killed by his mechanical slave,[37] as well as to Mumford's sorcerer's apprentice applied to modern machinery:[38]

> Our civilization has cleverly found a magic formula for setting both industrial and academic brooms and pails of water to work by themselves, in ever-increasing quantities at an ever-increasing speed. But we have lost the Master Magician's spell for altering the tempo of this process, or halting it when it ceases to serve human functions and purposes.[39]

Of course, how much one is gripped by the need to produce goods efficiently and properly depends on one's relationship to those goods. While packing pickles on an assembly line, I remember the foreman often holding up improperly packed bottles to us workers and trying to elicit shame at the bad job we

were doing. But his job depended on efficient production, which meant many bottles filled right the first time. This factory did not yet have any effective method of quality control, and as soon as our supervisor was out of sight, our efforts went toward filling as few bottles as we could while still concealing who had filled which bottle. In other factories, workers seem to express a certain grim pleasure when they can register objections to company policy by enacting imagery of machinery out of control. Noble reports an incident in which workers resented a supervisor's order to "shut down their machines, pick up brooms, and get to work cleaning the area. But he forgot to tell them to stop." So, like the sorcerer's apprentice, diligently and obediently working to rule, they continued sweeping up all day long.[40]

Perhaps one reason the negative image of failed production is attached to menstruation is precisely that women are in some sinister sense out of control when they menstruate. They are not reproducing, not continuing the species, not preparing to stay at home with the baby, not providing a safe, warm womb to nurture a man's sperm. I think it is plain that the negative power behind the image of failure to produce can be considerable when applied metaphorically to women's bodies. Vern Bullough comments optimistically that "no reputable scientist today would regard menstruation as pathological,"[41] but this paragraph from a recent college text belies his hope:

> If fertilization and pregnancy do not occur, the corpus luteum degenerates and the levels of estrogen and progesterone decline. As the levels of these hormones decrease and their stimulatory effects are withdrawn, blood vessels of the endometrium undergo prolonged spasms (contractions) that reduce the bloodflow to the area of the endometrium supplied by the vessels. The resulting lack of blood causes the tissues of the affected region to degenerate. After some time, the vessels relax, which allows blood to flow through them again. However, capillaries in the area have become so weakened that blood leaks through them. This blood and the deteriorating endometrial tissue are discharged from the uterus as

the menstrual flow. As a new ovarian cycle begins and the level of estrogens rises, the functional layer of the endometrium undergoes repair and once again begins to proliferate.[42]

In rapid succession the reader is confronted with "degenerate," "decline," "withdrawn," "spasms," "lack," "degenerate," "weakened," "leak," "deteriorate," "discharge," and, after all that, "repair."

In another standard text, we read:

The sudden lack of these two hormones [estrogen and progesterone] causes the blood vessels of the endometrium to become spastic so that blood flow to the surface layers of the endometrium almost ceases. As a result, much of the endometrial tissue dies and sloughs into the uterine cavity. Then, small amounts of blood ooze from the denuded endometrial wall, causing a blood loss of about 50 ml during the next few days. The sloughed endometrial tissue plus the blood and much serous exudate from the denuded uterine surface, all together called the *mentrum,* is gradually expelled by intermittent contractions of the uterine muscle for about 3 to 5 days. This process is called *menstruation.*[43]

The imagery of catastrophic disintegration: "ceasing," "dying," "losing," "denuding," and "expelling." is not neutral; rather, these terms convey failure and dissolution. Of course, not all texts contain such a plethora of negative terms in their descriptions of menstruation. But unacknowledged cultural attitudes can seep into scientific writing through evaluative words. Coming at this point from a slightly different angle, consider this extract from a text that describes male reproductive physiology. "The mechanisms which guide the *remarkable* cellular transformation from spermatid to mature sperm remain uncertain. . . . Perhaps the most *amazing* characteristic of spermatogenesis is its *sheer magnitude:* the normal human male may manufacture several hundred million sperm per day (emphasis added)."[44] As we see, this text has no parallel appreciation of female processes such as menstruation or ovulation, and it is surely no accident that this "remarkable" process involves precisely

what menstruation does not in the medical view: production of something deemed valuable. Although this text sees such massive sperm production as unabashedly positive, in fact, only about one out of every 100 billion sperm ever makes it to fertilize an egg: from the very same point of view that sees menstruation as a waste product, surely here is something really worth crying about!

When this text turns to female reproduction, it describes menstruation in the same terms of failed production we saw earlier.

The fall in blood progesterone and estrogen, which results from *regression* of the corpus luteum, *deprives* the highly developed endometrial lining of its hormonal support; the immediate result is *profound constriction* of the uterine blood vessels due to production of vasoconstrictor prostaglandins, which leads to *diminished* supply of oxygen and nutrients. *Disintegration* starts, and the entire lining (except for a thin, deep layer which will regenerate the endometrium in the next cycle) begins to slough. . . . The endometrial arterioles dilate, resulting in *hemorrhage* through the weakened capillary walls; the menstrual flow consists of this blood mixed with endometrial *debris.* . . . The menstrual flow ceases as the endometrium *repairs* itself and then grows under the influence of rising blood estrogen concentration. [Emphasis added.][45]

And ovulation fares no better. In fact part of the reason ovulation does not merit the enthusiasm that spermatogenesis does may be that all the ovarian follicles containing ova are already present at birth. Far from being *produced* as sperm is, they seem to merely sit on the shelf, as it were, slowly degenerating and aging like overstocked inventory.

At birth, normal human ovaries contain an estimated one million follicles, and no new ones appear after birth. Thus, in marked contrast to the male, the newborn female already has all the germ cells she will ever have. Only a few, perhaps 400, are destined to reach full maturity during her active productive life. All the others degenerate at some point in their development so that few, if any, remain by the time she reaches menopause at approximately 50 years of age. One result of this is that the ova which are released (ovulated) near menopause are 30 to 35 years older than those ovulated just after puberty; it has been suggested that certain congenital defects, much commoner among children of older women, are the result of aging changes in the ovum.[46]

How different it would sound if texts like this one stressed the vast excess of follicles produced in a female fetus, compared to the number she will actually need. In addition, males are also born with a complement of germ cells (spermatogonia) that divide from time to time, and most of which will eventually differentiate into sperm. This text could easily discuss the fact that these male germ cells and their progeny are also subject to aging, much as female germ cells are. Although we would still be operating within the terms of the production metaphor, at least it would be applied in an evenhanded way to both males and females.

One response to my argument would be that menstruation just is in some objective sense a process of breakdown and deterioration. The particular words are chosen to describe it because they best fit the reality of what is happening. My counterargument is to look at other processes in the body that are fundamentally analogous to menstruation in that they involve the shedding of a lining to see whether they also are described in terms of breakdown and deterioration. The lining of the stomach, for example, is shed and replaced regularly, and seminal fluid picks up shedded cellular material as it goes through the various male ducts.

The lining of the stomach must protect itself against being digested by the hydrochloric acid produced in digestion. In the several texts quoted above, emphasis is on the *secretion* of mucus,[47] the *barrier* that mucus cells present to stomach acid,[48] and—in a phrase that gives the story away—the periodic *renewal* of the lining of the stomach.[49] There is no reference to degenerating, weakening, deteriorating, or repair, or even the more neutral shedding, sloughing, or replacement.

The primary function of the gastric secretions is to begin the digestion of proteins. Unfortunately, though, the wall of the stomach is itself constructed mainly of smooth muscle which itself is mainly protein. Therefore, the surface of the stomach must be exceptionally well protected at all times against its own digestion. This function is performed mainly by mucus that is secreted in great abundance in all parts of the stomach. The entire surface of the stomach is covered by a layer of very small *mucus cells* which themselves are composed almost entirely of mucus; this mucus prevents gastric secretions from ever touching the deeper layers of the stomach wall.[50]

In this account from an introductory physiology text, the emphasis is on production of mucus and protection of the stomach wall. It is not even mentioned, although it is analogous to menstruation, that the mucus cell layers must be continually sloughed off (and digested). Although all the general physiology texts I consulted describe menstruation as a process of disintegration needing repair, only specialized texts for medical students describe the stomach lining in the more neutral terms of "sloughing" and "renewal."[51] One can choose to look at what happens to the lining of stomachs and uteruses negatively as breakdown and decay needing repair or positively as continual production and replenishment. Of these two sides of the same coin, stomachs, which women *and* men have, fall on the positive side; uteruses, which only women have, fall on the negative.

One other analogous process is not handled negatively in the general physiology texts. Although it is well known to those researchers who work with male ejaculates that a very large proportion of the ejaculate is composed of shedded cellular material, the texts make no mention of a shedding process let alone processes of deterioration and repair in the male reproductive tract.[52]

What applies to menstruation once a month applies to menopause once in every lifetime. As we have seen, part of the current imagery attached to menopause is that of a breakdown of central control. Inextricably connected to this imagery is another aspect of failed production. Recall the metaphors of balanced intake and outgo that were applied to menopause up to the mid-nineteenth century, later to be replaced by metaphors of degeneration. In the early 1960s, new research on the role of estrogens in heart disease led to arguments that failure of female reproductive organs to produce much estrogen after menopause was debilitating to health.

This charge is marked unmistakably in successive editions of a major gynecology text. In the 1940s and 1950s, menopause was described as usually not entailing "any very profound alteration in the woman's life current."[53] By the 1965 edition dramatic changes had occurred: "In the past few years there has been a radical change in viewpoint and some would regard the menopause as a possible pathological state rather than a physiological one and discuss therapeutic prevention rather than the amelioration of symptoms."[54]

In many current accounts, menopause is described as a state in which ovaries fail to produce estrogens.[55] The 1981 World Health Organization report defines menopause as an estrogen-deficiency disease.[56] Failure to produce estrogen is the leitmotif of another current text: "This period during which the cycles cease and the female sex hormones diminish rapidly to almost none at all is called the *menopause*. The cause of the menopause is the 'burning out' of the ovaries. . . . Estrogens are produced in subcritical quantities for a short time after the menopause, but over a few years, as the final remaining primordial follicles become atretic, the production of estrogens by the ovaries falls almost to zero." Loss of ability to produce estrogen is seen as central to a woman's life: "At the time of the menopause a woman must readjust her life from one that has been physiologically stimulated by estrogen and progesterone production to one devoid of those hormones."[57]

Of course, I am not implying that the ovaries do not indeed produce much less estrogen than before. I am pointing to the choice of these textbook authors to emphasize above all else the negative aspects of ovaries failing to produce female hormones. By contrast, one current text shows us a positive view of the decline in estrogen production: "It would seem that although menopausal women do have an estrogen milieu which is lower than that necessary for *reproductive* function, it is not negligible or absent but is perhaps satisfactory for *maintenance* of *support tissues*.

The menopause could then be regarded as a physiologic phenomenon which is protective in nature—protective from undesirable reproduction and the associated growth stimuli."[58]

I have presented the underlying metaphors contained in medical descriptions of menopause and menstruation to show that these ways of describing events are but one method of fitting an interpretation to the facts. Yet seeing that female organs are imagined to function within a hierarchical order whose members signal each other to produce various substances, all for the purpose of transporting eggs to a place where they can be fertilized and then grown, may not provide us with enough of a jolt to begin to see the contingent nature of these descriptions. Even seeing that the metaphors we choose fit very well with traditional roles assigned to women may still not be enough to make us question whether there might be another way to represent the same biological phenomena. . . . Here I suggest some other ways that these physiological events could be described.

First, consider the teleological nature of the system, its assumed goal of implanting a fertilized egg. What if a woman has done everything in her power to avoid having an egg implant in her uterus, such as birth control or abstinence from heterosexual sex. Is it still appropriate to speak of the single purpose of her menstrual cycle as dedicated to implantation? From the woman's vantage point, it might capture the sense of events better to say the purpose of the cycle is the production of menstrual flow. Think for a moment how that might change the description in medical texts: "A drop in the formerly high levels of progesterone and estrogen creates the appropriate environment for reducing the excess layers of endometrial tissue. Constriction of capillary blood vessels causes a lower level of oxygen and nutrients and paves the way for a vigorous production of menstrual fluids. As a part of the renewal of the remaining endometrium, the capillaries begin to reopen, contributing some blood and serous fluid to the volume of endometrial material already beginning to flow." I can see no reason why the menstrual blood itself could not be seen as the desired "product" of the female cycle, except when the woman intends to become pregnant.

Would it be similarly possible to change the nature of the relationships assumed among the members of the organization—the hypothalamus, pituitary, ovaries, and so on? Why not, instead of an organization with a controller, a team playing a game? When a woman wants to get pregnant, it would be appropriate to describe her pituitary, ovaries, and so on as combining together, communicating with each other, to get the ball, so to speak, into the basket. The image of hierarchical control could give way to specialized function, the way a basketball team needs a center as well as a defense. When she did not want to become pregnant, the purpose of this activity could be considered the production of menstrual flow.

Eliminating the hierarchical organization and the idea of a single purpose to the menstrual cycle also greatly enlarges the ways we could think of menopause. A team which in its youth played vigorous soccer might, in advancing years, decide to enjoy a quieter "new game" where players still interact with each other in satisfying ways but where gentle interaction itself is the point of the game, not getting the ball into the basket—or the flow into the vagina.

Notes

1. Lein 1979: 14
2. Guyton 1986: 885
3. Benson 1982: 129
4. Netter 1965: 115
5. Norris 1984: 6
6. Dalton and Greene 1983: 6
7. Mountcastle 1980: 1615
8. Guyton 1986: 885
9. Guyton 1986: 885
10. Lein 1979: 84
11. Evelyn Fox Keller 1985: 154-56 documents the pervasiveness of hierarchical models at the cellular level.
12. Norris 1984: 6
13. Giddens 1975: 185
14. McCrea 1983
15. Lein 1979: 79, 97
16. O'Neill 1982: 11
17. Vander et al. 1985: 598
18. Norris 1983: 181
19. Vander et al. 1985: 598
20. Norris 1983: 181
21. Netter 1965: 121
22. Netter 1965: 116
23. Vander et al. 1985: 580
24. Guyton 1986: 968
25. Vander et al. 1985: 576
26. Lein 1979: 43
27. Guyton 1986: 976
28. Vander et al. 1985: 577
29. Guyton 1986: 976; see very similar accounts in Lein 1979: 69, Mountcastle 1980: 1612, Mason 1983: 518, Benson 1982: 128-29.
30. Ganong 1985: 63
31. Winner 1977: 185, 187
32. Ewbank 1855: 21-22
33. Ewbank 1855: 23
34. Ewbank 1855: 27
35. Ewbank 1855: 141; on Ewbank, see Kasson 1976: 148-51.
36. Fisher 1967: 153
37. Fisher 1967: 153; 1966
38. Mumford 1967: 282
39. Mumford 1970: 180
40. Noble 1984: 312
41. Bullough 1975: 298
42. Mason 1983: 525
43. Guyton 1984: 624
44. Vander et al. 1980: 483-84. The latest edition of this text has removed the first of these sentences, but kept the second (Vander et al. 1985: 557).
45. Vander et al. 1985: 577
46. Vander et al. 1985: 567, 568
47. Mason 1983: 419; Vander et al. 1985: 483
48. Ganong 1986: 776
49. Mason 1983: 423
50. Guyton 1984: 498-99
51. Sernka and Jacobson 1983: 7
52. Vander et al. 1985: 557-58; Ganong 1985: 356
53. Novak 1944: 536; Novak and Novak 1952: 600
54. Novak et al. 1965: 642
55. See McCrea and Markle 1984 for the very different clinical treatment for this lack in the United States and the United Kingdom.
56. Kaufert and Gilbert 1986: 8-9; World Health Organization Scientific Group 1981
57. Guyton 1986: 979

58. Jones and Jones 1981: 799

References

Benson, Ralph C. 1982. *Current Obstetric and Gynecologic Diagnosis and Treatment*. Los Altos, CA: Lange Medical Publishers.

Bullough, Vern L. 1975. "Sex and the Medical Model." *The Journal of Sex Research* II (4):291-303.

Dalton, Katharina and Raymond Greene. 1983. "The Premenstrual Syndrome." *British Medical Journal* May: 1016-17.

Ewbank, Thomas. 1855. *The World a Workshop: or the Physical Relationship of Man to the Earth*. New York: Appleton.

Fisher, Marvin. 1967. *Workshops in the Wilderness: The European Response to American Industrialization, 1830-1860*. New York: Oxford University Press.

Ganong, William F. 1983. *Review of Medical Physiology*. 11th Edition. Los altos, CA: Lange.

Giddens, Anthony. 1975. *The Class Structure of the Advanced Societies*. New York: Harper and Row.

Guyton, Arthur C. 1981. *Textbook of Medical Physiology*. Philadelphia, W.B. Saunders.

——. 1984. *Physiology of the Human Body*. 6th Edition. Philadelphia: Saunders College Publishing.

——. 1986. *Textbook of Medical Physiology*. 7th Edition. Philadelphia: W.B. Saunders.

Jones, Howard W. and Georgeanna Seegar Jones. 1981. *Novak's Textbook of Gynecology*. 10th Edition. Baltimore, MD: Williams and Wilkins.

Kasson, John F. 1976. *Civilizing the Machine: Technology and Republican Values in America 1776-1900*. New York: Penguin.

Kaufert, Patricia A. and Penny Gilbert. 1986. "Women, Menopause and Medicalization." *Culture, Medicine and Psychiatry* 10(1): 7-21.

Keller, Evelyn Fox. 1985. *Reflections on Gender and Science*. New Haven, CT: Yale University Press.

Lein, Allen. 1979. *The Cycling Female: Her Menstrual Rhythm*. San Francisco: W.H. Freeman.

Mason, Elliott B. 1983. *Human Physiology*. Menlo Park, CA: Benjamin Cummings Publishing Co.

McCrea, Frances B. 1983. "The Politics of Menopause: The 'Discovery' of a Deficiency Disease." *Social Problems* 31(1): 111-23.

McCrea, Frances B. and Gerald E. Markle. 1984. "The Estrogen Replacement Controversy in the USA and UK: Different Answers to the Same Question?" *Social Studies of Science* 14: 1-26.

McNaught, Ann B. and Robin Callander. 1983. *Illustrated Physiology*. 4th Edition. Edinburgh: Churchill Livingstone.

Mountcastle, Vernon B. 1980. *Medical Physiology*. 14th Edition, V. II. St. Louis, MO: C.V. Mosby Co.

Mumford, Lewis. 1967. *The Myth of the Machine: Technics and Human Development*. V.I. New York: Harcourt, Brace and World.

——. 1970. *The Myth of the Machine: The Pentagon of Power*. V.2. New York: Harcourt, Brace and World.

Netter, Frank H. 1965. *A Compilation of Paintings on the Normal and Pathologic Anatomy of the Reproductive System*. The CIBA Collection of Medical Illustrations, V. II. Summit, NJ: CIBA.

Noble, David. 1984. *The Forces of Production*. New York: Berkeley Books.

Norris, Ronad V. 1984. *PMS: Premenstrual Syndrome*. New York: Simon and Schuster.

Novak, Edmund, Georgeanna Seegar Jones, and Howard W. Jones. 1965. *Novak's Textbook of Gynecology*. 7th Edition. Baltimore, MD: Williams and Wilkins Co.

Novak, Emil. 1944. *Textbook of Gynecology*. 2nd Edition. Baltimore, MD: Williams and Wilkins Co.

Novak, Emil and Edmund Novak. 1952. *Textbook of Gynecology*. Baltimore, MD: Williams and Wilkins Co.

O'Neill, Daniel J. 1982. *Menopause and Its Effect on the Family*. Washington, DC: University Press of America.

Sernka, Thomas and Eugene Jacobson. 1983. *Gastrointestinal Physiology: The Essentials*. Baltimore: Williams and Wilkins.

Vander, Arthur J., James H. Sherman, and Dorothy S. Luciano. 1980. *Human Physiology: The Mechanisms of Body Function* 3rd Edition. New York: McGraw Hill.

Vander, Arthur J., James H. Sherman, and Dorothy S. Luciano. 1985. *Human Physiology: The Mechanisms of Body Function*. 4th Edition. New York: McGraw-Hill.

Winner, Langdon. 1977. *Autonomous Technology: Technics-out-of-Control as a Theme in Political Thought*. Cambridge: MIT Press.

World Health Organization Scientific Group. 1981. *Research on the Menopause*. World Health Organization Technical Report Series 670. Geneva: World Health Organization.

Further Reading

George Lakoff and Mark Johnson. 1981. *Metaphors We Live By*. Chicago: University of Chicago Press.

Frances McCrea. 1983. "The Politics of Menopause: The Discovery of a Deficiency Disease." *Social Problems* 13: 111-123.

Sonja M. McKinlay, D. J. Brambilla, N.E. Avis, and John B. McKinlay. 1991. "Women's Experience of the Menopause." *Current Obstetrics and Gynaecology* 1:3-7.

Discussion Questions

1. What are the most significant metaphors Martin identifies? Why are they significant?

2. How have you used metaphors to think and talk about health, illness, and care?

3. How might metaphors reflect dominant socio-historical themes and trends?

29

The Rise of the Surgical Fix

Kathy Davis

In this selection, Kathy Davis notes changes in the development of plastic surgery from reconstructive uses to reshaping otherwise healthy bodies. Like Emily Martin, Davis refers to the body metaphorically in her discussion of plastic surgery. She draws a relationship between bodies and objects like automobiles and houses. Her metaphor of the body as an object allows us to imagine how bodies, like automobiles and houses, might be shaped, remodelled, transformed into better, more improved versions of the self. As with material objects, bodies, due to surgical technology and innovations, can now take a multitude of forms and figures. Consider what popularizing cosmetic surgery through TV talk shows and advertisements does for individual bodies and for the industry of cosmetic surgery. Bodies are embedded in social and cultural processes.

Cosmetic surgery has indeed become a business, and nearly ninety percent of all operations are performed on women. Think about the socio-cultural factors that make women's bodies better targets for surgeons than men's bodies. We see that cosmetic surgery as a market commodity is a peculiarly American form. Yet, when consumers request a particular kind of health care and have the resources to finance it, who becomes responsible for ensuring its safety? Given the high demand for cosmetic surgery in the United States and the cultural context in which it has developed, is it reasonable to expect medical professionals or policy makers to restrict the growth of the cosmetic surgery market? As you read this selection by Davis, consider the issues central to quality of care that are not being addressed by medical professionals or by policy makers.

Plastic Surgery in Retrospect

Plastic surgery has a long history. As early as 1,000 B.C., the first plastic surgery was reported in India, where a person's nose might be cut off as a form of punishment or, in the case of an adulterous Hindu wife, bitten off by the wronged husband. Procedures which displayed remarkable similarity to present rhinoplasties were developed to reconstruct the noses of such errant individuals (Gabke and Vaubel 1983: 29). Plastic surgery appeared on the European continent considerably later. In the early fifteenth century, the Sicilian physician Branca began doing nose surgery, using a flap of skin from the patient's arm which was immobilized by binding it to the nose until the graft could take. Other forms of plastic surgery began to appear around the early sixteenth century and were sporadically performed up until the late nineteenth century on individuals with congenital abnormalities or with deformities due to diseases like leprosy or syphilis. Harelips and cleft palates could be repaired, ears corrected, and breasts amputated in the case of tumors.

Although techniques for surgically altering the appearance of the human body have been available for centuries, the development of the field has nevertheless been slow. This is hardly surprising. The emergence of plastic surgery is linked to the development of medicine as well as to changing cultural notions about the alteration of the body. Prior to 1846 when ether and chloroform were discovered, surgery had to be done without anesthesia. Surgeries done under these conditions would have inevitably been traumatic for the patient and probably for the physician as well. If patients did not die from shock or loss of blood, the chance that they would perish from infection was imminent. Before the discovery of antisepsis in 1867, it is a wonder that patients managed to survive surgery at all.[1]

In addition, the body was thought to be the corporeal manifestation of the relationship between God and man, with disease a deformity being due to the consequences of immorality (Turner 1984; Finkelstein 1991). Leprosy or small pox were divine punishment for sins committed, a monstrous infant the result of the mother's promiscuous behavior. In this context, surgical intervention took on a slightly blasphemous character as it disturbed the natural order of things and eliminated the marks of punishment. Early facial surgery, a case in point, was frequently employed to repair the ravages of syphilis. The lowly status of the surgeon, who was up until the seventeenth century little more than a local barber, further accounts for plastic surgery being regarded as a slightly disreputable practice.

With the development of medicine as a science, surgery underwent a general rehabilitation. Surgeons were required to have a university education, setting them apart from other lay practitioners. Medical science replaced traditional beliefs linking the physical body to the person's moral character and propagated the merits of observation and classification. Under the all-encompassing medical gaze, every aspect of the body became a welcome object for scrutiny, including abnormalities in bodily appearance. While the status of surgery improved, it took the phenomenon of mass warfare to eliminate the moral onus attached to plastic surgery and to enable it to emerge as a full-fledged specialty.

The Crimean war and both world wars produced a large number of casualties. Thousands of young men were severely burned or disfigured during battle. Surgeons were sent to the front en masse to fix mutilated faces, reconstruct severed body parts, and repair burns, thereby gaining invaluable practice in their craft. Enormous strides were made in developing techniques for reconstructing limbs and hands and for repairing badly scarred or burned skin. In the process, plastic surgery underwent something of a moral face lift as well. It became associated with deserving heroes, injured in the course of doing their patriotic duty, rather than with the mere victims of an unkind fate who were expected to bear their suffering with fortitude. In short, plastic surgery became a respectable field of medicine.

In the years that followed, surgery continued to be performed for reconstructive purposes—that is, for restoring physical dysfunction or for minimizing disfigurement due to disease, congenital deformity, or accident. The emergence of cosmetic procedures in the mid-twentieth century dramatically altered the field of plastic surgery, marking a new phase in its history. Whereas nearly all plastic surgery in the first part of the century was done to alleviate deformities due to disease, birth, or mishap, in the second half of the century this was no longer the case. Plastic surgery began to be performed for the aesthetic improvement of otherwise healthy bodies and the number of operations increased dramatically.

The rise in cosmetic surgery was spurred on by improvements in surgical procedures and technologies. Air drills for cutting bone and planing skin, binocular magnifying lenses, precision instruments, and refined suturing materials all enabled surgical interventions to be performed with better results and less trauma for the patient (Meredith 1988). Improved technology is only part of the explanation, however. With the advent of cosmetic surgery, the rationale for surgical intervention in bodily appearance changed and along with it, the kinds of technologies being developed. It was not only done for different reasons, but the scale on which it was performed shifted. The extension of plastic surgery into the realm of body improvement has led to a veritable boom in cosmetic surgery—a kind of "Surgical Age" (Wolf 1991). Cosmetic surgery became, for the first time, a mass phenomenon. Today cosmetic operations make up well over forty percent of all plastic surgery, and where previously patients were men disabled by war or industrial accidents, now the recipients are overwhelmingly women who are dissatisfied with the way their bodies look.[2]

In this selection, I explore the rise of this surgical age. I consider how cosmetic surgery could become such a popular phenomenon as well as the risks and dangers associated with it. Finally, I examine how the tensions between the enormous expansion of cosmetic surgery and its shadow side are dealt with in public discourse, contrasting how the surgical fix is dealt with in the U.S. and abroad.

Plastic Bodies

The development of cosmetic surgery technology is inextricably connected to a market model of medicine, on the one hand, and to a consumer culture, on the other. With the rise of medicine as a profession, medical cures and services become something which could be obtained for a fee. In an open market system, the patient is a consumer and, like consumers of other products, free to choose any treatment, provided it can be paid for. The body is no longer simply a dysfunctional object requiring medical intervention, but a commodity not unlike "a car, a refrigerator, a house—which can be continuously upgraded and modified in accordance with new interests and greater resources" (Finkelstein 1991: 87). It can be endlessly manipulated—reshaped, restyled, and reconstructed to meet prevailing fashions and cultural values.

Modern cosmetic surgery technology sustains and is a product of the notion of the body as "cultural plastic"—"a construction of life as plastic possibility and weightless choice, undetermined by history, social location, or even individual biography" (Bordo 1990: 657). The technologies of cosmetic surgery assume the makeability of the human body, expanding the limits of how the body may be restyled, reshaped and rebuilt. A twin "disdain for material limits" and an "intoxication with change" (ibid., p. 654) make the possibilities for surgical intervention both desirable and endless. Nowhere is this more tellingly manifested than in the use of computer technology whereby potential recipients are given a preview of how they might look after a face lift, or breast augmentation. The patient is photographed and the image is duplicated on the screen. The surgeon (God and artist, all in one) uses an electronic pencil on a special board to make the desired changes while the patient watches. Flesh is added or taken away, wrinkles disappear, breasts are inflated, or body shape is transformed. The makeability of the body and the power of medical technology are visually sustained in each demonstration (Balsamo 1993).

Cosmetic surgery is the cultural product of modernity and of a consumer culture which treats the body as a vehicle for self-expression (Featherstone 1983; 1990; Turner 1984; Finkelstein 1991; Bordo 1990; Giddens 1991). By engaging in a wide array of available body maintenance routines, individuals are encouraged to seek their salvation through altering their appearance. ("You are the way you look.") Along with the beauty, fitness, and diet industries, medical technologies can be drawn upon to help turn back the biological clock—to combat the natural deterioration of the body which accompanies age and the rigors of everyday life. The notion of Nature-as-the-ultimate constraint is replaced by Nature-as-something-to-be-improved-upon. Whereas plastic surgery was formerly aimed at repairing bodily deficiencies which made a person noticeably different from the rest of the world, it increasingly came to be seen as a normal intervention for essentially normal bodies. Bodies no longer have to be damaged or impaired to merit surgical alteration. Growing older, gaining or losing weight, or simply failing to meet the transitory cultural norms of beauty are now sufficient cause for surgical improvement. Cosmetic surgery allows us to transcend age, ethnicity, and even sex itself.[3]

From Celebrity Junkie to the Girl Next Door

Cosmetic surgery has increasingly become a mass phenomenon, with the media playing an essential role in making it acceptable for an ever growing population. Initially, it was associated with the rich and famous (the jet set, celebrities, pop singers). Tales of the surgical exploits of Farah Dibah, Raquel Welch, Sophia Loren, Jane Fonda, Michael Jackson, Joan Collins, and others abounded as the media regaled us with descriptions of lavish clinics where they enjoyed gourmet meals and private suites, along with their face lifts and body sculpting.[4] Models, news commentators, or actresses whose work puts them in the public eye have come to consider cosmetic surgery part of the job. In Beverly Hills, plastic surgeons have their own publicity firms and even accept Visa and MasterCard[5]. The undisputed queen of cosmetic surgery is the pop singer and actress Cher, who has reputedly undergone dozens of operations. She has spent over seventy-five thousand dollars on altering her body ("My body is my capital."), having her stomach corrected to give her navel a "girlish look," her dimples enhanced with silicone, and, most dramatically, two ribs removed to emphasize her waist. By chronicling the operative histories of individuals who are already considered by the public to be beautiful, the media makes its message clear: no one is so beautiful that she cannot become even more so with the help of surgery.

The first articles on cosmetic surgery began to appear between 1965 and 1975, and the end of 1975 marked the beginning of a new era with an increase of nearly two hundred percent in the number published (Dull and West 1987: 3). Upscale glossies like *Vogue, Cosmopolitan*, or *Self* as well as most daily newspapers today regularly feature advertisements for clinics specializing in such surgery. Women's magazines frequently provide personal testimonies of the "before and after" variety, which depict women's experiences with various kinds of operations. A typical article describes an ordinary, young, professional woman who "just wants to feel a little better" by having her breasts augmented.[6] She is not portrayed as a celebrity ("My breasts never dominated my life, not like other women.") and her motives seem imminently reasonable—after all, who wouldn't want to feel better? The reader is subsequently taken behind the scenes as she goes through the procedure. Potential unpleasantness and difficulties are downplayed in pictures which show the patient lying bare-breasted and smiling on the operating table with circles drawn where the surgeon will cut. ("Here is C., right before the operation. . . [I]n just over an hour, the silicone implants will be sitting pretty.") Having a breast augmentation becomes a kind of adventure, something to look forward to in pleasant anticipation. The story has a happy ending, the patient emerging with a new body and a boost to her self-confidence as well.

Although magazines occasionally feature a personal testimony about a failed operation ("My life was ruined after having a nose job."), the mishap tends to be attributed to medical malpractice rather than to problems inherent in the operation itself. The patient is simply unfortunate in having run into the one bad apple in the otherwise exemplary bunch of plastic surgeons. In general, surgery is presented as a relatively harmless way to improve appearance—an acceptable path toward happiness and well-being.

There is, of course, the problem of the "plastic surgery junkie"— the individual who indulges in "plastic surgery the way some of us eat chocolate—compulsively.[7]" Undeterred by the cost, pain, or terrible bruising, those who are pathologically addicted to having their bodies remade or beautified through surgery cannot be stopped. Although cases of repeated cosmetic surgery receive considerable media attention, the addiction of the recipients tends to be normalized in such public discourse. In her discussion of television's treatment of the cosmetic surgery boom, Dull (1989) shows how "scalpel slaves" may be used to promote the advantages of cosmetic surgery to the general public. For example, in 1986 Oprah Winfrey invited people who had as many as nine cosmetic operations to share their surgical resumes on her show. As the program progressed, the audience's horror and skepticism were gradually transformed. They no longer viewed this involvement as a sign of addiction, but began to see it as simply a matter of being "prosurgery"—an imminently reasonable choice among all the other choices available to the modern individual.[8]

In short, the media constructs cosmetic surgery as an option which is not only available to everyone, but which bears the promise of an exalted life—one can partake in what was formerly available to the chosen few. Or, as Featherstone (1983) puts it:

[T]he imagery of consumer culture presents a world of ease and comfort, once the privilege of an elite, now apparently within the reach of all. An ideology of personal consumption presents individuals as free to do their own thing, to construct their own little world in the private sphere (p. 21).

In such a climate, it is not surprising that cosmetic surgery would seem to be more and more of an option for everyone. Despite its cost, it is available for even those who would normally doubt that they could afford it.

The Cosmetic Surgery Boom

Cosmetic surgery is big business. In the U.S., it takes its place alongside the twenty billion dollar cosmetics industry and the thirty-three billion dollar diet industry as one of the most rapidly expanding fields in the beauty system today (Wolf 1991). Three hundred million dollars are spent every year on cosmetic surgery and the amount is increasing annually by ten percent. Operations are expensive, ranging from two hundred fifty dollars for a chemical face peel to over five thousand dollars for an abdominoplasty, or tummy tuck.[9] The average plastic surgeon makes a profit of $180,000 a year, earning nearly double the income of a family practitioner, pediatrician, or internist and considerably more than what the average obstetrician or gynecologist would earn.[10]

In 1988, more than two million Americans underwent some form of cosmetic surgery. This figure was up from 590,550 in 1986 and it continues to skyrocket.[11] In the U.S., the number of operations doubled every five years, until it tripled between 1984 and 1986 (Wolf 1991: 251). The situation is no different in many European countries. Within the last decade, cosmetic surgery has doubled in Great Britain. As Wolf graphically describes it: "a city the size of San Francisco gets cut open every year in the United States; in Britain, a village the size of Bath." In Germany one hundred eighty million marks are spent annually on cosmetic surgery. More than one hundred thousand Germans have such surgery each year, including ten percent from East Germany (a "new face for a new boss from the West").[12] In the Netherlands it is estimated that between ten and twenty thousand cosmetic surgery operations are performed every year. Since 1982, operations have doubled in frequency and eyelid corrections and tummy tucks are up five hundred and three hundred percent respectively, since 1975 (Starmans 1988).

Nearly ninety percent of the operations are performed on women: all breast corrections, ninety-one percent of face lifts, eighty-six percent of eyelid reconstructions, and sixty-one percent of all nose surgery. In 1987, American women had 94,000 breast reconstructions, 85,000 eyelid corrections, 82,000 nose jobs, 73,230 liposuctions, and 67,000 face lifts—nine times more operations than men had (American Society for Plastic and Reconstructive Surgeons 1987). The only procedures which are performed primarily on men are hair transplants (ninety-five percent) and ear surgery (forty-four percent) (National Center for Health Statistics 1987). Despite reports that men are having faces and necks lifted and sagging eyelids corrected to give them a "competitive advantage" in the business world, women continue to be the primary objects of surgical intervention.[13] Whereas the majority of cosmetic surgery operations have been performed on white women, in 1990 it was estimated that twenty percent of the cosmetic surgery patients in the U.S. were Latinos, African Americans, and Asian Americans. Of these, over sixty percent were women (Kaw 1993).[14]

Cosmetic surgery is the fastest growing specialty in American medicine (Faludi 1991: 217). Whereas the total number of physicians has little more than doubled in the last quarter of a century, the number of plastic surgeons has increased fourfold. At the end of World War II, there were only about one hundred plastic surgeons in the U.S. In 1965, there were 1,133 plastic surgeons and in 1990, the number of plastic surgeons had reached 3,850.[15] In Southern California alone, there are 289 practitioners. By 1988, the caseload of registered surgeons had more than doubled, to 750,000 operations annually. Since at least ninety percent of cosmetic surgery is performed in a physician's office or a private clinic,[16] it is not necessary to be a plastic surgeon to be able to perform cosmetic surgery. Face lifts, eyelid corrections, or chemical peeling may be performed by a dermatologist, while otorhinolaryngologists (ENT-specialists) are engaging in nose and ear corrections. There are no standard procedures for preoperative screening and less concern for quality control than would be the case in a hospital setting.[17]

New Technologies

Cosmetic surgery began with the application of reconstructive procedures to recipients who were not disfigured through birth, disease, or accident, but were concerned with improving their appearance. Although this distinction is not always easy to make, plastic surgeons now emphasize the difference between surgery for reconstructive purposes and surgery for aesthetic or cosmetic reasons. In fact, plastic surgeons in the U.S. belong to separate professional organizations from cosmetic surgeons and have different access to medical insurance. Consequently, they have different kinds of patients as well as different status. Although reconstructive surgeons earn less money, their work does not carry the commercial taint attached to surgery for aesthetic purposes. Nor do they face the difficulties of having to justify doing surgery without a clear-cut medical indication.[18]

While much of the growth in plastic surgery has been in cosmetic surgery, it often seems to be a matter of taking earlier reconstructive technologies and putting them to new uses. For example, rhinoplasties, the oldest form of plastic surgery, are now performed in response to the patient's desire to meet a cultural ideal (Millard 1974)—creating "the nose best suited for the individual face."[19] Nose contouring is currently regarded as a solution for "teen angst" and is an increasingly popular graduation gift for adolescents concerned that their noses are too large/too flat/too ethnic to meet the current standards of facial appearance.[20] Ear surgery (otoplasty) has also expanded its horizons (Huffstadt 1981). A relatively simple operation which was frequently performed on the "jug ears" of school-age children is now being perfected to ever more refined interventions. Earlobe reductions have become the "latest nip-and-tuck": overly-long earlobes ("a much overlooked sign of aging") are trimmed down to twenty-five percent of the total ear (a more "ideal" format).[21] Once done to alleviate vision impairment due to sagging eyelids, double eyelid surgery is increasingly employed to westernize the eyes of Asian businessmen, consumer-conscious Korean housewives (Finkelstein 1991) and, more recently, Asian American women (Kaw 1993). Braces and the capping of teeth, which used to be the province of orthodontists, has now been transformed into cosmetic dentistry—a rising specialty which can involve a radical reconstruction of the entire face and jaw for aesthetic purposes. In each case, old techniques are refined or applied to different kinds of patients.

In addition, new medical technologies and procedures have been developed since the early sixties which belong exclusively to the domain of cosmetic surgery. For example, face lifts, breast augmentations, and fat removal or body contouring are the most frequently performed procedures. They are done almost exclusively on women for aesthetic or cosmetic reasons.[22] Because these newer procedures mark a shift in both the practice of surgically altering bodily appearance as well as in cultural discourses about the human body, I will discuss them in more detail.

Face Lifts

Although face lifting was first developed in France in 1919, it took another fifty years before it was done to any great extent (Huffstadt 1981). In the U.S., rhytodectomies (the word comes from the Greek word for wrinkle) are now the third most common form of cosmetic surgery. They are performed to smooth out wrinkles or eliminate the sags and puffiness associated with age or the ravages of sunbathing, poor nutrition, smoking, or excessive drinking. The operation involves making an incision from the temples to the front of the ear and then behind the ear to the back of the head. The facial and neck skin are then lifted from the underlying skin and pulled toward the incision. The overlapping skin is cut off and the new edge is sewed to the scalp. It has been compared to "lifting off a wrinkled piece of plastic wrap, smoothing it out and putting it back again."[23]

Face lifts are not the solution for everyone and, as Finkelstein (1991) notes, the ideal candidate often seems to be the one who least needs it. To be ensured of success, the patient should be "of slender build, with soft, smooth skin and minimal sub-cutaneous fat, with a family story of youthful aging, without serious illness, emotional trauma, or weight fluctuation after operation, and with the desire and skill to augment the surgical improvement by makeup, hairstyling, and enhancing clothes (Goldwyn 1980: 693). Surgeons, in fact, recommend that face lifts should only be performed on patients who already have demonstrated concern for their appearance. For those who do not display the "appropriate concern for their appearance," a trip to the local farm is recommended instead (Huffstadt 1981).

Despite these restrictions, more than sixty-seven thousand American women had their faces lifted in 1987—nearly ten times more than the seven thousand male recipients in the same year (American Society of Plastic and Reconstructive Surgeons 1987). The typical face-lift candidate is described as a well-to-do, fashionably-dressed, middle-aged woman between the ages of forty-five and sixty who anticipates having to attract a new mate after a divorce or simply wants to hold her own on the job in the face of younger competition.[24] However, face lifts are increasingly being done on younger women as well. Ever on the lookout for new recipients, one enterprising surgeon found prisons provided a new market for his services. Some female prisoners suffered from "premature aging of the skin due to extensive use of drugs and poor nutrition;" others wanted to have needle marks removed.[25]

Face lifts often go hand in hand with additional surgical procedures. Eyelid corrections take care of telltale sagging or eliminate puffiness associated with fatigue, heavy drinking, or depression. Silicone may be implanted into chin or cheeks to fatten up faces shrunken by age or simply not lush enough to meet current standards of beauty. Dimples can be created surgically in cheeks or a chin enhanced with a ruggedly handsome cleft (Rees and Wood-Smith 1973: 510-511). Collagen treatments which involve pumping a protein directly into the skin to plump out the fine lines are becoming increasingly popular.

Face lifts and associated procedures do take off years, but they are not permanent. They have to be redone. For example, surgeons recommend that the patient should have her or his first face lift in the early to mid-forties, the second in the fifties, and the third in the sixties and so on. (Rees and Wood-Smith 1973). Moreover, since collagen is quickly absorbed by the body, this kind of treatment is only of temporary benefit and has to be repeated, sometimes more than once a year. It becomes, literally, a form of body maintenance—not unlike getting a permanent or having a facial.[26]

For individuals who cannot afford this kind of maintenance—maintenance which can run up to a total of eight thousand dollars—less drastic procedures for rejuvenating the face are available. Chemical peeling (dissolving the top layers of the skin with acid) or dermabrasion (sanding down the skin with a machine-powered wire brush) can delay face lifts or be used to eliminate fine facial wrinkles caused by exposure to the sun or smoking, acne scars, and other blemishes (Meredith 1988).

Breast Augmentations

Breast corrections (mastopexy, reduction, argumentation) also have a long history. In medieval times, breasts were amputated for tumors and the first case of a breast reduction for aesthetic reasons was reported in 1560.[27] It wasn't until the late nineteenth century, however, that breast reductions were performed to any significant degree. The practice of enlarging breasts did not appear until mid-twentieth century.

Augmentations were first performed in the early 1950s in Japan, but it was not until the early sixties that they became a commercial success. A topless cocktail waitress working in San Francisco became an instant media star in the late fifties when she allowed twenty shots of silicone to be injected directly into her breasts. The press had a field day exploiting Carol Doda's—now forty-four double D—chest. Enthusiasm for this method waned when it was discovered that paraffin or silicone injected directly tended to migrate to other parts of the body, causing cysts and necrosis of the skin. Sponges made of terylene wool, polyvinyl or polyethylene were then introduced to replace the injections.

These new materials were an improvement but they often hardened, protruded or caused fluid to accumulate in the breasts, which then had to be drained.

By 1963, inflatable silicone implants were becoming increasingly popular as a way to enlarge small breasts or correct asymmetrical breast development. The implants consisted of bags containing silicone gel or, less commonly, saline solution. Some were coated with a polyurethane foam, although these were later taken off the market by the manufacturers themselves because of their possible carcinogenicity (*FDA Medical Bulletin* 1991). Silicone implants could be inserted by means of a small incision in the armpit, nipple, or underneath the breast. These implants had the advantage of feeling like real breasts and were less likely to be rejected by the body's immune system, particularly if used in conjunction with steroids. A pocket was created below or behind the chest muscle so that the implant could be inserted.

Although silicone implants also had drawbacks, breast augmentations became one of the most popular forms of cosmetic surgery (Meredith 1988). It is estimated that over one million women in the United States have had their breasts "enhanced," usually by means of silicone implants. Each year one hundred thirty thousand women embark on this operation in the U.S.—the single most commonly performed operation next to liposuctions. The situation is similar in other countries. In Britain, six thousand silicone implant operations are carried out every year. In The Netherlands, there has been a fifty percent increase in the number of augmentations performed since 1982 (van Ham 1990: 99)—more breast augmentations per one hundred thousand habitants than in any other country in the world.

Most breast augmentations are performed on women between the ages of twenty and thirty. However, increasingly younger women are having them (two percent of the breast augmentations in the US. are performed on women under the age of eighteen) as well as women well into middle age whose breasts have begun to sag after pregnancies and breast feeding. Breast augmentations are in-creasingly a prerequisite for any job which places a woman in front of the camera.[28]

Fat Removal and Body Contouring

In a culture which suffers under a "tyranny of slenderness" (Chernin 1981) and where the diet industry has reached epidemic proportions, an increasing number of people consider themselves overweight. In the U.S., for example, more than seventy-nine million Americans claim that they weigh too much (Spitzak 1990: 9). In this context, it is not surprising that various techniques in cosmetic surgery have been developed for eliminating fat and trimming overweight bodies. Procedures range from tightening abdominal skin that has lost its elasticity due to weight loss, pregnancy, or the normal aging process, to abdominoplasties that involve cutting off an apron of excess skin which has caused discomfort and irritation.

Originally, cosmetic surgery was not considered a substitute for dieting. In recent years, however, a technique has been developed which makes dieting a thing of the past. The lyposuction or suction lipectomy has been developed to remove fatty tissue. Imported from France in 1982, this procedure involves injecting a saline solution, which liquefies the fat, into the area in question. A small incision is then made and fatty deposits are sucked out with a kind of vacuum cleaner. The procedure may be performed in conjunction with abdominoplasties or locally to eliminate saddlebag thighs, trim hips and buttocks, and even get rid of "pudding knees."[29] The most extreme form of body contouring or sculpting involves trimming, tucking and remodeling the entire body in a series of nearly simultaneous operations. The advantage to the patient is that she only has to be put under anesthesia once (Pitanguy 1967). For example, fat can be removed from hips and ankles, sagging skin in upper arms and tummy tucked, and a neck lift performed—all in one sitting.

Liposuctions are the fastest growing form of cosmetic surgery in the U.S. In 1986 alone one hundred thousand operations were performed—a number which rose by seventy-eight percent between 1984 and 1986.[30] By

1989 one hundred thirty thousand women alone underwent liposuctions and more than two hundred thousand pounds of body tissue was suctioned out of them (Wolf 1991: 261).[31] Although liposuctions are far from safe and have even been known to cause death when too much body tissue is removed, they continue to enjoy an unprecedented popularity.[32]

Problems and Pitfalls

Without a doubt, cosmetic surgery is popular. It is, however, also painful and risky. The most minor intervention causes discomfort, ranging from the dead crust of skin left by a chemical peel to swelling and inflammation of a face lift. Other operations like abdominoplasties, breast corrections, and liposuctions fall under the category of major surgery, requiring hospitalization and sometimes even intensive care. Recovery periods can be long and arduous—painful drains and a slow healing process for breast corrections, wearing a tight girdle after a liposuction to keep the skin from sagging, or having the jaws wired together for two months following cosmetic dentistry are all routine postsurgical experiences. While these discomforts may force the recipient into hiding until her bruised and swollen body returns to some semblance of normalcy and she can show herself to the outside world, there is more involved, in most cosmetic surgery than just discomfort.

Most operations have side effects, many of which are serious and even permanent. Although statistics are not kept, the list of complications accompanying cosmetic operations is long (Goldwyn 1980). For starters, infections, wound disruption, and erosion of overlying skin are a routine byproduct of any operation. Scar tissue can harden or darken. There is no way to prevent this kind of disfigurement and it is estimated that over twenty percent of all cosmetic surgery involves repairing scar tissue left over from previous operations.[33] Negative reactions to anesthesia are so common that they are called routine complications, though in some cases they can be fatal.[34]

Each operation has its own specific dangers. Pain, numbness, bruising, discoloration, and depigmentation frequently follow a liposuction, often lingering up to six months after the operation. Face lifts can damage nerves, leaving the person's face permanently numb. More serious disabilities include fat embolisms, blood clots, hypovolemia (fluid depletion), and, in some cases, death. While a breast augmentation is relatively minor surgery, and can even be performed on an outpatient basis, it is, nevertheless, a risky undertaking. Health experts estimate that the chance of side effects is between thirty and fifty percent, some of which are very serious. The least dramatic and most common side effects include decreased sensitivity of the nipples, painful swelling or congestion of the breasts, hardening of the breasts which makes it difficult to lie down comfortably or to raise the arms without the implants shifting position, or asymmetrical breasts (Gurdin 1972). While such side effects are common, they are usually temporary and not health threatening. More serious is the problem of encapsulation, whereby the body reacts to the presence of foreign matter by developing an enclosing capsule of fibrous tissue around the implant. This happens in nearly thirty-five percent of the cases. The implant becomes doorknob-shaped, rock hard, and painful. In some cases, a firm massage on the part of the surgeon (euphemistically called "fluffing them up") will break up the tissue—at great pain to the patient. If this does not work, however, the implants have to be removed—a formidable procedure sometimes requiring that the hardened implants be literally chiseled from the patient's chest wall. More rarely, the implant's outer envelope ruptures or there is gradual leakage of silicone into the body ("gel bleed")—a process which can impair the woman's immune system permanently, leading to arthritis, lupus, connective tissue disease, respiratory problems, or brain damage (Walsh et al., 1989; Weiss 1991; Goldblum et al., 1992). There is still debate about whether the detection of cancerous abnormalities in mammograms is impaired by the presence of an implant or that the implants themselves can cause cancer.

Cosmetic operations often have to be redone. While face lifts fall and have to be repeated every five years, silicone breast implants need to be replaced after fifteen years. Fat which has been removed from thighs or buttocks may return, requiring another liposuction, or the skin may bag and have to be cut and redraped.

Finally, the recipient of cosmetic surgery faces the very real possibility that she may emerge from the operation in worse shape than she was before. Unsuccessful breast augmentations are disfiguring. They leave the recipient with unsightly scars instead of a bigger chest size. An overly tight face lift produces the zombie look—a countenance utterly devoid of expression.[35] Following a liposuction, the skin can develop a corrugated, uneven texture or dents so that the recipient looks worse than she did before the surgery.

Situated Critique

Making sense of both the popularity and the problems of the surgical fix requires situating cosmetic surgery in the cultural and social context from which it emerged. Cosmetic surgery belongs to the cultural landscape of late modernity: consumer capitalism, technological development, liberal individualism, and the belief in the makeability of the human body. It is in this context that cosmetic surgery could emerge as an acceptable means for altering or improving the appearance of the body.

In recent years, however, cosmetic surgery has become increasingly controversial as well. Cosmetic surgery involves a surgical intervention in otherwise healthy bodies. It is a painful and dangerous solution for problems which are rarely life threatening and seldom evoke physical discomfort. And, last but not least, cosmetic surgery is expensive. In an age when cutbacks in health-care expenditure are the order of the day, it is a problematic medical practice.

While cosmetic surgery has become a source of contention in both the U.S. and Europe, these controversies take a different form, depending upon the organization of health care and the political commitment to welfare in each country in question. The organization of health care delivery not only sets limits on who may or may not indulge in the surgical fix, but it shapes the cultural discourses through which the controversial dimensions of cosmetic surgery can be expressed. Like other controversial medical procedures and technologies (in vitro fertilization, fetal monitoring, organ transplants or even female genital excision), cosmetic surgery is justified and criticized for different reasons.[36]

To deepen our understanding of how cosmetic surgery is problematized (as well as of what is left out of the critique), I shall now take a look at two different models of medicine—a market model and a welfare model—and the discourses through which cosmetic surgery in each case tends to be criticized.

A Market Model: The Discourse of Risk

In a market model of medicine, health care is provided on the basis of fee-for-service (Cockerham 1992).[37] Government regulation of services and technologies is limited. Specialists are free to provide services, just as patients are free to choose the health care they desire, provided they can pay for it. Public access is not guaranteed. By encouraging competition, among providers, a market model is supposed to enhance the quality of health care. The issue of equality in the distribution of health care is largely unaddressed.[38] Patients see themselves as consumers, regarding health care as a privilege rather than an entitlement. However, as consumers, they expect value for their money. The medical profession is responsible for providing quality health care while keeping risks at a minimum.

In a market model of medicine, controversies about care tend to center around the problems of risk, informed consent, and malpractice. Patients are free to embark upon dangerous or even experimental medical practices, provided they know what they are getting into and can knowledgeably calculate the risks.[39] The medical profession, and more indirectly, the regulatory bureaucracy, are expected to keep patients posted concerning the advantages and disadvantages of medical services so that they can make informed decisions. Patients are not supposed to be exposed to medical experimentation unless they have had access to this information and their consent has been obtained in advance. The malpractice suit insists that the medical profession toe the line, giving patients the possibility of compensation in cases of medical failure.[40]

In the U.S., the drawbacks of cosmetic surgery have been discussed in terms of risk and informed consent. Nowhere is this more tellingly illustrated than the recent controversy concerning silicone implants for breast augmentation surgery. The development of breast implants has always been an enterprise fraught with difficulties (Pickering et al., 1980). In the 1960s, the Food and Drug Administration (the FDA) banned the direct injection of silicone into the breasts. By the early seventies, the rubbery implants of the sixties were succeeded by implants filled with silicone gels which were less likely to be rejected by the body. Silicone implants were on the market even before they were officially approved in 1976. Like in any other medical devices—for example, the infamous Dalkon shield—silicone implants were grandfathered by the FDA, meaning that manufacturers could continue to sell the implants while scientific data were being collected (*FDA Medical Bulletin*, 1991). It was known as early as 1965 that silicone might be carcinogenic. By 1972, information was available that silicone migration could cause serious damage to the immune system. However, this information was not made public and manufacturers—most notably, Dow Corning—continued to distribute silicone implants for breast augmentations to women on a large scale. The FDA ignored the matter for another twelve years, relying on drug companies to keep the public informed and on physicians, in turn, to advise women about the risk and benefits of implants before scheduling surgery.

In 1984, the silence surrounding the dangers of silicone implants was broken when a federal court awarded a Nevada woman one and a half million dollars in punitive damages after her implants had leaked silicone into her body. The manufacturer was held responsible for withholding information about the dangers of the implants. In the decade that followed, more successful law suits against implant manufacture followed. Atrocity stories about silicone began to accumulate.

Consumer-advocate groups filed complaints with the FDA regarding misleading information in the literature published by the makers of breast implants. Pressure ensued from congressional critics as well as the media. Allegations were made that Dow Corning—the primary manufacturer of silicone implants—had violated federal laws regarding the labeling of medical devices and had failed to warn consumers about risks which they had known of since 1968. In the decade which followed, negative test results continued to trickle in. Congressional committee hearings were held and, finally, in 1991, the FDA, by now a little hot under the collar about implants, demanded that they be taken off the market until the contradictory data could be more thoroughly evaluated. Since 1992, use of silicone implants has been limited to cases of "urgent need"—usually meaning reconstruction following mastectomies—and to candidates enrolled in clinical studies. It is unclear how many women will be able to get implants through these trials, and, indeed, how many will want to have them since the negative findings on silicone have been made available to the general public.

The crux of the silicone controversy was not that the implants were risky per se. Data about side effects has been contradictory and inconclusive.[41] Moreover, despite the drawbacks of the implants, studies abound which show a high level of patient satisfaction.[42] The controversy concerned how the implants had been made available. By withholding information, the manufacturers and, later, the FDA by association, made themselves guilty of fraud. Patients had not been able to weigh the risks against the benefits of the implants. It was argued that women as consumers had a right to be informed that the implants were risky and to decide whether or not they wanted to be guinea pigs for a procedure which was still being tested.

The case of the implant illustrates both the strengths and the weaknesses of a discourse of risk, and, by implication a market model of medicine, for coming to terms with the problems associated with cosmetic surgery.

On the one hand, it sustains—at least, in theory—the notion that the individual patient, including the woman who wants surgery, has the right to expect quality service (as long as she pays for it), is entitled to complete information about the service, and is capable of making her own decisions (Parker 1993). This right could be mobilized by consumers as a resource in their struggles for satisfactory health care, both individually through malpractice suits or actively through pressure from consumer organizations.

On the other hand, the issue of why silicone implants should have been available in the first place is more difficult to raise in a market model of medicine. Determining the safety or efficacy of a device after it has already been developed is not the same as deciding whether it is desirable or necessary, or why certain individuals feel that it is necessary for their well-being. When cosmetic surgery is treated as a private matter, the issue of why individuals might regard the surgical alteration of their appearance as a precondition for their happiness and well being is left unexplored. And, of course, the issue of why most cosmetic surgery recipients are women is not addressed.

In most European countries where a welfare model of medicine prevails, medical technology and procedures are evaluated within a discourse of need and scarcity of resources for public health services. Since cosmetic surgery tends to be limited to the private sector, just as it is in the U.S., it is not discussed within this discourse. The exception is The Netherlands where cosmetic surgery was, until recently, covered by national health insurance and included in the basic health care plan. I shall now turn to the welfare model of medicine with its discourse of need in order to explore another problematic dimension of cosmetic surgery—a dimension which tends to be ignored in a market model of medicine with its discourse of risk.

A Welfare Model: The Discourse of Need

Most industrialized European countries have a welfare model of medicine, ranging from socialized medicine to decentralized health care (Cockerham 1992). Despite differences—notably in how directly the government regulates services and payments to providers—welfare models of medicine offer comprehensive health care for all citizens. In theory, a patient has a right to any form of health care he or she needs. Health care is not simply a privilege to be enjoyed by those who can afford it, but an entitlement for every citizen, regardless of his or her social position.

In practice, however, many health care services are too expensive for the state to fund. The most common dilemma in the European welfare model of medicine is the increasingly articulated need for particular services and technologies and the equally pressing necessity to limit government expenditure on health care (Ginsburg 1992). A discourse of need shifts attention from risk to whether a particular medical service or procedure is really necessary in a context of scarcity. There is generally an implicit or explicit consensus that unnecessary services cannot be included in the basic health-care package and must, therefore, be abandoned or made available through other means.

Controversies about medical procedures and technologies center around the problem of equal distribution rather than the quality of the service itself. If quality is an issue, it tends to be raised in the context of attempts on the part of the welfare bureaucracy to cut costs. Patient organizations are less concerned with information about the risks of procedures and more concerned with filling up the holes in a crumbling welfare system by setting up support groups, hot lines, or alternative health care centers.

In most European welfare systems, cosmetic surgery is considered a luxury. It is performed in private clinics and is not covered by national health insurance unless there is clear-cut medical indication. Despite the increase in the number of cosmetic surgery operations performed in Europe, the expansion is often referred to as a "typically American" phenomenon. Wolf (1991), the leading American critic of the cosmetic surgery craze, echoes this sentiment:

> Procedures . . . we have come to tolerate in America still sound nauseating in Great Britain and revolting in The Netherlands,

but next year British women will be able to keep their gorge from rising and Dutch women feel merely queasy (p. 251).

European reactions to the implant controversy are a case in point. In Britain, for example, the FDA decision to ban silicone implants was denounced in the media as a "typical instance of Americans being frightened of malpractice suits."[43] In The Netherlands, plastic surgeons and policy makers reassured the public that there was no real evidence that silicone implants were dangerous. The Secretary of the Health, Education and Welfare Department was quoted as saying he saw no reason to conduct a large-scale follow-up on women with silicone implants as he had "full confidence that the plastic surgeons who use implants have fully informed the recipients of the risks involved."[44] Instead of generating a full-scale controversy, the problems associated with the silicone breast implant were minimized ("We don't have that problem here") or left to the medical profession and welfare bureaucracy, who predictably kept the problem under wraps. Thus, silicone implants continue to be distributed in Europe. In most European welfare states, the risks of cosmetic surgery tended to fall between the cracks of public discourse.

The Netherlands was the exception. Unlike the U.S. and most European countries, cosmetic surgery was not available only on a private basis. It became controversial precisely because it could be considered in terms of welfare as a medical service which was—at least in some cases—necessary for patients' health and well-being and, therefore, should be covered by national insurance.

The Discourse of Need Revisited: The Dutch Case

In The Netherlands, cosmetic surgery began as a small, but acceptable branch of plastic surgery. Like any other medical practice, it was included in the basic health care package, providing the surgeon thought it was necessary. Initially, plastic surgeons did not justify performing cosmetic surgery in terms of the patient's physical characteristics. Instead, they reiterated that appearance is a

source of psycho-social problems and can cause an unacceptable degree of damage to the person's happiness and well-being.[45] They defended cosmetic surgery patients against charges of vanity or hypochondria. On the contrary, there may be deep psychological reasons for wanting surgery. "Loss, feelings of inferiority, sexual frigidity, and other expressions of despair" were cited (Van de Lande and Lichtveld 1972: 428). Modern society imposes norms of appearance, so that children with "jug ears" run the risk of being teased by their classmates. Women with sagging breasts may be afraid to go swimming with their children. Problems with appearance can lead to antisocial or even suicidal behavior (Huffstadt et al. 1981). Thus, cosmetic surgery is not a luxury, according to this argument, but a necessity for alleviating a specific kind of problem. The term "welfare surgery" was born.

Cosmetic surgery became problematic, however, when, in the early eighties, the demand for operations began to double. For a welfare state already in crisis, this expansion was bad news. In an attempt to stem the flow of applicants for cosmetic surgery, the national health insurance system, together with plastic surgeons, decided that guidelines were necessary for deciding when and under what circumstances cosmetic surgery was necessary (Starmans 1988).

They began by establishing three categories of problems which merited cosmetic surgery and should be eligible for coverage by national health insurance:[46]

- A functional disturbance or affliction (for example, eyelids which droop to such an extent that vision is impaired).
- Serious psychological suffering (the patient is receiving psychiatric treatment specifically for problems with appearance).
- A physical imperfection which falls "outside a normal degree of variation in appearance" (the patient's appearance does not meet certain aesthetic standards as determined by the medical inspector).

The first two categories were straightforward. Functional or physical, disturbances could be unproblematically delineated within medical discourse. Recipients rarely applied for cosmetic surgery due to "severe psychologic suffering" because it meant bringing a report from a psychiatrist. In practice, the majority of the cosmetic surgery recipients fell under the third category: "outside a normal degree of variation in appearance."[47] It was also this category which proved something of a headache for the national health insurance system and, indirectly for the medical profession.

Initially, medical experts, together with the national health insurance system, attempted to develop guidelines for abnormal appearance. They looked for criteria which could be objectively observed, classified, and applied to candidates for cosmetic surgery. Undeterred by the adage that beauty is in the eye of the beholder, these men of science seemed convinced that appearance—as any other feature of the body—could be assessed scientifically.

Some problems did, indeed, seem to be amenable to classification. For example, ears could be measured in centimeters; i.e. how far they protruded from the side of the head. Other problems received more praxeological (rule of thumb) criteria. For example, a breast lift was indicated if the "nipples were level with the recipient's elbows." A "difference of four clothing sizes between top and bottom" was sufficient in that a breast augmentation or liposuction was in order. A sagging abdomen which "makes her look pregnant" was enough reason to perform a tummy tuck. For a face lift, the patient had "to look ten years older than his or her chronological age."

To be sure, these criteria seem to be based more on common sense than science. This was, however, only part of the problem. More seriously, the guidelines were inadequate in the practical context of deciding which kinds of cosmetic surgery should be covered by national health insurance. Attempts to develop general rules for applying guidelines to particular cases failed in the face of the myriad exceptions.Confronted with the exceptions, the medical profession was forced to go beyond its own discourse and draw upon subjective or commonsensical arguments. Or,

more problematically, it made use of the ideological discourses available to them which meant, at least in The Netherlands, liberal individualism and ethnocentrism.

Plastic surgeons began admitting publicly that cosmetic surgery was a subjective enterprise and that they often could not see what the problem was. Medical inspectors for the national health insurance system complained about having to make practical decisions on coverage without having adequate guidelines. And more seriously, after nearly a decade of trying to get cosmetic surgery under control, the rise in the number of operations showed no signs of abating.

The medical experts and welfare bureaucrats were forced to admit defeat. After a short, heated, but somewhat belated public debate, primarily among plastic surgeons, the proponents of welfare surgery were overruled. Since the medical profession was unable to back up the welfare argument with a plan for stemming the flow of operations, there was no other recourse but to hand the issue over to the government and let it decide. Unsurprisingly, the government allowed financial considerations to prevail and decided to limit the state's responsibility to those few cases which could be justified unproblematically within medical discourse—cases of functional or psychiatric disturbance. The solution to the problem of cosmetic surgery was, therefore, to drop it from the national health insurance system and limit cosmetic surgery for strictly aesthetic reasons to the private sector.[48]

In conclusion, the Dutch case, like the U.S. case, has left some pieces missing when it comes to understanding the rise in cosmetic surgery despite its drawbacks. In the U.S., the problem of risk became a matter of public concern and the importance of the individual being able to make an informed choice was acknowledged. The problem of why individuals would want to embark on such a risky undertaking to begin with, however, was not addressed. In The Netherlands, individual welfare and the necessity of making choices in the collective provision of health care were central concerns. Although no workable solution was found for making such decisions, the discussion itself raised the issue of need.

Problems with appearance were acknowledged as a source of such suffering that cosmetic surgery surgery could, in some cases, become necessary for the welfare of some individuals. Cosmetic surgery remained a problematic solution, however—something which should not be left to individual market economy, but should rather be treated as a matter of collective concern. Ironically, the Dutch discussion faltered because cosmetic surgery was treated as a strictly medical matter. It was left to medical practitioners to justify cosmetic surgery and, as we have seen, they were unable to come up with a convincing defense within their own discourse.

What is missing from debates about cosmetic surgery in both the U.S. and The Netherlands is the recipient. Little attention is paid to why patients are willing to take the risk of having cosmetic surgery. Nor have they been consulted in discussions about cosmetic surgery as a matter of welfare. Social policy tends to be made without enlisting the aid of those who are most affected by the outcome. Moreover, the debates have been noticeably silent about the fact that the recipients of cosmetic surgery are primarily women. Why are women so dissatisfied with their appearance that they are prepared to undergo a dangerous operation to have it altered? Why is it taken for granted by the medical profession, the welfare bureaucracy and, for that matter, the general public, that it is the female body which needs surgical alteration?

Notes

1. This did not prevent surgeons from performing operations. See, for example, Dally's *Women Under The Knife (1991)*.

2. The number of reconstructive procedures performed in 1990 was 1,250,000—nearly twice the 640,000 cosmetic surgery procedures. *The New York Times*, February 23, 1992.

3. As evidenced by recent strides in sex-change operations—the most radical form of cosmetic surgery.

4. Pitanguy, a well-known plastic surgeon for the jet set has his private clinic on his own island and is reputed to treat celebrities and society women at the rate of two a day ("I feel I should spend as much time as a painter with a paint-

ing would, or a sculptor with a statue."). *The New York Times*, July 8, 1983.

5. *TV Guide*, October 26, 1991.

6. Taken from a Belgian women's magazine, *Flair*, May 3, 1991, which is comparable to *Cosmopolitan*.

7. *Newsweek*, Jan 11, 1988.

8. For a discussion of how Oprah's representations of women's experiences with their appearance and the practices of the beauty system can work to empower women, albeit in a somewhat ambivalent mixture of fluff and gravity, sensationalism and social analysis, the reader is referred to Squire (1994).

9. The prices vary depending upon the extent of the surgery, whether or not the patient is hospitalized, the reputation and expertise of the surgeon, and the geographical region. *Consumers' Digest*, July/August 1986.

10. Quoted from "Medical Economics" in *The New York Times*, February 23, 1992.

11. It is virtually impossible to obtain accurate statistics on the actual number of cosmetic surgery operations performed each year. In both the U.S. and Europe, statistics are recorded for operations performed in hospitals by registered plastic surgeons. Since the majority of the operations are performed in private settings and many operations are not performed by registered plastic surgeons, such estimates do not begin to cover the actual incidence of operations.

In The Netherlands, for example, the official estimate was 6,060 cosmetic surgery operations between 1980 and 1989, of which 5,925 were women (more than ninety-seven percent). However, since there are thirty-nine private institutes in The Netherlands performing cosmetic surgery, the actual number of operations is considerably higher. National health insurance experts have suggested that twenty thousand might be a "modest estimate," i.e. nearly four times higher than the official figure!

12. *Der Spiegel* 32 (1992).

13. In addition to the difference in the number of cosmetic surgery operations performed on men and women, marketing strategies are very different for the sexes. For men, cosmetic surgery is presented as a means to enhance job performance and increase chances to compete, while women are targeted in terms of general attractiveness or changes in identity.

14. The types of cosmetic surgery are also ethnically specific. White women opt for liposuc-

tions, breast augmentations, or wrinkle removal procedures, whereas Asian women tend to have double-eyelid surgery or nose corrections (Kaw 1993).

15. *The New York Times*, February 23, 1992.

16. In the U.S., at least ninety percent of the cosmetic surgery operations are performed in the physician's office or in a private clinic (American Society of Plastic and Reconstructive Surgeons 1988).

17. *The Los Angeles Times*, December 23, 1991.

18. A similar situation exists in The Netherlands, as illustrated by a recent inaugural address by a plastic surgeon who had been appointed professor in a university department of plastic and reconstructive surgery. He defended his discipline, explicitly setting it apart from the cosmetic surgery craze. He explained that plastic surgery, in contrast, was primarily reconstructive and aimed at "real problems" like replacing hands which had been severed during industrial accidents or alleviating birth defects.

19. *Consumers' Digest*, July/August 1986.

20. Cosmetic surgery on teenagers is up as much as 300 percent, warns *The New York Times*, December 19, 1989. According to the American Society of Plastic and Reconstructive Surgeons, 73,250 nose jobs were done in 1988—the first year statistics we kept—and sixteen percent of those were performed on patients under eighteen.

21. *Self*, December 1991.

22. Breast augmentations are of course, also done following mastectomies. In 1984, breast reconstructions immediately following a mastectomy accounted for thirty-four percent of the ninety-eight thousand reconstructions. The rest were performed on healthy breasts for the improvement of appearance which makes breast augmentations one of the most common forms of cosmetic surgery. *Consumers' Digest*, July/August 1986. By 1990, the number of reconstructions for cosmetic reasons was up to eighty-five percent. *The Los Angeles Times*, December 10, 1990.

23. *The New York Times*, February 3, 1982.

24. ibid.

25. This was in response to the governor of California's proposal that in return for state-supported funds to reduce the cost of malpractice insurance, physicians would be required to treat indigent patients or patients for whom there was little medical care available. Grabbing his chance, this plastic surgeon proceeded to offer his services to female prisoners. By 1977, he had operated on more than seventy of them. *The New York Times*, July 25, 1979.

26. *Consumers' Digest*, July/August 1986.

27. Gabke and Vaubel (1983) refer to a barber surgeon who amputated the left breast of a maidservant, claiming that it had "assumed such great proportions that she could not support (it), neither standing up nor being seated" (p. 95).

28. *TV Guide*, October 26, 1991.

29. *The New York Times*, August 3, 1991 warns about a new "dilemma." "How to wear the new short skirts without being called pudding knees, cottage cheese knees and such?"

30. *The New York Times*, June 29, 1988.

31. As one surgeon with a feeling for alliteration explained to me in an informal conversation, the "typical" candidate for a liposuction is "Fat, Forty, and Female."

32. Early on, eleven deaths were reported as a result of liposuctions. When this number was brought to the attention of a U.S. Senate ad hoc committee, it was pointed out that this is a very low mortality rate for a surgical intervention (.01 percent). However, since the patients getting liposuctions are otherwise healthy, this rate is clearly too high. *The New York Times Magazine*, February 28, 1988.

33. Intermediar (1991): 67.

34. *The Los Angeles Times* reports of a case of a thirty-five- year-old mother of four who was discovered unconscious in the recovery room of the doctors office after a routine breast augmentation. She was taken by ambulance to a nearby hospital where she died four days later (December 24, 1991). There have been other fatalities, but statistics are not kept on deaths related to medical procedures.

35. *The New York Times*, February 3, 1982.

36. Genital excision is a case in point. Both The Netherlands and Great Britain are faced with the problem of Somalian and Ethiopian immigrants who want to continue the practice of infibulation on their daughters. In the Netherlands, a heated debate emerged when several Somalian mothers asked general practitioners to perform excision on their daughters. Worried that the intervention would be carried out under unsanitary conditions, many physicians and social workers argued that a "ritual" cut on the clitoris might be a humanitarian way to prevent more drastic forms of genital mutilation. In Great Britain, the issue was

tackled differently. Rather than advocating a medical solution to the problem of excision, grass-roots women's groups like the black Women's Health Organization set up discussion groups for the mothers, attempting the slower and often painful process of reeducation.

37. The U.S. and South Africa are the only major industrial countries which operate under a market model of medicine.

38. With the notable exception of the critics of capitalist medicine. See, for example, Ehrenreich (1976), Waitzkin (1983), and Navarro (1986).

39. See Abel (1982) for a thoughtful discussion of risk in a market model. He shows how the political philosophy of liberal individualism individualizes risk. Individuals are given the opportunity to minimize their own risk taking, while little attempt is made to equalize the exposure of all citizens to risk.

40. The malpractice suit could only emerge in the U.S., where the medical profession is almost completely free of external regulation. In this context, public awareness of medical mistakes has to be expressed juridicially. In the U.S., malpractice suits rose dramatically from a few hundred a year in the 1950s to ten thousand a year in the 1980s (Cockerham 1992, Chapter 13).

41. See Parker (1993: 63-64). For example, fibroid encapsulation—the single most common side effect—has been variously reported in fifteen percent (Meyer and Ringberg 1987) to seventy percent of implant recipients (Burkhardt 1988; Rheinstein and Bagley 1992). Pain or lack of sensation in the nipples ranges from ten percent (Meyer 1987) to thirty-eight percent (Ohlsen, Ponten, and Hambert 1978). Cancer due to "gel bleed" has been disputed (Berkel et al., 1992; Fisher 1992) as has the actual incidence of implant rupture. The FDA advisory committee suggested that this occurs in more than 1.1 percent of "asymptomatic women," whereas Kessler (1992) estimates that it may happen in up to six percent of the recipients.

42. Recent surveys indicate that ninety-five percent of the augmentation candidates and eighty-nine percent of the reconstruction candidates report being "very satisfied" with the outcome of the surgery (American Society of Plastic and Reconstructive Surgeons 1990; Iverson 1991; Fisher 1992).

43. *The Guardian*, January 8, 1992.

44. *De Volkskrant*, February 24, 1992. Interestingly, the Public Health Department did send a directive to all plastic surgeons, family physicians, and hospital directors, requesting them to inform breast augmentation patients of the risks involved in silicone implants and follow up any complaints involving contracture of fibrous tissue and autoimmune diseases (January 1992). Whereas the letter was not exactly covert, it was also not made public.

45. This is an additional possibility for justifying cosmetic surgery. Dull and West (1991) have shown that in the U.S., plastic surgeons are limited to defending surgery in cases where the patient has "realistic expectations" and her body is "objectively in need of repair."

46. It is worth noting here that eligibility meant that cosmetic surgery was one hundred percent deductible if the patient met one of the three criteria. Otherwise, the patient had to pay half of the costs of surgery. In practice, this made cosmetic surgery highly available, even for patients who had to shoulder some of the burden themselves. The ruling also did not affect privately insured patients who obtained operations in private clinics without going through these channels.

47. Nearly two-thirds of all applicants received 100 percent coverage, while one-third had to pay half of the costs of surgery themselves. Of the two-thirds, fifty percent fell under the heading "outside normal variation in appearance," thirty-four percent involved physical or functional disturbances, and only three percent severe psychological suffering. The rest involved second operations to repair scars—one of the most common cosmetic surgery interventions.

48. In 1991, a task force which had been set up by the Department of Health and Welfare (the Dunning Commission) published a report, *Kiezen en delen* (*Choosing and Sharing*) as an answer to the problem of an expanding medical technology and shrinking public resources. The report developed guidelines for setting limits to the development of medical technology and deciding how choices in the provision of health care could be made. The following criteria for decisions concerning which services should be included in the basic health-care package were suggested: Is the care necessary? Is the service effective? Does it do what it is intended to do? Could the care be provided through private means? It was assumed that by assessing the health care services presently covered by national health

insurance along these lines, unnecessary services could be removed from the basic health care package, thereby reducing expenditure. There is no reason, of course, that cosmetic surgery could not have been subjected to this kind of assessment and it is quite possible that it would have been rejected anyway. However, the Council of the National Health Insurance System had already thrown cosmetic surgery out before the Dunning Commission had published its criteria for assessment.

Recent developments show just how shortsighted and premature this decision was. Since the 1991 ruling, the number of individuals seeking psychiatric treatment for reasons of appearance has doubled and more than half of all patients contesting decisions concerning coverage by national health insurance are applicants for some form of cosmetic surgery. Appeals tend to be denied in one of two ways: either the patient is labeled so disturbed that surgery won't help her, or her problems are described as not serious enough to warrant surgery. This damned-if-you-do and damned-if-you-don't argument provides a good look at the unwillingness of the medical profession to take the needs of cosmetic surgery candidates seriously. I am indebted to Marianne van Kan for this information. See also Davis (1992).

References

Abel, Richard L. 1982. "A Socialist Approach to Risk." *Maryland Law Review* 41: 695-754.

American Society for Plastic and Reconstructive Surgeons. 1987.

American Society for Plastic and Reconstructive Surgeons. 1988. "Estimated Numbers of Cosmetic Procedures Performed by ASPRS Members." Arlington Heights, Illinois.

American Society of Plastic and Reconstructive Surgeons. 1990. "First National Survey Asks Women How They Feel About Breast Implants." Chicago.

Balsamo, Anne. 1993. "On the Cutting Edge: Cosmetic Surgery and the Technological Production of the Gendered Body." *Camera Obscura* 28: 207-237.

Berkel, Hans, Birdsell, Dale C., and Jenkins, Heather. 1992. "Breast Augmentation: A Risk Factor for Breast Cancer?" *New England Journal of Medicine* 326: 1649-1653.

Bordo, Susan. 1990a. "Feminism, Postmodernism, and Gender-Scepticism." In L.J. Nicholson (ed.), *Feminism/Postmodernism*. New York: Routledge. 133-156.

——. 1990b. " 'Material Girl': The Effacements of Postmodern Culture." *Michigan Quarterly Review* 653-677.

——. 1990c. "Reading the Slender Body." In Mary Jacobus, Evelyn Fox Keller and Sally Shuttleworth (eds.), *Body/Politics*. New York: Routledge. 83-112.

Burkhardt, Boyd R. 1988. "Breast Implants: A Brief History of Their Development, Characteristics, and Problems." In Thomas D. Gant and Luis O. Vasconez (eds.), *Postmastectomy Reconstruction*. Baltimore: Williams and Wilkins.

Chernin, Kim. 1981. *The Obsession: Reflections on the Tyranny of Slenderness*. New York: Harper and Row.

Cockerham, William C. 1992. *Medical Sociology*. Fifth Edition. Englewood Cliffs, N.J.: Prentice Hall.

Consumer's Digest. July/August 1986.

Dally, Ann. 1991. *Women Under the Knife*. London: Hutchinson Radius.

Davis, Kathy. 1992. "The Rhetoric of Cosmetic Surgery: Luxury or Welfare?" Paper presented at the Annual meeting of the American Sociological Association, Pittsburg, August 1992.

Department of Health and Welfare. 1991.

Der Spiegel. 32 (1992).

De Volkskrant. Feb. 24, 1992.

Dull, Diana. 1989. "Before and Afters: Television's Treatment of the Boom in Cosmetic Surgery." Paper presented at the Annual Meeting of the American Sociological Association. San Francisco, August 1989.

Dull, Diana and West, Candace. 1987. "'The Price of Perfection': A Study of the Relations Between Women and Plastic Surgery." Paper presented at the Annual Meeting of the American Sociological Association. Chicago, August 1987.

Dull, Diana and West, Candace. 1991. "Accounting for Cosmetic Surgery: The Accomplishment of Gender." *Social Problems* 38 (1): 54-70.

Ehrenreich, John (ed.). 1978. *The Cultural Crisis of Modern Medicine*. New York: Monthly Review Press.

Ehrenreich, Barbara and English, Deirdre. 1979. *For Her Own Good*. London: Pluto Press.

Faludi, Susan. 1991. *Backlash: The Undeclared War on American Women*. New York: Crown Publishers, Inc.

FDA Medical Bulletin. July 1991.

Featherstone, Mike. 1983. "The Body in Consumer Culture." *Theory, Culture & Society* 1: 18-33.

Featherstone, Mike. 1990. "Perspectives on Consumer Culture." *Sociology* 24 (1): 5-22.

Finkelstein, Joanne. 1991. *The Fashioned Self.* Cambridge: Polity Press.

Fisher, Jack. 1992. "The Silicone Controversy: When Will Science Prevail?" *New England Journal of Medicine* 326: 1696-1698.

Flair. May 3, 1991.

Gabke, Joachim and Vaubel, Ekkehard. 1983. *Plastic Surgery Past and Present: Origin and History of Modern Lines of Incision.* Basel: Karger.

Giddens, Anthony. 1991. *Modernity and Self-Identity: Self and Society in the Late Modern Age.* Cambridge: Polity Press.

Ginsburg, Norman. 1992. *Divisions of Welfare: A Critical Introduction to Comparative Social Policy.* London: Sage Publications.

Goldblum, Randall M., Relley, Ronald P. and O'Donnell, Alice A. 1992. "Antibodies to Silicone Elastomers and Reactions to Ventriculoperitoneal Shunts." *Lancet* 340: 510-513.

Goldwyn, Robert M. (ed.) 1980. *Long-Term Results in Plastic and Reconstructive Surgery.* 2nd edition. Boston: Little, Brown & Co.

Gurdin, Michael. 1972. "Augmentation Mammaplasty." In Robert M. Goldwyn (ed.), *Long-Term Results in Plastic and Reconstructive Surgery.* 1st edition. Boston: Little, Brown & Co.

Huffstadt, A.J.C. (In collaboration with F.G. Bouman, N.H. Groenman, and H.M.A. Marcus-Timmers). 1981. *Kosmetische Chirurgie.* Alphen a.d. Rijn: Stafleu's.

Intermediar. 1991.

Iverson, R. 1991. "National Survey Shows Overwhelming Satisfaction with Breast Implants." *Plastic and Reconstructive Surgery* 88: 546-547.

Kaw, Eugenia. 1993. "Medicalization of Racial Features: Asian American Women and Cosmetic Surgery." *Medical Anthropology Quarterly* 7 (1): 74-89.

Kessler, David A. 1992. "The Basis of the FDA's Decision on Breast Implants." *New England Journal of Medicine* 326: 1713-1715.

Meredith, B. 1988. *A Change for the Better.* London: Grafton Books.

Meyer, L. and Ringberg, A. 1987. "Augmentation Mammaplasty: Psychiatric and Psychosocial Characteristics and Outcome in a Group of Swedish Women. *Scandinavian Journal of Plastic Reconstructive Surgery* 21: 199-208.

Millard, D.R., Jr. 1974. "Aesthetic Rhinoplasty." In M. Saad and P. Lichtveld 9eds.), *Reviews in Plastic Surgery: General Plastic and Reconstructive Surgery.* New York: American Elsevier. 371-386.

National Center for Health Statistics. 1987.

Navarro, Vincente. 1986. *Crisis, Health, and Medicine: A Social Critique.* New York: Tavistock.

Newsweek. Jan. 11, 1988.

Ohlsen, L., Ponten, B., and Hambert, G. 1978. "Augmentation Mammapolasty: A Surgical and Psychiatric Evaluation of the Results. *Annals of Plastic Surgery* 2: 42-52.

Parker, Lisa (1993). "Social Justice, Federal Paternalism, and Feminism: Breast Implants in the Cultural Context of Female Beauty." *Kennedy Institute of Ethics Journal* 3(1): 57-76.

Pickering, P.P., J.E. Williams, T.R. Vecchione. 1980. "Augmentation Mammaplasty." In R.M. Goldwyn (ed.), *Long-Term Results in Plastic and Reconstructive Surgery.* Boston: Little, Brown & Company. 696-706.

Pitanguy, I. 1967. "Abdominal Lipectomy, an Approach to It, Through an Analysis of 300 Consecutive Cases. *Plastic Reconstructive Surgery* 40: 384.

Rees, R.D. and Wood-Smith, D. 1973. *Cosmetic Facial Surgery.* Philadelphia: Saunders.

Rheinstein, Peter H. and Bagley, Grant P. 1992. "Update on Breast Implants."*American Family Physician* 45: 472-473.

Self. Dec. 1991.

Spitzak, Carole. 1990. *Confessing Excess: Women and the Politics of Body Reduction.* Albany: State University of New York Press.

Squire, Corinne. 1994. "Empowering Women? The Oprah Winfrey Show." *Feminism & Psychology* 4 (1): 63-79.

Starmans, P.M.W. 1988. "Wat gebeurt er met de esthetische chirurgie?" *Inzet. Opinieblad van de ziekenfondsen* 1: 18-25.

The Guardian. Jan. 8, 1992.

———. Dec. 23, 1991.

———. Dec. 24, 1991.

The Los Angeles Times. Dec. 10, 1990.

The New York Times. Feb. 3, 1982.

———. July 8, 1983.

———. July 29, 1988.

———. Dec. 19, 1989.

———. Aug. 3, 1991.

———. Feb. 23, 1992.

The New York Times Magazine. Feb. 28, 1988.

Turner, Bryan S. 1984. *The Body & Society.* Oxford: Basil Blackwell.

TV Guide. October 26, 1991.

van de Lande, J.L. and Lichtveld, P. 1972. "Hypoplasia mammae, een psychosociaal lijden." *Nederlands Tijdschrift voor Geneeskunde* 116 (11): 428-431.

van Ham, I. 1990. "Borstvergroting en borstverkleining. Een literatuuronderzoek." *Huisarts en Wetenschap* 33: 98-102.

Waitzkin, Howard. 1983. *The Second Sickness: Contra- dictions of Capitalist Health Care*. New York: The Free Press.

Walsh, Frank W., Solomon, David A., and Espinoza, Luis R. 1989. "Human Adjuvant Disease: A New Cause of Chylous Effusions." *Archives of Internal Medicine* 149: 1194-1196.

Weiss, Rick. 1991. "Breast Implant Fears Put Focus on Biomaterials." *Science* 252: 1059-1160.

Wolf, Naomi. 1991. *The Beauty Myth: How Images of Beauty Are Used Against Women*. New York: Wil- liam Morrow and Company, Inc.

Further Reading

Diana Dull and Candace West. 1991. "Accounting for Cosmetic Surgery: The Accomplishment of Gen- der." *Social Problems* 38: 801-817.

Deborah Sullivan. 1993. "Cosmetic Surgery: Market Dynamics and Medicalization." *Research in the So- ciology of Health Care* 10: 97-115.

Bryan Turner. 1992. *Regulating Bodies: Essays in Medi- cal Sociology*. London: Routledge.

Discussion Questions

1. What factors most influenced the tran- sition from reconstructive to cosmetic surgery? Keeping these factors in mind, do you think that cosmetic surgery will be curtailed by medical professionals or policy makers?

2. Compare Davis' discussion of the body and plastic surgery to Martin's analysis of menopause. What sorts of themes are similar in Martin's and Davis' analyses? How are their discussions different?

3. What kinds of quality of care issues need to be addressed with regard to cosmetic surgery?

30

The Marketing of Rehabilitation Goods and Services

Gary L. Albrecht

Gary Albrecht portrays rehabilitation as a business and marketing strategies as a means of managing it. This perspective highlights the development and maintenance of a clientele and cooperation and conflict between professional (and corporate) groups. Albrecht's work presages the massive transition in medical care in the United States from entrepreneurial and corporate services to managed care plans. The rationale *for managed care is efficiency in distributing needed services without excess treatments and costs. The reality of managed care is managed profits. As such, services are trimmed, streamlined, and truncated. Services requiring extensive professional staff time are assessed for their consumer appeal and costs. Offering some access to rehabilitation services like occupational and physical therapy makes a particular managed care plan more attractive to consumers. Certainly claiming a range of rehabilitation services is a powerful marketing strategy for an aging population. Under managed care, controlled and limited access may give the illusion of more substantial coverage than consumers actually have and may learn that they want. Comprehensive rehabilitation programs raise health plan costs, lower profits and, thus, may not survive budget costs.*

Rehabilitation goods and services are marketed and managed and bought and sold. As Albrecht states, marketing practices define the growth and profit potential of the rehabilitation business and simultaneously affect the or-ganization of care. New markets are forecast and sought; old ones reassessed. Rehabilitation services rise in demand when consumers clamor for them and medical professionals prescribe them. Albrecht points out that health facilities carve out market niches by offering sophisticated specialized services. When the specialized market niche captures the territory, the sponsoring institution gains prestige, justifies higher fees, and promotes increased profits and investment potentials. Look for Albrecht's account of why and how rehabilitation markets have changed. Think about the kinds of rehabilitation goods and services your family and friends have had—they may range from a removable cast for a sports injury of a young athlete to a hip replacement and subsequent physical therapy of an aging relative.

Albrecht's analysis of marketing in physical rehabilitation can be applied to much of medical care in the United States today. Yet marketing strategies always exist within an economic, political, and cultural context. Shrinking insurance coverage, for example, affects what, how, why, and to whom certain services and products are marketed. Marketing strategies have become integral to organizational survival in the competitive business of medical care.

Marketing strategies and technologies are changing the character of health care delivery in the United States and perhaps worldwide. Until recently, health care institutions and medical professionals did not formally market or advertise their products and services. Increased competition, changes in laws and funding, new diseases, and modification in population demography, however, introduced more uncertainty into the environment and forced these institutions and professionals to take a more proactive stance in the marketplace to ensure their survival and growth. Health care managers responded by marketing goods and services to influence the level, timing, and character of demand and to meet their organizational or professional objectives. [1]

The delivery of rehabilitation goods and services provides an example of how market forces shape the definitions of *health prob-*

lems and *service delivery systems*. Marketing and advertising serve to support the reception of persons with disabilities as a social problem and to reinforce the need for goods and services that address the problem. Because *rehabilitation goods and services* are defined as "commodities that can be bought and sold" and consumers are able to pay for them, a new segment of the health care market has developed. Like other markets, the size and dynamism of the rehabilitation market is determined by a balance between supply and demand.[2] The market can be increased by a growth in demand due to larger numbers of persons with disabilities, including those with more serious disabilities, and by additional funding, which makes consumption possible.[3] The market can grow also because of increases in supply, represented by more rehabilitation professionals, specialized clinics, and more products that are desirable to the consumer. Although regulators and managers can control some of these market forces, they do not have much influence over others. In either instance, rehabilitation organizations must deal with these forces or risk failure.

Marketing effectively manages environmental forces by providing a coherent set of activities specifically designed to span the boundaries between organizations and their environments. Marketing employs needs assessment and feasibility analysis to direct an organization's buying and selling activities.[4] Although recognizing the importance of these assessments and studies, this chapter concentrates on the consequences of buying and selling in the rehabilitation marketplace. A business organization has to sell products and services to survive, while people or institutions in the external environment have needs and demands to be met. Marketing is the transactional activity that brings these parties together in completed social exchange processes, making the specialized division of labor in rehabilitation possible.[5] In principle, marketing activities are beneficial to all parties involved, whereas in practice, they may not always serve the consumers' best interests.

Conceptualizing rehabilitation as an industry, this chapter analyzes the marketing of rehabilitation goods and services in terms of their structural relationships to the larger health care industry, the growth and profit potential of the business, and the benefits to consumers, providers, and society. The central question addressed is, How have marketing activities, expressed in strategies and technologies, changed the structure and operation of health care systems, particularly those involving the delivery of rehabilitation goods and services? . . .

Rehabilitation Needs and Demands

Rehabilitation goods and services are products increasingly in demand that are delivered by a broad range of providers across institutional settings, age groups, and health conditions. Familiar forms of rehabilitation services include physical therapy aimed at improving mobility, and occupational therapy, designed to help white-collar workers who have experienced finger or arm amputations resume their performance in office duties. Because no single professional group, brand of therapy, institution, or treatment setting dominates the rehabilitation field, considerable room exists for competition among providers.[6] Rehabilitation products are important in the disability business because, appropriately delivered, they can reduce treatment costs and improve function in large groups of people who traditionally have gone without treatment altogether, received care on a limited outpatient basis, or consumed large quantities of expensive treatment as inpatients in hospitals.[7] The marketing of rehabilitation goods and services is consequential because these activities help sort out which persons with disabilities are most likely to receive treatment and determine which institutions and professional groups will flourish and which will succumb to competition.

Rehabilitation services here refers to any form of therapy or exercise that is performed on and by patients and that supports services that improve the level of functional independence for persons with disabilities. *Rehabilitation goods* include mechanical aids, modified vehicles, and architecture, prosthetics, orthotics, and pharmaceuticals that help achieve the same goals. Anticipated outcomes commonly are expressed in, but not limited to, improvements in performing activities of daily living.

Earlier systems for delivering a complex set of integrated rehabilitation goods and services had numerous deficiencies. The focus of the programs was on providing a modicum of help to individuals who had specific diagnoses and were covered by insurance, not on returning every person with a disability to his or her highest level of function regardless of ability to pay or earn income.[8] Indeed patients received treatment based primarily on their ability or government willingness to pay rather than on need.[9] Rehabilitation services were targeted primarily for those in the labor force or children in school. As a consequence, women, the poor, and older persons were underserved. In addition, rehabilitation treatment was delivered in institutions in which services were much more expensive than those delivered in ambulatory sites or at home. As a result, services were directed to selected portions of the population, unit costs of rehabilitation remained high, and many citizens in need were forced to become increasingly dependent because they were denied access to care.

Until recently, rehabilitation systems also were not well integrated into the larger medical care delivery process. The ensuing discontinuities in care often resulted in patients losing many of their functional gains as they moved from surgery to postoperative recovery, discharge, evaluation, rehabilitation, and home or to a less intensive care environment. Attempting to recover previous gains was both time-consuming and expensive.[10] The existing systems were relatively uncoordinated and inefficient.

In recent years, the rehabilitation marketplace has changed significantly. Payment sources for rehabilitation care have expanded and deepened. Insurance companies and the government realized that, over the course of a disease process, it is less expensive to bring individuals back to their highest level of function, given moderate intervention, than to provide support services for dependent individuals for life. For all of these reasons, the market is open for competition and growth.

The need for rehabilitation has increased as chronic illnesses, work-related injuries, and accidents have taken their toll in the last half of the 20th century. Furthermore, as advanced medical technology results in saving precarious lives (premature infants, burn and trauma victims), more survivors are in need of medical care and rehabilitation for their subsequent disabilities. In addition, while people are living much longer than their predecessors, they also are experiencing more disability. General population surveys indicate that at any one time 10–15 percent of the American noninstitutionalized adult population is limited in at least one functional activity such as walking independently, brushing teeth, or paying bills.[11]

Recent data from the Census Bureau suggest that 37 million Americans aged fifteen and over have difficulty in performing one or more basic physical activities.[12] Two of the most common problems are walking and lifting a weight equivalent to a bag of groceries. As the population ages, the numbers of people with limitations and the severity of the limitations increase. According to these national data, 14.1 percent of people between ages 15 and 64, and 58.5 percent of those aged sixty-five and over, experience some disability. In fact, 13.5 million people, or 7.5 percent of the entire population, have severe disabilities that prevent or seriously impede their ability to walk, lift, listen, or read. Emergent diseases such as AIDS, and debilitating "yuppie diseases" believed related to the Epstein-Barr virus, compound the disability problem.[13]

As the nation experiences a rapid rise in the number of people aged 85 and older, the demands for nursing home care and rehabilitation for these older people increase. Based on 1987 national data, the rate per 1,000 nursing home residents ranged from 10.8 for males and 13.8 for females of those aged 65–74, to 145.3 for males and 248.9 for females aged 85 and over.[14] Dependency levels also increase with age. Only 55 percent of nursing home residents under age 65 but more than 75 percent of those in nursing homes who are over age 85 require assistance in performing activities of daily living. Similar trends exist for those not in nursing homes or other institutions. In a 1984 survey of the noninstitutionalized who have worked since age 45, 29.5 percent of those aged 55–59 reported they had difficulty with or were unable to stoop, crouch, or kneel.[15] Yet 44.3 percent of those aged 70–74 related they had similar difficulties. As the population ages, the demand for such community services as homemaker services and meals on wheels for the noninstitutionalized population rises. Similar trends exist for inpatient and outpatient hospital rehabilitation services. As diminished function and increased demand for rehabilitation occur with age, total cost of care and utilization rates mount. A 1989 overview of the home health care crisis confirms these patterns and suggests that they will continue through the 1990s.[16] In fact, experts warn that if people desire a comfortable old age, they must plan for long-term care and rehabilitation.[17]

Individuals with such musculoskeletal disorders as swollen joints and low-back pain offer a specific example. More than 44 million people, or 19.9 percent of the United States noninstitutionalized population, in the 1980 National Medical Care Utilization and Expenditure Survey, reported at least one musculoskeletal disorder.[18] Many of these disorders are associated with loss in function. These individuals made almost twice the number of ambulatory visits (10.1) to health care providers as did the noninstitutionalized general population, at a cost of over $6 billion a year. These respondents made visits to a broad range of medical professionals, including chiropractors and physical therapists, from whom they sought rehabilitation services. . . .

Identification and Creation of Rehabilitation Markets

A *market* is the sum of the actual and potential constituents that are capable of purchasing the products and services available and can be encouraged to do so. Those in the market for rehabilitation services share an interest, an ability to transact the social exchange between provider and consumer, and an access to care.[19] Conceptually the marketing of rehabilitation services is a social exchange process expressed in completed transactions between consumers and service providers. For such exchanges to take place, communication between qualified buyers and sellers is required. Marketing provides this essential link in the transaction. The integration of the poor and the underinsured in the market is problematic, however, as they tend to be excluded from services due to lack of purchasing power. Today 37 million Americans have no health insurance at all, and 28 percent of the population is uninsured or underinsured.[20] People with disabilities within this group do not have full access to rehabilitation.

Traditional markets organized around the demand for physical rehabilitation to restore function after orthopedic surgery have remained vital and indeed even have expanded so that today almost everyone who undergoes surgery receives some rehabilitation. New and undiscovered markets involve concepts such as *preventive rehabilitation*, in which combined regimens of heat, cold, electrical stimulation, and extensive exercise therapy are used to reduce pain and swelling and to stabilize joints so that surgery is not necessary. Rehabilitation techniques are used also by exercise and corrective therapists working in health clubs and sports medicine clinics to strengthen potentially weak joints and muscles to prevent injuries among athletes. The American Hospital Association sees diversification into these markets as a key for increased hospital competitiveness and institutional growth, acknowledging that only the strong will survive.[21]

Changing disease, technological, and demographic processes create demand for rehabilitation goods and services and constitute new markets. Technological advances keep certain populations, such as ventilator-dependent children, alive who previously would have succumbed to a disease. The emergence of such conditions as AIDS presents novel challenges to the existing rehabilitation industry. Demographic shifts from a younger population toward an older population with disabilities open such new fields as geriatric rehabilitation.

Technological advances drive all aspects of modern rehabilitation. Indeed in 1990, a panel of experts reported that they judged rehabilitation facilities in large part on the level of technological sophistication and quality of nursing staff.[22] Entire specialties are constructed around CAT scanners, arthroscopic surgery, body contouring exercise programs, electrical stimulation in pain clinics, and joint replacement procedures.[23] Rehabilitation services grew with the popularity of health clubs and sports medicine clinics. Physical therapy departments of hospitals and clinics actually share equipment and facilities with health clubs.

Pediatric rehabilitation is another growth area that is rapidly expanding due to treatment advances that permit infants to live with birth defects and diseases that would have killed them a few years ago but now leave them in a disabled condition. In addition, surgical and pharmaceutical advances permit early intervention to reduce the level of impairment and consequently to offer increased rehabilitation potential. Such surgical procedures as rhizotomy, for example, are used with young cerebral palsy patients to alleviate spastic involvement.[24] As a result of this surgery, children with cerebral palsy have more functional potential and can be expected to consume increased amounts of rehabilitation services. Specialized pediatric rehabilitation programs for such youngsters have been developed at Children's Medical Center in Dallas and Children's Hospital in Seattle.

The rehabilitation market potential for persons with AIDS is growing because of increases in new cases and innovative technologies that prolong life. As of 1990, more than 200,000 AIDS cases from 152 countries have been reported officially to the World Health Organization's Global Programme on AIDS (GPA). Because of serious under-reporting, GPA estimates the cumulative total of actual AIDS cases to be more than 600,000. Because many cases are as yet undiagnosed and the disease is spreading rapidly, experts estimate that more than 1,500,000 will have AIDS worldwide by 1992. The United States will have an estimated 145,000 diagnosed individuals living with AIDS and a cumulative patient total of 365,000 by 1993.[25] If, as expected, AIDS and AIDS-related complex (ARC) disable individuals for years before resulting in death, an entirely new potential market for rehabilitation services is being created. AIDS and ARC are emergent chronic conditions that will require enormous rehabilitation resources and the development of new treatment techniques. . . .

Geriatric rehabilitation, focusing on individuals aged 70 and older with generalized weakness, is another burgeoning area in rehabilitation. Large numbers of individuals in this age cohort experience general weakness but otherwise are in good health. If their physical capacities and general level of function can be strengthened and maintained, they will be able to live independently at home for years without consuming expensive nursing home care.[26] This type of program can be developed on an outpatient basis as has been done at the Rusk Institute in New York and the Texas Rehabilitation Institute.

The Rehabilitation Industry

When businesses begin to manipulate rehabilitation markets for their own profit and growth, conflicts of interests arise among corporations, professionals, and those individuals with disabilities.[27] The Burroughs Welcome Company's announcements encouraging people to be tested for the AIDS virus, for example, seemed to be more concerned with generating a new market for an expensive AZT medication than with the consequences of arousing fear among those who might have been exposed to the virus.[28] Likewise when government controls the market so that it can control the professions and the industry, conflicts arise among government, business, and consumer interests.

. . . The rehabilitation industry today is driven by a mix of humanitarian, State, and profit-oriented values that shape the rehabilitation marketplace. Existing legislation disproportionately gives more benefits to military veterans, disabled workers, and others judged to be of more utilitarian value to the nation than the severely disabled, poor, and elderly. Many service delivery programs are specialized to treat special populations because federal money is available to pay for services. Private insurance companies and fee-for-service patients shape a different segment of the market. Here services that turn a profit are developed into strong product lines. . . .[29]

Methods Used to Market Rehabilitation Services

Managers of health facilities develop marketing to help their firms survive and grow.[30] These strategies range from the expansion of existing services, such as physical therapy, into new markets, such as geriatric rehabilitation, to the development of new services, such as nutritional and sexual counseling. Once such strategies are formulated, marketing techniques and advertising are employed to implement them. Open houses are held for new clinics, sports figures such as Magic Johnson are shown helping children with disabilities use the facility or equipment, and having a personal trainer is made to appear highly desirable for amateur athletes and persons with disabilities alike.

In the health business, most professionals and managers share the goals of survival and growth of the business, delivering high-quality care to those in need, providing access to medical care, and making a profit or return on investment. Rehabilitation facilities and professionals develop specific strategies through market analyses designed to help the institution meet these goals and related objectives.[31] In a formal marketing analysis, the institutional goals are specified, the external environment is assessed, an internal and external marketing audit is accomplished, and an internal capability analysis is completed before marketing strategies are developed. In such an analysis, the environment and organizational resources shape the successful interconnected set of marketing strategies. The *environment* includes existing markets, competition, and economic, political, legal, social, cultural, and technological forces that affect the organization's goals. The *market audit* identifies the target markets, service areas, service mix, competition, and exchange facilitators. The *internal capability analysis*

assesses the organization's strengths and weaknesses.

Health professionals increasingly develop and select strategies based on these formal marketing analyses.[32] Such strategies usually include (a) developing new products and markets based on the strengths of the organization and opportunities in the environment, (b) widening established service lines or areas, (c) the service specialization sometimes known as *market segmentation* or *niches*, (d) vertical and horizontal integration, (e) joint ventures, (f) diversification, and retrenchment. Given the resources and environment at hand, managers select strategies judged most likely to accomplish the organization's goals. Health professionals similarly employ expansion strategies to strengthen their practices. Physical therapists in private practice have increased their patient load and profits by constructing interlocking referral networks with surgeons, nutritionists, occupational therapists, and chiropractors in the community.[33]

The marketing strategies of managers and professionals most often are expressed through institutional plans. Sports medicine clinics, for example, are a spin-off of physical rehabilitation departments aimed at widening the service or product line.[34] Increased physical activity among Americans who jog, lift weights, bike, surf, sailboard, hike, golf, bowl, or play tennis or softball has produced stress fractures, muscle pulls, and tendon and joint problems. Hospitals were able to capitalize on present staff and facilities by reorganizing their house and therapy staffs around the new sports medicine market. Athletes and insurance companies are willing to pay for therapy to control pain and to return those injured to their previous activity levels. Athletic teams hire sports medicine specialists to condition athletes offseason in order to prevent injuries, to be present at games in order to control any damage incurred by injuries during competition, and to work, between contests, with those who have been injured. Sports medicine clinics market similar services to a large amateur athletic population.

Rush-Presbyterian St. Luke's Medical Center in Chicago is planning to build an entirely new clinic, dedicated to sports medicine, across the Eisenhower Expressway on the "L" line near the Chicago Stadium. The medical center has lobbied the city of Chicago and the Chicago Bulls, Bears, and Sting to develop a sports and shopping complex adjacent to the Medical Center. In addition, it has recruited highly visible athletes and community leaders to the Medical Center so that the general public is attracted by the quality of care and recognition of sharing the facility with such world-class athletes as Michael Jordan. Hero worship is used as a marketing tool. Advertising is done in newspapers and on TV. Celebrity benefit "runs for fun" are held to promote the institutional offerings and to sell services through identification with healthful activities and healthy celebrities. . . .

Other rehabilitation facilities have widened their established product lines to include services for the elderly, aimed at keeping the elderly functionally independent rather than placed in custodial institutions.[35] Emory University Medical and Rehabilitation Centers, for example, offer outpatient therapy services and medical clinics on-site for residents at Wesley Woods Homes, a residential facility for the elderly that is affiliated with the university. The centers also extended their service areas to encompass other community-based outpatient clinics, mobile therapy teams, freestanding clinics placed in shopping malls, and home visits. The elderly are encouraged to take care of themselves, to form support groups, to live in groups, to be politically active, and to demand quality medical care services. Other hospitals have amplified their return on investment in these rehabilitation product lines through advertising, offering reduced fees to senior citizens to increase volume, and effectively lobbying to alter insurance plans and DRG [Diagnostic Related Groups] reimbursement schedules so that delivering rehabilitation services to the elderly became a growing, profitable business.[36]

Rehabilitation organizations further widened their service lines by lobbying for expanded government and private insurance benefits for all people with disabilities. As a consequence of expanded benefit packages, institutions now can provide a wider range and depth of service for which they will be reimbursed. For instance, most patients are now eligible for physical and occupational therapy after surgery.

Rehabilitation departments and clinics also expanded by segmenting the market through specialization. Years ago therapists and physicians would work with any paying patient who walked into the clinic. Now entrepreneurial institutions and groups specialize in such conditions as spinal cord injury, fractured hips, low-back pain, and head injuries. The Shepard Spinal Cord Center in Atlanta, Georgia, and Craig Hospital in Englewood, Colorado, for example, specialize in treating spinal cord injured patients.[37] Both centers utilize a team approach in providing a wide range of integrated services with a strong emphasis on sports activities and community involvement to immerse patients in the world outside the hospital. New technologies and equipment are developed in these specialized settings. Shepard's EES (electro-ejaculation stimulation) clinic was the first in the Southeast to result in the birth of a child, to a nurse and her quadriplegic husband. Similarly the Baylor Institute for Rehabilitation in Dallas has an intensive amputee program, and the National Rehabilitation Hospital in Washington, DC, has a clinic to help people with traumatic head injuries.

The decision to specialize is influenced by institutional resources and community need. Providing housing for patients and their families during treatment and transition periods, for instance, is an innovation that makes specialized treatments possible for people who otherwise would not find these services accessible. The Mayo Clinic was a leader in providing subsidized housing for the families of patients while treatment was under way. The Rehabilitation Institute of Chicago and the National Rehabilitation Hospital in Washington, DC, offer transitional housing to help rehabilitated persons with spinal cord injuries reintegrate in the community. Such market segmentation claims a territory and eliminates competition that cannot offer similar services. In addition, specialization adds prestige to the institution, usually justifies higher fee structures, and offers increased profit potential. Specialization typically requires advanced equipment and training that can be used also for other purposes, thus increasing the return on investment. Institutions develop these markets by sponsoring training sessions and educational programs that tout their expertise and effectiveness, by contracting with insurance companies to take a set number of patients at preestablished fees, and by locating in large medical centers that attract specialists and difficult cases.

Rehabilitation units have grown also through strategies of vertical and horizontal integration.[38] *Vertical integration* refers to assimilation into a large medical complex in which patients can be sent from emergency room to surgery, medical-surgical nursing, and then rehabilitation and outplacement in the community. *Horizontal integration* is accomplished by offering a broader and more integrated range of services, often in coordination with other units in the medical center, to persons with disabilities. The Rehabilitation Institute of Chicago (RIC) provides an example of both types of integration. RIC grew in size and stature by moving from affiliate status in the Northwestern University Medical Center to full membership in the university's McGaw Medical Center. This organizational rearrangement coincided with a physical move from an old warehouse in an off campus location to a new seventeen-story building in the heart of the medical center. Vertical and horizontal integration occurred in the development of numerous joint programs in the university. The Department of Pediatrics and RIC developed a comprehensive program for youngsters with developmental disabilities. The Department of Surgery, RIC, and the Engineering School built a premier spinal cord injury system that was both vertically and horizontally integrated into the university medical center and the city of Chicago and state of Illinois regional trauma centers. Finally the university revitalized their School of Physical Therapy by moving it into RIC and increasing its financial support. Through these measures, treatment, education, and research programs were integrated and enhanced, thus strength-

ening the market position of the Rehabilitation Institute of Chicago. . . .

Physicians in practice and in medical institutions have used joint ventures to secure a strong position in the marketplace. Easter Seal of Bridgeport, Connecticut, for instance, entered a joint venture with Bridgeport Hospital that benefitted both institutions. The Easter Seal Society offered extensive outpatient rehabilitation services through a highly trained staff but had trouble maintaining consistent patient and cash flow in a rapidly changing external environment. Bridgeport Hospital, on the other hand, was a solidly established community hospital that did not have sufficient staff or space to offer extensive rehabilitation services. An ingenious solution was reached when the Easter Seal Society was built directly across the street from the hospital. The two institutions constructed a tunnel between the buildings so that patients could be moved easily from their rooms to comprehensive therapy programs and back. Both institutions gained from the joint venture. The hospital could market an integrated care system, including postoperative rehabilitation services, and the local Easter Seal Society had a guaranteed flow of paying patients.

Professionals and organizations also use diversification to expand their businesses. Sports medicine physical therapy clinics, for instance, now sell heavy-duty rubber bands and instructional booklets so that those with musculoskeletal problems can do rehabilitation exercises at home or on the road. Rehabilitation clinics have included juice bars and health club affiliations to entice new members. Separate rooms are set aside for men and women, to make them comfortable. Massage therapists, visiting home exercise therapists, and consultants are built into the panoply of services.

Other rehabilitation groups have moved into the instructional field through the sale and rental of audiotapes and videotapes designed to present model exercises for those disabled or injured. Similarly professionals now visit work sites to deal with specific occupation-related conditions. Preventive and restorative programs are designed specifically for these workers. Even computer-assisted skill development programs are available to those with learning disabilities and brain injuries. . . .

Finally *retrenchment* is a desirable strategy when analysis indicates that a traditional market is diminishing in size, no longer exists, or is unprofitable. Rehabilitation efforts aimed at leprosy, tuberculosis, and polio went through retrenchment as prevention and treatment regimens improved. The custodial and rehabilitation programs either retrenched, reorganized around other chronic conditions, or went out of business. Marketing analyses make planning and reorientation possible so that organizations and staff are not caught unaware of changes in the health marketplace. Astute managers have used these readjustments to move into a new market or business. TB sanatoria were converted to long-term care facilities. Polio experts emphasized their knowledge of degenerative orthopedic and neurological conditions. Rancho Los Amigos in Los Angeles, for instance, began as a county farm for the poor in 1887, became a center for polio patients in 1944, and reemerged as a comprehensive medical rehabilitation center in the mid 1950s.[39]

In practice, after an analysis of institutional strengths and environmental forces, professionals and organizations use interlocking sets of marketing strategies and techniques to achieve their goals by responding to and manipulating their environments. Organizational survival and growth depend on the provider's ability to accumulate valuable resources; to identify, respond to, and create demand; to offer quality products; and to anticipate the environment. Marketing provides these necessary tools.

The Consequences Of Marketing Rehabilitation Services

The marketing of rehabilitation services has both intended and unintended consequences for providers and consumers. The first major consequence of marketing is that rehabilitation services and products are considered commodities to be sold at a profit in the marketplace. This is true even for organizations that provide services under break-even conditions because they too need an operating safety margin. Traditionally, medical professionals and institutions had been perceived to operate on humanitarian values. Business principles presumably entered the decision-making process only in discussions of feasibility. Although this may only have been a fiction, public marketing, advertisement, and open competition for the rehabilitation dollar have disabused any previous illusions that observers may have had about the values driving the system.[40]

The open marketing of rehabilitation announces that health professionals are in competition for patients and dollars.[41] Survival and growth of the firm and robust salaries for health professionals are viewed as being as important to providers as the well-being of the patient. Such a modified free market system is constructive in that the consuming public is made acutely aware of the cost and quality of rehabilitation care. Providers are compelled by consumers and insurers to determine the actual costs of equipment and procedures. Rehabilitation formally has become a business heralded by public marketing and competition. As such, it is more fiscally accountable and public than ever before. . . .

This business orientation in rehabilitation reinforces a multi-tiered system of health and medicine in the United States. Providers of rehabilitation services are highlighting needs and marketing products principally to those potential customers who can recognize the need and pay for the services out-of-pocket or through insurance. The poor, unemployed, homeless, and poorly insured women, children, and elderly are not fully included in the market because they cannot pay for services except through Medicare and Medicaid. Thus the rehabilitation system serves to illustrate and reinforce a multi-tiered system detrimental to those most at risk. This system is incompatible with the American value system, which emphasizes helping those in need, as well as those who can pay.[42] At present, those without access and resources have little recourse.

A second consequence of marketing is an industry penchant for selling products irrespective of their benefits or risks to the consumer. Ciba-Geigy, for example, has run full page ads for Actigall, a pill to dissolve gallstones, under the caption, "Gallbladder Surgery. What to Do If You Can't or Won't Have It." The ad suggests that persons who are considering surgery and subsequent rehabilitation can take Actigall instead. Only later in the ad does the text state that the pills must be taken "for 6 to 24 months and dissolution may not occur in all cases."[43] Only in small print at the bottom of the page does the ad caution that most gallstones cannot be treated with pills and that Actigall is an expensive drug that usually must be taken twice daily for years. . . .

. . . The marketing of rehabilitation has interacted with a change in health ideology, resulting in a new conceptual approach to medical care. Professionals, insurance companies, and rehabilitation organizations are selling prevention and maintenance, as well as restoration and the retardation of functional decay.[44] The traditional rehabilitation model emphasized functional restoration so that people could return to work or at least take care of themselves. The new model of rehabilitation includes prevention and therapeutic activities designed to retard functional decay processes resulting from natural aging and chronic diseases. Thus rehabilitation that was previously seen as coming last in the medical care system . . . now fronts the system as well.

The reason for this successful marketing of preventive rehabilitation is that the therapies aimed at restoring function are the same as those that maintain and prevent. Diet and exercise programs supervised by rehabilitation professionals, for example, can prevent myocardial infarctions, as well as assist in recovery from cardiovascular accidents. Preventive outpatient rehabilitation services fit with the ideology of reducing medical costs through prevention activities and endorse the valued physically active lifestyles of today. This ideology, revised rehabilitation model, and lifestyle values are a basis for the successful marketing of rehabilitation services.

The new place of rehabilitation in the doctor-consumer relationship is a third consequence; it emphasizes consumers as active participants in health purchase decisions. Although a danger exists that preferences occasionally are manipulated, the consumer does take a more active, decision-making role in the rehabilitation process. The consumer is sold a service or product based on perceived need, availability and efficacy of the service, price, and ability to pay. Under these circumstances, consumers can make sound purchase decisions if they have good information. Likewise the nature of rehabilitation is such that the individual in need is the one who must work to improve function. Others cannot do this for them. Therefore the marketing of rehabilitation services has helped redefine the sick role from one of the uninformed passive patient to a purchasing and physically active consumer. . . .

The Effect of Marketing on the Structure of Health Care Delivery

Besides altering the social relationships between the consumers and producers of medical care, the marketing of rehabilitation services has helped change the structure of health care delivery. The business functions of marketing and strategic planning have been introduced formally into the medical business. Professional managers are replacing physicians as administrators of the nation's health care institutions. Experience with finance, accounting, cash flow management, and marketing are as important in the management of these organizations as knowledge of medicine.[45] In fact, in 1990 the American Hospital Association reported that an estimated 59 percent of hospitals in the United States have marketing departments or an individual who is responsible for marketing.[46] Public relations departments have a new role to play in presenting favorable images in the media and in keeping the institutions in the public eye. The reason for this effort is that health institutions that traditionally operated in local communities on a *pro bono* basis are increasingly operated as profit-generating, multiproduct firms that are expected to produce a healthy return on investment, in addition to serving the consumer.

Marketing symbolizes and intensifies competition among rehabilitation facilities. Competition for resources requires capturing a significant segment of the rehabilitation market.[47] Expansion into cardiac rehabilitation, sports medicine clinics, and large outpatient programs are efforts to control this growing market.[48] The latest in electrotherapy and hydrotherapy technology is used also to attract referring physicians and their patients.[49] Specialists who treat individuals with chronic illnesses were seen as a significant market resource. They have the power to refer patients into rehabilitation programs. Therefore rehabilitation facilities catered to these sources of patients by placing referring physicians and therapists on retainers, hiring them as consultants, or even offering them an ownership position in the business. Rehabilitation, then, became a part of a vertical monopoly in health institutions that ranged from inpatient medical-surgical care to rehabilitation services. As competition became fiercer, rehabilitation programs specialized and merged with larger and more powerful institutions. Rehabilitation marketing accelerated tertiary care in multi-institutional settings.

The marketing of rehabilitation also demonstrated how health care services can be delivered in many settings ranging from huge hospital complexes to freestanding clinics and the individual's home. Aggressive hospitals also market their services to insurance companies and the government. As a result, the government designated preferred treatment institutions as regional centers in burn treatment or stroke rehabilitation. In other instances, huge insurance companies, such as Prudential and Washington National, funneled seriously injured patients to only a few institutions with whom they had privileged relationships. The structure of medicine changed, in that health providers sold their services more to the government, private insurance companies, and referring physicians than to individual patients. Successful firms accumulated referral networks, treatment dollars, and diversified treatment facilities.

As competition for the rehabilitation dollar increased, individual providers moved outside hospital walls to establish new markets. Physicians, nurses, orthopedic surgeons, physical and occupational therapists, and sports medicine specialists went into business for themselves or in joint ventures with hospitals. The structure of the business developed from traditional non-profit forms to for-profit and hybrid forms. Humana and other large multi-institutional organizations set up franchise-type systems, including rehabilitation clinics in local communities where the need was greatest and clients could pay.

Aggressive marketing of rehabilitation services forced health institutions that wanted to compete with their neighbors to diversify and enter the rehabilitation business if they wanted to compete for the chronically ill or long-term care patient. For some institutions, rehabilitation became a marketing tool or loss leader item. Indeed no tertiary medical center can continue to operate without an extensive array of rehabilitation services.

Although competition through marketing established rehabilitation as a required part of large hospital services, informal arrangements between competing institutions in the same communities divided up the rehabilitation marketplace into niches. One institution would specialize in burn patients, while another would concentrate on children with developmental disabilities. In this way, coexisting institutions divided the market by geography and medical problem. Market niches were established and negotiated in the community.

The marketing of rehabilitation services is an excellent case study of orienting the growth of a specialty service around reimbursement mechanisms. A marketing analysis identifies the strengths of an institution and the reimbursable services in which the institution can make a profit. Today the structure of the rehabilitation business is greatly determined by the DRG, Medicare and Medicaid reimbursement schedules, and the number of visits and procedures allowable under private insurance and HMO [Health Maintenance Organization] agreements.[50] Institutions responded to these constraints by developing a business serving a market and by maximizing profit-making services. To make rehabilitation available for all, underinsured and uninsured persons with disabilities must have access to treatment through some expanded form of government health insurance. These issues add fuel to the debate over national health insurance.[51] Under present market conditions, rehabilitation institutions do not have incentives to provide services to this population.

In the current uncertain financial environment, some hospitals have contracted with outside agencies to provide rehabilitation services so that if times get bad, the contracts can be canceled without substantial loss to the larger institution. This subcontracting strategy also permits rapid response in number and type of services in a volatile environment.

The marketing of rehabilitation services has introduced new forms of cooperation and competition among the helping professions. Physicians are compelled to go into joint practice with physical and speech therapists. Occupational therapists compete with vocational counselors and sports medicine experts and are in joint practices with orthopedic surgeons. As a result, many forms of rehabilitation practice are emerging. Physicians, however, have kept a dominant position in this marketplace through judicious use of their referral power.[52] Only physicians have the power to refer large numbers of patients to other health facilities, medical specialists, and helping professions. Hospitals and therapists in private practice that recognize this resource market themselves to physicians. As the marketplace becomes more complex, persons with disabilities will experience increased difficulty in finding help and negotiating the system.

Summary and Conclusions

This chapter examined how the marketing of rehabilitation services has changed the structure and operation of established health care delivery systems. *Marketing* is the transactional process that makes contractual arrangements between buyers and sellers of rehabilitation services possible. Marketing is particularly valuable to health care professionals and institutions that operate in an increasingly complex, ambiguous, and changing environment in which identification and creation of markets is difficult. Marketing is

a catalyst that facilitates the transactions on which the rehabilitation business is built. Although marketing serves the survival and growth needs of institutions, it also changes the established relationships between providers and consumers of rehabilitation care and alters the social structure of the medical care delivery system.

Consumers are bombarded with incredible amounts of technology and information without knowing how to purchase intelligently. Although the volume of consumption has risen due to marketing, increased supply, insurance to pay for commodities, and growing demand, the benefit to consumers is not always clear. The rich panoply of goods and services available to the consumer with disabilities offers incredible potential for a better life. Yet because of the complexity of the purchase decisions and the volume of information to be processed, patients often are not in control of their own health care, nor do they know whether the goods and services consumed are needed or cost beneficial. If market forces primarily drive the business, profits and control of the market are likely to dictate goods and services sold, and not necessarily what is best for the persons with disabilities.

Institutions, health care providers, insurers, and government workers benefit because rehabilitation is a growth business insuring survival and generating jobs and profits. Even at that, however, anomalies exist in the system. Although professionals financially gain from the dynamism of the business, for example, they appear to lose some personal autonomy over their work as free market forces are unleashed. In sum, the political economic question remains: To whose benefit are these changes? Some are in the patient's best interest, but most benefit the providers of care and the State more than the individual in need. Certainly the poor, the elderly, and the disenfranchised do not necessarily profit by the commodification of rehabilitation goods and services.

Viewed from this perspective, marketing is a powerful tool that can be used for the good or the harm of the public. Although marketing can be used to bring the latest in health care to those in need, it can also be part of a larger exploitation process in which disabilities are produced and treated at a profit in a society. The value of marketing then, must be determined by its intended use and unintended consequences. If unregulated, marketing efforts are used to perpetuate a political economic system that benefits institutions and professionals at the expense of the individual citizen consumer. These trends are likely to continue in the near future because both the Reagan and Bush administrations openly promoted free market systems in the health care arena and in fact discouraged regulation.

Regardless of government regulation, marketing of rehabilitation services is an activity that is going to grow in importance in the health care system and affect all of the participants. Future studies and analyses should determine how different stakeholders benefit from marketing activities. These analyses should be extended to examine how marketing activities can be controlled and aimed at the good of the community and individual, not just the good of the firm, the professional, and the State.

Notes

1. Philip Kotler and Roberta N. Clarke, *Marketing for Health Care Organizations*. Englewood Cliffs, NJ: Prentice-Hall, 1987; and Philip Kotler and Alan R. Andreanson, *Strategic Marketing for Non-profit Organizations* 3rd ed. Englewood Cliffs, NJ: Prentice-Hall, 1987.

2. Paul J. Feldstein, *Health Care Economics* 2nd ed. New York: John Wiley, 1988.

3. Richard E. Verville, "Legislative Update," *Psychiatrist*, 1990, 6:3.

4. J. S. Rakich et al., *Managing Health Service Organizations*. Philadelphia: V. B. Saunders, 1985; and Brent England, Rita M. Glass, and Carole H. Patterson, *Quality Rehabilitation: Results-Oriented Patient Care*. Chicago: American Hospital Association, 1989.

5. Philip Kotler, *Principles of Marketing* 3rd ed. Englewood Cliffs, NJ: Prentice-Hall, 1988.

6. Glen Gritzer and Arnold Arluke, *The Making of Rehabilitation*. Berkeley: University of California Press, 1985.

7. Gary L. Albrecht (ed.), *The Sociology of Physical Disability and Rehabilitation*. Pittsburgh: Pittsburgh University Press, 1976.

8. Gary L. Albrecht (ed.), *Cross National Rehabilitation Policies*. Beverly Hills, CA: Sage, 1981.

9. Deborah A. Stone, *The Disabled State*. Philadelphia: Temple University Press, 1984.

10. L. W. Heal, D. E. Uis, and R. Norman, "Research on Community Residential Alternatives for the Mentally Ill," *International Review of Research in Mental Rehabilitation*, 1978, 9:209-247.

11. Department of Health and Human Services, Public Health Service, *Health United States 1986*. Washington, DC: Government Printing Office, 1986, p. 123.

12. Department of the Census, *Disability, Functional Limitations and Health Insurance Coverage*, 1985. Washington, DC: Government Printing Office, 1986; and Bob Griss, *Measuring the Insurance Needs of Persons With Disabilities and Persons With Chronic Illness Access to Health Care*, September 1988. Berkeley, CA: World Institute of Disability, 1988.

13. D. Thompson, "Stealthy Epidemic of Exhaustion," *Time*, June 29,1987, p. 52.

14. Department of Health and Human Services, "Use of Nursing Homes by the Elderly: Preliminary Data From the 1985 National Nursing Home Survey," *Advancedata*. Washington, DC: Government Printing Office, May 24,1987.

15. M. G . Kovar and A. Z. LaCroix,"Aging in the Eighties, Ability to Perform Work-Related Activities," *Advancedata*. Washington, DC: Government Printing Office, 1987.

16. Nancy M. Kane, "The Home Care Crisis of the Nineties," *Gerontologist*, 1989, 29:24-31.

17. Lisa W. Foderaro, "Want a Comfortable Old Acre? Plan Care, Experts Advise," *New York Times*, March 30, 1990, pp. 1, A10.

18. Department of Health and Human Services, *Disability, Utilization, and Costs Associated With Musculoskeletal Conditions, United States, 1980*. Washington, DC: Government Printing Office, 1986.

19. P. Kotler and A. Andreanson, *Strategic Marketing for Nonprofit Organizations*. Englewood Cliffs, NJ: Prentice-Hall, 1987.

20. See H. E. Frech III (ed.), *Health Care in America*, San Francisco: Pacific Research Institute for Public Policy, 1988; and Barbara Ehrenreich, "Our Health-Care Disgrace," *Time*, December 10, 1990, p. 112.

21. American Hospital Association, *Vision, Values, Viability*. Chicago: Author, 1988, p. 63.

22. "Reputations Are Made of These: How Physicians Judged Service," *U.S. News and World Report*, April 30, 1990, p. 83.

23. Indian Smith, "Electrotherapy in Action—A Market on the Move," *Rehab Management*, 1990, 3:23-28, 70-71.

24. Anne Framerose, "Pediatric Rehabilitation: Growing by Leaps and Bounds," *Rehab Management*, 1989, 2:51-57.

25. "Global AIDS: Patterns and Trends," *AIDS and Society*, 1990, 1:3; and Anne Framerose, "Coping With AIDS in the Rehab Environment," *Rehab Management*, 1989, 2:57-63.

26. "Industry News," *Rehab Management*, 1990, 3:20.

27. H. Kohlman, "Physicians as Business Partners in Healthcare Marketing," *Healthcare Financial Management*, December 1985, p. 10; and Fred H. Darner, Richard Barr, and Stephen L. Tucker, "Hospital Market Share: The Declining Share of Small Players in the Market," *Health Care Management Review*, 1990, 15:11-15.

28. Elizabeth Rosenthal, "Drug Makers Set Off a Bitter Debate With Ads Aimed Directly at Patients," *New York Times*, March 3, 1991, p. 17.

29. R. S. MacStravic, "Product-line Administration in Hospitals," *Health Care Management Review*, 1986, 35-43.

30. C.M. Pimlott, "Health-care Marketers Should Map Strategies," *Marketing News*, February 26, 1986, p. 23.

31. Rose D. Plelan, "Nursing: An Unrecognized Major Health Care Marketing Force for Hospitals," 1987, 7:45-49.

32. D. Gregory and D. Klegon, "The Value of Strategic Marketing to the Hospital," *Healthcare Financial Management*, December 1983, pp. 16-22.

33. A. F. Roy, "Strategic Alliances for PTs: Joining Forces," *Rehab Management*, 1989, 2:23-27.

34. William N. Zelman and Deborah L. Parham, "Strategic, Operational, and Marketing Concerns of Product-Line Management in Health Care," *Health Care Management Review*, 1990, 15:19-25.

35. Mary Ann Wharton, "Rehabilitation and the Elderly: Emphasizing Function," *Rehab Management*, 1989, 2:53-56.

36. D. G. Halide, "Healthcare Ads Shape Up as Big TV Growth Category," *Television/Radio Age*, August 19, 1985, pp. 55-56; and Nancy J. Scharmach, "Diversifying Into Skill-Nursing Care," *Modern Healthcare*, April 30, 1990, 20:30-31.

37. Curtis Pichell, "Shepard Spinal Center: A Dream Made Real," *Rehab Management*, 1989, 2:37-41; and John Callender, "Focusing on the Tough Cases: Craig Hospital, Englewood, Colorado," *Rehab Management*, 1989, 2:50-54.

38. B. H. Gray (ed.), *For Profit Enterprise in Health Care*. Washington, DC: National Academy, l986.

39. Edward D. Berkowitz, "Allocating Resources for Rehabilitation: A Historical and Ethical Framework," *Social Science Quarterly*, 1989, 70:40-52.

40. J. H. Reade and R. M. Ratzan, "Yellow Professionalism: Advertising by Physicians in the Yellow Pages," *New England Journal of Medicine*, 1987, 316:1315-1319; and H. Waitzkin, B. V. Akin, Luis M. de la Marja, and F Atlubell, "Deciding Against Corporate Management of a State-Supported Academic Medical Center," *New England Journal of Medicine*, 1986, 315:1299-1304.

41. R. M. Battistella, "Hospital Receptivity to Market Competition: Image and Reality," *Health Care Management Review*, 1985, 10:19-26.

42. See Cindy Jajich-Toth and Burns W. Roper, "Americans' View on Health Care: A Study in Contradictions," *Health Affairs*, 1990, 9:149-157, for a discussion of these contradictions.

43. Elizabeth Rosenthal, "Drug Makers Set Off a Bitter Debate With Ads Aimed Directly at Patients," *New York Times*, March 3, 1991, p. 417.

44. Vicki S. Freimuth, Sharon L. Hammond, and Judith A. Stein, "Health Advertising: Prevention for Profit," *American Journal of Public Health*, 1988, 78:557-561.

45. K. T. Higgins, "Health Industry Must Emulate Retail, Financial," *Marketing News*, April 11, 1986, p. 9.

46. American Hospital Association, *Visions, Values, Viability*. Chicago: Author, 1988, p. 62.

47. R. A. Reif, Patricia A. Bickett, and Donald G. Halberstad, "Case Study: Analyzing the Market Using DRGs and MDCs," *Healthcare Financial Management*, December 1985, pp. 44-47.

48. American Hospital Association, op. cit., p. 63.

49. Steven Findlay, Marjory Roberts, and Joanne Silberner, "The Best Hospitals, From AIDS to Urology," *U.S. News and World Report*. April 30, 1990, p. 83.

50. R. L. Ludke and G. S. Levitz, "Referring Physicians: The Forgotten Market," *Health Care*

Management Review, 1983, 8:13-22; Daryl P. Evans, "Burogenesis," *Social Science Journal*, 1985, 22:59-86; J. J. Pena, T. R. Jamison, and Bernard Rose, "Marketing: A Necessary Art Under DRGs," *Hospital and Health Services Administration*, 1986, 31:55-73; P D. Benz and J. Burnham, "Case Study: Developing Product Lines Using ICDA-CM Codes," *Healthcare Financial Management*, December 1985, pp. 38-41; and Michael R. Pollard, "Managed Care and a Changing Pharmaceutical Industry," *Health Affairs*, 1990, 9:55-65.

51. See Peter McMenamin, "What Do Economists Think Patients Want?" *Health Affairs*, 1990, 9:112-119, for a discussion of the inconsistencies in public support for national health insurance.

52. Roy, op. cit. (Note 33).

Further Reading

Gary Albrecht. 1992. *The Disability Business*. Thousand Oaks, CA: Sage.

J. Warren Salmon (ed.). 1990. *The Corporate Transformation of Health Care*. Amityville, NY: Baywood.

Donald W. Light. 1994. "Excluding More, Covering Less: The Health Insurance Industry in the United States." In Nancy F. McKenzie (ed.) *Beyond Crisis: Confronting Health Care in the United States*. New York: Penguin, pp. 310-320.

Discussion Questions

1. What do you see as the effects of these strategies upon consumers both individually and collectively?

2. In which ways do marketing strategies affect the organizational environment in medical care?

3. What marketing strategies do health plans use in your area?

31

Robust Resistance

Alexandra Dundas Todd

What happens when patients and practitioners view health, illness, and healing differently? In this account of healing cancer, Alexandra Dundas Todd critically reflects on the consequences of merging eastern medicine with western practices of care. Todd points out that physicians cling to what they know, in spite of genuine evidence that another approach, definition, or treatment regimen could have better effects. Modern medicine's emphasis on warfare provides its practitioners with a design for fighting cancer and other diseases chemically. Consider the assumptions of disease based on the notion of medicine as chemical warfare. Now consider the status of a person with the disease. Where is the patient in western medicine? How do patients fit into "disease as enemy" models of treatment? In this selection, Todd contrasts western models of treatment with eastern philosophies, suggesting that models of disease prevention cannot be based on the warfare analogy. Consider the differences she articulates between western and eastern notions of health, illness, and healing.

"Well, I guess this is it." Dr. R smiled on the last day of Drew's radiation treatment. I had come along on this momentous day to discuss long-range plans for follow-up. Dr. R was the doctor we had seen the most. Drew saw him regularly for over two months. I had come to the center occasionally. Dr. R was the only doctor we encountered who consistently had time to talk and to listen. In the beginning he had chatted with all of us. What did we do? Where did we come from? How were we coping? He gave us large chunks of his time, he was never rushed, he asked about Drew's life as well as his health, and he listened carefully. His research and practice limited him to a few carefully chosen patients. These lucky few got his full attention.

Although I didn't go with Drew for most of his radiation, when I did, Dr. R commented on how well Drew was doing physically and psychologically with the program. Certainly, compared to his fellow patients, Drew was a marvel of health.

Of all of the people Drew had worked with in the past months, Dr. R was the most open to different points of view and to being questioned. He seemed the doctor most likely to be interested in the alternative methods Drew had experienced. Since the Japanese studies on radiation and diet seemed the most convincing and since Dr. R, a radiotherapist, might find them intriguing, Drew decided to start with these articles. He took me along, all of the studies at my fingertips. Dr. R and I had discussed our medical research interests at some length. Drew and I were optimistic that he could use some of what we had learned to help others cope with the myriad problems of radiation therapy.

Drew started explaining about how well he felt, connecting it to miso soup, seaweed, umeboshi plums. I, in my most academic voice, inserted scientific data, study after study. Drew had decided to start small—a few easily used, inexpensive remedies accessible to all.

Dr R listened carefully, smiling at Drew's references to his initial reactions to seaweed. Dr. R was unfailingly polite. But the longer Drew talked, the less this expert communicator listened. Something had switched off. I told him I had all of the references if he was interested. He smiled his broad, sincere smile, looked Drew right in eye and said, "Drew, the main thing is it made *you* feel better to do it. For that I'm happy. The main thing here is your great attitude."

In other words, do what works for you. You believe it, do it; it'll work. Placebo effect. Nothing generalizable here. Of course, Dr. R was right about Drew's attitude—it is great. But attitude is not enough. He'd always had a great attitude. That didn't stop his getting cancer. And how great would his outlook have remained if he'd had to live with piercing headaches or extreme nausea and fatigue? No, Dr. R was not interested. He was interested in Drew; he was genuinely happy that he was doing so well. He had no curiosity at all about alternative treatments, even those embedded in careful, suggestive research.

Lack of curiosity. It always surprises me, especially in such clever people. Ten years ago doctors were likely to try to dissuade, to dismiss as quackery, to rage against the absurdity of anything other than conventional medical treatment. That still happens occasionally but is far less common. No one objected to what Drew was doing. No doctor stormed into Drew's hospital room demanding that he eat the hospital's food. Doctors, nurses, and staff either thought it a good idea to avoid hospital cuisine or were indifferent to what he ate. No one treated Drew as deviant when he mentioned visualization or acupuncture. He was, in fact, consistently treated with respect. The attitude was, "If it works for you, do it, but I don't need to know about it. This is your thing."

People writing about healing themselves report the same phenomenon. . . . If so many doctors, when presented with evidence of potentially successful treatment plans in the face of such devastation from cancer, show no curiosity, then the salient questions are why, how come, how can this be.

Many medical watchers and writers focus on the roles of power, greed, and money in our health care system. Doctors cling to what they know, excluding the new, in order to maintain control. The more outsiders who emerge, the more control is required to keep them out. The medical power base, expressed through the American Medical Association (AMA), is increasingly in jeopardy from such institutional factors as rising costs and threats in the form of national health coverage and big-business, for-profit hospital takeovers, as well as from growing public dissatisfaction with current medical care. In response it tries to tighten its hold and control the increasingly uncontrollable. A lot is at stake: self-regulation, a free market profession, and tremendous amounts of money in the form of corporate profits (to pharmaceutical and insurance companies, for example) and physician incomes. . . .

Individual doctors and medicine as a whole are described by one writer as "pursu-

ing economic self-interest just like everyone else, and arrangements that maximize income are always going to be looked upon favorably by those whose incomes are maximized. But the high costs of maintaining that self-interest and our burdened medical system are astronomical, and no one, including orthodox medicine, is happy about it. In 1930, 3.5 percent of the American gross national product went to health care; by 1990, 12.2 percent did. Everyone—doctors, hospitals, the public—agrees change is necessary. The controversy arises only when it comes to what the changes will look like, where to cut.

These economic critiques are relevant for what ails our health care system as well as what keeps medicine an empire. After all, only in the early 1990s did the United States administratively move toward a national health plan, the last industrialized country to do so.

Money and power are clearly parts of the problem. Yet shocking as some of the economic arguments are, they are not enough; such explanations don't account for behaviors of individual doctors. Dr. R was not thinking of money or power when his eyes glazed over after two minutes of alternative talk. Nussbaum's friendly, even supportive oncologist, welcoming her with a cheerful "Here comes my miracle," was not afraid macrobiotics would put her out of business. No, the problem goes deeper than money. Belief systems also play a crucial role. A friend recently gave her internist a copy of Sherry Roger's *Tired or Toxic*, a book that looks at our current environment, how it causes disease, and what to do about it. Although conventionally trained, Rogers is by no means a conventional doctor. My friend's internist said he would read it; he didn't. He sent it back to her with a note explaining that if he read it he might have to completely change his orientation to health and illness, a change he couldn't face making.

People in general and institutions in particular are slower to change. We all hold on to what we know to make sense of our lives and worlds. And as worlds change ever faster, more chaotically, the more strongly we are apt to hold onto what we understand until we can incorporate changes into our knowledge base with the least disruption. Historically, this has been particularly true of medicine. The germ theory, the cornerstone of modern medicine, had as hard a time being accepted in the nineteenth century as holistic or alternative understandings do today. The very idea of bacteria, germs as microscopic organisms that could make people sick, was foreign to medical men. . . .

Why did the germ theory generate such resistance? In part it challenged the status quo, the known, the illusion of certainty in one's belief system. The new approach was not yet well understood—unseeable germs, much like meridians, required a leap of faith. Knowledge of the role of bacteria and viruses was limited, and to suggest that cleanliness and health might be related probably seemed farfetched. As Thomas Kuhn has discussed, we have a long legacy of resistance to new ideas in science that require great bounds, and the same can be seen in medicine. Furthermore, doctors are trained to be healers, not harmers. For them to reconceptualize the death of patients as iatrogenic (doctor induced) was not an easy task. Whenever doctors feel challenged, the implication is that what they do is not enough. To question their brand of medicine is to question their ability to heal. It is only a short step to the slippery slope of questioning whether they are harming as well as healing. Many find it easier to dismiss the challenging and the challenger rather than face the shock of the new. In the case of germs, as has been true with modern challenges such as the changing role of nutrition in heart disease, resistance decreased as times changed and evidence piled up. . . .

The increasingly sophisticated discovery of microorganisms and methods of treatment in this century have led to massive campaigns against disease. After World War II, as these campaigns grew more successful, optimism for the end of disease abounded in the medical profession and the general public. And indeed, great strides in health care were made—polio vaccines, antibiotic cures, more recently the field of imaging (such as MRI), and so forth. Modern medicine, derived in part from chemical warfare, was applied to eradicate disease, and medical metaphors, in fact, became deeply militaristic: "the war on

AIDS," "the eradication of the enemy," and the like. The body became (and remains) a battlefield, with good doctors fighting the good fight against bad bugs. The ill find themselves in a unique position. Perri Klass, in her book on her medical education, sums up this fight:

> If we are at war, then who is the enemy? Rightly the enemy is disease, and even if that is not your favorite metaphor, it is a rather common way to think of medicine: we are combatting these deadly processes for the bodies of our patients. They become battlefields, lying there passively in bed while armies of pathology and the resplendent forces of modern medicine fight it out. . . . The real problem arises because all too often the patient comes to personify the disease, and somehow the patient becomes the enemy.

In this war, the asumption is that all diseases can be conquered. First, the enemy is defined and then cordoned off. An active doctor and passive patient agree "the doctor knows best." Specific etiology (causation), with an emphasis on the cell or a particular organ rather than the whole person, is the focus. Even as some researchers start to expand the germ theory model with explorations of strengthening the body's immune system as a means to create balance and thus health, the battlefield image remains intact. One team of researchers writing on, what else, the "war on cancer," addresses the "immune surveillance system." Instead of doctors playing gunmen attacking—germs—these writers suggest the need to stimulate the body's own, "defensive system by which immune cells patrol silently throughout the body, attacking foreign invaders." Activate those "killer cells." In this newer landscape of the body, a continuous defend-and-conquer scenario unfolds in each of us, sick or well, all of the time. Reflections of military strategies against disease show up in literature as well as medical discussion. In Jeanette Winterson's *Written on the Body*, the narrator mourns a lover's diagnosis of chronic lymphocytic leukemia,

> In the secret places of her thymus gland Louise is making too much of herself. Her faithful biology depends on regula-

tion but the white T-cells have turned bandit. They don't obey the rules. They are swarming into the bloodstream, over-turning the quiet order of spleen and in-testine. . . . It used to be their job to keep her body safe from enemies on the out-side. They were her immunity, her cer-tainty against infection. Now they are the enemies on the inside. The security forces have rebelled. Louise is the victim of a coup.

Despite many advances in medicine using such war-based metaphors, optimism that aggressive, scientific medicine can eradicate or cure all diseases has diminished by the late twentieth century.

Repeatedly, polls show public dissatisfac-tion with health care in the United States; the costs are too high, doctors don't listen, and so forth. At the same time, the public, each day, places inordinate trust in this system. And the breakthroughs such as imaging, proton beam radiation, and laser surgeries *are* stunning. Doctors find themselves in a paradoxical situation: On the one hand, they face enough failure and criticism to make them defensive (and in need of enormous amounts of mal-practice insurance); on the other, they expe-rience enough success and devotion to pro-mote arrogance. Neither posture is condu-cive to change or openness to new paradigms. Alternative models of health care, while per-haps complementary with orthodox medi-cine, may be only perceivable as threats, based on their differences, their otherness, from the safety of the known, even if the known changes daily. Certainly, the alterna-tives I've discussed in this book *are* different. From their conceptual roots to actual prac-tice they are as *other* to Western medical thought as possible. For example:

- Where Western medicine looks for the single cause, Eastern medicine assumes multiple ones.

- Where Western medicine's focus is on curing illness, Eastern medicine at-tempts to prevent it. When Western medicine does go for prevention, the ap-proach is still quintessentially Western. For example, a controversial experi-ment is under way whereby healthy women at high risk of developing breast

cancer are to be given a drug—an anti-estrogen, tamoxifen—to see if it pre-vents the disease. Rita Arditti, a sociolo-gist specializing in women and cancer, writes about this experiment's critics: "The criticisms center around the fact that tamoxifen causes liver cancer in rats, liver changes in all species tested, and that a number of endometrial can-cers have been reported among ta-moxifen users." Do healthy women al-ready at higher than average risk for breast cancer need to add possible liver or endometrial cancer to their fears? If the West is going to shift to a prevention model, it will have to do better than this.

- Where Western medicine defines knowledge hierarchically, with the doc-tor the knower and the patient the known—the former active, the latter passive— Eastern medicine centers on a partnership of knowers. In this part-nership each has a different kind of knowledge, and all of the players are ac-tive participants. Patients become peo-ple responsible for making decisions about their treatment and recovery. Ex-perts offer guidance and information, treatments and support, but ill people decide what they are willing or able to do to cease their situation. This is not a blame-the-victim message of total re-sponsibility but rather a means to feel in power, in control of one's own life decisions instead of being a helpless vic-tim of disease processes and the experts that tend to them.

This Western inequality between doctor and patient is powerfully summed up in Alan Bennett's play about the medical miseries of and ministrations to King George III. In a stark scene, King George sits pitifully strapped into a chair, barefoot and dishev-eled, clothed in a tattered, stained nightdress, having been leeched, burned, purged, and pierced. He musters a shred of strength to proclaim to one of his overbearing physi-cians: "King: (Howling) I am the King of Eng-land."

His doctor, grandly dressed, elegantly erect, booms with authority to King George and to the audience: "No, sir. You are the patient."

- Where Western medicine does battle against the enemies of disease with big guns, Eastern medicine seeks peace through balance. Disease rather than being an invader, is a messenger from the body, signaling for help, change, and harmony. Elizabeth Kubler-Ross, well known to many for her help in coping with dying, says, "If one is in pain, comfort must be sought. The body is asking for something. Don't keep denying it."

Vivien Newbold, talking about her own shifts in perspective as a Western doctor incorporating some Eastern values, tells a story of her experience with a lump in her breast.

Was this lump going to turn out to be a cancer to pay me back for all my bad habits? After obtaining a mammogram which indicated that the possibility of cancer was very remote and seeking macrobiotic counseling, I went on a strict diet. The lump disappeared; however whenever I overindulged in rich food, the lump would reappear and be very painful. For the first few months, I was angry and resentful. I could not overindulge in the foods I enjoyed so much without a rude reminder from this wretched little thing. Then, one day, I woke up and realized how precious that little lump was. It was my warning light which signaled that I was really harming myself.

Newbold went from fear to anger to gratitude. We are all familiar with the fear—fear of cancer, fear of pain, fear of death; and the anger—anger at our bodies for betraying us, anger at something or someone for letting such terrible things befall us. The idea of gratitude where illness is concerned is indeed a stretch for the imagination. But it is all more complicated than I used to think. I'm not grateful, per se, that I developed environmental sensitivities, but I'm glad that what I learned from that experience helped Drew. None of us is grateful that Drew got cancer. In fact, we are still coping with the fear and the anger—a fear and anger that are appropriate and probably will never fully disappear. But Drew had no control over developing a tumor. He only had changes to make

once he knew he had it. So why not, along with all of the enormous variety of emotions, treasure some of the close moments, delight in the new sense of one's own courage? The importance of every moment is fresh in Drew's mind regardless of how long or short his life may be. No one, no disease can take this away from him. He has been given a terrible gift. The Chinese philosophy that holds that buried in the seeds of danger are the seeds of opportunity helps to steady the nerves and build strength out of the ashes of weakness.

- Where Western medicine seeks proof and tangible evidence, striving for a practice based on experiments, validity, and controlled studies, Eastern medicine looks to clinical and historical experience, empirical knowledge passed down for thousands of years.

- Where the West looks to parts of the body, the individual organ or cell, utilizing skills that zero in on the part, separating the mind from the body, the East expands to the entire person, both body and mind considered part of the whole organism. In an obviously extreme but telling example in Western medicine of the part becoming more important than the whole (taken from an "AIDS Quarterly" segment on PBS television), one doctor advocated continuing an experimental AIDS drug despite the patients worsening condition on the medication. His reason: the blood work showed improvement. Luckily for the ill man, the principle investigator (P.I.) of the experiment discontinued the drug. In an argument with his colleague, the P.I. pointed out that the blood work didn't matter; the patient was dying. The junior doctor reluctantly agreed to stop the experiment on this person and on others. But he wasn't convinced. After all, as he kept repeating, the blood work looked good.

Such an approach in which a test result can become more important than the empirical evidence and a part of the body can be weighted over the person's well-being, would be unusual in an Eastern orientation to health and illness. Here the person is connected to the larger environment in a series of expansions and contractions, a push and pull relationship between matter and energy. Deep in its theoritical roots, modern Western physics is similar to the Eastern philosophy of expansion and contraction, yin and yang. The very structure of the atom is based on attraction and repulsion, an ongoing interplay of opposition and integration. Modern medicine, however, is not based on current physics, with its emphases from Werner Heisenberg and Albert Einstein on uncertainty and relativity. Rather it is embedded in the more graspable, concrete biological sciences.

Anthony Sattilaro, grappling with the differences between (1) his own scientific training as a scientific physician and experiences as a patient in the Western mind's eye and (2) his introduction to and healing from the Eastern perspective, found himself challenging and changing his own assumptions.

> I went from focusing my attention on viruses and cells under a microscope to sitting back and contemplating the vast interwoven mosaic of the universe. For example, when my back pain had returned, ... I immediately believed the cancer had reawakened along my spinal column. The macrobiotic view was quite different. ... According to [Eastern theory], the origin of my back pain was stagnation in a meridian that ran along my back, preventing energy . . . earth from freely passing along this meridian and nourishing my body. The two points of view are good examples of Western and Eastern thinking. The former addresses the effects, while the latter attempted to understand the correct causes. Once I accepted the Eastern view as possible, I began to gain a new appreciation of the vast interconnectedness of the universe.

Sattilaro was indeed grateful for his expanded view of health and healing; " In treating my own cancer, I put this holistic view to the ultimate test and it saved my life."

Aesthetically and logically, Eastern methods of health and healing appeal to me more than the take-charge Western model does. The idea of a holistic approach to treatment, the shift from passive patient to active participant, the ideal prevention, all make sense to me. I prefer a movement toward a preventative, socially, and environmentally aware model of health promotion rather than our current medical model of waiting for disease. But no one would argue that Eastern medicine saved Drew's life. In fact, Western medicine did. Heroic medicine, doing what it does best, isolating the affected area and attacking it, rode into town and indeed was heroic. Careful, scientific studies of bodily parts and technical fixes over the past decade radically improved the surgical techniques and radiation used. Without theses innovations, Drew's chances of survival were slim. Western medicine was crucial. Eastern medicines played a less obvious role. The help derived from such modalities as acupuncture were important but secondary. . . .

So why not seek a blended model of medicine that allows for varied mixtures of treatments, depending on the problem? . . .

Drew benefitted from the best of both. He used Eastern methods to be a more active patient in the Western model. He energetically set a course toward health that served him well. Acupuncture was used to stimulate his immune system, help diffuse his stress, and thus contribute to his physical and mental well-being. By daily visualizing the tumor's being replaced by healthy, glowing cells, he was reclaiming his body, making both the unhealthy and the healthy cells a part of himself that he could navigate, instead of suffering rage at his own body. Rather than feeling betrayed, he could offer himself sympathy and constructive action. By eating foods that made him feel stronger during all of the curing by taxing events—surgeries, radiation, hospital procedures—he could feel an active partner in the process rather than a passive pawn. His rapid recoveries can be credited in part to these strengthening activities.

By feeling better, he could better tolerate the medical procedures and appreciate how much all of these processes were helping him. Radiation may be saving your life, but if you are too ill to eat or your head is pounding, it doesn't feel that way. Better to feel good while you're getting well. Drew believed he was working with the doctors to make himself well.

Here perhaps we can find some overlap between East and West. Both agree that attitude, while by no means the decisive element some would have us believe, is important to quality of life during the illness and important to getting over the illness. Judith Glassman, in her study of terminal cancer survivors, found that "the most striking thing about all of these people is that each engineered his or her own recovery and each had an enormous will to live." A feeling of control and participation in health care, so integral to Eastern medicine, is slowly inching its way into some Western practices.

In a review of thirty-four controlled studies, researchers found that when surgical or coronary patients were given information, support, or both to help them get through medical procedures, they did better than patients who received routine care. Hospital stays were reduced, and recovery time was decreased. Similar results on information giving, mainly from the psychology and nursing literatures, have been shown in childbirth, in difficult or painful physical exams, and when the patient is a child.

When Drew first entered the hospital, a nurse came to his room, did the usual vital-signs routine, and them whipped out a questionnaire. She explained that they had recently started asking how much people wanted to know. Did Drew want to be informed about the procedures? How detailed did he want the discussion to be? And so forth. She explained that some patients want to know nothing: "Just do what you have to do and get me out of here." Others want a sketchy picture but not too detailed. Still others want the full score; they want to know everything. Drew wanted the full score. She gave it to him, at least a technical one. She put his request in his file, and it seemed that every time we turned around, at least before the first surgery, he got it again. Frightening as it was, Drew found that knowing what to expect was easier than facing what his imagination could do with the unknown. There were already enough unknowns.

Increased patient control and participation lead to better understanding of the problem and the necessary treatment, which then come full circle to deliver more patient control. Rather than telling the ill to shape up, improve their attitudes, and assume total individual responsibility, research suggests that medical forces can help people develop the strength to face procedures by encouraging feelings of control.

Informing and thus activating ill people and utilizing alternative programs are recent developments in this country, incorporated by some, rejected by others. Despite ongoing changes, however, there are concrete and subtle obstacles to fundamental change within the medical community. An interpretation of modern scientific views within medicine offers perhaps one last note for understanding the whys of these obstacles. As discussed earlier, doctors want studies. They want proof. They want certainty. . . .

The scientific method is rooted in a vision of pure, objective inquiry in which observed facts confirm or deny hypotheses. Once a hypothesis is tested repeatedly and confirmed, it becomes a law, a workable fact. Controlled studies in medicine require one group to be tested with the new procedure, test, or drug; the other group, not. If it is the preferred double-blind study, no one knows which group any patient is in. The mind is banished from the activities. Sounds good: neat, clean, compact, a method that delivers truth. And sometimes it does. Much of medical progress in the form of dazzling technology is a result of this method—careful studies, whether blind or not. Proton beam radiation, primarily zapping the tumor instead of the healthy tissue, owes its origins to medicine marching ahead. Just a decade ago these techniques were not a refined for chondrosarcomas, the outcome more a danger than an opportunity.

Some scientists, however, like Stephen Jay Gould, are questioning too rigid, too concrete a perception of science: "I believe that science must be understood as a social phenomenon, a gutsy human enterprise, not the work of robots programmed to collect pure information." Just because no one has yet thought of the hypothesis or tested its validity doesn't mean something doesn't exist or isn't useful. Just because questions haven't been asked doesn't mean there are no answers. What I interpret Gould calling for is more imagination, to use science as a means to broaden the landscape, not narrow it. If scientists were more sensitive to the multifaceted aspects of life, the uncertainties as well as the absolutes, different questions could be asked and methods developed to study medicines such as acupuncture.

Furthermore, as already pointed out, medical practice is based at least as much on clinical experience as on scientific inquiry. Despite this reality, doctor's responses to unknown areas are often to assume they don't exist. The problem (such as environmental illness) or the treatment (macrobiotics or acupuncture) can be dismissed. "Where are the studies?"" Where is the proof?" These may be appropriate questions, but if the studies haven't been done and the proof doesn't exist, then the rational response to questions about unknowns is "I don't know" or "I'd like to know more." In fact, scientific inquiry, by its own internal logic, focuses on asking questions, knowing that the answers shift like grains of sand. Modern medical thought all too often dismisses the unknowns, clings to the known answers, forgetting about the questions. To focus on the answers at the expense of the questions invites a rigidity that short-circuits the very knowledge medical science seeks. Thus, science, narrowly defined, can become a cloak behind which established health care hides, as well as a pathfinder with innovative research. A scientific cosmology can serve as a blinder. And it is exactly behind this cloak, these blinders, that many doctors remain when it comes to the unknown, in this case complementary treatments for cancer.

But not all doctors adhere to this strict a code. It is through the work of mavericks that we see the other side of a scientific worldview, a side that enlightens and encourages new visions. People, including scientists, may cling to the known, but the scientific enterprise in its deepest philosophical roots assumes change. In fact, the scientific revolutions of the sixteenth and seventeenth centuries opened doors to critical, rational inquiry—even of science itself. An open, excited mind, always looking for new, unexplored questions, should be integral to any scientific enterprise, even if that means changing the form of the inquiry as well as the content.

Thus, it is no surprise that some doctors, trained in scientific medicine, are at the forefront of pushing the borders of the medical model, expanding horizons. It is, after all, doctors trained in conventional medicine who have written the majority of books on visualization and meditation methods for healing. Environmental medicine is a new discipline—physicians interested in expanding medicine out from the cell to the environment, drawing on a variety of holistic understandings to do so. Although not recognized by the AMA as a speciality, interest in environmental illness is slowly showing up in mainstream medicine. Massachusetts General Hospital, often ahead of its time, has opened a new group practice to treat "sick building syndrome," focusing on how materials in our environment can make us ill. The practice emphasizes diagnosis and treatment, and prevention and education as well. Acupuncture, still foreign to many if my students are indicators, was brought to this country by American doctors who had visited China, and it is increasingly being studied in hospitals here for a variety of diseases, as well as for pain and substance detoxification. And macrobiotics, still considered the most obscure of these methods, is drawing a small but interested following in medical circles. When I asked a holistic doctor in California why he had incorporated alternative methods into his practice, he responded:

> I began to feel that all I did was push pills. I wasn't making enough people feel better; I was often making them sicker. It was a gradual change for me from cure to prevention, from invasive procedures to gentler measures. I still prescribe drugs when necessary. I haven't abandoned my training. I've just added to it.

. . . In my own research I have talked with physicians who have been ill themselves; surgeons needing surgery, gynecologists experiencing difficult births. It can be a sobering ordeal for a doctor to face another doctor, often a stranger, from that far side of the room where the sick live. They are shocked at how helpless they feel, how indifferent the doctor often is, how little information they receive even when they put their questions in doctor-talk. One surgeon who underwent a traumatic surgery told me, disbelief still in his voice two years later, "I'm a surgeon and he treated me this way. I couldn't believe it. I hate to think how he treats the guy off the street." Did this experience change how he treats patients? "Oh yes," he assured me. "Yes indeed. For one thing, I'll never again tell a patient 'You'll be jogging in two days.' "

Recently I visited Drew's grandfather in Washington, D.C. A retired physician and loyal AMA member for sixty-some years, he was in the hospital following a harrowing surgery with multiple complications. I asked, "Do you like your doctors?"

"They saved my life," he responded quickly. "Yes," I agreed. "So you would kiss their feet and you love them. But do you like them? Are you pleased with how they treat you?"

"I don't know," he replied with a tired laugh. "I've never seen one of them for more than sixty seconds. Doctors don't have time for people anymore. It's a serious problem. . . ."

Eastern practices can soften the harsh edges of the technologies so often needed to help cure—in Drew's case MRIs, blood tests, X-rays, surgeries, radiation. For these treatments can be distancing and painful, making ill people feel alienated from their own bodies as well as their illness. Anatole Broyard, writer and former editor of the *New York Times Book Review*, sums this up eloquently, remarking that "since technology deprives me of the intimacy of my illness, it makes it not mine but something that belongs to science. I wish my doctor could somehow repersonalize it for me. It would be more satisfying to me, it would allow me to feel that I *owned* my illness." Broyard wants more from his doctors; he wants help to reconnect himself to his body once the machines and bureaucracies have done their work. "Just as he orders blood tests and bone scans of my body, I'd like my doctor to scan *me*, to grope for my spirit as well as my prostate. Without some such recognition, I am nothing but my illness." Broyard doesn't require that his doctors love him or wallow in his miseries. He just wishes his doctors would "brood on my situation for perhaps five minutes." But his doctor wouldn't brood on his illness, nor

would the doctor "survey [his] soul as well as [his] flesh." Anatole Broyard reports that his doctors groped only for his prostate.

I used to think it was possible to change doctor-patient relationships, educating doctors to probe deeper than the prostate, the brain, the womb. And maybe it is. Rita Charon, a physician at Columbia Medical School, requires students in her classes to write narratives in their patients' voices to get closer to what the patient, the ill person, the other, experiences. But her excellent teaching techniques were not in time for Anatole Broyard, who died medically unrequited in 1990.

Neither were her ideas in time for Drew, at least not this time around. He did indeed have excellent medical care, with occasional "groping for his soul" by some doctors. Even the great surgeon fleetingly reached out to him, tentatively but with tenderness. The antidote, however, for the alienation of all the high tech, all of the tests, even those endless arm punctures when there seemed to be no more veins to tap, resided for Drew in the alternatives. He had to do the equivalent of switching computer programs in midstream. Meditations, visualizations, relaxation breathing techniques, seeing the inside of his head with his mind's eye, and later counseling, all retrieved him and his illness in one piece from the MRI chamber, the piercing radiating beam, and all of those tubes and gadgets. In fact, he could incorporate the curative powers of these technologies into his imagination, making them less alienating, more healing. Relaxation techniques soothed his soul as well as his body. He had Val, not a doctor but a practitioner, someone to "brood" on his illness with him on a regular basis. Everything mingled in his body and his mind to make him feel in the center of this full catastrophe rather than peripheral to it. . . .

If only the many practitioners working in these areas would recognize each other. It would have been wonderful, for example, if Val and Dr. T had discussed what each was doing to help Drew, had made joint adjustments, whether in physical or psychosocial care, to enhance each other and thus maximize their efforts.

This doesn't mean each would have to become an expert in the other's work. After all, Dr. T works in surgery with and trusts anesthesiologists each day without being able to do what they do. Imagine that Dr. R's staff included a nutritionist learned in foods and vitamins to ease the radiation process—perhaps serving soothing bancha tea and vegetable dip or miso broth and rice balls in the waiting room rather than cake and coffee. People might leave with more spring in their step, the spring they were surprised that Drew had and were sorry they lacked. Such rapport and mutual acceptance would broaden public imagination of what health care can be. Such mainstreaming of alternative medicines would make them more accessible to people of all classes and more likely to be covered by insurance companies and government programs.

In fact, East and West are getting closer, at least in theory if not yet in practice, despite their many differences. Dietary recommendations of the heart and cancer associations, along with various government agencies, are basically what macrobiotic experts have been advocating for years. The power of the mind to contribute to illness, long acknowledged by modern medicine (perhaps overly so), is increasingly recognized as a power that can also heal. Instead of banishing the mind from healing in double-blind, placebo-effect studies, some are trying to cultivate this energy in beneficial ways. A recent *Time* magazine cover story on alternatives described acupuncture as on the verge of becoming a mainstream approach to illness. And the National Institutes of Health have recently allocated funds for a grand-scale study into alternative methods to better understand how they work and where they help the most. After all, macrobiotics literally means "long life" and who can argue with that?

Not Drew. He walked down two parallel roads: first, the Western way of surgeons, drugs, blood tests, MRIs and radiation— the world of the body; second, the Eastern path of macrobiotics, meditations, acupuncture— the world of the body drenched in the mind. At the level of theory and practitioners the roads never met. At the level of experience they became integrally entwined in Drew's body, his life, and his recovery. East and West meshed, enhancing each other, offering Drew unique ways of healing and coping. He cultivated calmness and strength from eating a balanced diet, doing visualizations, going to acupuncture. Counseling gave him a sense of sureness about himself, increased his self-knowledge and introduced yet another learning experience. Surgery and radiation saved his life, giving him a profound appreciation for sophisticated technology and acute medical care.

In the end so many modalities came together, turning a dreadful time into a productive one. Drew learned more than he thought possible, at times more than he ever wanted to know. There are so many experiences, so many feelings, so much new information to sort out. Although at times perplexed that his life was ever so at risk, Drew's grateful he's alive to ponder the matter. And ponder the matter, he does, when he's not too busy savoring every moment, taking all and nothing for granted.

Further Reading

Sandra Butler and Barbara Rosenblum. 1991. *Cancer in Two Voices*. San Francisco: Spinsters.

Cai Jingfeng. 1988. "Integration of Traditional Chinese Medicine with Western Medicine—Right or Wrong?" *Social Science and Medicine* 27:521-29.

Michio Kushi. 1991. *Macrobiotics and Oriental Medicine*. New York: Japan Publications, Inc.

Discussion Questions

1. What are the principal conceptions of disease that underlie and distinguish eastern and western models of medicine? What are their views of the patient?

2. Given your understanding of acute care models, explain how eastern conceptions of health and illness are distinguished from acute models of care. How might they inform models of chronic care?

3. How might eastern models of care inform preventive care strategies in the United States?

From *Double Vision: An East-West Collaboration for Coping with Cancer*. Pp. 116-137. Copyright © 1994 by Alexandra Todd and John Andrew Todd, Jr., Wesleyan University Press. Reprinted by permission of University Press of New England. ✦

The Distribution of Health and Illness

32

Race and Infant Mortality

*David U. Himmelstein
Steffie Woolhandler*

In the following graphs, David Himmelstein and Steffie Woolhandler depict the rates of infant mortality by race within the United States and show mortality rates between the United States and six other industrialized countries. As you review these infant mortality rates, speculate why they might be so high for African Americans in the United States Consider your

explanations for infant mortality rates within the United States in terms of disparities between the United States and other countries.

The black:white infant mortality gap has widened substantially over the past 20 years and currently stands at an all-time high. This racial disparity fell precipitously during World War II, coincident with the increase in integration and improved opportunities for African-Americans. This ratio rose again during the 1950s and early 60s. It fell quite sharply in the late 60s and early 1970s, at the time of the landmark civil rights legislation, affirmative action, and implementation of many social programs in response to the civil

Figure 32-1
Black:White Infant Mortality Ratio
1940–1989

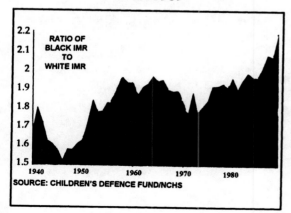

SOURCE: CHILDREN'S DEFENCE FUND/NCHS

Figure 32-2
Infant Mortality, 1990

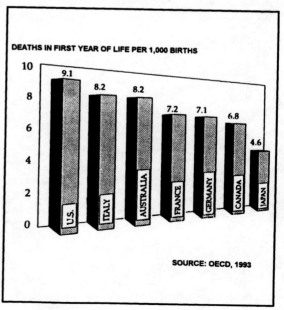

SOURCE: OECD, 1993

rights movement. With the retrenchment of the late 70s and the 1980s the racial gap has once again widened, and now stands at the highest level ever recorded.

The U.S. trails many other nations in infant mortality. Even some developing nations such as Singapore have substantially lower rates of infant death. Moreover, many nations have achieved low infant mortality rates among ethnic and racial minority groups. Thus, infants of non-native-born Swedes (10 percent of all Swedes) have almost the same low death rates as the infants of native-born Swedes.

Further Reading

Centers for Disease Control. *Mortality and Morbidity Weekly Report*.

Robert A. Hummer. 1993. "Racial Differences in Infant Mortality in the U.S.: An Examination of Social and Health Determinants." *Social Forces* 72:529-554.

Vicente Navarro. 1990. "Race or Class Versus Race and Class: Mortality Differentials in the United States." *Lancet* 336: 1238-40.

The World Bank. 1991. *World Development Report*. Oxford: Oxford University Press.

Discussion Questions

1. What factors account for differences in infant mortality between whites and blacks in the United States?

2. What explanations can you offer for gaps in infant mortality between the U.S. and other industrialized countries?

3. Can you think of feasible policies that might address these gaps?

33

U.S. Socioeconomic and Racial Differences in Health: Patterns and Explanations

David R. Williams
Chiquita Collins

While there has been much debate about the influence of race on health and other concerns, social scientists have argued persistently that matters of race are complicated by matters of social class. David Williams and Chiquita Collins suggest that socio-economic differences between racial groups in the United States are largely responsible for differences in health statuses between racial groups. Williams and Collins look at the differences in health between African Americans and whites due to widening disparities in socio-economic inequalities. Recognizing the importance of racism, acculteration, occupation, and childhood social class, they illuminate the effects of intersecting social forces on health and illness.

Social class, measured in terms of socioeconomic status, has not only been a significant contributor to differential health statuses in the United States, but the association between social class and health is strong. Consider some of the explanations these authors present for the increasing disparities in the health outcomes of African Americans and whites. Think about the characteristics of infant mortality depicted by David Himmelstein

and Steffie Woolhandler as you read this discussion of the widening differences in health status. Consider Williams' and Collins' argument regarding social classifications of race in the United States and issues of biological distinctiveness.

Problems in the construction of race obscure problems in the organization of health care more generally. The issue of biology obscures our understanding of what causes racial disparities in health; focus on biology emphasizes individuals as responsible for illness. Contrary to this notion, Williams and Collins argue that emphasis on social structures and population groups clarifies the causes of illness. Think critically about the issues raised by Williams and Collins. See how these issues might apply to other readings in this section. See how their evidence resonates with the claims of Vicente Navarro that the U.S. health care system does not respond to people's needs.

Introduction

Class is a very widely used concept in the social sciences in general, and sociology in particular. Although no consensus exists on exactly what it means and how it should be measured, class, however defined, has proven to be remarkably robust in elucidating the complexities of social and historical processes and in predicting variations within and between social groups in living conditions and life chances, skill levels and material resources, relative power and privilege. Health status is one arena where the effects of class are readily evident.

Similarly, race is one of the major bases of division in American life, and throughout U.S. history racial disparities in health have been pervasive. The vast majority of studies focus on the black-white contrast, but a rapidly growing literature describes variations in health status within and between America's increasingly diverse racial populations. The U.S. government requires all federal statistical reporting agencies to recognize four racial groups (American Indian or Alaskan Native, Asian or Pacific Islander, black, and white) and one ethnic category (Hispanic). Given that racial taxonomies are socially constructed and arbitrary, we treat all of these categories as racial groups. Moreover, since group designations should reflect generally recognized definitions as well as individual dignity, and there are varying views within racial groups with regard to terminology, we treat the following paired categories as alternative labels: American Indian or Native American, Hispanic or Latino/Latina, and black or African American.

This selection reviews the evidence for persisting inequalities in health by socioeconomic status (SES) and race. We focus on the magnitude of the differences, the trends over time, and the major explanatory factors invoked to account for these variations. Methodological issues are also discussed, and directions for future research are outlined. We begin with a consideration of SES differences in health.

Socioeconomic Status and Health

SES is widely used as a proxy for social class in studies that examine variations in the distribution of disease, and it continues to be a remarkably robust determinant of variations in the rates of illness and death. The terms SES and social class are used interchangeably in the literature, but we treat SES as the preferred term except when explicit theories of social class are invoked. SES is typically assessed more in line with Weberian notions of stratification (income, education, occupation, and ownership of property) than with the Marxist emphasis on relationship to the system of production.

Recent reviews reveal that SES remains a persistent and pervasive predictor of variations in health outcomes (Bunker et al.. 1989, Haan and Kaplan 1986, Marmot et al.. 1987, Wilkinson 1986, Williams 1990, Adler et al.. 1993, Adler et al.. 1994, Feinstein 1993, Krieger and Fee 1994, Krieger et al.. 1993). A robust inverse association between SES and health status dates back to our earliest records and exists in all countries where it has been examined. Some of the clearest recent evidence for the United States comes from studies of mortality rates. Descriptive data from the National Longitudinal Mortality Study (NLMS) reveal, for example, that higher levels of both income and education are associated with

lower rates of mortality (Rogot et al.. 1992). For blacks and whites, males and females, the mortality ratios for persons with a total family income of less than $5,000 (1980 dollars) per year were at least twice those of persons with incomes greater than $50,000 per year. Other recent studies have also found a strong inverse relationship between SES and mortality (Mare 1990, Feldman et al.. 1989, Duleep 1989, Pappas et al.. 1993, Haan et al.. 1987).

Research interest in the association between SES and mental health status has been declining over time (Dohrenwend 1990), but recent findings continue to demonstrate a powerful role for SES. The Epidemiologic Catchment Area study (ECA), the largest study of psychiatric disorders ever conducted in the United States, found that low SES predicted elevated rates of a broad range of psychiatric conditions (Holzer et al.. 1986, Robins and Regier 1991). Moreover, this inverse association between SES and psychiatric disorders was evident for both blacks and whites (Williams et al.. 1992).

The direction of causality between SES and health has been debated in the literature. The positive association between SES and health could reflect selection or "drift" processes where poor health is the cause of low SES. The competing social causation hypothesis views the elevated rates of illness among low SES populations as a consequence of their low socioeconomic circumstances. The direction of influence cannot be assessed in the typical study, but a growing number of cohort studies suggest that although health-driven downward social mobility occurs, it makes only a minor contribution to SES differences in health (Power et al.. 1990, Fox et al.. 1985, Wilkinson 1986).

Widening Inequality

The extent to which the association between SES and health has been widening in recent decades has emerged as a major issue in the SES literature. Three U.S. studies have compared SES differences in mortality in recent studies with those reported by Kitagawa and Hauser (1973) from the 1960 Matched Records Study. Feldman et al.. (1989) found that mortality differentials by education increased substantially for white men between 1960 and 1984. Duleep (1989) noted that the observed mortality differentials by education and income in the late 1970s for men aged 25-65 years old were not smaller than those in 1960. A comparison of 1960 mortality differentials with those from the 1986 National Mortality Follow-back Survey found evidence for an increase in socioeconomic disparity (Pappas et al.. 1993).

Much of the widening disparity in health status reflects more rapid gains in the health status for high SES than for low SES groups, but for some health indicators, evidence suggests a worsening health status at the low end of the socioeconomic spectrum. A recent study by Wagener and Shatzkin (1994), for example, documents that although the SES differential in breast cancer narrowed between 1969 and 1989, breast cancer mortality has been declining for women in high SES counties in the United States, but rising for women in low SES counties.

Differences between SES groups in accessibility, utilization, and quality of care, or differences in the benefits derived from medical care, are contributing factors to the widening inequality. Mandinger (1985) shows that in the wake of the large budget cuts in health and social service spending early in the Reagan administration, an increase occurred in the number of pregnant women not receiving prenatal care, in the incidence of anemia in pregnant women, and infant mortality rates among poverty populations in 20 states. Similarly, Lurie et al (1984) found evidence of significant deterioration in access to care, satisfaction with care, and health status in a population of medically indigent adults in California six months after their termination from Medicaid. For example, their mean diastolic blood pressure increased by 10 points (mm Hg).

However, an increase in economic inequality is apparently the major driving force behind widening health disparities. Since the mid-1970s in the United States, there have been an increase in income inequality, a growing concentration of wealth among the highest income groups, and a worsening of the economic conditions of a substantial portion of the population (Danziger and Gottschalk 1993). The economic expansion of the 1980s was accompanied by a deterioration in the standard of living for a majority of households. Compared to the 1970s, more American adults in the 1980s fell from middle- to low-income status, and low-income families found it increasingly difficult to climb into the middle class (Duncan et al.. 1993). This polarization of the income distribution may have resulted from changes in the economy that led to a decline in manufacturing jobs and simultaneous increases in both low-wage (service industry and low-skilled) and high-wage (high technology industries) employment.

Income inequality has also increased in Western European countries (Danziger and Gottschalk 1993), and a pattern of widening socioeconomic differentials in mortality is also evident in England, France, Finland, Norway, and the Netherlands (DHSS 1980, Kunst and Mackenbach 1994). A study of mortality trends over time in England, Wales, and the Netherlands documents most clearly for England and Wales, although the pattern for the Netherlands is consistent, that a widening of mortality differences between SES groups is partly due to differences in the decline of mortality from conditions amenable to medical intervention. However, the contribution of medical care is limited. The higher SES groups also experienced larger improvements in mortality than did their lower SES counterparts from those causes of death where medical care does not play a major role (Mackenbach et al.. 1989).

Nature of the Gradient

The nature of the SES gradient in health status has generated considerable interest. Some studies indicate a stepwise progression of risk in the relationship between SES and health status, with each higher level of SES associated with better health status. The most impressive evidence of this pattern comes from the Whitehall Study of civil servants in England (Marmot et al.. 1984, Marmot et al.. 1991). This study population consists of adults mainly from one ethnic group, residing in one geographic area, stably employed in white-collar jobs, with limited exposure to industrial hazards. Workers in the lowest occupational grades had a rate of mortality three times higher than those in the highest occupational grades. However, each higher grade of employment had lower levels of mortality and better health status than the prior grade. Further, homeowners engaged in professional employment who own two cars have lower mortality than their counterparts who own only one car (Goldblatt 1990). Thus, elevated rates of disease and death are not restricted to the low occupational grades but are evident even for privileged groups, when compared to those of highest SES.

Some recent reviews have noted a similar pattern in at least some studies conducted in the United States, and they have concluded that this finely graded pattern is characteristic of the association between SES and health status (Adler et al.. 1993, Adler et al.. 1994). Accordingly, there has been great interest in understanding the determinants of this finely stratified mortality difference that appears to run from top to bottom of the social hierarchy. Several studies document that the gradient is nonetheless characterized by a threshold that predicts a weakening of the association between SES and health. That is, beyond some level of SES, usually around the median for income, additional increases in SES have little or a greatly diminished effect in reducing mortality and morbidity rates. For example, both the Kitagawa and Hauser (1973) and the Pappas et al.. (1993) studies of mortality document diminishing returns to increases in socioeconomic status after a certain level of income. House et al.. (1990) also report a similar pattern for morbidity indicators. The health gains due to income are small for households above $20,000 per year. Recent analyses of the association between income and mortality in the Panel Study of Income Dynamics (PSID) also find large reductions in the mortality rate associated with increases in income at low levels of SES, but smaller declines in mortality linked to additional income at higher levels of SES (McDonough et al.. 1995). Wilkinson (1986) reports a similar pattern for income data in Great Britain.

Evidence suggests that even in a single study, patterns of association vary for different indicators of SES. For example, Rogot et al.. (1992) found in the NLMS a continuous linear gradient between income and mortality for African Americans and whites, males and females, aged 25–64. In contrast, although an inverse association exists between education and mortality, a graded pattern of association was not evident for all of the four race-sex groups. Clearly needed now are more systematic efforts to identify the conditions under which particular indicators of SES manifest patterns of linear or nonlinear associations with health outcomes. We need to identify the thresholds after which weaker effects of SES are observed, and we also need to identify the social, psychological, material, and especially occupational resources and risks that characterize each level of SES.

Measuring Socioeconomic Position

Numerous variables are used to measure SES: Income, education, and occupational status are the most common. Although SES tends to be related to health outcomes irrespective of the indicator used, each SES measure has its own set of advantages and limitations. Some researchers suggest that education is the most stable and robust indicator of SES (Kitagawa and Hauser 1973, Liberatos et al.. 1988) or the most practical and convenient in some contexts (Williams et al.. 1994).

However, the education measure suffers from several limitations (Krieger and Fee 1994). First, in at least some national data, inequalities in health associated with income are larger than those associated with education, such that using education as a measure of SES may minimize estimates of social inequalities in health. Second, the lack of volatility in education levels for most adults precludes assessing how health status is affected by changes in SES. Third, many studies that use education as an indicator of SES are individualistic in approach and do not incorporate information about the education level of other members of the household. Fourth, as discussed in greater detail later, the return for a given level of education varies importantly by race and gender.

Numerous problems appear with the measure of income. Analyses using income are more likely than those of some other SES indicators to be open to reverse causation arguments. That is, poor health can lead to declines in income such that the association between low income and health status can be a cause rather than a consequence of poor health. In addition, income information may be especially sensitive for some, resulting in higher nonresponse for income questions than for other SES indicators. Measuring income well can also be costly and time-consuming. Income is probably best measured in the Survey of Income and Program Participation, which uses 50 questions to assess annual income. Moreover, the poverty measure, a widely used indicator of income, is almost 40 years old and of questionable current applicability (Sheak 1988, Ruggles 1990).

Income is also a more unstable measure of SES than is either education or occupation. Family incomes throughout the life cycle are characterized by considerable volatility, with many households experiencing sharp losses in income, and a substantial portion of the population is at risk of experiencing such losses. Duncan (1988) shows, for example, that between 1969 and 1979 in the United States, between 20 percent and 35 percent of women between the ages of 25 and 75 experienced poverty at least once. The rates of poverty were higher among women than among men. Persistent poverty, defined as living in poverty for more than half of the eleven-year period, increased with age from 5 percent among women aged 25-45 to 11 percent among those in the 66-75 year age group. Thus, volatility of income also was patterned by age. Measures of education miss this dynamic component of SES, and although highly educated persons are not completely shielded from the volatility of income, they tend to be protected from income drops to near-poverty levels.

Rather than using the volatility of income as a reason not to collect income information, the dynamic nature of income highlights the importance and potential contribution of indicators of long-term economic well-being. Three longitudinal studies have documented that measures of average income capturing long-term exposure to economic deprivation are more strongly related to childhood health outcomes than are single-year indicators of economic status (Miller and Korenman 1994, Takeuchi et al.. 1991, Duncan et al.. 1994). These findings highlight the importance of having longitudinal data with multiyear or long-term measures of income. This larger effect for long-term economic deprivation may reflect the fact that families may use assets or credit to cushion the impact of short-term economic losses.

Permanent income or wealth may thus be better measures of economic status than is annual household income. In addition, wealth may be more strongly linked to social class location than is earned income. In a study of 100,000 black, white, and Hispanic youth between 1973 and 1990, parental home ownership had a large effect on both school dropout and college entry independent of parental income, education, and occupational status (Hauser 1993). More health studies should include indicators of assets or wealth. In the National Longitudinal Survey of the Labor Market Experience of Mature Men (NLS), Mare (1990) found that family assets were strongly related to mortality independent of the effects of education and first occupation. Studies in Britain also find that home and car ownership are predictive of decreased mortality risk (Goldblatt 1990). The extent to which traditional measures of economic consumption such as the monthly cost of housing and food are predictors of health status is another important but neglected issue.

Occupational status is likely to be a better indicator of long-term income than is income at a single point in time. Nonetheless, there is some volatility to occupational status, and this may also have consequences for health. A national study of black and white male workers found that one third of the sample changed their occupational class over the 7-13 years of follow-up (Waitzman and Smith 1994). Compared to whites who remained in professional and technical jobs between baseline and follow-up, African American and white males who remained in the lower occupational classes or made certain transitions, especially into lower occupational classes, had significantly higher rates of new cases of hypertension.

Considering multiple measures of occupational status can also shed light on underly-

354 Section 5 ◆ *Social and Cultural Structures of Care*

ing processes. Mare (1990) studied the association of father's occupation, first occupation, and current occupation to mortality in the NLS. Father's occupation was inversely related to mortality, but the effects of first occupation on mortality were stronger than those of father's occupation, and they appeared to be due to the ability of sons from higher SES origins to acquire more schooling. Current occupation and family assets were also linked to mortality. The association between multiple measures of occupation and mortality can be complex. Moore and Hayward (1990) found in the NLS data that the occupational category with the highest mortality risk for longest occupation was different from that for most recent occupation.

A practical barrier to the use of occupation for analyses of national mortality data in the United States is that the numerator and denominator do not use the same units of measurement. Denominator data comes from the census, which collects information about current occupation. The 21 states that record occupational information on death certificates collect information about usual, instead of current, occupation (Krieger and Fee 1994). The collection of uniform data about both current and usual occupation could alleviate this problem.

Krieger and Fee (1994) emphasize that social class should be measured at the level of the individual, the household, and the neighborhood. At the individual level, class-based (occupational) measures can capture exposure to occupational health risks, while household SES measures can provide information regarding standards of living and cultural patterns. Community level measures of SES can provide information about neighborhood-related conditions such as exposure to environmental hazards and levels of neighborhood violence. Two California studies have found that measures of deprivation based on area characteristics were associated with mortality independent of individual socioeconomic status indicators (Haan et al.. 1987, Krieger 1991). Moreover, Krieger (1991) found that a deprivation measure based on census block characteristics (smaller unit of analysis) explained more variance than did the one based on the char-

acteristics of the census tract. These studies document that area characteristics provide additional information about social inequalities in health that are not captured by individual level data. Similarly, British studies have found a robust relationship between area-based measures of social deprivation and health status (Townsend et al.. 1988, Carstairs and Morris 1989). Future research needs to identify the specific characteristics of residential environments that are deleterious to health.

Greater attention also needs to be given to theoretically driven measures of social class. Krieger (1991) found that a relational measure of social class (that emphasizes social class location based on relationship to others and to property through employment) was more strongly related to women's reproductive history outcomes than was a measure of household poverty. The three class categories utilized were working class, not working class, and other class. An alternative measure for assessing objective class location distinguishes social class based on the possession of productive assets: property assets, skill assets, and organizational assets (Baxter 1994). There is growing awareness that SES, as well as social class, attempts to capture a dynamic multidimensional process, and greater attention needs to be given to modeling the joint effects of SES variables.

Other Emerging Issues

The age patterning of the association between SES and mortality has been addressed in recent studies. Early studies noted that SES differentials in health status tend to be largest during middle age but are relatively small at older ages (Antonovsky 1967). Analyses of the NLMS data found that although the association between education and mortality exists for persons aged 65 or older, it was not as strong as at the younger ages (Rogot et al.. 1992). Similarly, House et al.. (1990), using two national probability samples, document that the association between SES and morbidity (chronic conditions, functional status, and activity limitation) is most marked between ages 45–64, but narrows with increasing age. Replications and extensions of these cross-sectional findings with short-term longitudinal data provide further support for this pattern with both income and education (House et al.. 1994). However, the evidence is not uniform. Recent analyses by Wu and Ross (1994) found the opposite pattern. Using two nationally representative telephone samples, they found that educational differences for three measures of health (physical functioning, self-reported health, and physical well-being) widens with increasing age. It is not clear if these findings reflect differences in the measurement of health status or the coverage of the population.

Women are overrepresented among the poor, but the nature of the association between SES and women's health status is not well understood. The measurement of occupation has been particularly problematic for women. Findings are inconsistent for the few studies that have assessed the association between occupation and women's health. Strong linear SES gradients have been found in some studies, while others report relatively weaker associations than those obtained for men (Arber 1987, 1991). In some studies occupation has been unrelated to mortality risk for women (Passannante and Nathanson 1985, Hibbard and Pope 1991, Moen et al.. 1989).

It is likely that these inconsistencies reflect, at least in part, the limitations of the measurement of SES. Frequently, married women are assigned to the occupational class of their husband, while single women are given their own or their father's class position. The assignment of women to the occupational status of male relatives is increasingly problematic given the growing number of women who are employed outside of the home and the increasing number of female-headed households (Liberatos et al.. 1988). Most of the widely used classification systems are based on the occupational patterns of men. Gender-based differences in income and education within occupations and the gender segregation of employment suggest that the inclusion of women may require modifications in occupational classification schemes (Haug 1977, Powers and Holmberg 1982).

Evidence from the United Kingdom reveals that for married women, social class based on the husband's occupation predicts mortality better than does social class based upon the woman's own occupation (Moser et al.. 1990). For single women, own social class is a powerful predictor. A recent study of the relationship between objective class location and subjective class identification for men and women in the United States, Sweden, Norway, and Australia found that husbands' class location is a major determinant of subjective class identity for women (Baxter 1994). Thus, women's increasing independence from men appears not to undermine the conventional view of class analysis. These findings also suggest the importance of studying social class at the household level, as opposed to only the individual level, for women.

There is growing interest in understanding the contribution of biological factors to human behavior in general and processes of social stratification in particular. Ellis's review (1993) suggests that genetic and physiological factors account for a substantial portion of the variation in both adult education and earning levels. For example, sex hormone levels, especially testosterone, are associated with individuals' career choices, and some twin studies suggest that as much as 40-50 percent of the variation in vocational interest can be attributed to genetic factors. However, cause and effect remain problematic because a person's experiences also affect hormone levels. In addition, the determinants of individual risks of disease are often different from those of population risks of disease (Rose 1985). It is likely that genetic factors play a larger role in the causes of individual variations in disease than they do in socioeconomic group differences in health status. While guarding against biological determinism is important, social scientists need to give greater attention to the biological mechanisms and processes through which social factors affect health and to the interrelationships between genetic factors and social variables. Much remains to be understood about the ways in which genetic susceptibilities combine additively or interactively with exposures in the social and physical environment to affect health at different stages of the life cycle and for persons living under varying environmental conditions.

Racial/Ethnic Differences in Health Status

The United States is relatively unusual among industrialized countries in that it reports the health status of its population based on race (Navarro 1990). Most other countries focus on social class differences. For most of this century, the contrast between whites and nonwhites (a category that consisted almost exclusively of blacks) was the basis of differentiation. Since the late 1970s there has been a growing emphasis on collecting more data on the racial and ethnic minority populations that constitute an increasing proportion of the American population. Recent reviews reveal that race and ethnicity remain potent predictors of variations in health status (Braithwaite and Taylor 1992, Furino 1992, Livingston 1994, Zane et al.. 1994).

The most recent report card on the health of the U.S. population presents infant and adult mortality rates by race (National Center for Health Statistics 1994a). Infant mortality rates are reported for major subgroups of the Asian and Pacific Islander American (APIA) and the Hispanic population, but subgroup differences were not available for adult mortality. The infant mortality rate for blacks is twice that of whites, and American Indians also have elevated infant mortality rates compared to the white population. The APIA population and its four major subgroups have rates that are lower than those of whites, while the rate for Hispanics is equivalent to that of whites. However, variation occurs within the Hispanic category: Puerto Ricans have higher infant mortality rates than do the other Hispanic groups and the white population. The report also revealed that the age-adjusted death rate for the entire black population is dramatically higher than that of whites, but all of the other racial/ethnic populations have death rates lower than the white population, with the APIA population having the lowest death rates.

These overall data mask important patterns of variation for subgroups of these populations and for specific health conditions, a point readily evident in recent overviews of the health of the Hispanic population (Sorlie et al.. 1993, Vega and Amaro 1994). While Latinos have lower death rates for the two leading causes of death (heart disease and cancer) than do non-Hispanics, they also have higher mortality rates than do non-Hispanic whites for tuberculosis, septicemia, chronic liver disease and cirrhosis, diabetes, and homicide. Death rates of Hispanics also exceed those of whites in the 15-44 age group (Fingerhut and Makuc 1992). Moreover, Hispanics have elevated rates of infectious diseases such as measles, rubella, tetanus, tuberculosis, syphilis, and AIDS. The prevalence of obesity and glucose intolerance are also particularly high, especially among Mexican Americans. Similar to the findings for infant mortality, adult mortality rates for Puerto Ricans are higher than the other Hispanic groups. However, even among Puerto Ricans, the mortality rate is lower than for white non-Hispanics and considerably lower than for African Americans.

Specific subgroups of the APIA population have elevated rates of morbidity and mortality across a number of health indicators. The Native Hawaiian population has the highest cancer rates of any APIA population in the United States (Lin-Fu 1993) and the highest death rates due to heart disease of any racial group in the United States (Chen M.S. 1993). Rates of stomach cancer are high among Japanese Americans, and Chinese Americans have an incidence of liver cancer that is four times higher than that of the white population (Lin-Fu 1993). Very high rates of obesity are evident for Native Hawaiians and Samoans, and these populations, along with Asian Indians, Japanese Americans, and Korean Americans, have prevalence rates of diabetes that are more similar to those of the black population than of the white population (Crews 1994). Death rates for Native Americans are high for the under-45 age group, and suicide rates for American Indian youth are two to four times higher than those of any other racial group (Fingerhut and Makuc 1992). Native American youths also have higher levels of alcohol and other drug use than does any other racial group (Smith 1993).

Worsening Health Status

As part of the increasing income inequality in the United States, the gains in economic status of blacks relative to that of whites have stagnated in recent years (Smith and Welch 1989). Moreover, for several economic indicators there has been an absolute decline in the economic status of African Americans. For example, unlike the pattern for white families, low-income black and Hispanic families have experienced absolute declines in family income since 1973, and weekly wage and salary income declined for all black and Hispanic males below the 90th percentile of income between 1979 and 1987 (Karoly 1993). Similarly, the percentage of black children living in poverty increased from 41 percent to 44 percent between 1979 and 1988 (Hernandez 1993). Similar to the findings noted earlier for SES, this decline in black economic well-being and increase in black-white inequality is associated with worsening black health across a number of health status indicators.

The gap in life expectancy between blacks and whites widened between 1980 and 1991 from 6.9 years to 8.3 years for males and from 5.6 years to 5.8 years for females (NCHS 1994b). Moreover, for every year between 1985 and 1989, the life expectancy for both African American men and women declined from the 1984 level, although an upturn has been reported in the most recent data (NCHS 1994a). A slower rate of decline among blacks than whites for heart disease is the chief contributor to the widening racial gap in life expectancy, while HIV infection, homicide, diabetes, and pneumonia are major causes of decreasing life expectancy for blacks (Kochanek et al., 1994).

The age-adjusted death ratios for blacks and whites were greater in 1991 than in 1980, and the annual number of excess deaths for the African American, compared to the white population, increased from 60,000 in 1980 to 66,000 in 1991 (NCHS 1994b). During this period, the overall age-adjusted death rate decreased more rapidly for white males and females than for their black counterparts. Under the age of 70, three causes of death—cardiovascular disease, cancer, and problems resulting in infant mortality—account for 50 percent of the excess deaths for black males and 63 percent of the excess deaths for black females. Homicide accounts for 19 percent of the excess deaths for black males and 6 per-

cent for black females. An analysis of death rates between 1900 and the present reveals that black-white health inequality among men is currently at an all-time high for this century (Cooper 1993). In some depressed urban environments there has been no improvement in the health status of the black population over time. For example, Freeman (1993) shows that, in contrast to a steady decline in national mortality rates for both blacks and whites between 1960-1980, there was no change in mortality for African Americans in Harlem over this 20-year period. However, the potential contribution of selection processes via migration to this pattern was not assessed.

The gap in infant mortality rates for white and black babies widened for each sex between 1980 and 1991 (NCHS 1994b). Rates of both preterm delivery (Rowley et al., 1993) and low birth weight (NCHS 1994b) have remained stable for white women but have been increasing among African Americans. A widening differential between African Americans and whites is also evident for rates of sexually transmitted diseases (Castro 1993). Between 1986 and 1989, cases of gonorrhea and syphilis decreased by 50 percent and 11 percent, respectively, for whites. In contrast, gonorrhea declined by only 13 percent for blacks while syphilis increased by 100 percent. The increase in syphilis is thought to be associated with increases in the use of crack cocaine and related increases in prostitution.

Major Historical Events

This recent evidence of the deterioration in the health of the African American population emphasizes the importance of considering the larger historical context in understanding the health status of population groups. Mullings (1989) has suggested that the Civil Rights Movement, for example, has had important positive effects on black health. By reducing occupational and educational segregation, it improved the SES position of at least a segment of the black population and also influenced public policy to make health care accessible to larger numbers of people. Consistent with this hypothesis, one study found that between 1968 and 1978 blacks experienced a larger decline in mortality rates (both on a percentage and absolute basis) than whites (Cooper et al.. 1981).

More recently, the presidential campaign of Jesse Jackson may have had a positive short-term impact on the health of the African American population. Using four-wave data from the National Study of Black Americans that span the period 1979-80 to 1992, Jackson et al.. (1995) found that during the third wave of data collection (1988), the reported levels of physical and mental well-being were at their highest. In addition, the proportions of respondents reporting that they had experienced racial discrimination and that they perceived whites as wanting to keep blacks down were at their lowest levels. Contemporaneously, Jesse Jackson, a black male, was making the most successful run for the presidency of the United States that had ever been made by an African American in the history of the United States. These researchers suggest that this political event may have had spillover effects for black adults' perceptions of America's racial climate and their health status.

The massive internal migration of blacks in the United States earlier this century has been an important influence on the African American population. Although the initial economic and longer-term political gains linked to migration may have had positive health consequences, the black migration may have also had profound adverse effects on health (Williams 1995a). First, the black migration disproportionately distributed the African American population to urban residential areas where living conditions are hostile to life and health. Unlike the white urban poor who are dispersed throughout the city, with many residing in relatively safe and comfortable neighborhoods, the black poor are concentrated in depressed central-city neighborhoods (Wilson 1987) where the stress of poor urban environments can lead to illness (Harburg et al.. 1973, Haan et al.. 1987). A recent study in Harlem, one of the poorest areas of New York City, documented that black males between the ages of 25-44 in Harlem are six times more likely to die than are their white counterparts in the United States (McCord and Freeman 1990). More-

over, the life expectancy of blacks in Harlem is lower than that of persons in Bangladesh, one of the poorest countries in the world.

Wilson (1987) suggests that the concentration of black poverty in the inner city is due to the out-migration of middle class blacks to other areas. In contrast, Massey and Gross (1993) found that three complementary mechanisms were responsible: the wholesale abandonment of black and racially mixed areas by middle class whites, the selective migration of poor people into black neighborhoods, and the net movement into poverty of blacks living in segregated areas. Living conditions in inner-city areas are also deteriorating over time. The economic status of central-city African Americans has declined relative to other urban blacks. In 1940, central-city blacks earned 10 percent more than did other black urban dwellers, but by 1980 they were receiving 10 percent less (Smith and Welch 1989). There is also growing concern about the health consequences of stress in residential environments such as the high level of community violence in many depressed urban environments (Gabarino et al.. 1992).

The internal migration of the African American population also affected health by changing health behaviors in ways that lead to high risks of disease and death. With the great migration and urbanization of black Americans came a dramatic rise in their use of alcohol and tobacco, and a reversal in the racial distribution of alcohol and tobacco use (Williams 1991). During the first half of this century, the prevalence of cigarette smoking and alcohol abuse was higher for whites than for blacks. The great migration shifted a considerable portion of the black population from the relatively "dry" rural South, where social life revolved around churches and family associations, to the "wet" areas of the urban North, where taverns and associated alcohol use were an integral part of social life (Herd 1985). Moreover, by producing feelings of alienation, powerlessness, and helplessness, life in urban settings created the need for individuals to mask these feelings or obtain temporary relief from them by consuming tobacco and alcohol. African Americans have been special targets of the advertising of both the tobacco and the alcohol industries

(Davis 1987, Singer 1986), targeting that dates back to the 1950s (Levin 1988).

A recent provocative theory designed to account for the high rates of hypertension among African Americans also gives a central role to historical factors (Wilson and Grim 1991). According to the "slavery hypothesis" the historic conditions of slavery, especially those linked to capture in Africa and the transatlantic slave voyage, resulted in the preferential survival of those Africans who had a genetic propensity to conserve sodium and water. Contemporary African Americans have inherited this trait, which is responsible for the elevated rates of high blood pressure. Despite its deceptive simplicity and intuitive appeal, like earlier biological explanations, it locates racial disparities in health inside of the individual and pays scant attention to current living conditions. Serious questions have been raised regarding the plausibility of a historic genetic "bottleneck" being a key determinant of current genetic characteristics (Jackson 1991), and about the validity of the historic data that have been invoked to support this theory (Curtin 1992). Moreover, there is abundant evidence that the current social circumstances of African Americans play a major role in accounting for their elevated rates of high blood pressure (Williams 1992).

Race and SES

Socioeconomic differences between racial groups are largely responsible for the observed patterns of racial disparities in health status. Race is strongly correlated with SES and is sometimes used as an indicator of SES. For example, while 11 percent of the white population is poor, poverty rates for the African American and Hispanic population are 33 percent and 29 percent, respectively. Not surprisingly, differentials in health status associated with race are smaller than those associated with SES. For example, in 1986 persons with an annual household income of $10,000 or less were 4.6 times more likely to be in poor health than those with income over $35,000, while blacks were 1.9 times more likely to be in poor health than whites (Navarro 1990). Thus, race differentials were less than half of the SES differentials.

Researchers frequently find that adjusting racial disparities in health for SES substantially reduces these differences. In some cases the race disparity disappears altogether when adjusted for SES (Baquet et al.. 1991, Rogers 1992). Two recent studies provide striking evidence of the contribution of SES to observed racial differences in violence and illegal drug use. Greenberg and Schneider (1994) showed that rates of violent deaths in New Jersey were associated not with race per se, but with residence in urban areas with a high concentration of undesirable environmental characteristics such as waste incinerators, landfills, and deserted factories. Violent deaths from homicide, poisoning/drug use, falls, fires, and suicide in these marginal areas were ten times higher for males and six times higher for females than for their counterparts in the rest of New Jersey. Moreover, deaths in these marginal areas were high for whites and Hispanics as well as blacks, females as well as males, and middle-aged and elderly populations as well as youthful populations. Lillie-Blanton et al.. (1993) also found that a twofold higher prevalence of crack cocaine use for blacks and Hispanics compared to whites was reduced to nonsignificance when adjusted for census indicators of social environmental risk factors. Thus, failure to adjust racial differences for SES can reinforce racial prejudices and perpetuate racist stereotypes, diverting both public opinion and research dollars from the underlying social factors that are responsible for the pattern of risk distribution.

More frequently, it is found that adjustment for SES substantially reduces but does not eliminate racial disparities in health (Cooper 1993, Otten et al.. 1990, Krieger and Fee 1994). That is, within each level of SES, blacks generally have worse health status than whites. One recent study found higher infant mortality rates among college-educated black women than among their similarly situated white peers (Schoendorf et al.. 1992). Moreover, some studies find that the black-white mortality ratio actually increases with rising SES. This is clearly the case for infant mortality where the black-white gap is narrowest among women who have not completed high school, and highest among women with a college education (Krieger et al. 1993).

Kessler and Neighbors (1986) emphasize the importance of systematically testing for interactions between race and socioeconomic status. They reanalyzed data from eight epidemiologic surveys and demonstrated that, although controlling for SES reduced to nonsignificance the association between race and psychological distress, low-SES blacks had higher rates of distress than did low-SES whites. However, the findings have not been uniform. Analyses of data from the large ECA study found that low-SES white males had higher rates of psychiatric disorders than did their black peers (Williams et al. 1992).

Among women, low-SES black females had higher levels of substance abuse disorders than did their white peers. These findings suggest the importance of distinguishing distress from disorder, as well as the need to understand the interactions among race, gender, and class.

One reason for the persistence of racial differences despite adjustment for SES is that the commonly used SES indicators do not fully capture the economic status differences between households of different races. For example, racial differences in wealth are much larger than those for income. There are large racial differences in the inheritance of wealth and intergenerational transfers of wealth. Table 33-1 shows that while white households have a median net worth of $44,408, the net worth was $4,604 for black households and $5,345 for Hispanic households (Eller 1994). Compared to white households, black households had a significantly greater percentage of their net worth in durable goods such as housing and motor vehicles, and a significantly lower percentage of their net worth in financial assets. Moreover, at every income level, the net worth of black and Hispanic households is dramatically less than that of white households. Thus, in studies of racial comparisons, measures of assets are necessary for the identification of the economic status of the household.

In some cases where blacks are more exposed to particular risk factors, these risk factors appear to have weaker effects for the black population. In a national study in which black children constituted 75 percent of those in the category of lowest long-term income, persistent poverty was unrelated to either stunting or wasting for blacks, unlike the strong pattern evident for non-Hispanic whites and Hispanics (Miller and Korenman 1994). Similarly, although black infants have twice the low-birth-weight risk of whites, low birth weight is more strongly linked to infant mortality in the neonatal period for blacks than for whites (Hogue et al. 1987).

Table 33-1
Median net worth in 1991 by monthly household income quintiles for whites, blacks, and Hispanics

Household income	White	Black	Hispanic
All	$44,408	$4,604	$5,345
Lowest quintile	$10,257	$1	$645
Second quintile	$25,602	$3,299	$3,182
Third quintile	$33,503	$7,987	$7,150
Fourth quintile	$52,767	$20,547	$19,413
Highest quintile	$129,394	$54,449	$67,435

(Source: Eller 1994)

Racism

Another reason for the failure of SES indicators to completely account for racial differences in health is the failure of most studies to consider the effects of racism on health. A growing body of theoretical and empirical work suggests that racism is a central determinant of the health status of oppressed racial and ethnic populations (King and Williams 1995, Williams et al. 1994, Williams 1995b, Krieger et al 1993, Cooper 1993). Racism is viewed as incorporating ideologies of superiority, negative attitudes and beliefs toward racial and ethnic outgroups, and differential treatment of members of those groups by both individuals and societal institutions. Racism can affect health in at least three ways (Williams et al. 1994, Cooper 1993).

First, it can transform social status such that SES indicators are not equivalent across race. There are large differences related to race in the quality of elementary and high school education, so that blacks bring fewer basic skills to the labor market than do whites (Maxwell 1994). In addition, as Table 33-2 indicates, whites receive higher income returns from education than blacks and Hispanics. These racial differences are larger among males than among females, and the black-white income gap for males does not become narrower with increasing years of education. In addition, although Hispanic males do better than their black peers at the higher levels of education, the same is not true for Hispanic females. These data indicate that simply equalizing levels of education would still leave a large racial gap in earned income.

Table 33-2
Median earnings in 1990 by education (years of school completed) for white, black, and Hispanic, male and female full-time workers

	MALES		
Education level	White	Black	Hispanic
8 Years or less	16,906	16,961	13,913
9-11 Years	21,048	16,778	17,868
12 Years	26,526	20,271	20,932
Some college	31,336	25,863	26,380
College degree	38,263	30,532	33,074
Graduate	47,787	36,851	42,315
	FEMALES		
Education level	White	Black	Hispanic
8 Years or less	11,826	11,364	11,231
9-11 Years	14,010	13,643	12,586
12 Years	17,552	16,531	16,298
Some college	21,547	19,922	20,881
College degree	26,822	26,881	22,555
Graduate	31,991	31,119	30,133

(Source: US Bureau of the Census 1991)

Dressler (1993) also indicates that the pattern of income production varies for black and white households. Black households are more likely than white ones to rely on several wage earners to contribute to total household income. Middle class blacks are also more likely than their white peers to be recent and tenuous in that class status (Collins 1983). College-educated blacks, for example, are almost four times more likely than their white peers to experience unemployment (Wilhelm

1987). Researchers have also emphasized that the purchasing power of a given level of income varies by race (Cooper 1984, King and Williams 1995), with blacks paying higher prices than whites for a broad range of goods and services in society, including food and housing. African Americans also have higher rates of unemployment and underemployment than do whites. Moreover, employed blacks are more likely than their white peers to be exposed to occupational hazards and carcinogens, even after adjusting for job experience and education (Robinson 1984).

Second, racism can restrict access to the quantity and quality of health-related desirable services such as public education, health care, housing, and recreational facilities. Recent studies have found a positive association between residential segregation and mortality rates for both adults (Polednak 1993) and infants (LaVeist 1989, Polednak 1991). The relationship between segregation and infant mortality exists for blacks but not for whites. A recent review of racial differences in medical care found that even after adjusting for severity of illness, SES and/or insurance status, blacks are less likely to receive a wide range of medical services than are whites (Council on Ethical and Judicial Affairs 1990).

Third, the experience of racial discrimination and other forms of racism may induce psychological distress that may adversely affect physical and mental health status, as well as the likelihood of engaging in violence and addiction. Recent reviews reveal that a small but growing body of evidence indicates that the experience of racial discrimination is adversely related to a broad range of health outcomes (Krieger et al. 1993, Williams et al. 1994). In addition, the internalization of racist ideology is also adversely associated with morbidity (Williams et al. 1994).

In color conscious American society, skin color may be an important determinant of the degree of exposure to racial discrimination, access to valued resources, and the intensity of the effort necessary to obtain them (Dressler 1993). Dressler (1993) has employed darker skin color as an objective indicator of low social status within the black population and found that status inconsistency based on the relation of skin color to life-style (ownership of material goods and engaging in status enhancing behaviors) is associated with elevated rates of hypertension. Independent of education level, persons with darker skin color and higher life-style had the highest levels of blood pressure. Klag et al. (1991) also found an interaction between skin color and SES in a sample of blacks. Darker skin color was associated with elevated rates of hypertension for low but not high SES blacks. Consistent with the notion that darker skinned African Americans may experience higher levels of discrimination, analyses of data from the National Study of Black Americans found that skin color was a stronger predictor of occupational status and income of blacks than was parental SES (Keith and Herring 1991).

Age may be a proxy for the cumulative exposure to racism and adverse living conditions. There is an intriguing age patterning of at least some of the racial disparities in health. For both obesity and high blood pressure, racial differences are absent in childhood but emerge in early adulthood (Williams 1992, Kumanyika 1987). Similarly, neonatal mortality rates increase with age of the mother from the teens through the twenties for blacks and Puerto Ricans, while an opposite pattern is evident for whites and Mexican Americans (Geronimus 1992). These patterns may reflect a lagged effect of environmental exposure or a marked change in health status, as young adults are forced to confront restricted socioeconomic opportunities and truncated options (Williams 1992). Geronimus (1992) has proposed a "weathering hypothesis" to account for this pattern: for disadvantaged populations, age is a proxy for chronic exposure to adverse living conditions, with older age reflecting cumulative exposure to environmental assaults and the consequent increase in biological vulnerability.

Acculturation

The health profile of the Hispanic population in general and Mexican Americans in particular has seriously questioned the dominant paradigm that focuses heavily on SES and medical care as key explanatory factors for racial differences in health. Although Mexican Americans are low in SES and have low rates of health insurance, utilization of medical care and preventive health care, they have rates of infant mortality, overall mortality, and many chronic illnesses that are lower than those of African Americans and comparable to those of Anglos (Furino 1992). Moreover, several recent studies have noted that unlike the pattern for other racial groups, SES is unrelated to health outcomes such as blood pressure and low birth weight for Mexican Americans or foreign-born Mexican Americans (e.g. Sorel et al. 1992, Collins and Shay 1994). It is unclear whether this pattern reflects a healthy immigrant effect, protective effects of host cultures, or differences in the historical time period across societies in the secular distribution of disease. For example, SES has opposite effects in the earlier versus the later periods of the heart disease epidemic. A role for acculturation is suggested by the fact that foreign-born Hispanics have a better health profile than do their counterparts born in the United States. Rates of infant mortality, low birth weight, cancer, high blood pressure, adolescent pregnancy, and psychiatric disorders increase with length of stay in the United States (Vega and Amaro 1994). Migration studies of the Chinese and Japanese show that rates of some cancers such as prostate and colon increase when these populations migrate to the United States, while the rates of other cancers such as liver and cervix decline (Jenkins and Kagawa-Singer 1994).

It has been hypothesized that the cultural factors resident in traditional Mexican culture enhance the health of Mexican immigrants (James 1993). However, exactly what these protective cultural symbols, attitudes, or experiences are has not been clearly identified. As groups migrate from one culture to another, immigrants often adopt the diet and behavior patterns of the new culture. At the same time the transition to a new culture can also generate stress that may have adverse consequences for health. Several behaviors that adversely affect health status increase with acculturation. These include decreased fiber consumption, decreased breast feeding, increased use of cigarettes and alcohol especially in young women, driving under the influence of alcohol, and the use of illicit drugs (Vega and Amaro 1994). Acculturation also brings declines in caloric intake and fat, and reduced rates of diabetes and obesity.

Earlier studies of acculturation and heart disease among the Japanese immigrants to the United States provide a useful model for identifying and studying the health consequences of different aspects of culture (Marmot and Syme 1976). Rogler et al. (1991) have also outlined directions for improvement in the conceptualization and measurement of acculturation and for assessing its relationship to health.

Conceptualization of Race

Researchers have recently emphasized that we need to give more attention to what race is and why it is related to health status. They emphasize that our fundamental assumptions about what race is will shape the research questions developed to understand racial disparities in health (Dressler 1993, Krieger et al. 1993, King and Williams 1995, Williams et al. 1994). Historically, explanations for differences in health between the races focused on biological differences between racial groups. The biological approach views racial taxonomies as meaningful classifications of genetic differences between human population groups. The available scientific evidence shows that such a view of race is seriously flawed. Our current racial categories do not capture biological distinctiveness. Racial groups are more alike than different in terms of biological characteristics and genetics, and no specific scientific criteria distinguish different racial groups. Williams et al. (1994) note that unlike the social sciences, medicine and epidemiology have been slower in rejecting the now scientifically discredited biological view of race. They argue that an emphasis on biological sources of racial variations in health are least threatening to the status quo. Biological explanations focus on factors that reside within the individual and develop solutions that target individuals. They can effectively divert attention from current societal arrangements and policies that shape the health status of population groups.

Diseases that have a clear genetic component account for only a tiny part of racial disparities in health. For example, sickle cell anemia in African Americans accounts for three tenths of one percent of the total number of excess deaths in the black population (Cooper 1984). Thus, racial differences in biology are not the primary cause of racial variations in health and disease. Although the genetic contribution to racial variations in health status is likely to be small, researchers should be attentive to interactions between biological variables and environmental ones.

Studies that have examined the ways in which race is used in health and medical research document that race and ethnicity are widely used in the health literature to stratify or adjust results and to describe the sample or population of the study (Jones et al. 1991, Williams 1994). However, the terms used for race are seldom defined, and race is frequently employed in a routine and uncritical manner to represent ill-defined social and cultural factors. Researchers seldom specify how race is measured. A more deliberate, purposeful, and theoretically informed explication of race is needed (Williams 1994). Race is a proxy for specific historical experiences and a powerful marker of current social and economic conditions that determine exposure to pathogenic factors. Advances in our understanding of the role of race in health are contingent on efforts to directly assess the critical aspects of race that are implicated in health outcomes.

Problems with Racial Data

There is growing awareness of serious reliability and validity problems with the measurement of race and ethnicity (Hahn 1992). One study of a large national population found that fully one third of the U.S. population reported a different racial or ethnic status one year after their initial interview (Johnson 1974). There is also considerable discrepancy, especially for American Indians, Hispanics, and APIAs, between interviewer-observed race and respondent self-report. Massey (1980) found, in a large national sample, that 6 percent of persons who reported themselves as black, 29 percent of self-identified APIAS, 62 percent of self-identified

American Indians, and 80 percent of persons who self-identified with an "other" category (70 percent of whom were Hispanic) were classified by the interviewer as white. Given that racial status on death certificates is typically based on observer identification, the undercount problem in the numerator for mortality rates may be especially acute for some minority populations. Variations in the classification of race by different administrative systems can affect reported rates of health conditions, and this has also emerged as a major concern (Hahn 1992).

The implications of census undercount for the quality of health data for racial and ethnic populations have also been receiving increasing attention (Williams et al. 1994, Notes and Comments 1994). Census data are routinely used to construct sampling frames for population-based epidemiologic studies, to adjust obtained samples for nonresponse, and to calculate denominators for mortality and selected morbidity rates. Any rate that uses an undercounted denominator is overestimated in exact proportion to the undercount in the denominator. For all five-year age groups of black men ages 30-54, the estimated net undercount is almost 20 percent. Estimates of undercount based on demographic analysis are only available at the national level, and rates are probably even higher in selected geographic areas.

There is growing awareness that the Latino, APIA, and Native American populations are characterized by considerable heterogeneity in sociodemographic characteristics as well as the distribution of disease and risk factors for disease (Vega and Amaro 1994, Zane et al. 1994). Failure to attend to the variations in health indicators within a racial category can prevent the identification of health needs for some specific groups. Increasing attention has also been given to the heterogeneity of the black population (Williams et al. 1994). The major white ethnic groups are also characterized by distinctive histories and cultures, but little recent attention has been given to exploring ethnic variations in health for the non-Hispanic white population.

The classification of persons of mixed racial parentage is a significant issue facing data collection agencies, and American society more generally. The numbers of interracial couples and children from these unions have been increasing steadily over time. The health risks associated with multiracial status have not been systematically studied. Morton et al. (1967) studied the birth weight of infants of mixed race in Hawaii and found that such infants had birth weights intermediate between those of their parents' racial groups. A recent study suggests that the relationship between multiracial status and health may be complex, e.g. infants born to black mothers and white fathers were more likely to be low in birth weight than those born to white mothers and black fathers (Collins and David 1993).

The noncoverage of selected racial/ethnic subgroups in population-based epidemiologic surveys is a matter of continuing concern. In addition to precluding our understanding of the distribution of disease in certain populations, the unavailability of data also has policy implications. For example, due to the lack of baseline data, there were fewer objectives in Healthy People 2000 for the APIA population than for any other racial group (Chen M.S. 1993). Healthy People 2000 is a national health planning initiative that has defined a set of measurable health targets to improve the health status of the American population by the year 2000. Because it has increasingly become a basis for the allocation of funds to support public health programs, lack of objectives can importantly determine the distribution of economic resources.

Mechanisms Underlying SES and Racial Differences in Health

Research on the determinants of health has suggested that a broad range of factors such as stress in family home and work environments, health practices, social ties and attitudinal orientations are important determinants of health. Typically, inadequate attention is given to the ways in which the social distribution of risk factors and resources for health is constrained by societal norms and structures. A growing body of evidence suggests that risk factors for health outcomes are related to SES and race (Mirowsky and Ross

1989, Williams 1990, House et al. 1990; 1994). The distribution of risk factors and resources are shaped by the conditions under which people live and work. Researchers should also be attentive to interactions between social status and risk factors because evidence suggests that comparable stressful events, for example, have stronger negative effects on lower SES persons than on those of higher status (Kessler 1979).

Medical Care

Inadequate use of medical care, especially preventive medical care, by the poor and members of racial/ethnic minority populations is generally viewed as an important determinant of their health status. There are racial and socioeconomic status differences in the quantity and quality of medical care (e.g. Blendon et al. 1989). A study of deaths of blacks and whites in Alameda County, California (Woolhandler et al. 1985) found that deaths due to causes amenable to medical intervention accounted for about one third of the excess total death rate of blacks relative to whites. Recent reviews of the evidence on the contribution of medicine to health status indicate that the role of medicine is frequently overstated and that the removal of economic barriers alone will not eliminate social disparities in health care utilization (Williams 1990, Adler et al. 1993).

However, equitable access to medical care is important and crucial to preventing further deterioration of the health status of disadvantaged populations (Williams 1990). For many disease conditions such as cancer, tuberculosis, and hypertension, the higher incidence rates among African Americans do not account for the higher mortality rates (Schwartz et al. 1990). The higher mortality rate may result from later initial diagnosis of disease, comorbidity, delays in treatment, or other gaps in the quality of care. Thus, preventive medical care, appropriate early intervention in the course of an illness, and medical management of chronic disease can play important roles in enhancing the quantity and quality of life. Some evidence indicates that medical care has a greater impact on the health status of vulnerable racial and low SES groups than on their more advantaged counterparts (Williams 1990). For disadvantaged groups faced with multiple deficits, medical care may be a critical health-protective resource, while the incremental contribution of medicine is more limited for groups that already enjoy many social advantages.

Health Behavior

Health behaviors are important determinants of health. A U.S. Surgeon General's Report indicated that unhealthy behavior or life-style account for half of the annual number of deaths in the United States (U.S. Department of Health, Education and Welfare 1979). In comparison, 20 percent are due to environmental factors, 20 percent to genetics, and 10 percent to inadequate medical care. Health practices such as better nutrition and eating habits, diminished tobacco, alcohol, and drug abuse, and more exercise can dramatically improve health. The federal report on black and minority health (U.S. Department of Health and Human Services 1985) also identified health behaviors as the major determinants of the excess levels of mortality in minority populations in the United States.

Cigarette smoking is responsible for more than one in six deaths annually in the United States, for a total of 430,000 deaths (V.W. Chen 1993). A growing body of evidence suggests that smoking is increasingly concentrated among the lowest socioeconomic groups and minority populations. The prevalence of smoking is higher for black and Hispanic men than for whites. There is a paradox to black rates of smoking. Compared to whites, African American smokers start smoking later and smoke fewer cigarettes per day, but they are more adversely affected by smoking (Sterling and Weinkam 1989). In particular, there has been a sharper rise in lung cancer incidence among blacks than whites. Part of this difference may reflect differences in occupational exposures (Sterling and Weinkam 1989). A much greater proportion of blacks than whites work in occupations where they are exposed to occupational hazards such as toxic chemicals, dust, and fumes. Another factor accounting for this difference is the tendency for blacks to smoke cigarettes with higher tar content than those smoked by whites. More than 75 percent of black smokers use high tar cigarettes compared to 56 percent of whites and 69 percent of other races. Blacks are also three times more likely than other groups to smoke menthol cigarettes (V.W. Chen 1993). In general, blue collar and service workers are more likely to smoke nonfilter cigarettes than are professional managerial workers, and blacks are disproportionately represented in the former category.

Working Conditions

In one of the earliest sociological treatises on the association between social class and health, Engels ([1844] 1984) noted that the average longevity of the upper classes in Liverpool in 1840 was 35 years, compared to 22 years for business men and better-placed craftsmen, and only 15 years for operatives and day-laborers. He identified conditions of work including machine-paced employment, long hours, exposure to dust, fumes, other bad atmospheric conditions, and having to maintain uncomfortable body positions as major mechanisms responsible for excess mortality. Most recent U.S. studies utilize income and education as indicators of SES and neglect the role of occupational conditions. Low SES persons are more likely to be employed in occupational settings where there is an elevated risk of exposure to toxic substances and bad working conditions, but the role of occupational conditions tends to be neglected. Moore and Hayward (1990) is an exception to this pattern. They used data from the NLS and found that the aspects of the occupational environment that accounted for the association between occupation and mortality varied with the occupational indicator utilized. For longest occupation, the substantive complexity of the job (routinization and autonomy) is the major factor, while social skills and physical and environmental demands are the major factors accounting for the effects of the most recent occupation. In a study of over 5613 persons aged 15-75 in Sweden, Lundberg (1991) found that the physical working conditions were the major source of SES differences in physical illness, although economic hardship during upbringing and health-related behav-

iors also played a role. Bad working conditions were defined as heavy work, and daily contact with poisons, dust, smoke, acid, explosives, vibration, and the like.

Environmental Exposure

Concerns have also been raised about the extent to which low SES persons in general and racial minorities in particular are disproportionately exposed to environmental risks in residential environments. One early study found that treatment, storage, and disposal of hazardous waste sites were disproportionately located in areas where the surrounding residential population was black, and a study by the United Church of Christ (Commission for Racial Justice 1987) found that race was the strongest predictor of the location of hazardous waste sites in the United States. However, a recent industry-funded national study found that there is no significant relationship between the racial or ethnic composition of census tracts, and the presence of commercial hazardous waste facilities (Anderton et al. 1994).

The Economy and Health

Brenner (1995) has recently reviewed the evidence linking changes in the economy to health status. Rates of suicide and admissions to psychiatric hospitals increase during economic recessions. Cirrhosis mortality increases substantially one to two years after a national economic recession. Instructively, it is the consumption of distilled spirits, rather than wine or beer, that is a significant factor in the increase in cirrhosis mortality. Blacks are estimated to purchase half of all the rum sold in the United States, 41 percent of the gin, 50 percent of scotch whiskeys, and 77 percent of Canadian whiskeys (Djata 1987).

In Britain, higher mortality rates are also found for the unemployed compared to the employed (Brenner 1995). The wives of unemployed men had higher mortality rates during the follow-up period in some studies. This literature also indicates that economic stress induces divorce and separation in families, and adversely impacts friendship networks.

Personality

A number of personality variables have emerged as major risk factors for health status or as buffers or moderators of the impact of stressful experiences on health. These include self-esteem, perceptions of mastery or control, anger or hostility, feelings of helplessness and hopelessness, and repression or denial of emotions (Kessler et al. 1995). The distribution of at least some health enhancing personality characteristics varies by SES (Williams 1990, Mirowsky and Ross 1989), and future research must seek to identify the ways in which individual dispositions are shaped by the larger social context. Research on John Henryism illustrates the interaction between personality characteristics and socioeconomic status (James 1994). The John Henryism scale measures an active predisposition to master stress. Research with this measure suggests that John Henryism acts to increase blood pressure among lower SES blacks while simultaneously decreasing it among their higher SES black counterparts. It is interesting that the limited evidence available indicates that John Henryism is unrelated to blood pressure in whites.

Early Life Conditions

Most studies of SES and racial differences in health focus on current socioeconomic status. However, an adult's health status is a function not only of current SES but of the SES conditions experienced over the life course (Williams 1990, Mare 1990). Elo and Preston (1992) have provided a comprehensive review of the evidence suggesting that early life socioeconomic and health conditions have long-term consequences for an adult's health status. Several mechanisms appear to be at work. It appears that some diseases acquired in childhood, such as tuberculosis and typhoid, can be harbored for decades and manifest themselves later in life. Infection with the Hepatitis B virus can impair liver functioning and lead to cirrhosis of the liver and liver cancer. Living in a crowded household can increase one's risk of streptococcal infection and acute rheumatic fever, which in turn become major risk factors for rheumatic heart disease later in life. Infection plays a major role in growth retardation,

and malnutrition as reflected in height may adversely affect the immune system. Diarrhea in childhood can also affect child growth.

In other instances a childhood disease may impair an individual's organ system, which can create a chronic debility that leads to worse health status and earlier mortality. Some childhood illnesses and conditions can lead to changes in adult health status. Nutritional intake in childhood and exposure to and host resistance to infections play a major role in determining adult height. Respiratory tract infections in childhood as well as height (a proxy for early environmental influences) are related to the development of chronic bronchitis, asthma, and emphysema in adulthood. Several studies have also noted an association between height and mortality. Shorter persons have higher mortality rates than do their taller counterparts. However, some of these connections between height and adult mortality can be linked indirectly through SES status achieved in adulthood. There is a positive relationship between height and SES.

There is growing evidence that conditions related to the intrauterine environment during the fetal period and patterns of behavior acquired in early childhood are major risk factors for cardiovascular disease in adulthood (Elo and Preston 1992). Several of these factors appear to have direct relevance for the health status of the African Americans as population. For example, some studies have found that growth retardation during the fetal period or low birth weight is associated with high blood pressure in later life. Rates of low birth weight are twice as high for African Americans as for whites, and low birth weight is believed to be a crude indicator of growth retardation.

Using infant weight up to age one as a proxy for nutritional deprivation in early childhood, a study of over 5000 British boys documented a strong association between nutritional deprivation in childhood and heart disease in adulthood (Barker et al. 1989). Death rates for heart disease were 2.6 times higher for those in the lowest weight category at age one than for those in the highest category. Interestingly, breast-fed children were also at lower risk of heart disease. Breast-feeding is positively associated with SES, and blacks are less likely to breast-feed than whites; rates of breast-feeding also decline for Hispanic and Asian immigrants with assimilation (Jeffrey 1993). Infant formula companies aggressively market their product to low income and minority women, who may be less aware of the benefits of breast-feeding, and the WIC program (a federal program that provides nutritional support to poor women) accounts for 40 percent of the sale of infant formula in the United States (Jeffrey 1993).

Power

The proliferation of studies of socioeconomic status and health needs to be placed within an appropriate framework to enhance our understanding of the underlying dynamics. Some studies tend to reify the categories of SES such as education or income by addressing what it is about these specific factors that are linked to health outcomes. Rather, SES measures are crude indicators of location in social structure. A return to the sociological construct of social class can serve to inform and structure our understanding of inequalities in health. Social classes are hierarchically arranged, socially meaningful groupings linked to the structure of society. Systematic inequality will flow from membership in one class rather than another. The Marxist view of class, in particular, emphasizes that antagonistic and contradictory relations would exist between classes as they mobilize and struggle over economic and political power. Class membership leads to differential political and economic power, and inequality in power is a neglected but important construct for enhancing our understanding of the consequences of class for health (Packham 1991).

Power is differentially distributed in society, and location in social structure determines the degree of power and influence that social groups have with regard to the decisions that have a differential impact on all members of society. Good health status is one product of the power of the class to which one belongs. The power of social classes in a given community can be inferred from an analysis of which groups occupy important institutional positions, who takes part in important decisions made over private and public issues, and ultimately who benefits or is harmed by these decisions and policies (Packham 1991). Packham (1991) illustrates this process in the case of the location of hazardous waste sites and hazardous production. Similarly, Brenner (1995) argues that because of blue collar workers' relative lack of power (knowledge of occupational health risks and political influence to change their work environments) they are less able to affect the development of occupational safety and health codes. Also, Rice and Winn (1990) emphasize that those with the most power and influence have greater impact on decision-making and the allocation of benefits for themselves. Groups with less influence are less competitive in policy and decision-making processes, and therefore they experience inequities in a broad range of societal outcomes linked to this deficit in power. Rice and Winn argue that governmental involvement and advocacy are necessary to reduce the natural tendency for the higher social classes to exert greater control and extract greater benefit from the allocation and distribution of valued benefits and services.

The concept of power along with the related concept of control can serve to integrate major findings in the literature on inequalities in health and point to promising directions for future research. LaVeist (1992) found a strong inverse relationship between black political power and post-neonatal mortality rates, and outlines some pathways through which political empowerment may enhance health. Syme (1991) also indicates that control may be the key determinant of the SES gradient in health. He argues the effects of social support, Type A behavior, and stressful life events can all be interpreted to reflect the presence or absence of different aspects of control (Syme 1991). Other evidence suggests that the ability to understand, predict, and control daily life experiences can determine both the level of stress to which persons are exposed and the impact of stress on them (Sutton and Kahn 1987). Control may facilitate the management of uncertainty, which can be a key determinant of the stressfulness of many social situations. Lack of control in occupational environments has also been shown to predict increased risks of disease (Karasek and Theorell 1990).

Differences in power may also undergird the greater awareness of health risks by higher SES persons and their greater responsiveness to health education campaigns. Coleman (1974) indicates that access to and control of valuable information in society is a key manifestation of power. High SES persons are among the first to be exposed to new information and have the necessary economic and other resources to capitalize on new information and to develop alternatives to behaviors that have been shown to be health damaging.

Are Inequalities in Health Inevitable?

International comparisons of inequality in health and trends in social inequalities over time provide compelling data to address the issue of reducing health inequalities. National mortality rates are not strongly related to a country's overall economic status but are closely linked to the level of inequality within each country (Wilkinson 1992b). Countries with the least inequality have the best health profiles (Smith et al. 1990, Wilkinson 1992a). Differences in income distribution alone account for two thirds of the variation in national mortality rates for the 23 countries belonging to the Organization for Economic Cooperation and Development. Trends in income inequality are also related to SES variations in health over time within a given country. An analysis of SES differences in mortality in England and Wales between 1921 and 1981 revealed that they widened or narrowed to correspond with increases or decreases in relative poverty (Wilkinson 1989).

A study of the relationship between education and mortality in nine industrialized countries also suggests that a country's level of egalitarian social and economic policy is linked to the nature of SES differentials in health within that country. Inequalities in mortality were twice as large in the United States, France, and Italy as in the Netherlands, Sweden, Denmark, and Norway (Kunst and Mackenbach 1994). Finland,

England and Wales occupied intermediate positions. Vagaro and Lundberg (1989) have shown that the lowest social classes in Sweden have lower mortality than the highest social classes in Great Britain. Thus, the benefits of income redistribution within a society may affect the health status of the majority of the population.

A clear illustration of the link between economic inequality and health is found in the comparison of the trends in life expectancy and income for Japan and Great Britain over the past two decades (Wilkinson 1992a). In 1970, Japan and Great Britain were similar in average life expectancy and income distribution. During the last two decades SES differentials in Japan became the narrowest in the world, while the income distribution widened in Great Britain. During this same period Japan's life expectancy rapidly increased to become the highest in the world while Britain's relative international ranking in life expectancy has declined. Changes in Japanese nutrition, health services, or prevention policies do not account for these differences (Marmot and Smith 1989).

Further evidence that the health status disadvantage of low SES groups is not driven by an absolute standard of economic well-being comes from comparisons of the African American population in the United States with their counterparts in the Caribbean. Although the average annual income in Barbados is under U.S. $3000, life expectancy among black men in Barbados was 71 years in 1988, while it was 65 years for black men in the United States. Infant mortality in Barbados was similar to that of U.S. blacks—19 per 1000 live births (Cooper 1993).

The evidence is fairly clear that reductions in inequalities in health are closely linked to reductions in societal inequality. Factors such as medical care, even if equally provided to all, are unlikely to diminish SES differentials. Improved access to health enhancing resources may improve health for both high and low social status groups without reducing the health disparity between them. Reducing the SES gradient in health will require more fundamental changes. Freeman (1993) suggests that Third World communities in the United States (geographically and culturally defined areas of extreme excess mortality) should be identified and designated as chronic disaster areas. Special federal, state, and local resources should then be provided to such designated areas as is done in the case of natural disasters. Conditions such as substandard housing, low educational levels, poor social support and unemployment, as well as insufficient access to preventive health services should then be improved.

Income is probably the component of SES that is most amenable to change through redistributive policies such as tax credits or direct income supplementation. Two studies have documented that changes in household income can enhance health. In a study of expanded income support, Kehrer and Wolin (1979) found that the birth weight of the infants of mothers in the experimental income group was higher than those of mothers in the control group, although neither group experienced any experimental manipulation of health services. Improved nutrition, probably a result of the income manipulation, appeared to have been the key intervening factor. Similarly, Wilkinson (1990) found in analysis of mortality over a ten-year period that changes in the proportion of workers with low earnings in specific occupational categories were significantly associated with changes in occupational mortality.

Conclusion

One of sociology's most enduring contributions to the health field is the documentation that social class position is a key determinant of variations in the distribution of disease. Researchers in diverse disciplines recognize that SES is so strongly linked to health that they must statistically control for it in order to study their phenomena of interest. However, familiarity has bred complacency, and an opportunity exists for sociologists to provide leadership and direction to enhance understanding of the pathways by which social structure affects health.

The evidence reviewed indicates that large-scale societal factors are the primary determinants of health status. They determine not only the social categories to which people are assigned but their exposure to risk factors and resources. However, the ways in which location in social structure constrains and shapes daily life experiences in ways that adversely affect health is not well understood. Studies that seek to identify these pathogenic factors and mechanisms are urgently needed. Research on racism, acculturation, and power are fruitful places to begin. However, research and policy aimed at understanding the determinants of, and ensuring improvements in, health must recognize that intervening mechanisms and risk factors can be understood and effectively modified only in the context of the larger social environment in which they occur. For example, the high levels of low birth weight among African Americans are regarded as the prime risk factor for elevated rates of infant mortality. However, the mean birth weight for blacks in the United States is similar to that in Japan, but Japan has the lowest rate of infant mortality in the world (Wise and Pursley 1993). Not surprisingly, the available evidence indicates that interventions aimed at altering known risk factors without addressing fundamental social causes have had very limited success (Syme 1994). Thus, improvement in the health of vulnerable populations appears to be contingent on altering the fundamental macrosocial causes of inequalities in health.

Racial and socioeconomic inequality in health is arguably the single most important public health issue in the United States. The evidence reviewed indicates that SES inequalities in health are widening, and the health status of at least some racial groups has worsened over time. The ranking of the United States relative to other industrialized countries in terms of health has been declining over time, while America continues to spend more on medical care per capita than any other country in the world. The evidence reviewed suggests that a serious and sustained investment in reducing societal inequalities can enhance the quantity and quality of life of all Americans and create the necessary liberty for the pursuit of health and happiness.

References

Adler, N. E., T. Boyce, M. A. Chesney, S. Folkman, and S. L. Syme. 1993. "Socioeconomic inequalities in health: no easy solution." *J. Am. Med. Assoc.*, 269:3140-45.

Adler, N. E., T. Boyce, M. A. Chesney, S. Cohen, and S. Folkman et al.. 1994. "Socioeconomic status and health: the challenge of the gradient." *Am. Psychol.*, 49:15-24

Anderton, D.L., A. B. Anderson, J. M. Oakes, and M. R. Fraser. 1994. "Environmental equity: the demographics of dumping." *Demography*, 31:229-48.

Antonovsky, A. 1967. "Social class, life expectancy and overall mortality." *Milbank Q.*, 45:31-73.

Arber, S. 1987. "Social class, non-employment and chronic illness: continuing the inequalities in health debate." *Br. Med.*, 1. 294:1069-73.

Arber, S. 1991. "Class, paid employment and family roles: making sense of structural disadvantage, gender and health status." *Soc. Sci. Med.*, 32:425-36.

Baquet, C. R., J. W. Horm, T. Gibbs, and P. Greenwald. 1991. "Socioeconomic factors and cancer incidence among blacks and whites." *J. Natl. Cancer Inst.*, 83:551-57.

Barker, D. J. P., C. Osmond, P. D. Winter, B. Margetts, and S. J. Simmonds. 1989. "Weight in infancy and death from ischaemic heart disease." *Lancet*, 9:578-80.

Baxter J. 1994. "Is husband's class enough? Class location and class identity." *Am. Sociol. Rev.*, 59:220-35.

Blendon, R., L. Aiken, H. Freeman, and C. Corey. 1989. "Access to medical care for black and white Americans." *J. Am. Med. Assoc.*, 261:278-81.

Braithwaite, R. L. and S. E. Taylor. 1992. *Health Issues in the Black Community.* San Francisco: Jossey-Bass.

Brenner, M. H. 1995. "Economy, society, and health: theoretical links and empirical relations." In *Society and Health: Foundation for a Nation*, ed. S. Levine, D. C. Walsh, B. C. Amick, and A. R. Tarlov. New York. Oxford Univ. Press. In press.

Bunker, J.P., D. S. Gomby, and B. H. Kehrer, eds. 1989. *Pathways to Health: The Role of Social Factors.* Menlo Park, CA: Kaiser Family Found.

Carstairs, V. and R. Morris. 1989. "Deprivation and mortality: an alternative to social class?" *Commun. Med.*, 11:210-19.

Castro, K. G. 1993. "Distribution of acquired immunodeficiency syndrome and other sexually transmitted diseases in racial and ethnic populations, United States: influences of life-style and socioeconomic status. *Ann. Epidemiol.*, 3:181-4.

Chen, M. S. 1993. "A 1993 status report on the health status of Asian Pacific Islander Americans: comparisons with *Healthy People 2000* objectives." *Asian Am. Pacific Islander J. Health*, 1:37-55.

Chen, V. W. 1993. "Smoking and the health gap of minorities." *Ann. Epidemiol.*, 3:159-64.

Coleman, J. S. 1974. *Power and the Structure of Society.* New York: Norton.

Collins, J. W. Jr., and R. J. David. 1993. "Race and birthweight in biracial infants." *Am J. Pub. Health*, 83:1125-29.

Collins, J. W. Jr., and D. K. Shay. 1994. "Prevalence of low birth weight among Hispanic infants with United States-born and foriegn-born mothers: the effect of urban poverty." *Am. J. Epidemiol.*, 139:184-92.

Collins, S. M. 1983. "The making of the black middle class." *Soc. Prob.*, 10:369-82.

Commission for Racial Justice. 1987. *Toxic Wastes and Race in the United States: A National Report on the Racial and Socioeconomic Characteristics of Communities with Hazardous Waste Sites.* New York: United Church of Christ.

Cooper, R. 1984. "A note on the biological concept of race and its application in epidemiologic research." *Am. Heart J.*, 108:715-23.

Cooper, R. S. 1993. "Health and the social status of blacks in the United States." *Ann. Epidemiol.*, 3:137-44.

Cooper R. S., M. Steinhauer, A. Schatzkin, and W. Miller. 1981. "Improved mortality among U.S. blacks, 1968-78: the role of antiracist struggle." *Int. J. Health Serv.*, 11:511-22.

Council on Ethical and Judicial Affairs. American Medical Association. 1990. "Black-white disparities in health care." *J. Am. Med. Assoc.*, 263:2344-46.

Crews, D. E. 1994. "Obesity and diabetes." In *Confronting Critical Health Issues of Asian and Pacific Islander Americans*, ed. N. W. S. Zane, D. T. Takeuchi, and K. N. J. Young, pp. 174-208. Thousand Oaks, CA: Sage.

Curtin, P. D. 1992. "The slavery hypothesis for hypertension among African Americans: the historical evidence." *Am. J. Pub. Health*, 82:1681-86.

Danziger, S., and P. Gottschalk P, eds. 1993. *Uneven Tides: Rising Inequality in America.* New York: Russell Sage.

Davis, R. M. 1987. "Current trends in cigarette advertising and marketing." *New Engl. J. Med.*, 316:725-32.

Department of Health and Social Security. 1980. *Inequalities in Health: Report of a Research Working Group* (The Black Report). London: Dep. Health Soc. Security.

Djata. 1987. "The marketing of vices to black consumers." *Bus. Soc. Rev.*, 62:47-49.

Dohrenwend, B. 1990. "Socioeconomic status (SES) and psychiatric disorders." *Soc. Psychol. Psychiatr. Epidemiol.*, 25:41-47.

Dressler, W. W. 1993. "Health in the African American community: accounting for health inequalities." *Med. Anthropol. Q.*, 7:325-45.

Duleep, H. O. 1989. "Measuring socioeconomic mortality differentials over time." *Demography*, 26:345-51.

Duncan, G. 1988. "The volatility of family income over the life course." In *Life Span Development and Behavior*, Vol. 9, ed. P. Bates, D. Featherman, and R. Lerner, pp. 317-58. Hillsdale, NJ: Lawrence Erlbaum Assoc.

Duncan, G. J., J. Brooks-Gunn, and P. K. Klebanov. 1994. "Economic deprivation and early childhood development." *Child Dev.*, 65:296-318.

Duncan, G. J., T. Smeeding, and W. Rodgers. 1993. "W(h)ither the middle class?: a dynamic view." In *Poverty and Prosperity in the USA in the Late Twentieth Century*, ed. D. Papadimitriou, and E. Wolff, pp. 240-271. London: MacMillan.

Eller, T. J. 1994. *Household Wealth and Asset Ownership: 1991. US Bureau of the Census, Current Population Reports, P70-34*. Washington DC: U.S. Govt. Printing Off. (USGPO).

Ellis, L, ed. 1993. *Social Stratification and Socioeconomic Inequality*, Vol. 1. Westport, CT: Praeger.

Elo, I. T. and S. H. Preston. 1992. "Effects of early-life conditions on adult mortality: a review." *Pop. Index*, 58:186-212.

Engels, F. 1984. [1844] *The Condition of the Working Class in England*. Chicago: Academy Chicago.

Feinstein, J. S. 1993. "The relationship between socioeconomic status and health." *Milbank Q.*, 71:279-322.

Feldman, J. J., D. M. Makuc, J. C. Kleinman, and J. Cornoni-Huntley. 1989. "National trends in educational differentials in mortality." *Am. J. Epidemiol.*, 129:919-33.

Fingerhut, L. A. and D. M. Makuc. 1992. "Mortality among minority populations in the United States." *Am. J. Pub. Health*, 82:1168-70.

Fox, A., P. O. Goldblatt, and D. R. Jones. 1985. "Social class mortality differentials: artifact, selection or life circumstances?" *J. Epidemiol. Commun. Health*, 39:1-8.

Freeman, H. P. 1993. "Poverty, race, racism, and survival." *Ann. Epidemiol.*, 3:145-49.

Furino, A., ed. 1992. *Health Policy and the Hispanic*. Boulder: Westview.

Gabarino, J., N. Dubrow, K. Kosteiney, and C. Pardo. 1992. *Children in Danger. Coping with the Consequences of Community Violence*. San Francisco: Jossey-Bass.

Geronimus, A. T. 1992. "The weathering hypothesis and the health of African-American women and infants: evidence and speculations." *Ethnicity & Disease*, 2:207-21.

Goldblatt, P. 1990. *Longitudinal Study: Mortality and Social Organisation*. London: HMSO.

Greenberg, M. and D. Schneider. 1994. "Violence in American cities: young black males is the answer; but what was the question?" *Soc. Sci. Med.*, 39:179-87.

Haan, M. N. and A. G. Kaplan. 1986. "The contribution of socioeconomic position to minority health." In *Report of the Secretary's Task Force on Black and Minority Health*, 2:69-103. Washington, DC: U.S. Dep. Health Hum. Serv.

Haan, M., G. Kaplan, and T. Camacho. 1987. "Poverty and health: prospective evidence from the Alameda County Study." *Am. J. Epidemiol.*, 125:989-98.

Hahn, R. A. 1992. "The state of federal health statistics on racial and ethnic groups." *J. Am. Med. Assoc.*, 267:255-58.

Harburg, E., J. Erfurt, C. Chape, L. Havenstein, W. Scholl, and M. A. Schork. 1973. "Sociological stressor areas and black-white blood pressure: Detroit." *J. Chron. Dis.*, 26:595-611.

Haug, M. 1977. "Measurement on social stratification." *Annu. Rev. Sociol.*, 3:51-77.

Hauser, R. M. 1993. "Trends in college entry among blacks, Hispanics, and whites." In *Studies of Supply and Demand in Higher Education*, ed. C. Clotfelter and M. Rothschild, pp. 61-119. Chicago: Univ. Chicago Press

Herd, D. 1985. "Migration, cultural transformation and the rise of black liver cirrhosis mortality." *Br. J. Addict.*, 80:397-410.

Hernandez, D. J. 1993. *America's Children: Resources from Family, Government and the Economy*. New York: Russell Sage.

Hibbard, J. and C. Pope. 1991. "Effect of domestic and occupational roles on morbidity and mortality." *Soc. Sci. Med.*, 32:805-11.

Hogue, C. J. R., J. W. Buehler, L. T. Strauss, and J. C. Smith. 1987. "Overview of the national infant mortality surveillance (NIMS) project: design, methods, results." *Pub. Health Rep.*, 102:126-38.

Holzer, C., B. Shea, J. Swanson, P. Leaf, J. Myers et al.. 1986. "The increased risk for specific psychiatric disorders among persons of low socioeconomic status." *Am. J. Soc. Psychiatr.*, 6:259-71.

House, J. S., R. C. Kessler, A. R. Herzog, R. P. Mero, A. M. Kinney, and M. J. Breslow. 1990. "Age, socioeconomic status, and health." *Milbank Q.*, 68:383-411.

House J. S., J. M. Lepkowski, A. M. Kinney, R. P. Mero, R. C. Kessler, and A. R. Herzog. 1994. "The social stratification of aging and health." *J. Health Soc. Behav.*, 35:213-34.

Jackson, F. L. C. 1991. "An evolutionary perspective on salt, hypertension, and human genetic variability." *Hypertension*, 17 (1, Suppl. I):129-32.

Jackson, J. S., T. N. Brown, D. R. Williams, M. Torres, S. L. Sellers, and K. Brown. 1995. "Perceptions and experiences of racism and the physical and mental health status of African-Americans: a thirteen year national panel study." *Ethnicity and Disease*, 5(1).

James, S. A. 1993. "Racial and ethnic differences in infant mortality and low birth weight." *Ann. Epidemiol.*, 3:130-36.

James, S. A. 1994. "John Henryism and the health of African-Americans." *Culture Med. Psychiatry*, 18:163-82.

Jeffrey, C. 1993. "Formula for failure." *Chicago Reporter*, 22:1,6-11.

Jenkins, C. N. H., M. Kagawa-Singer. 1994. "Cancer." In *Confronting Critical Health Issues of Asian and Pacific Islander Americans*, ed. N. W. S. Zane, D. T. Takeuchi, and K. N. J. Young, pp. 105-47. Thousand Oaks, CA: Sage.

Johnson, C. E. 1974. *Consistency of Reporting Ethnic Origin in the Current Population Survey. U.S. Dep. Commerce Tech. Pap. No. 31* Washington, DC: Bur. Census.

Jones C. P., T. A. LaVeist, and M. Lillie-Blanton. 1991. "Race in the epidemiologic literature: an examination of the *American Journal of Epidemiology, 1921-1990*." *Am. J. Epidemiol.*, 134:1079-84.

Karasek R. A. and T. Theorell T. 1990. *Healthy Work*. New York: Basic Books.

Kehrer, B. H. and C. M. Wolin. 1979. "Impact of income maintenance on low birth weight: evidence from the Gary experiment." *J. Hum. Resour.*, 14:434-62.

Keith, V.M. and C. Hening. 1991. "Skin tone and stratification in the black community." *Am. J. Sociol.*, 97:760-78.

Kessler, R. C. 1979. "Stress, social status, and psychological distress." *J. Health Soc. Behav.*, 20:259-72.

Kessler, R. C., J. S. House, R. Anspach, and D. R. Williams. 1995. "Social psychology and health." In *Sociological Perspectives on Social Psychology*, ed. K. Cook, G. Fine, and J. S. House, pp. 548-70. Boston: Allyn and Bacon.

Kessler R. C. and H. W. Neighbors. 1986. "A new perspective on the relationships among race, social class, and psychological distress." *J. Health Soc. Behav.*, 27:107-15.

King, G. and D. R. Williams. 1995. "Race and health: a multi-dimensional approach to African American health." In *Society and Health: Foundation for a Nation*, ed. S. Levine, D. C. Walsh, B. C. Amick, and A. R. Tarlov. New York: Oxford Univ. Press.

Kitagawa E. M. and P. M. Hauser. 1973. *Differential Mortality in the United States: A Study in Socioeconomic Epidemiology*. Cambridge: Harvard Univ. Press.

Klag M. H., P. K. Whelton, J. Coresh, C. E. Grim, and L. H. Kuller. 1991. "The association of skin color with blood pressure in U.S. blacks with low socioeconomic status." *J. Am. Med. Assoc.*, 265:599-602.

Kochanek, K. D., J. D. Maurer, and H. M. Rosenberg. 1994. "Why did black life expectancy decline from 1984 through 1989 in the United States?" *Am. J. Pub. Health*, 84:938-44.

Krieger N. 1991. "Women and social class: a methodological study comparing individual, household, and census measures as predictors of black/white differences in reproductive history." *J. Epidemiol. Commun. Health*, 45:35-42.

Krieger, N. and E. Fee. 1994. "Social class: the missing link in U.S. health data." *J. Health Serv.*, 24:25-44.

Krieger, N., D. L. Rowley, A. A. Herman, B. Avery, and M. T. Phillips. 1993. "Racism, sexism, and social class: implications for studies of health, disease, and well-being." *Am. J. Prev. Med.*, 9(supp.):82-122.

Kumanyika, S. K. 1987. "Obesity in black women." *Epidemiol. Rev.*, 9:31-50.

Kunst, A. E. and J. P. Mackenbach. 1994. "The size of mortality differences associated with educational level in nine industrialized countries." *Am. J. Pub. Health*, 84:932-37.

LaVeist, T. A. 1989. "Linking residential segregation and infant mortality in U.S. cities." *Social Soc. Res.*, 73:90-94.

LaVeist, T. A. 1992. "The political empowerment and health status of African-Americans: mapping a new territory." *Am. J. Sociol.*, 97:1080-95.

Levin, M. 1988. "The tobacco industry's strange bedfellows." *Bus. Soc. Rev.*, 65:11-17.

Liberatos, P., B. G. Link, and J. L. Kelsey. 1988. "The measurement of social class in epidemiology." *Epidemiol. Rev.*, 10:87-121.

Lillie-Blanton, M., J. C. Anthony, and C. R. Schuster. 1993. "Probing the meaning of racial or ethnic group comparisons in crack cocaine smoking." *J. Am. Med. Assoc.*, 269:993-97.

Lin-Fu, J. S. 1993. "Asian and Pacific Islander Americans: an overview of demographic characteristics and health care issues." *Asian Pacific Islander J. Health*, 1:20-36.

Livingston, I. L. 1994. *Handbook of Black American Health: The Mosaic of Conditions, Issues, and Prospects*. Westport, CT: Greenwood.

Lundberg, O. 1991. "Causal explanations for class inequality in health—an empirical analysis." *Soc. Sci. Med.*, 32:385-93.

Lurie, N., N. B. Ward, M. F. Shapiro, and R. H. Brook. 1984. "Termination from Medi-Cal—does it affect health?" *New Engl. J. Medicine*, 311:480-84.

Mackenbach, I. P., K. Stronks, and A. Kunst. 1989. "The contribution of medical care to inequalities in health: differences between socio-economic groups in decline of mortality from conditions amenable to medical intervention." *Soc. Sci. Med.*, 29:369-76.

Mandinger, M. O. 1985. "Health service funding cuts and the declining health of the poor." *New Engl. J. Med.*, 313:44-47.

Mare, R. D. 1990. "Socio-economic careers and differential mortality among older men in the United States." In *Measurement and Analysis of Mortality—New Approaches*, ed. J. Vallin, S. D'Souza, and A. Palloni. pp. 362-87. Oxford: Clarendon.

Marmot, M. G., M. Kogevinas, and M. A. Elston. 1987. "Social/economic status and disease." *Annu. Rev. Pub. Health*, 8:111-35.

Marmot, M. G., M. J. Shipley, and G. Rose. 1984. "Inequalities in death-specific explanations of a general pattern?" *Lancet*, 1:1003-06.

Marmot, M. G. and D. G. Smith. 1989. "Why are the Japanese living longer?" *Br. Med. J.*, 1547-51.

Marmot M. G., G. D. Smith, S. Stansfeld, C. Patel, F. North et al. 1991. "Health inequalities among British civil servants: the Whitehall II Study." *Lancet*, 337:1387-93.

Marmot, M. G. and S. L. Syme. 1976. "Acculturation and coronary heart disease in Japanese-Americans." *Am. J. Epidemiol.*, 104:225-47.

Massey, D. S. and A. B. Gross. 1993. "Black migration, segregation, and the spatial concentration of poverty." *Irving B. Harris Graduate School of Public Policy Studies Working Paper Series: 93-3*. Chicago: Univ. Chicago.

Massey, J. T. 1980. *A comparison of interviewer observed race and respondent reported race in the National Health Interview Survey*. Presented at Ann. Meet. Am. Statis. Assoc., Houston, Texas.

Maxwell, N. L. 1994. "The effect on black-white wage differences in the quantity and quality of education." *Indust. Labor Relat. Rev.*, 47:249-64.

McCord, C. and H. P. Freeman. 1990. "Excess mortality in Harlem." *New Engl. J. Med.*, 322:173-77.

McDonough, P., G. Duncan, D. R. Williams, and J. S. House. 1995. *Income Dynamics and Adult Mortality in the U.S., 1972-1989*. Unpublished ms. Survey Res. Ctr. Inst. for Soc. Res. Ann Arbor, MI.

Miller, J. E. and S. Korenman. 1994. "Poverty and children's nutritional status in the United States." *Am. J. Epidemiol.*, 140:233-43.

Mirowsky, J. and C. E. Ross. 1989. *Social Causes of Distress*. New York: Aldine de Gruyter.

Moen, P., D. Dempster-McClain, and R. Williams R. 1989. "Social integration and longevity: an event history analysis of women's roles and resilience." *Am. Sociol. Rev.*, 54:635-47.

Moore, D. E. and M. D. Hayward. 1990. "Occupational careers and mortality of elderly men." *Demography*, 27:31-53.

Morton, N. E., C. S. Chung, and M-P Mi. 1967. *Genetics of Interracial Crosses in Hawaii*. Basel, Switzerland: S. Karger.

Moser, K. A., H. Pugh, and P. Goldblatt P. 1990. "Mortality and the social classification of women." In *Longitudinal Study: Mortality and Social Organization*, Ser. LS, no. 6, ed. P Goldblatt, pp. 146-62. London: Her Majesty's Stationery Off.

Mullings. L. 1989. "Inequality and African-American health status: policies and prospects." In *Twentieth Century Dilemmas—Twenty-First Century Prognoses*, ed. W. A. VanHome and T. V. Tonnesen, pp. 154-182. Madison: Univ. Wisc. Inst. on Race and Ethnicity.

National Center for Health Statistics. 1994a. *Health United States 1993*. Hyattsville, MD: USDHHS.

National Center for Health Statistics. 1994b. *Excess Deaths and Other Mortality Measures for the Black Population: 1979-81 and 1991*. Hyattsville, MD: Pub. Health Serv.

Navarro, V. 1990. "Race or class versus race and class: mortality differentials in the United States." *Lancet*, 336:1238-40.

Notes and Comments. 1994. "Census undercount and the quality of health data for racial and ethnic populations." *Ethnicity and Disease*, 4:98-100.

Otten, M. C., S. M. Teutsch, D. F. Williamson, and J. S. Marks. 1990. "The effect of known risk factors on the excess mortality of black adults in the United States." *J. Am. Med. Assoc.*, 263:845-50.

Packham, J. 1991. *Power as a neglected variable in the assessment of the class/health relation*. Presented at Ann. Meet. Am. Soc. Assoc.

Pappas, G., S. Queen, W. Hadden, and G. Fisher. 1993. "The increasing disparity in mortality between socioeconomic groups in the United States, 1960 and 1986." *New Engl. J. Med.*, 329:103-15.

Passannante, M. K. and C. Nathanson. 1985. "Female labor force participation and female mortality in Wisconsin 1974-78." *Soc. Sci. Med.*, 21:655-65.

Polednak, A. P. 1991. "Black-white differences in infant mortality in 38 standard metropolitan statistical areas." *Am. J. Pub. Health*, 81:1480-82.

Polednak A. P. 1993. "Poverty, residential segregation, and black/white mortality rates in urban areas." *J. Health Care Poor Underserv.*, 4:363-73.

Power, C., O. Manor, A. J. Fox, and K. Fogelman. 1990. "Health in childhood and social inequalities in health in young adults." *J. Royal Statist. Soc.*, 153 Part 1:17-28.

Powers, M. and J. Holmberg. 1982. "Occupational status scores: changes introduced by the inclusion of women." In *Measures of Socioeconomic Status: Current Issues*, ed. M. Powers, pp. 55-81. Boulder, CO: Westview.

Rice, M. F. and M. Winn. 1990. "Black health care in America: a political perspective." *J. Natl. Med. Assoc.*, 82:429-37.

Robins, L. N. and D. A. Regier, eds. 1991. *Psychiatric Disorders in America: The Epidemiologic Catchment Area Study.* New York: Free Press.

Robinson J. 1984. "Racial inequality and the probability of occupation-related injury or illness." *Milbank Q.,* 62:567-90.

Rogers, R. G. 1992. "Living and dying in the U.S.A.: sociodemographic determinants of death among blacks and whites." *Demography,* 29:287-303.

Rogler, L. H., D. E. Cortes, and R. G. Malgady RG. 1991. "Acculturation and mental health status among Hispanics." *Am. Psychol.,* 46:585-97.

Rogot, E. 1992. *A Mortality Study of 1.3 Million Persons by Demographic, Social and Economic Factors: 1979-1985 Follow-up: U.S. National Longitudinal Mortality Study.* Bethesda: Natl. Inst. Health, Natl. Heart, Lung, and Blood Inst.

Rose, G. 1985. "Sick individuals and sick populations. *Int. J. Epidemiol.,* 14:32-8.

Rowley, D. L., C. J. R. Hogue, A. C. Blackmore, C. D. Ferre, K. Hatfield-Timajchy et al.. 1993. "Preterm delivery among African-American women: a research strategy." *Am. J. Prev. Med.,* 9(supp.):1-6.

Ruggles, P. 1990. *Drawing the Line: Alternative Poverty Measures and their Implications for Public Policy.* Washington DC: Urban Inst.

Schoendorf, K. C., C. J. R. Hogue, J. C. Kleinman, and D. Rowley. 1992. "Mortality among infants of black as compared with white college-educated parents." *New Engl. J. Med.,* 326:1522-26.

Schwartz, E., V. Y. Kofie, M. Rivo, and R. V. Tuckson. 1990. "Black/white comparisons of deaths preventable by medical intervention: United States and the District of Columbia 1980-1986." *Int. J. Epidemiol.,* 19:591-98.

Sheak, R. 1988. "Poverty estimates: political implications and other issues." *Sociol. Spectrum,* 8:277-94.

Singer, M. 1986. "Toward a political economy of alcoholism." *Soc. Sci. Med.,* 23:113-30.

Smith, D.G., M. Bartley, and D. Blane. 1990. "The black report on socioeconomic inequalities in health 10 years on." *Br. Med. J.,* 301:373-77.

Smith, E.M. 1993. "Race or racism? Addiction in the United States." *Ann. Epidemiol.,* 3:165-70.

Smith, J. P. and F. R. Welch. 1989. "Black economic progress after Myrdal." *J. Econ. Lit.,* XXVII:519-64.

Sorel, J. E., D. R. Ragland, S. I. Syme, and W. B. Davis. 1992. "Educational status and blood pressure: the Second National Health and Nutrition Examination Survey, 1976-1980, and the Hispanic Health and Nu-

trition Examination Survey, 1982-1984." *Am. J. Epidemiol.,* 135:1339-48.

Sorlie, P. D., E. Backlund, N. J. Johnson, and E. Rogot. 1993. "Mortality by Hispanic status in the United States." *J. Am. Medical Assoc.,* 270:2464-68.

Sterling, T. D. and J. J. Weinkam. 1989. "Comparison of smoking-related risk factors among black and white males." *Am. J. Industr. Med.,* 15:319-33.

Sutton, R. and R. L. Kahn. 1987. "Prediction, understanding and control as antidotes to organizational stress." In *Handbook of Organizational Behavior,* ed. J. W. Lorsch, pp. 272-85. Englewood Cliffs, NJ: Prentice Hall.

Syme, S. L. 1991. "Control and health: a personal perspective." *Advances,* 7:16-27.

Syme, S. L. 1994. "The social environment and health." *Daedalus,* 123:79-86.

Takeuchi, D. T., D. R. Williams, and R. I. C. Adair. 1991. "Economic stress in the family and children's emotional and behavioral problems." *J. Marriage Fam.,* 53:1031-41.

Townsend, P., P. Phillimom, and A. Beattie. 1988. *Health and Deprivation: Inequality and the North.* London, England: Croom Helm.

U.S. Bureau of the Census, Current Population Reports, Series P-60, No. 174. 1991. *Money Income of Households, Families, and Persons in the United States.* Washington DC: USGPO.

U.S. Department of Health, Education, and Welfare. 1979. *Healthy People: The Surgeon General's Report on Health Promotion and Disease Prevention.* Washington DC: USGPO.

U.S. Department of Health and Human Services. 1985. *Report of the Secretary's Task Force on Black and Minority Health.* Washington,DC: USGPO.

Vagaro, D. and O. Lundberg. 1989. "Health inequalities in Britain and Sweden." *Lancet,* II(8653):35-36.

Vega, W. A.and H. Amaro. 1994. "Latino outlook: good health, uncertain prognosis." *Annu. Rev. Pub. Health,* 15:39-67.

Wagener, D. K. and A. Schatzkin. 1994. "Temporal trends in the socioeconomic gradient for breast cancer mortality among U.S. women." *Am. J. Pub. Health,* 84:1003-06.

Waitzman, N. J. and K. R. Smith. 1994. "The effects of occupational class transitions on hypertension: racial disparities among working class men." *Am. J. Pub. Health,* 84:945-50.

Wilhelm, S. M. 1987. "Economic demise of blacks in America: a prelude to genocide?" *J. Black Stud.* 17:201-54.

Wilkinson, R. G., ed. 1986. *Class and Health: Research and Longitudinal Data.* London: Tavistock.

Wilkinson, R. G. 1989. "Class mortality differentials, income distribution and trends in poverty 1921-81." *J. Soc. Policy,"* 18:307-35.

Wilkinson, R. G. 1990. "Income distribution and mortality: a 'natural' experiment." *Soc. Health and Illness,* 12:391-412.

Wilkinson, R. G. 1992a. "Income distribution and life expectancy." *Br. Med. J.,* 304:165-68.

Wilkinson, R. G. 1992b. "National mortality rates: the impact of inequality?" *Am. J. Pub. Health,* 82:1082-84.

Williams, D. R. 1990. "Socioeconomic differentials in health: a review and redirection." *Soc. Psychol. Q.,* 53:81-99.

Williams, D. R. 1991. "Social structure and the health behavior of blacks." In *Aging, Health Behaviors and Health Outcomes,* eds. K. W. Schaie, J. S. House, D. Blazer, pp. 59-64. Hillsdale, NJ: Erlbaum.

Williams, D. R. 1992. "Black-white differences in blood pressure: the role of social factors." *Ethnicity and Disease,* 2:126-41.

Williams, D. R. 1994. "The concept of race in *Health Services Research,* 1966-1990." *Health Serv. Res.,* 29:261-74.

Williams, D. R. 1995a. "Poverty, racism and migration: the health of the African American population." In *Immigration, Race, and Ethnicity in America: Historical and Contemporary Perspectives,* ed. S. Pedraza and R. G. Rumbaut. Belmont, CA: Wadsworth.

Williams, D. R. ed. 1995b. "Special issue on racism and health." *Ethnicity and Disease,* 5: In press.

Williams, D. R., R. Lavizzo-Mourey, and R. C. Warren. 1994. "The concept of race and health status in America." *Pub. Health Rep.,"* 109:26-41.

Williams, D. R., D. Takeuchi, and R. Adair. 1992. "Socioeconomic status and psychiatric disorder among blacks and whites." *Soc. Forces,* 71:179-94.

Wilson, T. W. and C. E. Grim. 1991. "Biohistory of slavery and blood pressure differences in blacks today." *Hypertension,* 17(suppl. I): 122-28.

Wilson, W. J. 1987. *The Truly Disadvantaged.* Chicago: Univ. Chicago Press.

Wise, P. H. and D. M. Pursley. 1992. "Infant mortality as a social mirror." *New Engl. J. Med.,* 326:1558-60.

Woolhandler, S., D. U. Himmelstein, R. Silber, M. Bader, M. Harnly, and A. A. Jones. 1985. "Medical care and mortality: racial differences in preventable deaths." *Int. J. Health Serv.,* 15:1-11.

Wu, C.I. and C. E. Ross. 1994. *Education, Age, and Health.* Presented at Annu. Meet. Am. Sociol. Assoc., Los Angeles.

Zane N. W. S., D. T. Takeuchi, and K. N. S. Young eds. 1994. *Confronting Critical Health Issues of Asian and Pacific Islander Americans.* Thousand Oaks, CA: Sage.

Acknowledgements

Preparation of this paper was supported by grant AG-07904 from the National Institute of Aging. We wish to thank Greg Duncan, James S. House, and Sherman James for helpful comments on an earlier version of this paper.

Further Reading

Ronald L. Braithwaite and Sandra E. Taylor (eds.) 1992. *Health Issues in the Black Community.* San Francisco: Jossey-Bass.

Thomas A. LaVeist. 1992. "The Political Empowerment and Health Status of African Americans: Mapping a New Territory." *American Journal of Sociology* 97: 1080-95.

S. Leonard Syme. 1994. "The Social Environment and Health." *Daedalus* 123: 79-86.

Discussion Questions

1. What are the most significant problems in considering the relationship between race and health status?

2. Describe the relationship between socio-economic status and health.

3. In what ways does consideration of socio-economic factors and social structure move us beyond individualistic explanations of illness?

34

Pathways of Health and Death

Lois M. Verbrugge

Despite current trends to include women in clinical research, epidemiologists and health services researchers know little of what there is to know about the relationship between gender and health. What they do know is that there is a gap between the incidence and prevalence of disease by sex when we examine men's and women's rates of health and illness. In this selection, Lois Verbrugge investigates this gap for the physical health of adults, providing detailed information and analyses for why differences in men's and women's rates of health and illness exist. Using national level data for the United States, Verbrugge looks at trends in health by sex. She finds, for example, that across the life-span, men have higher rates of acute disease that lead to death; women, higher rates of disease that lead to illnesses less likely to lead to death. Women tend to have more chronic physical health conditions than do men. Look for other differences in health and illness between men and women that Verbrugge describes. Examine her explanations for these differences carefully. Pay attention to her claims about the social versus biological differences in health between men and women. Think about the relevance of this issue for race differences in health. Could you apply Williams' and Collins' argument about race and health to sex and health as well?

Go back to Verbrugge's initial question about the contradiction between sex differentials in health and mortality. When you are finished reading her article, you should be able to address this question and challenge biological assumptions related to health and illness. What kinds of explanations might you come up with regarding the dynamics of sex differentials and health through time in the United States?

Introduction

In contemporary health statistics, the largest differentials in rates of illness, disability, and death are related to age. Typically, rates rise across adult ages, and especially steeply at older ages (65+). Sex ranks second: women's experience of daily symptoms, their prevalence rates for many chronic conditions, their experience of short- and long-term disability due to health problems, and their use of professional health services exceed men's within each age group. Nevertheless, women's rates of mortality are strikingly lower than men's.

What causes these sex differentials has much to do with prior personal and social histories. The health status of any individual and any society at a given time is the consequence of past exposures and therapies as well as current ones. Whether we are able to understand the precise causes of sex differentials, or only able to see their distilled outcome in rates and other health-status measures, depends on scientific sophistication and energy.

Advances in the collection and processing of health information over the past century mean we now see levels and differentials that were only intuited or scantily recorded before. We now regularly report the health status of women and men with good accuracy and precision. Still, what we know descriptively about sex differentials is sparse compared to social needs and future scientific capabilities. How health information is interpreted has also changed greatly. Viewed as the "weaker sex" only a century ago, women are now considered the sturdier sex by most biologists and health scientists, with regard to longevity potential and intrinsic vulnerability to fatal pathologies.[1] Interpretations of sex differentials will continue to change, hopefully in ever more veridical directions. In short, our knowledge about population health is always bounded empirically and culturally—ideally less so as time goes on. As scientists, we strive to recognize those limitations and then proceed to tell the truth as accurately and fairly as possible.

Contents

This selection begins with contemporary statistics to highlight differences in health and death experiences of women and men. I concentrate on enduring rather than evanescent differences. Explanations for the differences are stated and evaluated. Then trends in health and mortality during the twentieth century and trends in sex differences are presented. Health and mortality prospects for women and men in the twenty-first century and forecasts of their position relative to each other are discussed. I note the shift from a young to an aged population and the rising importance of older women as a social force and as a concern for medicine and rehabilitation. Finally, the failure of statistics to see the dynamics of health—the health pathways that individuals take over their lifetimes—is considered.

Some basic features of the article should be mentioned:

(1) I discuss adults (ages 18+) rather than the whole age span since chronic morbidity and death are infrequent in childhood and youth. Although sex differences do exist in pre-adult years (poorer health for boys up to adolescence, and higher mortality for them at all pre-adult ages), they are relatively small compared to adult ages.[2]

(2) The rates summarized and discussed are age-specific ones (for age groups) unless otherwise noted. In health statistics, age groups are commonly split into young (18–44), middle-aged (45–64), and older (65+) persons. The total adult population's health is a function of both age specific rates and age distribution (percents of people in each age group). When studying trends, demographers prefer age-standardized rates (applying age-specific rates of various years to a fixed age distribution, thus allowing only rates to change and pretending age distribution does not).

(3) We will focus on physical health. Physical ailments are the dominant propellers of disability, and mortality, though mental diseases and cognitive deficits do increase in their causal importance with age. Besides this, national health surveys have long separated physical and mental health, studying one but not both. (A key data source for this selection is the National Health Interview Survey, which virtually excludes mental disorders.) In short, issues of pertinence and data lead us to examine physical health alone.[3]

(4) Health statistics provide aggregate estimates of ill and dead people. These are needed for health-services planning and policy for the whole nation. The statistics can legitimately be used to state probabilities for individuals or average profiles for subgroups. These are never meant to convey stereotypes. Thus, sex differentials discussed here indicate tendencies of men and women to differ, but do not imply completely, different health experiences for men versus women.

(5) The only way to demonstrate that women are special is to compare them to men, and vice versa. Studying just women leads to thinner empirical and less steady theoretical results. This comparative stance is a standard one in sociology. Readers will find that this selection says as much about men as women.

A few terms need definition: (1) I shall use the term "health" broadly to encompass both morbidity and disability.[4] *Morbidity* refers to symptoms, diseases, and impairments. *Disability* refers to consequences of morbidity for physical and social functioning. (2) The term "sex" is used in a demographic manner, simply to indicate the two groups being compared.[5]

Contemporary Health Profiles

Health surveys repeatedly show that women have higher rates of illness and disability than men. This excess appears in every adult age group, being most pronounced for acute conditions and short-term disability in reproductive ages (18–44), and for chronic conditions and associated disability in mid- or late life. Despite their lower levels of well-being throughout life, women tend to live longer than men. Two questions rise immediately: Why is there apparently a contradiction between sex differentials in health and mortality? And why do sex differences exist at all in health and mortality?

We begin this section with a summary of contemporary health and mortality levels for both sexes, and the general size of sex differentials.[6,7] The contradiction is then untangled. Lastly, reasons why sex differences in health and mortality exist are considered.

Morbidity

Acute conditions are transient. (In national health statistics, they can last no more than three months). Women's incidence rates of acute conditions overall are 20–30 percent greater than men's. A female excess appears in all main categories: infective/parasitic diseases, respiratory conditions, digestive system conditions, injuries (at ages 45+, but not 18–44), and the residual "all other acute conditions." The last category contains reproductive conditions, ear diseases, headache, genital tract and urinary disorders, and skin/musculoskeletal conditions. Even when reproductive conditions are excluded, a sizable sex difference still persists for this last category.

Chronic conditions are long-term health problems; they can be diseases or structural/sensory impairments. They are essentially permanent in a person's life, though their symptoms and progression can sometimes be controlled by drugs, lifestyle changes, and other therapeutic regimens. The key distinction for our discussion is between fatal (life-threatening) and nonfatal conditions. Prevalence rates for nonfatal chronic conditions are typically higher for women. Women 's disadvantage is especially large for some musculoskeletal problems, most digestive disorders, thyroid diseases, anemias, migraine headache, urinary conditions, and varicose veins. A special comment is needed about arthritis, since it is the leading chronic problem for women in mid- and late life, and the first or second rank one for men those ages. Women's prevalence rates for this often painful and limiting condition exceed men's by about 50 percent. Men have higher rates for relatively few nonfatal conditions, mostly some sensory and skeletal impairments. Altogether these data offer striking evidence of women's greater burden from nonfatal diseases, the conditions that bother but do not kill. The situation completely re-

verses for fatal chronic conditions. Here, men consistently have excess rates.

Incidence and prevalence rates tell us simply about the presence of conditions, but not the suffering they cause for people. Health-diary studies in which respondents record symptoms and health actions daily for several weeks or months show how health problems penetrate everyday life. Not surprisingly, daily symptoms are more frequent for women than men at all ages.

The incidence, prevalence, and symptom rates all point toward greater frequency of illness for women day by day, year by year. More time is spent feeling unwell. But women's illness burden also adds up in another way: Higher risks of experiencing most illness conditions, with the exceptions noted, imply that women end up with more chronic problems (this is called comorbidity) at any age. Thus, their health problems are more extensive both over time and at any given time.

In the midst of these differences, there is nevertheless a striking similarity. Even though rates differ so much, women and men tend to suffer from fundamentally the same health problems. And this similarity increases with age. The evidence: (1) Men's and women's lists of leading acute ailments are very similar. Flu and the common cold dominate the list for both young men and women. The roster of other leading titles is essentially the same (though injuries tend to rank higher for men than women). For ages 45+, when rates of acute conditions fall sharply and pregnancy vanishes from women's lives, the leading titles and ranks become almost identical. (2) Women's and men's lists of leading chronic conditions are also very similar. Respiratory problems top the list for young adults of both sexes. Fatal conditions are essentially absent for both. In midlife, the lists for both women and men become a more diverse mix of nonfatal problems, precursors to fatal ones (high blood pressure), and just a few fatal conditions (ischemic heart disease for men, diabetes for both women and men). At older ages, fatal circulatory problems become more prominent for both sexes. Still, their lists remain dominated by nonfatal impairments and diseases, especially women's. For both sexes, skeletal impairments diminish in importance with age, and sensory ones rise. In sum, women and men are distinguished more by their frequency of morbidity than by the conditions they typically suffer. I shall continue to emphasize women's excess rates for nonfatal conditions and men's for fatal conditions, but these tendencies lie within a context of basic similarity in the problems experienced by both groups.

Disability

Acute and chronic problems often induce people to restrict their activities. The impact of acute conditions generally goes no farther than reducing daily activities for a while or staying in bed. But chronic conditions pose long-term threats for physical and social functioning; for example, making walking a painful and difficult enterprise, or forcing people to quit their jobs.[8]

Statistics split disability into short-term versus long-term impact. Short-term disability is due to both acute and chronic problems. Women consistently have higher rates: They restrict their activities for health problems about 25 percent more days each year than men do, and spend about 40 percent more days in bed per year on average. The differences are largest during women's reproductive years (ages 18–44). But even when reproductive problems are removed, a sizable sex difference in disability remains at these ages.[9]

Long-term disability refers to compromised physical and social activities, due largely to chronic conditions. For physical disability, women have notably higher rates of difficulty for all indicators (mobility, other motions, strength, endurance). Their disadvantage is especially pronounced in tasks requiring strength or involving the lower extremities.[10] For social disability, sex differences are more mixed and also harder to interpret: (1) In working ages (defined as 18–69), men are more likely to report severe limitations in their major role, but women surpass them for mild and moderate limitations.[11] ("Severe" means unable to do one's major role, whether it is paid employment or housekeeping; "moderate" is limited in amount/kind of major activity; "mild" is limited in other secondary activities such as

shopping or church attendance.) It is hard to see direct reflections of illness in these rates because the physical demands that men and women face in their main roles probably differ on average. (Women still choose housekeeping more often than men, and even in the very same role there can be differences in physical demand.) Thus, social as well as morbidity aspects penetrate the disability statistics. Still, though the differences are hard to interpret precisely, they are genuine measures of the ultimate social impact of health problems. (2) It is currently conventional to measure social disability for older people by their ability to do basic personal care and household-management activities. Among people living in the community (noninstitutional), women are more likely to have difficulty doing routine personal and household tasks. (Examples of personal tasks are dressing self and getting to/using toilet; examples of household tasks are doing light housework and managing money.) The sex differences tend to increase with age; thus, women's problems are especially obvious among very elderly persons (85+). Some people have so much trouble they must rely on another person to help them get the job done. This is called dependency. Rates of dependency are much lower than rates of difficulty, but the sex differentials look the same. Women are more likely than men to be dependent for household tasks at all ages, and for personal-care tasks at advanced ages (80+; no difference at ages 65–79).[12] (3) Institutional residence is considered a form of disability since it signals inability to function adequately in the community for medical or social reasons. Institutional residence is more common for older women than older men. Among residents, women residents typically have higher disability levels for personal care than same-age men residents.[13]

Mortality

An ultimate disadvantage for males surfaces in death. Males' overall mortality rate is currently 70 percent higher than females' (1985; age-adjusted). The male excess appears at all ages. For example, the sex mortality ratio (M/F) for 1985 is 1.80 for ages 45–54, 1.84 at 55–64, 1.81 at 65-74, 1.63 at 74–85, and

1.28 at 85+.[14] Life expectancy portrays these rates in a compact manner: The average number of years of life for a newborn boy was 71.2 in 1985, compared to 78.2 for a girl.[15] Even at age 85, female life expectancy is higher: 6.4 years versus 5.1.[16] Males have higher mortality from all leading causes of death (diseases of heart, malignant neoplasms, cerebrovascular diseases, accidents, chronic obstructive pulmonary diseases, pneumonia/influenza, suicide, chronic liver disease/cirrhosis, atherosclerosis).[17]

Despite the pronounced sex differences in mortality rates, there is fundamental similarity in causes of death. The lists of leading causes, and the ranks of those causes, are very similar for men and women.[18]

Summary

Women's lives are filled with more health problems—higher incidence of acute conditions, higher prevalence of most nonfatal chronic ones, more frequent botheration by health problems. Their higher levels of disability are an understandable consequence. Compared to men, women's symptoms are more likely to be bothersome but not life-threatening, and their limitations are mild or moderate rather than severe until advanced ages. The conjunction of more nonfatal problems and fewer fatal ones means more total years of life—and also more years of sickness and dysfunction. By contrast, men's lives are freer of illness, discomfort, and disability. But when ill health does strike, it is more likely to be via fatal chronic diseases. These abbreviate men's lives. Which sex pays the higher price? There is no single answer. Women's compromised life quality and men's compromised longevity are both high prices.

Nevertheless, behind these profound differences lies a basic similarity that should not be overlooked. Women and men encounter largely the same health problems in their lifetimes. Our comparisons of leading titles (for acute conditions, chronic conditions, causes of death) always show fundamental similarities. What differs for women and men are the *paces* of these health problems, with fatal conditions entering men's lives earlier and nonfatal ones entering women's lives earlier.

A Contradiction Is Untangled

The seeming contradiction of "higher female morbidity, but higher male mortality" vanishes in face of the data above. Men have higher age-specific prevalence rates for fatal conditions, and it is these which ultimately drive their earlier mortality. Women have higher rates of transient ailments and of chronic conditions that bother but do not kill, and these largely account for their higher levels of discomfort and restriction during life.

Morbidity statistics focus on current problems and recent disability, so they are well-suited to showing women's excess in that regard. If instead morbidity statistics captured longitudinal health experiences of individuals, they would show not only a larger cumulative burden among women but also—and importantly—the earlier onset and possibly faster progression of fatal diseases among men. We can only hypothesize about such longitudinal differences now. Mortality statistics are the only overt signal of men's ultimate disadvantage, offering minimal insight into men's significant health decrements while living.

Reasons for Sex Differences

There are five categories of explanations for sex differences in health and mortality: (1) biological risks; these are intrinsic genetic and hormonal differences between males and females, (2) acquired risks; these are risks of illness and injury encountered in one's work and leisure activities, (3) psychosocial aspects of symptoms and care; called "illness behavior" in medical sociology, (4) health-reporting behavior; this concerns how men and women talk about their health problems to others, and (5) prior health care; or how one's care for health problems affects future health. Biological and acquired risks determine the occurrence of disease, injury, and impairment. Psychosocial factors then come into play—in perception of symptoms, evaluation of their cause and severity, choice and continuation of therapeutic actions, and short- and long-term disability. Willingness to discuss health problems becomes pertinent when people are interviewed. Lastly, health care for a prior problem can influence one's current and future health experiences.[19,20]

It is widely held by researchers, and increasing scientific evidence suggests, that men are disadvantaged by both biological and acquired risks for the development of fatal diseases and for experience of injuries. What lies behind women's greater tendency to develop nonfatal diseases has not been discussed, and it is a real mystery. The diseases are so diverse, no small array of risk factors (acquired or biological) is plausible. Far less epidemiologic and biomedical research has been devoted to etiology of nonfatal diseases than fatal ones. When the answers finally come, they will illuminate this aspect of sex differences. Similarly, women's higher rates of acute conditions are not yet explained. Symptom perception and predispositions to take care of symptoms are thought to be stronger among women. But the research evidence to date shows only small sex differences, in the direction just stated. Thinking about the matter in a theoretical way: sex differences in symptom-response are more likely when people confront "nonserious" health problems (nonfatal chronic conditions and mild acute ones) than "serious" ones (fatal diseases or severe acute conditions). For the latter, the illness is so overt and threatening, men and women are likely to respond similarly. Even if psychosocial differences prove rather small, their repeated expression does add up toward more health attentiveness, more care, and more accommodation over a lifetime for women. For reporting factors, it is often claimed that women are more willing to talk about their health problems and that they remember health events better. But the research evidence on this issue is scant; the evidence to date shows no sex differences. Finally, women's more attentive care for health problems may lead to earlier diagnosis of serious conditions, earlier and more persistent management for them, and ultimately longer lifetimes, compared to men. If supported by data, this hypothesis will show that women's higher morbidity actually contributes to lower mortality by prompting more care! The evidence is not yet in.

Summing up, I offer some judgments about the relative importance of the five factors. (1) What lies behind sex differences in diseases, impairment, and injury? Acquired risks rank first; social and recreational activities, stresses, and environmental exposures during life are the prime causes of health problems for each sex, and for differentials between them. Prior health care may rank next, giving a cumulative advantage to women. Biological risks come last. (Where do psychosocial and reporting factors fit in? They become pertinent when the data are obtained from health surveys. I hypothesize that their importance is lower than the other three factors.) (2) For mortality, the three principal reasons stack up in the same manner. Although biology ranks last, it is not negligible. The contribution of hormonal and genetic factors to sex mortality differences is hard to guess (my own is that 10–20 percent of the contemporary difference is due to biology) and will be very difficult to estimate quantitatively. (3) What lies behind sex differences in disability? Women's higher levels of day-to-day, year-to-year morbidity are the principal factor. (Morbidity, in turn, is the net product of acquired risks, prior health care, and biological factors.) Psychosocial factors rank second; they are pervasive aspects of illness experience and behavior in life, and they operate to boost women's responses to symptoms. Health-reporting factors come in last, maybe increasing women's survey reports of disability a little.[21]

These are hypotheses. The relative importance of the five factors in explaining sex differentials in morbidity, disability, and mortality is not known yet quantitatively. What has been accomplished in recent years are careful and comprehensive statements of the factors that must be considered, theoretically and empirically, in finding the answers. The basic scientific task ahead is to locate specific factors that influence health and mortality, and also differ in their presence among males and females. Both aspects are necessary for an explanation; neither suffices alone. High interest in sex differences assures us that coming decades will bring forth many detailed answers, which together will produce broad conclusions about the relative importance of social and biological factors. The most intriguing questions of all—"Are women intrinsically sturdier than men? In what biological ways? How much sturdier?"—will not be answered soon. But I believe that scientific imagination and intelligence will eventually produce firm responses.

Health and Mortality Trends in the Twentieth Century

The sex differentials in health and mortality evident in the late twentieth century are not new. This section considers their persistence and course over the past century.

All countries establish a vital registration system (for births, deaths, marriages) long before a national health survey program. Our knowledge of mortality trends is thus much richer than of morbidity trends, so we start with mortality.

Mortality Trends

Mortality data for the entire United States are available since 1933 (for selected states, 1880 to 1932). Demographers typically place confidence in figures starting at the century mark, 1900.

A profound epidemiological transition occurred in the twentieth century: Deaths, initially dominated by external and infectious/parasitic causes, are now due largely to chronic diseases (especially cardiovascular and neoplastic). Short-term perturbations in mortality rates, typically due to wars or epidemics, have largely disappeared. Death rates have fallen substantially in all age groups for both sexes. But the locus of gains has shifted; initially larger for children in this century, they are now (since the late 1960's) concentrated among older people.[22]

Sex differentials in mortality widened in the twentieth century, particularly since 1930. In 1900, females had only a slight advantage over males: Their life expectancy at birth was 50.9, compared to 47.9 for males. The ratio of male to female mortality rates was 1.10 (age-adjusted). In 1985, the sex difference was far larger: Life expectancies at birth were 78.2 and 71.2, respectively, and the sex mortality ratio was 1.75.[23] It is important to recognize that widening of the sex differential—that is, increasing the male excess—can come about by (a) mortality rates rising faster for males than for females, (b) rates falling faster for females than males, or (c) rising rates for males but falling ones for females. Thus, one must always turn back to mortality levels for each sex and note their trends in order to explain changes in the differential. Stated very generally, the principal reason for the widening gap in the twentieth century has been smaller mortality improvements overall and in most leading causes for men, than for women. This is (b) above. An additional factor in the decades before 1940, but not important since then, was the decline in reproduction-related mortality for women. This is also (b); being a sex-specific cause, it amounted to zero change for men but marked gain for women.[24] In short, for most of the century, women's advantage became larger and larger.

In the late 1970s, the situation began to change.[25] Although both sexes continue to experience mortality improvements, their gains are more comparable than before, and this acts to stabilize the sex differential. Quite certainly, a new era is before us in which the mortality gap will hold steady or even narrow. Some journalists have advanced a short-sighted explanation for this—that women are reaping pernicious consequences from stresses in multiple work and family roles due to their increased labor-force participation in recent years. But the truth is complex and longer-sighted, having more to do with (a) changes made by women decades ago such as increased smoking after World War II, or (b) their reaching limits of possible gain from medical and lifestyle improvements sooner than men.[26,27]

Morbidity and Disability Trends

From the late 1920's to the mid-1950's, a number of population-health surveys were sponsored by the United States government.[28] These yielded painstakingly-produced tables with rates of illness and restricted activity by age, sex, and condition. Pressure to have an ongoing survey covering the entire population mounted in the 1950's, and Congressional legislation in 1956 authorized it. The National Health Interview Survey (NHIS) was launched in July 1957 and has been collecting health data for the civilian noninstitutional population continuously since then.

The early surveys consistently show higher acute and chronic morbidity and higher disability days for females. The excess is smallest for children (sometimes it is a small male excess) and largest for reproductive ages. Males have higher accident/injury rates.[29] The NHIS has shown similar differentials since its inception, and it has provided clearer distinctions of the morbidity areas that disfavor women (acute conditions, chronic nonfatal ones) versus those which disfavor men (injuries at young adult ages, impairments, chronic fatal diseases). Notions of disability have expanded to include activities of daily living for older people, and these augment the evidence of excess female disability.

What has happened to population health over the century? And have sex differences changed so women report more, or fewer, problems relative to men than decades ago? The questions are impossible to answer easily for the whole century since the early surveys do not match up easily with NHIS. But NHIS itself has changed relatively little since 1957, so the period since then can be readily studied for trends.[30]

Since the late 1950's, age-specific prevalence rates have increased for most fatal diseases and also for some prominent nonfatal ones, especially arthritis and other musculoskeletal conditions. Short-term disability rates have increased for middle-aged and older people, largely since 1970. Long-term disability rates have increased sharply among middle-aged women and men, and less obviously for older people. These rises occur at all levels of disability, severe to mild. Overall, the bulk of empirical evidence points toward worsening health among U.S. adults.[31]

A number of reasons can account for this: (a) improved medical and lifestyle management of fatal chronic conditions, so ill people stay alive longer; (b) people's increased awareness of their chronic diseases due to improved diagnostic techniques, more frequent visits to physicians, and more frankness by physicians toward patients; (c) more willingness and ability to adopt the sick role

for both short and long periods; and (d) improvements in survey techniques, so fuller reports of illness and disability are elicited.[32] Debate over the importance of these factors, and even the direction of the health trends, is very active. My own judgment, shared by most other observers of the data, is that the rising morbidity and disability rates are intimately tied to falling mortality rates, which began a sharp downward turn in 1968. This is (a) above. Deaths have been delayed by secondary prevention; namely, control of fatal diseases so they advance less rapidly. This leads to lower case-fatality rates. The marginal survivors gain some years of life but are already ill and very vulnerable to acquiring new diseases. The subpopulation of marginal survivors is numerous because the mortality gains have been striking, especially for cardiovascular diseases. Simultaneously, people with less advanced disease have made gains too, and their symptoms and limitations are milder than otherwise (i.e., if the secondary prevention successes had not occurred). This subpopulation is very large, far greater than the number of marginal survivors. In short, prevalence rates have risen but the average severity of conditions has probably become milder.

I also believe that better and earlier diagnosis has increased awareness of existing disease, and that positive incentives for disability have increased. These are genuinely social reasons that also boost illness and disability rates. I do not think that survey techniques are an important factor behind the trends. Methodology changes influence data discontinuously, in the same year as the changes. Yet the observed trends are essentially continuous over time.[33]

The trends noted have occurred for both women and men. Have sex differences changed? Since it is hard enough to ascertain the trends in rates with certainty, review of the data for trends in sex differentials is a delicate endeavor. One study, for the 1957 to 1972 period, shows larger increases in chronic morbidity and severe disability for men than women.[34] As the data series lengthens, it will be able to sustain close scrutiny for changes in sex differentials, and discussion of their compatibility with changes in sex-mortality differentials.

In sum, we cannot trace the course of women's and men's health over the century easily. We must rely on occasional surveys until the mid-1950's and the good stream of NHIS data since then. The surveys to mid-century need more attention from demographically-inclined historians, and the NHIS from 1957 on needs more quantitative analysis to locate trends with certainty.

Health and Mortality Futures in the Twenty-First Century

The unprecedented and unanticipated mortality declines since the late 1960's have urged more thinking about potentials of population health and longevity.[35] What is our direction for the next 50 to 100 years? Will recent mortality improvements be sustained? Will the social burden of illness revealed in health surveys continue to rise? How fast will changes occur? Is it feasible to attain a life expectancy at birth of 100 by 2040, or 2090?

Future scenarios of health and mortality hinge on assumptions about three forms of prevention: (a) tertiary; this is saving people at the brink of death by costly medical measures, (b) secondary; this is controlling fatal diseases by medical and lifestyle interventions so they advance less rapidly, and (c) primary; this is reducing the incidence (clinical onset) of diseases. Strides in tertiary prevention happened in mid-century, and there is increasing public and even clinician resistance to furthering this kind of prevention. Contemporary medicine is distinctive for its emphasis on secondary prevention. Little is known about primary prevention, how to prevent chronic diseases from occurring at all to individuals.

Forecasts now being made are based largely on careful thinking and guesses about the three types of prevention, rather than formal quantitative models about presence of risk factors in the population, morbidity incidence and prevalence, and their implications for mortality. Lacking the foundation of such models, I shall state in narrative fashion

a plausible course for coming decades, in my judgment.

The twenty-first century holds not just one health future but several sequenced in time. The near future will continue recent trends in health and mortality, with secondary prevention the lead actor. Despite rising prevalence rates of chronic disease and disability, measures of severity will show a "shift toward mildness." Diseases, though present, will have less impact on people's lives. Five or six decades ahead, there will be an intermediate period with powerful pushes from both secondary and primary prevention. We may then see a larger percent of older people in vigorous health, as well as a larger percent in very poor health. A century hence, disease onsets may be delayed until near life's end for many people. But complete prevention, meaning that people avoid disease in their lifetimes and ultimately die from "natural aging" processes, is not likely to be common.[36]

Thus, we can anticipate continuing advances in disease control and gradually increasing ones in primary prevention. Population-health statistics, focused on prevalence rates, will "worsen" for the next several decades but then slowly turn around to show improving health. (The shift toward mildness that is occurring now and that will continue may be missed by statistics, since severity is seldom ascertained.) Accompanying these health trends, mortality rates will continue to fall. Some scientists think the advances will be swift and widespread, and that life expectancy at birth in 2040 will far surpass the Social Security Administration projection of 83.4 for females and 75.7 for males.[37] Others think that continuing degradation of outdoor and indoor environments, impact of AIDS, and violent deaths will offset medical/lifestyle gains, and those projections are too optimistic.

Sex differentials in mortality and health are likely to narrow over the next century, exchanging their twentieth century course for a very different one. The narrowing will come about by greater similarity between men and women in risk factors and psychosocial ones pertinent to health. Is it too much to anticipate that men will adopt more caretaking attitudes toward self and others, and more enthusiasm about regular medical contacts and preventive health behaviors? And that women will become increasingly engaged in renumerative and satisfying jobs, feel happier and less stressed, and pursue more strenuous leisure activities?[38] If these occur, the results will be improved physical well being, less disability, lower mortality—and smaller sex differences.

Some popular hypotheses must be felled: It is often claimed that women's mortality rates will *rise* to meet men's as they "behave more like men." This is unreasonable. More plausibly, one might assert that both sexes will continue to experience mortality declines, but women's may be slower than men's in coming decades. Even this is overly simplistic and ignores the extensive benefits women stand to accrue from fuller participation in productive and political roles. There is a general lesson here: Any forecast about future sex differentials must make some explicit assumptions about (a) how women and men change in personal behaviors and exposures, receipt of medical and rehabilitation advances, social attitudes about sickness and disability or even biological stamina; and (b) what the ensuing effects are on rates and the sex difference. Forecasts without assumptions should inspire doubt and be viewed as prophecy rather than science.

An Aging Society

At any time, the aggregate burden of illness and disability in a population depends on age-specific rates for each sex and the population distribution by age-sex. Simply put, it is a function of "rates times weights." So far in this article, we have discussed rates in the past, present, and future. Now we consider population dynamics; that is, the weights.

The U.S. population has aged considerably in the twentieth century. In 1900, 4.0 percent of the total population were ages 65+, and just 0.2 percent were ages 85+. In 1985, the figures were 12.0 and 1.1, respectively. This general aging is accompanied by two important features, called "aging-within-aging" and "feminization of the elderly." The 65+ group is itself aging, with increasing percents

among them being very old (85+). And the percent female is increasing in the 65+ group. Table 34-1 shows both of these features, comparing 1900 with 1980.

Aging has been a persistent feature of U.S. population dynamics throughout the century, fueled initially by secular declines in fertility rates and in recent decades by large mortality declines concentrated at older ages.[39] Aging-within-aging has been especially rapid in this recent period of mortality decline. Feminization of the elderly has been ongoing since the 1930's.

The twentieth century will stand out as the era in which the U.S. population aged. All of the above dynamics will continue into the twenty-first century but at a slower pace than before.[40] Table 34-1 shows current projections for 2040 and 2080, adjacent to figures for the twentieth century.

Table 34-1
Aging of the United States Population, 1900–2080.[a]

Aging	1900	1980	2040	2080
Percent of population ages 65+	4.0	11.3	21.1	22.1
Percent of population ages 85+	0.2	1.0	4.1	5.3
Aging Within Aging				
Among persons 65+, percent ages 85+	4.0	8.8	19.3	23.9
Feminization of the Elderly				
Among persons 65+, percent female	49.5	59.7	58.8	58.4
Among persons 85+, percent female	55.6	69.6	69.7	68.6

Source: For 1900: Cynthia M. Taeuber. America in Transition: An Aging Society. *Current Population Reports*, Series P–23, No. 128. Bureau of the Census, U.S. Department of Commerce. Washington, D.C. 1983; and Forrest E. Linder and Robert D. Grove. *Vital Statistics Rates in the United States*, 1900–1940. Bureau of the Census, U.S. Department of Commerce. Washington, D.C.: Government Printing Office. 1943. For 1980: Taeuber, America in Transition; and Jacob S. Siegel and Maria Davidson. "Demographic and Socioeconomic Aspects of Aging in the United States," *Current Population Reports*, Series P–23, No. 138. Bureau of the Census, U.S. Department of Commerce. Washington, D.C. 1984. For 2040 and 2080: John C. Wilkin. Social Security Area Population Projections, 1983. *Actuarial Study*, No. 88. SSA Publ. No. 11–11535. Office of the Actuary, Social Security Administration, Department of Health and Human Services. 1983.

a. Projected figures for 2040 and 2080, using Alternative II.

Increasing percents of old people, especially very old ones and women, will change both the volume and composition of population health over the long run. The shifting age distribution alone will push upward rates of illness, disability, and mortality for the whole population. (This is because weights will increase at the ages with highest rates.) Feminizing will augment the importance of chronic conditions that are symptomatic and disabling, but not themselves life-threatening, such as arthritis, osteoporosis, incontinence, varicose veins, and digestive disorders. Social and economic problems—loneliness, poverty, and feelings of helplessness and insecurity—will also ascend, often reflecting blunted opportunities and socialization for women in their earlier years. But if women use their "power of numbers," the views and attitudes expressed by very elderly people will be largely women's, and this can open political and social opportunities for those who were very dependent before. All of the changes just stated ensue directly from changes in age-sex composition of the population.

If age-specific rates change as well, as proposed in the prior section, then the needs for symptom relief, special aids, medical and rehabilitation services, home assistance, congregate housing, and nursing beds will rise dramatically for a number of decades, before the power of primary prevention acts to lower those rates.

Thus, the pronounced declines in mortality of the twentieth century, with their special relationship to secondary prevention and older ages, have both welcome and unwelcome consequences. They provide more years of life to individuals on average, but also increase the percent of ill older people. This pattern of events is not unique to the United States; it is a typical phase that developed societies will pass through at some point.

Individual and Societal Trajectories

Health and mortality statistics tell us a population's state of health at a calendar time. They say little about the dynamics of health actually experienced by individuals over their lives.

For individuals, health has many important dimensions besides simple presence or absence of a problem. First, there are movements "to and fro"—acute condition onsets and recoveries spread throughout a year, flares and remissions of chronic conditions, insidious development of dysfunction and welcome returns of function. Second, there is multiplicity to health problems. Chronic ailments tend to accrete over life, and dysfunctions also show a net increase, even though specific ones may vary from year to year. Lastly, there is synergism. Multiple conditions interact to hasten disability, and multiple disabilities interact to sap stamina and spirit. Health statistics have little to say about these three aspects of individual health. Yet they are perceived clearly by people and are fundamental components of physical well being and life quality.

For most people, chronic illnesses and death come in middle or older ages. Their timing and type are explained by risks extending over the individual's whole life, not just contemporary risks. People now 90 were born in the nineteenth century. People who will be 90 in 2040 are Baby Boomers, and everyone who will be 65+ in that year is already alive. Health attitudes, lifestyle behaviors, and stress responses are enduring features for individuals, and they are largely set in place in the first twenty to twenty-five years of one's life. Thus, states of health for individuals and society at any time bear immense, quiet imprints of personal and social history. The lags between risk factors and their health/mortality outcomes, and the accretion of risks over a lifetime into those outcomes, must always be recognized.

The pathways that women and men take differ somewhat: Women's lives are more filled with sickness and disability, due to greater tendencies to acquire nonfatal chronic problems plus lesser ones to acquire fatal problems. The longer average lifetimes earned by the second feature can be undone by the first. Men die sooner, having suffered fewer years of trouble while alive.

There is no "contradiction" whatsoever in females' higher morbidity rates and males' higher mortality rates, and the label should be abandoned. Those empirical facts emerge from differences in health pathways traced by the sexes; women tend to tarry, while men exit with undue swiftness. Exposures during life are the main reason for this, though biology also plays some part. Finding the causes of fatal diseases and ways to alleviate their progression will keep men with us longer. But it is just as important to find causes and controls for nonfatal diseases, so that women and men can in comfort and vigor tarry together.

Notes

1. For example, see Ashley Montagu, *The Natural Superiority of Women* (New York: Collier Books, 1978); David T. Purtilo and John L. Sullivan, "Immunological Bases for Superior Survival of Females," *American Journal of Diseases of Childhood* 133 (1979): 1251–53; Estelle R. Ramey and Peter Ramwell, "The Relationship of the Sex Hormone/ Prostaglandin Interaction to Female and Male Longevity," in *The Changing Risk of Disease in Women: An Epidemiologic Approach*, ed. E. B. Gold (Lexington, MA: D. C. Heath and Co., 1984), pp. 25–36.

2. John H. Dingle, George F. Badger, and William S. Jordan, *Illness in the Home* (Cleveland, OH: Case Western Reserve University Press, 1964); Mary Grace Kovar, "Health Status of U.S. Children and Use of Medical Care," *Public Health Reports* 97 (1982): 3–15; Lois M. Verbrugge, "Sex differentials in Health," *Public Health Reports* 97 *(1982): 17–37*.

3. See "Historical Perspectives on Women and Mental Illness" by Nancy Tomes.

4. This article will not review sex differences in health-services use and other preventive and therapeutic health behaviors. Many of the reviews cited herein have ample data and references on the topic.

5. By contrast, in sociology the terms "sex" and "gender" are used to suggest causes. Sex refers to features due solely to biology, and gender to features caused by an array of biological, social, and cultural factors.

6. Reviews and ample data on sex differentials in health are in Esther Hing, Mary Grace Kovar, and Dorothy P. Rice, "Sex Differences in Health and Use of Medical Care: United States, 1979." *Vital and Health Statistics*, series 3, no. 24. DHHS publ. no. (PHS) 83–1408. (Hyattsville, MD: National Center for Health Statistics, 1983); Con-

stance A. Nathanson, "Sex, Illness, and Medical Care: A Review of Data, Theory, and Method," *Social Science and Medicine* 11 (1977): 13–25; "Sex Roles as Variables in the Interpretation of Morbidity Data: A Methodological Critique," *International Journal of Epidemiology* 7 (1978): 253–62; Constance A. Nathanson and Gerda Lorenz, "Women and Health: The Social Dimensions of Biomedical Data," in *Women in the Middle Years*, ed. J. Z. Giele (New York: Wiley, 1982), pp. 37–87; Lois M. Verbrugge, "Sex Differentials in Morbidity and Mortality in the United States," *Social Biology* 23 (1976): 275–96; "Females and Illness: Recent Trends in Sex Differences in the United States," *Journal of Health and Social Behavior* 17 (1976): 387–403; "Sex Differentials in Health," *Public Health Reports* 97 (1982): 417–37; "Women and Men: Mortality and Health of Older People," in *Aging in Society: Selected Reviews of Recent Research*, eds. M. W. Riley, B. B. Hess, and K. Bond (Hillsdale, NJ: Lawrence Erlbaum ., 1983), pp. 139–174; "A Health Profile of Older Women with Comparisons to Older Men," *Research on Aging* 6 (1984): 291–322; "Gender and Health: An Update on Hypotheses and Evidence," *Journal of Health and Social Behavior* 26 (1985): 156–82; "From Sneezes to Adieus: Stages of Health for American Men and Women," in *Health in Aging: Sociological Issues and Policy Directions*, eds. R. A. Ward and S. B. Tobin (New York: Springer, 1987), pp. 17–57; "Gender, Aging, and Health," in *Aging and Health: Perspectives on Gender, Race, Ethnicity, and Class*, ed. K. S. Markides (Newbury Park, CA: Sage, 1989), pp. 23–78; Lois M. Verbrugge and Deborah L. Wingard, "Sex Differentials in Health and Mortality," *Women and Health* 12 (1987): 103–45; Ingrid Waldron, "An Analysis of Causes of Sex Differences in Mortality and Morbidity," in *The Fundamental Connection Between Nature and Nurture*, eds. W. R. Gove and G. R. Carpenter (Lexington, MA: D.C. Health and Co., 1982), pp. 69–115; "Sex Differences in Illness Incidence, Prognosis and Mortality: Issues and Evidence," *Social Science and Medicine* 17 (1983): 1107–23; Deborah L. Wingard, "The Sex Differential in Morbidity, Mortality, and Lifestyle," in *Annual Review of Public Health*, vol. 5, eds. L. Breslow, J. E. Fielding, and L. B. Lave (Palo Alto, CA: Annual Reviews, 1984): pp. 433–58.

7. Reviews and data on sex differentials in mortality, with emphasis on the United States, are in Eileen M. Crimmins, "The Changing Patterns of American Mortality Decline, 1940–77, and Its Implications for the Future," *Population and Development Review* (1981):229–54; "Life Ex-

pectancy and the Older Population," *Research on Aging* 6 (1984):490–514; Lois A. Fingerhut, "Changes in Mortality Among the Elderly, United States, 1978," *Vital and Health Statistics*, series 3, nos. 22 and 22a. DHHS publ. no. (PHS) 82–1406. 84–1406a. (Hyattsville, MD: National Center for Health Statistics, 1982, 1984); A. Joan Klebba, Jeffrey D. Maurer, and Evelyn J. Glass, "Mortality Trends: Age, Color, and Sex, United States, 1950–69." *Vital and Health Statistics*, series 20, no. 15. DHEW publ. no. (HRA) 74–1852. (Rockville, MD: National Center for Health Statistics, 1973); Metropolitan Life Insurance Co., "New High for Expectation of Life," *Statistical Bulletin* 68, no. 3 (1987): 8–14; "Women's Longevity Advantage Declines," *Statistical Bulletin* 69, no. 1 (1988): 18-23. Readers are encouraged to scan across years of the *Statistical Bulletin*, since it frequently presents data on health and mortality of U.S. women and men. Constance A. Nathanson, "Sex Differences in Mortality," in *Annual Review of Sociology*, vol. 10, eds. R. H. Turner and J. F. Short (Palo Alto, CA: Annual Reviews, 1984), pp. 191–213; S. Jay Olshansky and A. Brian Ault, "The Fourth Stage of the Epidemiologic Transition: The Age of Delayed Degenerative Diseases," *Millbank Memorial Fund Quarterly/Health and Society* 64 (1986): 355–91; Ira Rosenwaike, *The Extreme Aged in America* (Westport, CT: Greenwood Press, 1985); Lois M. Verbrugge, "Sex Differentials in Morbidity and Mortality in the United States"; Verbrugge, "Recent Trends in Sex Mortality Differentials in the United States," *Women and Health* 5 (1980): 17–37; Verbrugge and Wingard, "Sex Differentials in Health and Mortality"; Ingrid Waldron, "Why Do Women Live Longer Than Men?" *Social Science and Medicine* 10 (1976): 3,49–62.

8. General introductions to disability are in Joan C. Cornoni-Huntley et al., "Epidemiology of Disability in the Oldest Old: Methodologic Issues and Preliminary Findings," *Milbank Memorial Fund Quarterly/Health and Society* 63 (1985): 350–76; Lawrence D. Haber, "Disabling Effects of Chronic Disease and Impairment," *Journal of Chronic Diseases* 24 (1971): 469–87; Kenneth G. Manton and Beth J. Soldo, "Dynamics of Health Changes in the Oldest Old: New Perspectives and Evidence," *Milbank Memorial Fund Quarterly/Health and Society* 63 (1985): 206–85; Saad Z. Nagi, "An Epidemiology of Disability Among Adults in the United States," Milbank Memorial Fund Quarterly/ Health and Society 54 (1976): 439–67; World Health Organization, *International Classification of Impairments, Disabilities, and Handicaps* (Geneva, 1980). Readers are cau-

tioned that the terms used in disability research vary widely now and do not necessarily match the ones used in this selection.

9. Selected data on short-term disability are in Verbrugge, "Gender and Health." Readers who want to see the most recent disability rates should consult *Vital and Health Statistics*, series 10, annual issue on "Current Estimates From the National Health Interview Survey, United States" for a given year.

10. Data on physical disability by sex are in Daniel J. Foley et al., "Physical Functioning," in *Established Populations for Epidemiologic Studies of the Elderly: Resource Data Book*, ed. J. Cornoni-Huntley et al., NIH publ. no. 86–2443. (Bethesda, MD: National Institute on Aging, 1986), pp. 56–94; Lawrence D. Haber, "Disabling Effects of Chronic Disease and Impairment 11. Functional Capacity limitations," *Journal of Chronic Diseases* 26 (1973): 127–51 (data are for work-disabled people); Alan M. Jette and Laurence G. Branch, "The Framingham Disability Study: II. Physical Disability Among the Aging," *American Journal of Public Health* 71 (1981): 1211–16; Alan M. Jette and Laurence G. Branch, "Musculoskeletal Impairment Among the Noninstitutionalized Aged," *International Rehabilitation Medicine* 6 (1984): 157–61.

11. Summary data are in Verbrugge, "Gender and Health," and Verbrugge, "Gender, Aging, and Health." See also Mitchell P. LaPlante, *Data on Disability from National Health Interview Survey, 1983–85.* (Washington, D.C.: National Institute on Disability and Rehabilitation Research, U.S. Department of Education, 1988); Nagi, "An Epidemiology of Disability."

12. The concept of basic activities of daily living (personal care) is discussed in Sidney Katz and C. Amechi Akpom, "A Measure of Primary Sociobiological Functions," *International Journal of Health Services* 6 (1976): 493–507; and of instrumental activities of daily living (household management) in M. Powell Lawton and Elaine M. Brody, "Assessment of Older People: Self-Maintaining and Instrumental Activities of Daily Living," *The Gerontologists* 9 (1969): 179–86. Data on difficulty and dependency for these tasks are in Deborah Dawson, Hendershot, and John Fulton, "Aging in the Eighties: Functional Limitations of Individuals Age 65 Years and Over," *Advance Data*, no. 133. (Hyattsville, MD: National Center for Health Statistics, 1987); Barbara A. Feller, "Americans Needing Help to Function at Home," *Advance Data*, no. 92 (Hyattsville, MD: National Center for Health Statistics,

1983); Jette and Branch, "Framingham Disability Study"; Candace L. Macken, "A Profile of Functionally Impaired Elderly Persons Living in the Community," *Health Care Financing Review* 7 (1986): 33–49; Ethel Shanas, "Health and Incapacity in Later Life," in *Older People in Three Industries*, ed. E. Shanas et al. *(New York: Atherton Press, 1968).*

13. National data come from the National Nursing Home Survey (National Center for Health Statistics) and the decennial population census (U.S. Bureau of the Census). For the first, see Esther Hing, Edward Sekscenski, and Genevieve Strahan, "The National Nursing Home Survey: 1985 Summary for the United States." *Vital and Health Statistics*, series 13, no. 97. DHHS publ. no. (PHS) 89-1758. (Hyattsville, MD: National Center for Health Statistics, 1989); Esther Hing and Beulah K. Cypress, "Use of Health Services by Women 65 Years of Age and Over, United States, 1979." *Vital and Health Statistics*, series 13, no. 59. DHHS publ. no. (PHS) 81-1720. (Hyattsville, MD: National Center for Health Statistics, 1981). Data for the 1985 NNHS are forthcoming in issues of Series 13. For census data, see the special volume published on institutional residents subsequent to each census.

14. Note the decline from middle to advanced ages. The sex-mortality ratio follows a curvilinear pattern across age, with lowest values at the beginning and end of life, and highest values at ages 15–24. Data for 1985 are from *Monthly Vital Statistics Report*, vol. 36, no. 5, Supplement (Hyattsville, MD: National Center for Health Statistics, 1987), and *Vital Statistics of the United States*, 1985, vol. 2, part A (Hyattsville, MD: National Center for Health Statistics). Annual mortality statistics can be found in these two publications (the first for advance data, the second for detailed final data).

15. Life expectancy condenses age-specific mortality rates of a given year. It serves as a forecast of the average number of years remaining for individuals at an index age, x, assuming they experience the current rates. If rates actually change as they age, the forecast will be surpassed (mortality rates fall) or not achieved (mortality rates rise).

16. Life-table data for 1985 are from *Vital Statistics of the United States, 1985, Life Tables, volume 2, section 6.* DHHS publ. no. (PHS) 88-1104. (Hyattsville, MD. National Center for Health Statistics, 1988).

17. These titles are in rank order (1–6,8–10) by total number of deaths in the U.S., 1985. Diabetes (rank 7) is an anomaly; it has virtually equal rates for males and females since the 1970's. For most of the century, female rates were slightly higher.

18. See tables in Verbrugge, "Gender, Aging, and Health."

19. Reasons for sex differences in mortality are discussed in Marshall J. Graney, "An Exploration of Social Factors Influencing the Sex Differential in Mortality," *Sociological Symposium* 28 (1979): 1–26; William R. Hazzard, "The Sex Differential in Longevity," in *Principles of Geriatric Medicine*, eds. R. Andres, E. L. Bierman, and W. R. Hazzard (New York: McGraw Hill, (1984), pp. 72–81; G. Herdan, "Causes of Excess Male Mortality in Man," *Acta Genetica et Statistica Medica* (now called *Human Heredity*) 3 (1952): 351–76; Constance Holden, "Why Do Women Live Longer Than Men?", *Science* (October 9, 1987): 158–60; Alan D. Lopez and Lado T. Ruzicka, eds., *Sex Differentials in Mortality: Trends, Determinants, and Consequences*. Miscellaneous series, no. 4. (Canberra, Australia: Department of Demography, Australian National University, 1983) (the book contains Proceedings of a WHO conference on sex differentials in mortality); Francis C. Madigan, "Are Sex Mortality Differentials Biologically Caused?" *Milbank Memorial Fund Quarterly* 35 (1957): 202–23; Nathanson, "Sex Differences in Mortality"; Verbrugge, "Sex Differentials in Morbidity and Mortality in the United States"; Verbrugge and Wingard, "Sex Differentials in Health and Mortality"; Waldron, "Why Do Women Live Longer Than Men?"; Waldron, "An Analysis of Causes of Sex Differences"; Ingrid Waldron, "Sex Differences in Human Mortality: The Role of Genetic Factors," *Social Science and Medicine* 17 (1983): 321–33; "What Do We Know About Causes of Sex Differences in Mortality? A Review of the Literature," *Population Bulletin of the United Nations* 18 (1986): 59–76; "The Contribution of Smoking to Sex Differences in Mortality," *Public Health Reports* 101 (1986): 163–73.

20. For explanations of sex differences in health, readers are referred especially to David Mechanic, "Sex, Illness, Illness Behavior, and the Use of Health Services," *Social Science and Medicine* 12B (1 976): 207–14; Constance A. Nathanson, "Illness and the Feminine Role: A Theoretical Review," *Social Science and Medicine* 9 (1975): 57–62; Nathanson, "Sex, Illness, and Medical Care: A Review"; Verbrugge, "Females and Illness: Recent Trends"; Lois M. Verbrugge, "Female Illness Rates and Illness Behavior: Testing Hypotheses About Sex Differ-

ences in Health," *Women and Health* 4 (1979): 61–79; Verbrugge, "Gender and Health." The last reference is a comprehensive review of hypotheses and research evidence.

21. The same ranking of factors can explain women's more frequent use of health services.

22. For the epidemiologic transition, see Abdel R. Omran, "The Epidemiologic Transition: A Theory of the Epidemiology of Population Change," *Milbank Memorial Fund Quarterly* 49 (1971): 509–38; "Epidemiologic Transition in the United States," *Population Bulletin* 32, no. 2, 1977 (Washington, D.C.: Population Reference Bureau). For mortality trends, see references at the beginning of the Contemporary Health Profiles section; and Jacob A. Brody, Dwight B. Brock, and T. Franklin Williams, "Trends in the Health of the Elderly Population," in *Annual Review* of *Public Health*, vol. 8, eds. L. Breslow, J. E. Fielding, and L. B. Lave (Palo Alto, CA: Annual Reviews, 1987), pp. 211–34; Monroe Lerner and Odin W. Anderson, *Health Progress in the United States* (Chicago: The University of Chicago Press, 1963).

23. For sex-mortality ratio, 1900: Metropolitan Life Insurance Co., *Statistical Bulletin*, 1980, 61 no. 2, 1985: *Monthly Vital Statistics Report, 1987*, 1987, 36 no. 5, supplement (Hyattsville, MD: National Center for Health Statistics). For expectation of life, 1900–1985: Joseph F. Faber and Alice H. Wade, "Life Tables for the United States: 1900–2050," *Actuarial Study* no. 89. SSA publ. no. 11–11536 (Washington, D.C.: Office of the Actuary, Social Security Administration).

24. Trends in the sex-mortality differential in the twentieth century are examined in Philip E. Enterline, "Causes of Death Responsible for Recent Increases in Sex Mortality Differentials in the United States," *Milbank Memorial Fund Quarterly* 39 (1961): 312–28; Ellen M. Gee and Jean E. Veevers, "Accelerating Sex Differentials in Mortality: An Analysis of Contributing Factors," *Social Biology* 30 (1983): 75–85; Allan Johnson, "Recent Trends in Sex Mortality Differentials in the United States," *Journal of Human Stress* 3 (1977): 22–32; S. L. N. Rao, "On Long-Term Mortality Trends in the United States, 1850–1968," *Demography* 10 (1973): 405–19; Robert R. Retherford, "Tobacco Smoking and the Sex Mortality Differential," *Demography* 9 (1972): 203–16; Retherford, *The Changing Sex Differential in Mortality* (Westport, CT: Greenwood Press, 1975); Verbrugge, "Recent Trends in Sex Mortality Differentials." Earlier studies on sex-mortality differentials that permit an historical perspective are in Antonio Ciocco, "Sex Differences in Morbidity and Mortality," *Quarterly Review of Biology* 15 (1940): 59–73, 192–210; L. I. Dublin, A. J. Lotka, and M. Spiegelman, *Length of Life* (New York: Ronald Press, 1949); Wilson T. Sowder, "Why is the Sex Difference in Mortality Increasing?," *Public Health* 69 (1954): 860–64; Wilson T. Sowder and James O. Bond, "Problems Associated With the Increasing Ratio of Male Over Female Mortality," *Journal of the American Geriatrics Society* 4 (1956): 956–62; George J. Stolnitz, "A Century of International Mortality Trends: II," *Population Studies* 10 (1956): 17–42; Dorothy G. Wiehl, "Sex Differences in Mortality in the United States," *Milbank Memorial Fund Quarterly* 16 (1938): 145–55. Global (multi-national) analyses of patterns in sex-mortality differentials are in Alan D. Lopez, "The Sex Mortality Differential in Developed Countries," in *Sex Differentials in Mortality*, eds. Lopez and Ruzicka, pp. 53–120; Samuel H. Preston, "Older Male Mortality and Cigarette Smoking—A Demographic Analysis." *Population Monograph* no. 7 (Berkeley: Institute of International Studies, University of California, 1970); "An International Comparison of Excessive Adult Mortality," *Population Studies* 24 (1970): 5–20; *Mortality Patterns in National Populations* (New York: Academic Press, 1976), chapter 6; Samuel H. Preston and James A. Weed, "Causes of Death Responsible for International and Intertemporal Variation in Sex Mortality Differentials," *World Health Statistics Report* 29 (1976): 144–214.

25. First noted in Verbrugge, "Recent Trends in Sex Mortality Differentials." Since then, various issues of the *Statistical Bulletin* (Metropolitan Life Insurance Co.) have reported on the new situation.

26. With regard to the second point: A disadvantaged group typically gains more in the presence of medical and social improvements. Their higher rates drop farther in absolute and often relative terms compared to the advantaged group (in this instance, women).

27. For discussions of women's roles and health, Debra Froberg, Dwenda Gjerdingen, and Marilyn Preston, "Multiple Roles and Women's Mental and Physical Health: What Have We Learned?," *Women and Health* 11 (1986): 79–96; Mary Ann Haw, "Women, Work, and Stress: A Review and Agenda for the Future," *Journal of Health and Social Behavior* 23 (1982): 132–44; Glorian Sorenson and Lois M. Verbrugge, "Women, Work, and Health," in *Annual Review of Public Health*, vol. 8, eds. L. Breslow, J. E. Fielding, and L. B. Lave (Palo Alto, CA: Annual Reviews, 1987), pp. 235–51;

Lois M. Verbrugge and Jennifer H. Madans, "Social Roles and Health Trends of American Women," *Milbank Memorial Fund Quarterly/Health and Society* 63 (1985): 691–735. All three articles have extensive reference lists.

28. For descriptions of these surveys, see Selwyn D. Collins, "Sickness Surveys," in *Administrative Medicine*, ed. H. Emerson (New York: Nelson, 1951). pp. 511–35; Commission on Chronic Illness, *Chronic Illness in a Large City: The Baltimore Study*, vol. 4 of *Chronic Illness in the United States* (Cambridge, MA: Harvard University Press, 1957), chapter 1; Mortimer Spiegelman, *Introduction to Demography* (Chicago, IL: The Society of Actuaries, 1955); Kenneth R. Wilcox, *Comparison of Three Methods for the Collection of Morbidity Data by Household Survey*, Ph.D. dissertation (Ann Arbor, MI: Department of Epidemiology, School of Public Health, 1963), Chapter 1. Besides such broad health surveys, well-known community-based studies for special topics are discussed in 1.1. Kessler and M.L. Levin, eds., *The Community as an Epidemiologic Laboratory* (Baltimore: Johns Hopkins University Press, 1970). Other community-based studies have been started since then, especially under the aegis of the National Institute on Aging and the National Institute of Mental Health.

29. Ciocco, "Sex Differences in Morbidity and Mortality;" Selwyn D. Collins, "Cases and Days of Illness Among Males and Females, with Special Reference to Confinement to Bed," *Public Health Reports* 55 (1940): 47–94; "A Review and Study of Illness and Medical Care." *Public Health Monograph* no. 48. PHS publ. no. 544. (Washington, D.C.: Public Health Service, 1957); Selwyn D. Collins, Katharine S. Trantham, and Josephine L. Lehmann, "Sickness Experience in Selected Areas of the United States." *Public Health Monograph* no. 25. (Washington, D.C.: Public Health Service, 1955); Commission on Chronic Illness, *Chronic Illness in a Rural Area: The Hunterdon Study*, vol. 3 of *Chronic Illness in the United States* (Cambridge, MA: Harvard University Press, 1959); Commission on Chronic Illness, *Chronic Illness in a Large City* (cited above); David E. Hailman, "The Prevalence of Disabling Illness Among Male and Female Workers and Housewives." *Public Health Bulletin* no. 260. (Washington, D.C.: Public Health Service, 1941); Lemer and Anderson, *Health Progress in the United States*, Chapter 10; Milbank Memorial Fund, *Morbidity Survey in Baltimore, 1938–1943*. (New York: Milbank Memorial Fund, 1957), see esp. chapters by Collins,

Phillips, and Oliver; Downes; Downes and Keller; Jackson, "Morbidity Among Males, and Females"; Jackson, "Duration of Disabling Acute Illness"; Sally Preas and Ruth Phillips, "The Severity of Illness Among Males and Females," *Millbank Memorial Fund Quarterly* 20 (1942): 221–44; Edgar Sydenstricker, "The Illness Rate Among Males and Females," *Public Health Reports* 42, (1927): 1939–57; "Sex Differences in the Incidence of Certain Diseases at Different Ages," *Public Health Reports* 43 (1928): 1259–76.

30. Changes were made in 1967–68 and 1982. See National Center for Health Statistics, Health Interview Survey Procedure, 1957–1974. *Vital and Health Statistics*, series 1, no. 11. DHEW publ. no. (HRA) 75–1311. (Rockville, MD: 1975); The National Health Interview Survey Design, 1973–1984, and Procedures, 1975–83. *Vital and Health Statistics*, series 1, no. 18. DHHS publ. no. (PHS) 85–1320. (Hyattsville, MD: 1985).

31. Trends toward worsening health are also reported for children in Paul W. Newacheck, Peter P. Budetti, and Neal Halfon, "Trends in Activity-Limiting Chronic Conditions Among Children," *American Journal of Public Health* 76 (1986): 178–84; Paul W. Newacheck, Peter P. Budetti, and Peggy McManus, "Trends in Childhood Disability," *American Journal of Public Health* 74 (1984): 232–36.

32. Comprehensive reviews of research on recent health trends are in Steven H. Chapman, Mitchell P. LaPlante, and Gail R. Wilensky, "Life Expectancy and Health Status of the Aged," *Social Security Bulletin* 49, no. 10 (1986): 24–48; Lois M. Verbrugge, "Recent, Present, and Future Health of American Adults," in *Annual Review of Public Health*, vol. 10, eds. L. Breslow, J. E. Fielding, and L.B. Lave (Palo Alto, CA: Annual Reviews, 1989), pp. 333–61. Reasons for worsening population health are discussed in Jacob A. Brody, "Prospects for an Ageing Population," *Nature* 315 (1985): 463–66; Chapman, LaPlante, and Wilensky, "Life Expectancy and Health Status"; Alain Colvez and Madeleine Blanchet, "Disability Trends in the United States Population 1966–76: Analysis of Reported Causes," *American Journal of Public Health* 71 (1981): 464–71; Jacob J. Feldman, "Work Ability of the Aged Under Conditions of Improving Mortality," *Milbank Memorial Fund Quarterly/Health and Society* 61 (1983): 430–44; Dorothy P. Rice and Mitchell P. LaPlante, "Chronic Illness, Disability, and Increasing Longevity," in *Ethics and Economics of Long-Term Care*, eds. S. Sul-

livan and M. Ein Lewin (Washington, D.C.: American Enterprise Institute, 1988); Edward L. Schneider and Jacob A. Brody, "Aging, Natural Death, and the Compression of Morbidity: Another View," *New England Journal of Medicine* 309 (1983): 854–56; Lois M. Verbrugge, "Longer Life But Worsening Health? Trends in Health and Mortality of Middle-Aged and Older Adults," *Milbank Memorial Fund Quarterly/Health and Society* 62 (1984): 475–519; Verbrugge, "Recent, Present, and Future Health"; Martynas A. Yeas, "Recent Trends in Health Near the Age of Retirement: New Findings from the Health Interview Survey," *Social Security Bulletin* 50, no. 2 (1987): 5–30.

33. For a contrasting view, see Ronald W. Wilson and Thomas F. Drury, "Interpreting Trends in Illness and Disability: Health Statistics and Health Status," in *Annual Review of Public Health*, vol. 5, eds. L. Breslow, J. E. Fielding, and L. B. Lave (Palo Alto, CA: Annual Reviews, 1984), pp. 83–106.

34. Verbrugge, "Females and Illness: Recent Trends."

35. Kenneth G. Manton, "Changing Concepts of Morbidity and Mortality in the Elderly Population," *Milbank Memorial Fund Quarterly/Health and Society* 60 (1982):183–244; "Past and Future Life Expectancy Increases at Later Ages: Their implications for the Linkage of Chronic Morbidity, Disability. and Mortality," *Journal of Gerontology* 41 (1986): 672–81; Verbrugge, "Recent, Present, and Future Health."

36. This notion is called the "compression of morbidity"; it assumes both complete disease prevention and a fixed upper limit to average life expectation for humans. See James F. Fries, "Aging, Natural Death, and the Compression of Morbidity," *New England Journal of Medicine* 303 (1980): 130–35; "The Compression of Morbidity," *Milbank Memorial Fund Quarterly/Health and Society* 61 (1983): 397–419.

37. Joseph F. Faber and Alice H. Wade, Life Tables for United States: 1900–2050. *Actuarial Study*, no. 89. SSA publ. no. 11–11536. (Washington, D.C.: Office of the Actuary, Social Security Administration: 1983).

38. For viewpoints about forthcoming change in sex differentials, see Michel A. Ibrahim, "The Changing Health State of Women," *American Journal of Public Health* 70 (1980): 120–21; Charles E. Lewis and Mary Ann Lewis, "The Potential Impact of Sexual Equality on Health," *New England Journal of Medicine* 297 (1977): 863–69; Constance A. Nathanson and Alan D. Lopez, "The Future of Sex Mortality Differentials in Industrialized Countries: A Structural Hypothesis," *Population Research and Policy Review*, 6 (1987): 123–36, Lois M. Verbrugge, "Unveiling Higher Morbidity for Men: The Story," in *Social Structures and Human Lives*, vol. I of *Social Change and the Life Course*, ed. M. W. Riley (Newbury Park, CA: Sage Pub., 1988), pp. 138–60.

39. Eileen M. Crimmins, "The Changing Pattern of American Mortality Decline"; Ira Rosenwaike, "A Demographic Portrait of the Oldest Old,"*Milbank Memorial Fund Quarterly* 63 (1985): 187–205; Rosenwaike, *The Extreme Aged in America* (Westport, CT: Greenwood Press, 1985); Jacob S. Siegel and Maria Davidson, "Demographic and Socioeconomic Aspects of Aging in the United States," *Current Population Reports*, series P–23, no. 138. (Washington, D.C.: Bureau of the Census, 1984); Beth J. Soldo, "America's Elderly in the 1980s," *Population Bulletin*, vol. 35, no. 4. (Washington, D.C.: Population Reference Bureau, 1980); Cynthia M. Taeuber, "America in Transition: An Aging Society." *Current Population Reports*, series P–23, no. 138. (Washington, D.C: Bureau of the Census, 1983); Barbara Boyle Torrey, Kevin Kinsella, and Cynthia M. Taeuber, "An Aging World," *International Population Reports*, series P–95, no. 78. (Washington, D.C.: Bureau of the Census, 1987); Paul E. Zopf, Jr., *America's Older Population* (Houston, TX: Cap and Gown Press, 1986).

40. When the Baby Boom cohort born between 1946 and 1959 reaches older ages, there will be some added propulsion to aging. But this will occur in a general context of slowed aging.

Further Reading

Ason, Ofra, Sara Carmel, and Mordechai Levin. 1991. "Gender Differences in the Utilization of Emergency Department Services." *Women and Health*. 17: 91–104.

Charlotte F. Muller. 1990. *Health Care and Gender*. New York: Russell Sage Foundation.

Sheryl B. Ruzek, Virginia L. Olesen, and Adele E. Clarke. 1997. *Women's Health: Complexities and Differences*. Columbus, OH: Ohio State University Press.

Richard M. Steingart. 1991. "Sex Differences in the Management of Coronary Artery Disease." *New England Journal of Medicine*. 325: 226–230.

Ingrid Waldron. 1994. "What Do We Know About the Causes of Sex Differences in Mortality? A Review of the Literature." In *The Sociology of Health and Illness: Critical Perspectives*, P. Conrad and R. Kern (eds.). New York: St. Martin's Press, pp. 42–54.

Discussion Questions

1. Lois Verbrugge notes that women use health services more than men. Why do you think this is the case?

2. What kinds of implications do Verbrugge's findings have for (re)structuring health services in the United States?

3. What benefits does the specific study of gender and health have for women? For men? For the health of the entire U.S. population?

From *Women, Health, and Medicine in America.* Pp. 41-79. Copyright © 1990 by Garland Publishing. Reprinted by permission. ✦

35

Latina and African American Women: Continuing Disparities in Health

Marsha Lillie-Blanton
Rose Marie Martinez
Andrea Kidd Taylor
Betty Garman Robinson

These authors examine disparities in health based on race, gender, and social class experiences. Like previous authors in this section, Lillie-Blanton and her co-authors claim that race, gender, and social class experiences cannot be disentangled from health and illness outcomes. With reference to a variety of large data sets, they locate health and illness within socio-cultural experience of group membership. These authors show that minority women are more likely than nonminority women to face circumstances that put them at risk for illness and injury. Environmental and occupational factors, access to health services, self-perceived health, and lifestyle all contribute to disparities in health and illness between nonminority and minority women.

Because little is known about the complex disparities in health and illness between nonminority and minority women, not much has been done in the way of medical intervention or health services provision. Based on what you discovered as you read this selection and
as you think about previous ones, think about the most effective intervention strategies to bridge the gap Lillie-Blanton and her co-authors report. What kinds of interventions would you devise? What sorts of health services would you offer? Which points would you investigate further? Keep your answers to these questions in mind as you read through the section on the future of health and illness.

Race and gender are powerful determinants of life experiences in the United States. A legacy of racial discrimination and segregation continues to affect the quality of life of U.S. racial and ethnic minority populations. Similarly, discrimination based on gender has affected the life experiences of women. As members of both population subgroups, Latina and African American women have encountered discrimination based on their gender and race. Blatant and subtle barriers have affected minority women's access to educational and employment opportunities. Moreover, racism affects where individuals live and the quality of resources available within those neighborhoods. Both gender and race have historically triggered social relations (i.e., in the family and work environment) that are risk factors for diminished health.

Social class stratification in the United States also shapes the life experiences of women of color. Social class status, sometimes referred to as socioeconomic status (SES), is generally measured by an individual's family resources and/or the occupation and educational attainment of the head of household (1). These indices, however, are affected by discriminatory policies and practices that persist despite legislation and judicial decisions prohibiting discrimination based on race and gender. Thus, social class status is socially determined and inseparably linked to this nation's history of social inequalities. As such, the burden of illness and injury facing minority women reflects the common life experiences they share as a consequence of their race, gender, and social class.

Women represent about half of the 30.8 million African Americans and 21.4 million Latino Americans identified in the 1990 Census. Although stereotypically portrayed by contrasting profiles, Latina and African American women represent a diversity of socioeconomic and psychosocial backgrounds. For example, African American women often are described as disproportionately poor, single heads of household who are dependent on public welfare programs such as AFDC (Aid to Families with Dependent Children). The profile is one of women who are irresponsible and a financial burden on society. In contrast, there is an abundance of research—some disputed—on the "black matriarchy" (2). Sociologists have portrayed African American women as the "rocks of Gibraltar" who provide the stabilizing and nurturing foundation for the black family (3,4). Latina women are often characterized as submissive, self-denying, and self-sacrificing (5). Within the family environment, the profile is one of women who place the needs of children and husband first and ask little for themselves in return. Their submissiveness and self-denial are said to contribute to their general lack of power and influence within American society.

As with most women, Latina and African American women have had what paradoxically could be considered both the good fortune and ill-fortune of being the primary caretaker of the family's children and elderly. While caretaking roles expand the depth of compassion women feel for others, they also compromise women's ability to compete in a rapidly evolving market economy. While there is substantial evidence for their portrayal as pillars of strength, the health consequences of being a primary caretaker in a frequently hostile social environment deserve investigation.

The meaning of racial/ethnic classifications is a subject of intense debate and controversy. In U.S. census and survey data, respondents are generally asked to report their racial group as: white; black; Asian or Pacific Islander; Aleut, Eskimo, American Indian; or other. In another question, information about Hispanic national origin is asked and persons of Hispanic origin may be of any of the racial categories. When individuals have an opportunity to self-define their race, a small but sizable percentage report their race as "other" rather than one of the four major racial groups. We recognize that these categories oversimplify race/ethnic origin, but they are the social designations used for U.S. census and survey purposes.

Racial/ethnic classifications denote group membership in which there is some assumed commonality of inheritance and contemporary life experiences. Nonetheless, women classified by U.S. census or survey data as of Hispanic origin are a tremendously heterogeneous group ethnically, consisting primarily of individuals with Mexican, Puerto Rican, Cuban, and South and Central American ancestry. These ethnic groups share a common bond of language and culture, but there are major subgroup differences in terms of their inclusion in society and access to resources. African American women are a more homogeneous group but are also ethnically diverse, including individuals with African, Caribbean, Indian, and European ancestry. Latina and African American women, as evidenced by their varying shades of color, have experienced considerable cross-generational mixing of racial/ethnic groups. As a consequence, racial/ethnic classifications are more a measure of the sociocultural experience of being a member of a particular racial/ethnic group than a marker of biological inheritance. Although a number of biological explanations for racial differences in health have been advanced, there is little scientific evidence to support these theories (6,7).

Scope of the Investigation

In an effort to assess the quality of life experienced by Latina and African American women, this selection provides descriptive information on racial/ethnic differences in women's social conditions, health status, exposure to occupational and environmental risks, and use of health services. We examine indices of the quality of life using a framework that considers life experiences associated with being female, a racial/ethnic minority, and a member of a particular social class. This assessment attempts to address some of the limitations of past research but, at most, represents an initial exploration into an issue that deserves more in-depth review.

Framework for the Study of Minority Women's Health

Several articles assisted us in establishing a framework for examining the health of minority women (8–10). Zambrana (8) provides a thoughtful and poignant critique of the research on the health of minority women, noting that even authors sensitive to women's issues have failed to address social class and racial/ethnic differences among women. She proposes a conceptual model for studying the health of minority women that considers health status as an interactive relationship among socioeconomic, behavioral, and environmental factors. Focusing on reproductive health issues, Zambrana applies this conceptual model while illustrating the limitations of existing research. Asserting that adolescent sexuality and childbearing are influenced by sociocultural background and SES, Zambrana also sees their consequences for the mother's education and employment opportunities and the child's health. In reviewing data on pregnancy outcomes, she notes that Mexican American women have high childbirth mortality rates and African American women have high rates of low birthweight infants. Zambrana advances the premise that poorer outcomes are due to differences in use of prenatal care, social class, and psychosocial factors such as chronic stress and social support.

Bennett (9) and Bassett and Krieger (10) have examined minority women's health from a perspective that acknowledges the impact of social class on health. Bennett explores the premise that life stressors associated with poverty are risk factors for emotional distress and even mental illness. The relation between social class and mental health has been well documented (11); research, however, is limited regarding the impact of race, gender, and SES on mental health (12, 13). Bennett asserts that social strata are not necessarily comparable across racial/ethnic groups because who is considered poor is relative, depending on the wealth among one's peers. Using clinical case studies, Bennett describes some of the economic circumstances of African American single women that potentially exacerbate life stressors associated with loneliness or parenting.

The author argues that, depending on a woman's problem-solving skills, poor resolution of problems could lead to diagnosable emotional distress. Bassett and Krieger (10) examine the impact of race and social class on breast cancer survival in a population-based sample. After adjusting for social class, in addition to age and other medical predictors of survival, the authors found that black-white differences in breast cancer survival rates diminished greatly. The results provide strong evidence that racial differences in today's breast cancer survival rates are largely attributable to the poorer social class standing of black women.

Data Sources and Key Measures

Data on health indices of minority women are presented from a number of sources, including the 1990 U.S. Census, the National Health and Nutrition Examination Survey II (NHANES; 1976–1980), and the Hispanic Health and Nutrition Examination Study (HHANES, 1982–1984). We also analyze and present original data on women aged 18 to 64 from the 1988 Health Interview Survey (HIS).

When possible, this selection presents data on mutually exclusive racial/ethnic categories. In most of the analyses, women are classified as white American, not of Hispanic origin; African American, not of Hispanic origin; or Latina.[1] Although these categories inadequately capture the racial/ethnic diversity within a population subgroup, they are used to yield a more accurate comparison of the indices of racial/ethnic minority women with those of nonminority women. Since most Latinos are classified racially as white (in the 1990 census, 96 percent of the 21.4 million persons of Hispanic origin are identified as white), analyses in which they are not examined as a distinct population group could diminish the magnitude of the race/ethnicity differentials.

Additionally, health and access indices from the HIS are stratified by family income categories of: below $10,000; $10,000 to $19,999; $20,000 to $34,999; and $35,000 and above. Stratifying by income is intended to limit the confounding effects of social class on the comparison of racial differences and also to gain some insight into the impact of income differences on the health indices of racial/ethnic minority women. When racial differences in health are presented, questions inevitably arise about the extent to which disparities can be attributed to racial differences in poverty, or more broadly, to differences in social class. Despite the imprecision of family income as a measure of social class, we considered it the best of the readily available indicators.

Social Conditions of Latina and African American Women

Social environmental conditions are recognized as one of several determinants of a population's health. The term "social condition" is used to refer to socio-demographic factors (e.g., employment) and to physical surroundings (e.g., neighborhood of residence). Factors such as these, individually and in combination with more personal factors, are determinants of health status. Employment, for example, is not only a source of income, it is often important to an individual's sense of self-worth and is a potential source of life stress. Additionally, it is the means by which most Americans obtain health insurance. Social conditions also affect other determinants of health such as physiological factors, lifestyle behaviors, and access to and use of health services.

For racial/ethnic minority women, the social environment has undergone tremendous change during the last three decades (1960s through 1980s). Progress has been achieved in legally and socially challenging traditional male-female gender roles. Minority women have benefited from policies that foster greater inclusion of women in all sectors of society. Enforcement of antidiscrimination laws helped to assure minority women greater equity in access to educational and employment opportunities. Nonetheless, data on indicators of life conditions continue to suggest that minority women encounter barriers that prevent full participation in the opportunities available in society.

Income, Poverty, and Family Structure

A disproportionate share of racial/ethnic minority women face circumstances of low-wage jobs and/or poverty. After a sharp decline in poverty rates between 1960 and 1970, the percentage of the population with incomes below the federal poverty level has remained relatively unchanged in the last two decades.[2] In 1990, about three times as many African Americans (32 percent) and Latino Americans (28 percent) as white Americans (11 percent, including whites of Hispanic origin), had family incomes below poverty (14). (The rate for whites not of Hispanic origin was 8.8 percent). While the poverty rate is similar for Latino and African Americans, families headed by women represent 75 percent of all poor African American families, as compared with 46 percent of all poor Latino families.

Family composition has major implications for the economic resources and social support available to a family. Nearly one-third (31 percent) of African American and 19 percent of Latino American families were headed by women in 1990. In contrast, only 9 percent of white American families were headed by women. About half of Latino and African American families headed by women had incomes below poverty. High rates of poverty among minority populations have been attributed to the shift in the number of families with a female head of household.[3] However, the National Research Council's report on the Status of Black Americans (16) found that if family structure in 1984 were the same as in 1973, the percentage of children and/or persons in poverty would have changed only modestly. The report concluded that the decline in wages, not an increase in female-headed households, accounts for persistently high poverty rates.

Median income, another measure of a person's economic condition, shows continuing disparity between men and women, as well as racial/ethnic differences among women. Despite greater opportunities, the 1988 median income for households headed by women barely approached two-thirds of the median income for households headed by men. For Latina and African American families headed by women, the median income was slightly more than half that reported for white American families headed by women. Findings are somewhat better for single women (i.e., nonfamily households headed by women), with median incomes for African American and Latina American women being about three-quarters of the income for white American women. Thus, even with considerable growth in employment opportunities, the earnings of women of color are still lower than those of whites.

The increasing number of African American families headed by women is a recurring subject of policy debate. A number of factors, such as increasing rates of divorce and separation among all racial/ethnic groups, contribute to the rise in families headed by women; however, the small and declining pool of marriageable black males is one factor that cannot be overlooked. In 1989, the ratio of males to females aged 25 to 44 years was 87 per 100 for blacks, compared with 101 and 107 per 100 for whites and Latinos, respectively (17). These statistics reflect, in part, the high rates of incarceration and premature mortality among young African American males.[4] The difficulties facing minority males are directly linked to the options and resources of minority families.

Demographic and Housing Patterns

Racial and ethnic minority populations are primarily concentrated in densely populated large urban areas. In 1988, over half (57 percent) of African Americans resided in central cities of metropolitan areas, compared with 27 percent of whites. Similarly, 90 percent of Latinos reside in urban areas, with the largest concentration living in four cities: New York, Los Angeles, Chicago, and San Antonio. African Americans and white Americans live primarily in racially segregated neighborhoods. Using an index in which 100 means a racially homogenous neighborhood, Jaynes and Williams (16) found that although residential segregation declined during the 1970s, the average index for black-white neighborhoods in 1980 was about 80 points. Indices for Latino and Asian American neighborhoods, however, averaged about 45 points. It is likely that the impact of residential segregation varies depending on the qual-

ity of life in a particular neighborhood. However, the life experiences of minority women living in urban ghettos and barrios or in rural slums differ considerably from those of minority women living in more affluent, although segregated, neighborhoods.

Education and Employment

Educational achievement, as measured by years of completed school, provides some of the explanation for income differentials by race/ethnicity. Table 35-1 shows that in 1989, twice as many Latina American as white American women aged 25 and older had not completed high school (49 versus 22 percent). For African American women, the percentage not completing high school (35 percent) was somewhat less than the percentage for Latin American women but was still about 60 percent more than that for white American women. Women without a high school degree, or its equivalent, are more likely to enter the work force in low-wage, dead-end positions.

Employment patterns also help to explain the lower income of minority women. Over half of African American (58.7 percent), Latina American (53.5 percent), and white American (57.2 percent) women were in the labor force in 1989. Government enforcement of antidiscriminatory policies, however, has occurred in an era when there are fewer employment and business opportunities for those with less technically sophisticated skills. Data from the Bureau of Labor Statistics indicate that in 1989, African American women were less likely than white American women to work in managerial, professional, and technical positions and more likely to be employed in service occupations (17). Almost twice as many African American as white American women were employed in service positions such as food service, health service, and private household work (28 versus 15 percent). Additionally, 60 percent more African American women than nonminority women were employed in positions classified by the U.S. census as operators or fabricators (e.g., machine operators and assemblers). Current statistics are not stratified by gender for Latino Americans, although statistics similar to those of African American women probably hold true.

Due to long-standing inequities in education and training, minority women face difficulty taking advantage of new opportunities. As a consequence, the economic benefits of the transitions occurring in society have been shared unevenly across racial/ethnic groups.

Linking Health and Social Conditions

Latina and African American women have lower median incomes than white American women, and nearly half of Latino and American families headed by women have faced conditions of poverty for the last two decades. Also, minority populations live primarily in inner cities that lack the economic resources to address the varied problems associated with high rates of poverty. Many factors contribute to disparities in health; however, inadequate financial resources, limited education, and the stress of life in densely populated inner cities are important contributing factors that cannot be discounted. Furthermore, when illness or injury occurs, it not only raises a family's health care costs but can compromise an income earner's ability to work. Our society recognizes airline pilots, combat soldiers, and police officers, for example, as individuals who face life circumstances that place them at risk for stress-related illnesses and premature mortality. Yet we fail to recognize the similar impact of having inadequate resources to live, being perceived as inferior, or being part of a marginal, expendable workforce. Many racial/ethnic minority women, irrespective of their status as parents, experience life conditions that place them at risk for ill-health and injury. Measurement tools for the impact of these factors are not yet well developed, but statistics capturing the social environments of minority women are objective indications of the risks.

Minority Health: A Dearth of Research

In our review of the literature, we found that most reports addressing the health status of racial/ethnic minority population groups did not provide data by gender and race or were limited in the ethnic groups included (18–24). Also, research involving the health of women in general, and of minority women in particular, is limited (15, 25), and few studies have explored the effects of race and social class on health (24, 26–29). The Secretary's Task Force on Black and Minority Health (18), reporting in 1985, was a first attempt at providing a national perspective on the health of racial/ethnic minority groups. In many cases, data were disaggregated by gender. However, information on the health of Latinos was not included in this report due to the lack of data specifically identifying ethnic origin.

Since 1960, U.S. racial/ethnic minority population groups have experienced considerable gains in health status (18–21). The magnitude of racial disparities, however, has changed little in the last two decades. In some cases, the gap has widened. Mortality statistics, one of the most dramatic and reliable indicators of a population's health are evidence of continuing racial disparities.

The Secretary's Task Force contributed significantly to our understanding of the differences in mortality between African Americans and white Americans. As an indicator of the severity of racial disparities in health, the Task Force computed the number of "excess deaths" that occur among racial/ethnic minority women and men. Excess deaths reflect the number of deaths that would not have occurred if racial/ethnic minority populations experienced the same death rates, by age and sex, as whites. The measure reflects a standard of health that presumably could be achieved given the current state of knowledge and use of comparable resources. Using this approach, six health problems were identified as accounting for most of the excess deaths among African Americans of both genders.[5] The health problems that contributed most to the average annual excess deaths among female African Americans under the age of 70 were: cardiovascular disease (41 percent), infant mortality (12 percent), cancer (10 percent), homicide (6 percent), diabetes (5 percent), cirrhosis (3 percent), and accidents (1 percent). All other deaths continued to account for the remaining 22 percent of excess deaths for females in this age group.

More current information on the mortality experience of African American and Latino Americans as compared to white Americans is presented in Table 35-1 (22). Although the data are not gender specific, they provide an indication of the causes of death experienced more frequently among racial/ethnic minority groups than among white Americans. In 1990, African Americans of all age groups showed higher rates of mortality than white Americans for almost all causes of death examined. However, death rates for homicide, cerebrovascular disease (ages 45 to 64), HIV infection, and diseases of the heart (ages 25 to 44) were substantially higher for African Americans than for white Americans.

The mortality experience of Latino Americans differs greatly from that of African Americans. For the majority of causes, Latino American mortality rates are similar to or lower than those of white Americans. Two exceptions are the higher death rates for homicide and HIV infection. It should also be noted that death rates for malignant neoplasms, diseases of the heart, and cerebrovascular disease were lower for Latinos than for white Americans.

Several recent articles have examined the effects of race and social class on health (26–29). Navarro (26) estimated mortality rates for heart disease using data from the 1986 National Mortality Followback Survey and the 1986 U.S. Occupational Census. Blue-collar workers such as operators, fabricators, and laborers had mortality rates for heart disease that were 2.3 times higher than those of managers and professionals. Navarro found that class differentials in mortality were larger than race differentials. Lerner and Henderson (27, 28), using Baltimore, Maryland, census tract data on neighborhood characteristics, found that both race and income were significant factors in mortality due to cerebrovascular disease and cancer, but race was not independently associated with mortality due to heart disease. Since both of these studies analyzed aggregate population-based indicators (e.g., occupational group and census tract median income) rather than person-specific data, rela-

Table 35-1
Ratio of African American and Latino American to white American death rates for selected causes and age groups, 1988*

Age group/ selected causes	African Americans	Latino Americans
Age group 1–14		
Total	1.6	1.0
Injuries	1.5	0.9
Homicide	5.0	2.0
Malignant tumors	1.0	1.0
Other	1.6	1.1
Age group 15–24		
Total	1.5	1.2
Injuries	0.7	0.9
Homicide	7.4	3.5
Suicide	0.6	0.7
Other	2.0	1.2
Age group 25–44		
Total	2.5	1.2
Injuries	1.4	1.2
Homicide	7.0	3.1
Diseases of the heart	2.6	0.7
HIV infection	3.6	2.3
Other	2.3	1.1
Age group 45–64		
Total	1.7	0.8
Injuries	1.7	1.2
Diseases of the heart	1.7	0.7
Malignant neoplasms	1.4	0.5
Cerebrovascular disease	3.0	1.1
Other	2.1	1.1
Age group 65+		
Total	1.1	0.7
Diseases of the heart	1.1	0.6
Malignant neoplasms	1.2	0.6
Cerebrovascular disease	1.2	0.6
Other	1.1	0.8

*Source: reference 22.

tions among variables must be interpreted with caution. Using multivirate analytic techniques and person-specific data, Otten and associates (29) found that about one-third (31 percent) of the mortality differential by race could be explained by six well-established risk factors and that 38 percent could be accounted for by family income. This left 31 percent of the mortality differential by race unexplained.

Table 35-2
Health status measures by race/ethnicity and family incomes,
women aged 18 to 64 (weighted), 1988

Health status measure/ family income	African Americans	Latina Americans	White Americans	Ratio AA:WA	Ratio LA:WA
Fair or poor health, %					
All income groups	17.2	13.0	8.5	2.02	1.53
Under $10,000	29.5	24.4	21.0	1.40	1.16
$10,000–19,999	18.0	16.7	12.7	1.42	1.31
$20,000–34,999	9.2	9.6	7.5	1.23	1.28
$35,000+	7.8	5.0	4.2	1.86	1.19
Any activity limitation, %					
All income groups	15.6	10.3	12.9	1.21	0.80
Under $10,000	24.6	20.2	27.6	0.89	0.73
$10,000–19,999	17.8	9.7	18.0	0.99	0.54
$20,000–34,999	8.4	7.7	12.1	0.69	0.64
$35,000+	8.9	5.0	8.2	1.09	0.61
Unable to work due to activity limitations, %					
All income groups	8.2	5.3	4.8	1.71	1.10
Under $10,000	14.4	12.1	14.5	0.99	0.83
$10,000–19,999	9.3	4.9	7.1	1.31	0.69
$20,000–34,999	3.4	3.6	3.8	0.89	0.95
$35,000+	3.6	1.1	2.2	1.64	0.50

*Source: Analysis of data from the 1988 HIS.

Health Indices of Latina and African American Women

It is generally known that women have a longer life expectancy, report more symptoms of acute illness, and are more likely to make a physician visit than men; very little is known, however, about the extent to which women vary by race/ethnicity in patterns of illness and risk factors for ill-health. In this section, we provide descriptive information on several health indicators and risk factors for ill-health. The health measures (perceived health status, percentage with activity limitations due to chronic conditions, and percentage unable to work due to activity limitations) are indicators of the quality of life experienced by Latina and African American as compared with white American women. Data on risk factors (e.g., smoking, being overweight) reflect lifestyle behaviors that, while generally described as personal choices, also reflect sociocultural patterns, historic dietary practices, and financial resources.

Perceived Health Status

Self-assessment of health status has been found to correlate reasonably well with objective measures of health, including mortality and physician ratings of health (30). As such, it is a good indicator of the extent of health problems in a population. About one in ten women assess their health as fair or poor. As expected this finding varies by race and by income (Table 35-2). Twice as many African American (17.2 percent) as white American women (8.5 percent) reported their health as fair or poor in the 1988 HIS, and 1.5 times as many Latina American (13.0 percent) as white American women reported their health as fair or poor.

The proportion reporting their health as fair or poor is inversely related to income, with nearly one in four women with incomes under $10,000 feeling that their health was fair or poor, compared with one in 25 women with incomes of $35,000 or more. When examining self-reports of health by race and income, some racial differences persist but they are modest. For example, among women with incomes under $10,000, there are small differences by race/ethnicity in the percentage reporting fair or poor health (21 percent of white Americans, 24 percent of Latina Americans, 30 percent of African Americans). Similarly, among women with incomes of $35,000 or more, the percentage in fair or poor health is less than 10 percent irrespective of race/ethnicity, even though there is an almost twofold difference in the percentage of African Americans and white Americans reporting their health as fair or poor. In each income category, a larger percentage of Latina and African American women than white American women reported their health as fair or poor. Differences across racial groups, however, are smaller than the differences by income within a racial group.

Limitation of Activity

One frequently used indicator of a population's health is the percentage with limitation of major activity due to a chronic condition. The prevalence of reported chronic conditions is higher among older (aged 45 to 64) than younger (under age 45) women; however, heart disease, high blood pressure, orthopedic impairments, arthritis, sinusitis, and migraine headaches ranked among the leading chronic conditions for women of both age groups (31). Table 35-2 includes information on the percentage of women that reported limitation of the major activity associated with their age group in the 1988 HIS. For persons aged 18 to 64, the major activity is considered working or keeping house. As noted earlier, over half of women in each racial/ethnic group work outside the home.

Of women aged 18 to 64, 13 percent reported limitation of activity due to chronic conditions. This estimate includes individuals reporting they were (*a*) unable to perform the major activity, (*b*) able to perform the major activity but limited in the kind or amount of this activity, or (*c*) not limited in the major activity but limited in the kind or amount or other activities. Small differences by race/ethnicity are observed, with about 20 percent fewer Latinas (10.3 percent) than white Americans (12.9 percent) reporting

limitation of activity. Differences by income are striking. Three times as many low-income women (25.7 percent) as upper-income women (7.9 percent) reported limitation of activity. When stratified by income and race, the effects of race observed among all women persist only for women in the highest income category. Data suggest that lower-income and middle-income racial minority women are as likely as or less likely than their white counterparts to report activity limitations. For example, in the $20,000 to $34,999 income group, about 30 percent fewer Latinas (7.7 percent) and African Americans (8.4 percent) reported limitation of activity than did white Americans (12.1 percent).

Inability to Work Due to Activity Limitations

Another measure used to assess health status is the degree to which health problems limit one's ability to work. Table 35-2 shows the percentage of women who reported they were unable to work due to activity limitations, a subset of those reporting any activity limitation. Health problems limited the working capacity of more African American women than Latinas or white Americans. The percentage of African Americans who were unable to work is 1.7 times greater than that for white Americans and 1.5 times greater than that for Latinas. The proportion of women unable to work is inversely related to income levels, with nearly one of every seven women (13.9 percent) with incomes below $10,000 unable to work because of their health problems. At the higher spectrum of the income level (more than $35,000), one of every 45 women was unable to work (2.2 percent) due to health problems.

When income and race/ethnic group are considered, there are some differences across racial groups within each income level, but these are modest compared with the differences within a racial/ethnic group by income. For example, among women with incomes below $10,000, a similar percentage of African Americans and white Americans were unable to work (14.4 and 14.5 percent, respectively). When considering African American women by income, those with incomes under $10,000 were four times more

Table 35-3
*Age-adjusted prevalence rates for specific health risk factors for women,
by race/ethnic group, percentages*

Health risk factor	Mexican American	Puerto Rican	Cuban	Non-Hispanic black	Non-Hispanic white
Overweight	41.6	40.2	31.6	44.4	23.9
Hypertension	20.3	19.2	14.4	43.8	25.1
High cholesterol	20.0	22.7	16.9	25.0	28.3
Smoking	15.5	23.4	20.2	29.1	28.6

*Sources: For all factors except smoking, data for Hispanics are from the 1982-84 Hispanic HANES; data for non-Hispanic blacks and whites from the 1976-80 National HANES. For smoking, data are from the 1988 HIS.

likely to be unable to work than those with incomes above $35,000. Among white American women, those in the lowest income group were close to seven times more likely to be unable to work due to health problems than women in the highest income group. In general, a lower percentage of Latina women than both African American and white American women were unable to work. However, differences by income are more striking. Latinas in the lowest income level were 11 times more likely to be unable to work than were those in the highest income level.

Lifestyle Behaviors

The health profiles of racial/ethnic minority women often include characteristics of risk factors that are known to be associated with specific states of ill-health and are modifiable. Four common risk factors—overweight, hypertension, high cholesterol, and smoking—are noted in Table 35-3 for racial/ethnic minority women, with Latina women grouped according to their country of origin.

Being overweight is one of the most common nutritional problems among racial/ethnic minority women. It is an indicator of dietary practices and often signals a diet poor in quality and variety. In the NHANES, almost twice as many African American (44.4 percent) as white American women (23.9 percent) were overweight. A sizable percentage of Latina women in the HHANES were also overweight. The rate varies, however, by ethnic group. Cuban Americans had the lowest percentage of overweight women, and Mexican Americans the highest. The disproportionate number of overweight racial/ethnic minority women is disturbing given the strong associations between obesity and such diseases as diabetes, hypertension, and breast and uterine cancer.

The prevalence of hypertension, an important risk factor for cardiovascular disease, differs considerably among the various racial/ethnic minority groups. Cuban American women, for example, had the lowest rate of hypertension (14.4 percent), compared with 25.1 percent for white women. African American women had the highest rate, 1.7 times that of white American women. Hypertension rates for Latina women of Puerto Rican and Mexican ancestry were about 20 percent lower than that of white women. Higher rates of hypertension among African Americans are believed to be related to environmental factors (e.g., diet and stress) and genetic predisposition (21,32).

High serum cholesterol level and cigarette smoking are important risk factors for several chronic diseases including heart disease, stroke, and lung cancer. Data from the HIS (Table 35-3) show Latinas as having a lower prevalence of high serum cholesterol levels and fewer smokers than white American women. Data from the HHANES provide estimates of smoking rates among subgroups of Latinas that are higher than the HIS estimates but are still lower than the rates for white American women. Prevalence rates for high serum cholesterol level and cigarette smoking do not differ substantially for African American and white American women. This finding suggests that these risk factors, although very important to healthy living, are unlikely to be major contributors to the excess heart disease and lung cancer mortality of African American women when compared with white American women.

Another behavior pattern that affects the health of racial/ethnic minority women is drug abuse. In addition to the adverse physiological effects of the drugs used, users today are at higher risk of ill-health due to behaviors related to drug acquisition and use. For example, women who engage in sexual activity in exchange for cocaine are at a higher risk of exposure to sexually transmitted diseases, including HIV infection. Data from the Centers for Disease Control (33) indicate that African American and Latina women represent 86 percent of the AIDS cases among women (13 years and older) reported in 1991. Annual AIDS case rates were 14.5 times higher among African American women and 7.4 times higher among Latinas than among white American women. The high risk of AIDS among minority women is also reflected in the rising number of pediatric AIDS cases among minority children. Children born to minority women make up 81 percent of the cumulative pediatric AIDS cases reported through December 1991.

The risks of HIV infection are enormous for racial/ethnic minority populations because drug use, which can compromise one's judgment, is one of the major modes of transmission. Intravenous drug use was the mode of transmission in 48 percent of the AIDS cases among women in 1991, and having sex with an intravenous drug user exposed another 22 percent of the women to the virus. The high rates of transmission related to intravenous drugs could be an indicator of the prevalence of such drug use in minority communities or reflect racial/ethnic differences in the use of clean needles. For either case, changing the behavior of persons addicted to drugs is one of the greatest challenges facing society. Efforts to reduce HIV infection in racial/ethnic minority women will depend, in part, on the effectiveness of drug abuse prevention and treatment programs.

Occupational and Environmental Risks

The work and home environments, where individuals spend most of their waking hours, often contribute to the experience of ill-health. Hazards in the work place such as exposures to noxious agents, the pace of work, and general safety concerns, among others, have been found to be associated with higher rates of injury, disease, and death. Additionally, some ill-health experiences are localized within a geographic area. In such cases, surrounding environmental conditions may be suspect in contributing to ill-health. Combining information on occupational and environmental hazards with information on health indicators helps us to construct a profile of the health of Latina and African American women.

Occupational Safety and Health

One legacy of discrimination in the United States has been the percentage of Latino Americans and African Americans employed in the lowest paid and least desirable jobs. When racial minorities gained entrance into many industries and skilled trades, they often were assigned the most dangerous jobs (34). Even after controlling for racial differences in years of education and work experience, the disproportionate representation of African American workers in more hazardous jobs and occupations remains strong (35).

The devastating fire that occurred in 1991 in a Hamlet, North Carolina, poultry plant is one example of the dangerous working conditions of minority women. Twenty-five workers (men and women) were killed in the fire because locked safety doors kept them from escaping. Although the majority of the persons fatally injured were white, two-thirds of the plant workforce were African Americans. This tragedy increased the public's awareness of the magnitude of the problems in the workplace and the lax enforcement of Occupational Safety and Health Act (OSHA) guidelines. Over 240 such poultry plants exist today, employing 150,000 workers, the majority of whom are women. Nearly 75 percent of these industries are located in the south, in predominantly poor and African American neighborhoods. The health and safety conditions within these plants are abhorrent. Each year, almost 28,000 workers in poultry plants lose their jobs or become disabled due to work-related accidents or injuries. Icy temperatures, dull knives and scissors, fat and grease build-up, line speed-up, and hand and wrist injuries are only a few of the health and safety problems (36). The majority of these plants are nonunionized, pay minimum wages, and offer no health care benefits to their employees.

A large proportion of Latina American women are employed in the semi-conductor and agricultural industries. Studies show that workers in the semiconductor industry experience occupational illness at three times the rate of workers in the general manufacturing industries (37). Farmworkers and their families are exposed to dangerous pesticides, and occupational injuries occur at an alarming rate as the result of using faulty equipment.

The garment industry is another industry in which women of color constitute the majority of workers. Although conditions have improved somewhat with the passage of the OSHA standards regulating exposure to cotton dust, many hazards, similar to the sweatshop conditions of the nineteenth century, remain. Many garment shops are poorly lit working areas with inadequate ventilation. These conditions are similar to those that existed in New York's Triangle Shirtwaist Factory, where in 1911, a tragic fire killed 146 immigrant women (36). Workers suffer from formaldehyde exposure, carpal tunnel syndrome, and other ergonomic problems.

The majority of office employees are women. For minority women, many of whom are employed in lower level clerical positions, the health risks are substantial (38). The occupational hazards of office work are well known; however, current OSHA standards apply poorly to these hazards. The production line pace of most office settings and the modernization of offices with video display terminals, along with poor office design and inadequate ventilation, have increased employees' risk of developing job-related health problems. Ergonomic problems related to the hands and back (i.e., carpal tunnel syndrome, tendinitis, and back strain), vision problems, headaches, fatigue, colds and allergies due to poor indoor air quality, and job stress are among the most frequently re-ported health problems of office workers (39).

Environmental Exposures

Three of every five Latino Americans and African Americans live in areas with uncontrolled toxic waste sites (40). The most infamous dumping grounds are to be found in rural areas in the South. "Cancer Alley" located in Louisiana, along the Mississippi River between Baton Rouge and New Orleans, is among the worst. The area is lined with oil refineries and petrochemical plants, and its residents are predominantly African American and poor. The abnormally high cancer rates of the alley's residents have prompted one health official to call the alley a "massive human experiment"(41).

From the landfills of rural America to the "fly dumpsites" and toxic incinerators of urban America, the lives and health of racial minority populations are threatened. For example, excess cancer rates, respiratory problems, and birth deformities have been identified in Altgeld Gardens of Chicago, Illinois, and in East Los Angeles, California. These predominantly African American and Latino American communities have toxic dumpsites and incinerators located literally in residents' backyards (42). In Warren County, North Carolina, residents of a predominantly African American community protested against the proposed site of a polychlorinated biphenyl (PCB) landfill (43). In spite of their protest, however, the community became a dumping site for these cancer-causing agents. PCBs not only cause cancer, but also can affect the reproductive system of adults and may pass to a child through the mother's breast milk. Repeated and high exposure to PCBs can also cause liver and nervous system damage.

In a study conducted by the Commission for Racial Justice (40), investigators analyzed a cross section of U.S. commercial hazardous waste facilities and uncontrolled toxic waste sites, and correlated them with the ethnicity of the communities in which they were located. The study found that race/ethnicity is the most significant variable associated with the location of hazardous waste facilities and that African Americans are overrepresented in the populations of metropolitan areas with the largest number of uncontrolled toxic waste sites. The study also found that even though socioeconomic status plays an important role in the location of hazardous waste sites, race is more significant. Bullard and Wright (44) explain that because of housing patterns and limited mobility, middle-income and lower-income blacks, unlike whites, often cannot "vote with their feet" and move when a polluting facility arrives.

Access to Health Services

Dramatic changes have occurred in the U.S. system of financing and delivery of health services during the last three decades. New initiatives improved the availability of health resources (providers and facilities) within inner city and rural communities. Additionally, with enactment of Medicaid and Medicare in 1965 and federal enforcement of antidiscrimination laws, health care services have become more financially accessible for low-income, elderly, and ethnic minority populations. Yet inequities in access to health care persist, and there are indications that barriers to care have increased for some populations (45, 46). In the last decade, access to care has been threatened by rising uncompensated care (i.e., bad debt and charity care) as well as the increasing costs of medical care.

Blendon (45) and Freeman (46) and their colleagues, analyzing data from a 1986 national survey on access, provide evidence of continuing disparities for racial/ethnic minority populations. Blendon and associates (45) found that the proportion making a physician visit and the average number of visits are significantly lower for African Americans than white Americans. The gap is experienced by all income levels. Racial differences persisted even after using multiple regression analysis to take into account respondent differences in age, gender, health status, and income. In addition to lower rates of use, African Americans reported greater dissatisfaction than white Americans with the care received. Freeman and associates (46) compared access indicators of Latino Americans with those of African Americans and white

Americans. This study found that Latino Americans, on average, saw physicians at about the same rate as white Americans, but were less likely to receive hospital care, despite a larger proportion reporting poorer health.

With approximately 38 million people uninsured for their medical costs (47), access to care is problematic for many Americans. Problems are particularly acute for racial/ethnic minority populations. Barriers of language, cultural insensitivity, and the lack of health providers in minority communities compound problems in financial access for the uninsured and underinsured. Moreover, national policy emphasis during the 1980s shifted from expanding access to containing costs.

Table 35-4 presents information on racial/ethnic differences in indicators of women's access to ambulatory and hospital care (i.e., percentage without a physician visit, average number of physician visits, and hospital discharges per 100 persons), derived from HIS data. Health services utilization is an indicator of a population's health status as well as its access to health services. In general, individuals in poorer health may require more medical care and use services at higher levels than those who are healthier. However, financial and physical barriers to care could reduce utilization. Since many factors determine use of services, the most important of which is health status, measures of utilization, at most, provide suggestive evidence of barriers to care.

Ambulatory Care

The percentages of African American and white American women not visiting a physician in the last year do not differ (Table 35-4), with about one in five reporting no contact with a physician. Among Latina women, on the other hand, a larger percentage were without a physician visit (24.8 percent). When income is considered, women with incomes between $10,000 and $19,999 were the least likely to visit a physician among all racial/ethnic groups. This finding could reflect gaps in health coverage that are particularly severe for the working poor. Regardless of the reason, it is a disturbing finding that the population group with the largest percentage

Table 35-4
*Utilization measures by race/ ethnicity and family incomes,
women aged 18 to 64 (weighted), 1988[a]*

Utilization measure/ family income	African Americans	Latina Americans	White Americans	Ratio	
				AA:WA	LA:WA
No physician visit in last year, %					
All income groups	19.8	24.8	19.2	1.03	1.29
Under $10,000	19.0	23.3	18.4	1.03	1.27
$10,000–19,999	21.3	27.8	21.0	1.01	1.32
$20,000–34,999	19.9	23.7	19.3	1.03	1.23
$35,000+	14.6	22.4	17.2	0.85	1.30
Physician contacts, per person per year					
All income groups	4.8	4.1	4.8	1.00	0.85
Under $10,000	6.0	5.3	6.9	0.87	0.77
$10,000–19,999	5.1	4.3	5.2	0.98	0.83
$20,000–34,999	4.3	3.8	4.7	0.91	0.81
$35,000+	4.0	3.7	4.6	0.87	0.80
Short-stay hospital discharges, per 100 persons per year[b]					
All income groups	10.7	7.2	9.6	1.11	0.75
Under $10,000	14.9	11.4	17.9	0.83	0.64
$10,000–19,999	12.4	8.3	10.8	1.15	0.77
$20,000–34,999	7.5	5.3	9.3	0.81	0.57
$35,000+	7.4	4.4	7.1	1.04	0.62

[a]Source: Analysis of data from the 1988 HIS.
[b]Excluding childbirth.

in fair or poor health has the smallest percentage making contact with our health care system.

Latina American women in all income groups were less likely than either white American or African American women to report contact with a physician. For example, 23.3 percent of Latinas were without a physician visit in 1988, compared with 19 percent of African American and 18.4 percent of white American women with incomes under $10,000. At the higher end of the income spectrum, more Latina American (22.4 percent) than African American (14.6 percent) or white American (17.2 percent) women were without a physician visit. The data suggest that factors other than income may be important determinants of whether Latina women obtain health care services.

The average number of physician visits per person per year also varies by race/ethnicity and income (Table 35-4). Low-income women in each racial/ethnic group reported more physician contacts than women in higher income groups. This is likely a consequence of their poorer health status. However, when comparing women of similar income, Latina and African American women made fewer physician visits than white American women. Racial/ethnic differences are greatest between Latinas and white American women. The finding provides some evidence that minority women use health services less frequently than non-minority women of comparable income.

Hospital Care

Short-stay hospital discharge rates, unadjusted for health status, show higher annual rates of hospitalization for African American women (10.7 per 100 persons) and lower rates for Latinas (7.2 per 100) than for white American women (9.6 per 100) (Table 35-4). When hospital discharges are examined by family income, an inverse relation is observed for all racial/ethnic groups. Women in the lowest income groups had close to double the number of hospital discharges compared with women in the highest income category. Given the larger percentage of African American and low-income women in fair or poor health, higher rates may reflect their greater need for care.

Hospitalization rates also were found to vary by race and income. Among women with incomes below $10,000, fewer Latinas (11.4 per 100 persons) and African Americans (14.9 per 100) than white Americans (17.9 per 100) were hospitalized, even though a larger percentage of minority women reported being in poorer health. Also, fewer African American than white American women with incomes of $20,000 to $34,999 received hospital care. Latina women, on the other hand, had lower overall hospitalization rates than white American women and lower rates of hospital care in each income group. The data suggest that racial/ethnic barriers to hospital care exist for Latina women regardless of income; whereas for African American women, possible racial barriers are evident in only two of the four income groups.

Discussion

Latina and African American women, when compared with nonminority women, are more likely to face social environments (e.g., poverty and hazardous work conditions) that place them at risk for illness and injury. Although persistent racial disparities in health are often attributed to the lifestyle behaviors of racial minority populations, they are also a consequence of poorer social conditions as well as barriers in access to quality health services. The complex interplay of racial, economic, and gender-specific barriers has resulted in many minority and poor women experiencing social conditions that adversely affect their health. The health effects of these barriers may be cumulative across generations, with cause and effect difficult to disentangle.

This selection provides evidence that low-income women, regardless of race/ethnicity,

have poorer health indices than their higher income racial/ethnic peers. Moreover, racial disparities in health are reduced when considering a measure of social class such as family income. Nonetheless, within most income categories, African American women have poorer health indices than whites. The unexpected finding, however, is that Latina and African American women experience similar social environments, yet Latinas have health indicators that more closely resemble those of white America women. Many studies have documented a positive relation between socioeconomic conditions and health status, an association that generally holds true for U.S. racial groups. White Americans and Asian Americans, as a group, complete more years of school and have higher incomes and better health indices. In contrast, African Americans and Native Americans, as a group, complete fewer years of school and have lower incomes and poorer health indices. Latinas, for some reason, may be the exception.

Health indicators of Latina women must be considered with caution given the difficulties in accurately identifying ethnic origin. Mortality ratios showing lower or modest differences in death rates between Latinos and whites, for example, may reflect a problem of misclassification of ethnicity. As late as 1988, only 30 states included a Hispanic identifier on their death certificate. Misclassification has been found to be a significant problem plaguing infant mortality statistics. A recent study showed that 30 percent of infants assigned a specific Hispanic origin at birth were assigned a different origin at death (48). Another hypothesis is that the indicators we analyzed do not truly capture the health experiences of Latinas. It is also possible that the indicators are not sufficiently sensitive to detect racial/ethnic health differences for Latinas in aggregate. The inability to disaggregate Latinas into subgroups based on their country of origin or ancestry (due to the small number of cases) is one of the limitations of the HIS data and thus a limitation of this effort. For example, HHANES health indicators for Cuban-American women differed from those for Puerto Rican women. One must consider whether these differences are related to culture or to the social histories of the population subgroups. Cuban women living in the United States may disproportionately represent white Cubans (of Spanish origin), while Puerto Ricans and Mexican Americans may disproportionately represent black Puerto Ricans (of African descent) and Mexican Indians, respectively. Thus efforts to understand Latina health will require sample populations of sufficient size and clarity of definition to examine differences in population subgroups.

Utilization indicators suggest that racial/ethnic barriers to care persist, particularly for low-income women. The finding that Latinas are less likely to visit a physician, make fewer visits per person, and receive less hospital care than white women across income groups is an indication of possible barriers in access to care. Latinas who are primarily Spanish-speaking, for example, may prefer to use alternative healers than face the language barriers encountered in the general health care system. For African American women, data suggest that while entry into the health care system may be approaching levels that are somewhat comparable to those for nonminority women, some differences persist in the amount of care women receive. However, an assessment of whether levels of use are appropriate cannot be made without considering health needs. This analysis shows that low-income (under $10,000) and middle-income ($20,000 to $34,999) African American women receive less hospital care than nonminority women, but overall racial differences in receipt of hospital care as reported by Blendon and associates (45) are not evident from this analysis. One possible explanation for the varying findings is the effect of gender on insurance coverage and thus access to care. Since a larger percentage of minority women than men have health coverage (because of their eligibility for Medicaid through AFDC), they may experience fewer barriers to care than minority men even if problems persist in the quality of care received.

Gaps in Knowledge Hinder Policy and Interventions

Knowledge about the relative impact of race/ethnicity and social class on women's health and use of services is limited. Given the interrelated nature of economic, racial/ethnic, and gender-specific barriers, debate on the primary nature of one factor over the other is, to some extent, an academic exercise. Future research, however, should strive to improve our knowledge about the health effects of all three factors so as to develop interventions that will more precisely target causal factors. Disentangling the interrelated factors is complicated methodologically, but the limited progress to date is more a function of the lack of effort than the complexity of the task.

Much of the published research on the health of minority populations has been descriptive, with few studies exploring causal or contributing factors for ill-health. There are many reasons that could account for the lack of etiologic research, including a dearth of researchers interested in exploring such issues. Also, many epidemiologic studies exclude nonwhites from study populations because of concern about the confounding effects of race, even though there is little scientific evidence to support biological differences among racial/ethnic groups (6, 49). However, the lack of data by race/ethnicity is undoubtedly one major factor accounting for the lack of research. Although vital statistics and national surveys now routinely collect and report data by race/ethnicity, a paucity of national data persists for Latino, Asian, and native Americans. Vital statistics are collected by state agencies, which vary considerably in definition and data quality. Several national surveys have oversampled racial/ethnic minority populations in the last decade, but the number of observations is generally too small for analyses of specific ethnic groups (e.g., Mexican Americans, Puerto Ricans) or for analyses of nonwhite/nonblack racial groups (e.g., Native Americans and Asian Pacific Islanders) with any confidence.[6]

Moreover, health and safety hazards that largely affect women on the job, including women of color, have not been thoroughly investigated even by the Occupational Safety and Health Administration. Since OSHA's passage in 1970, considerable improvements have been made in occupational safety and health. However, regulating exposures to occupational hazards in jobs traditionally held by women has been slow. As a result of a recent Congressional mandate, in 1991 the Occupational Safety and Health Administration issued a standard covering occupational exposure to bloodborne pathogens. The issuance of this standard is a major step forward and should improve protections available to health care employees, the majority of whom are women.

Limited knowledge about the factors associated with racial disparities in health has hindered the development of policies and programs that could seek to reduce these disparities. In the absence of more precise knowledge, public health interventions can only vaguely address rather than specifically target factors contributing to the greater burden of illness and injury among racial minority women. Future research must move beyond descriptive analyses and investigate causal and contributing factors to ill-health, particularly those associated with modifiable social environmental conditions. Such investigations are critical for identifying risk factors and developing more effective preventive interventions.

The recent National Institutes of Health policy (50) requiring inclusion of "women and minorities in study populations for clinical research, unless compelling scientific or other justification for not including them is provided" is important if this nation is to advance its knowledge of the nature of health problems and the most effective interventions for reducing the health problems of racial/ethnic minority populations. Navarro's (26) urging federal research agencies to collect and analyze information on indicators of social class, such as occupation and income, is also critically important. In order to help us in moving toward a more egalitarian society, our data collection systems and analytic methods should have the capability of monitoring progress in reducing differentials by race/ethnicity and by social class.

Improving Minority Women's Health Provides Challenge and Opportunity

Further gains in the health of minority women will require a recognition of the role of the socioeconomic environment in facilitating or hindering improvements in health.

From generation to generation, minority women's worth has been devalued because of their race/ethnicity and their gender. This has resulted in conditions of poverty and powerlessness. With limited financial resources and minimal political influence, minority women have faced conditions of life defined by others. As is apparent from this study, poorer health indices of minority women are due in part to the disproportionate share of minority women living in poverty, but a disproportionate share live in poverty because of racial and gender-specific barriers that persist in this country.

The major health problems facing minority and nonminority women (e.g., lung cancer, breast cancer, heart disease, AIDS, substance abuse, violence) have behavioral and psychosocial etiologic components that affect their prevention and treatment. Having an impact on these conditions will require multidisciplinary, community-based programmatic efforts. This perspective may result in fewer expenditures on health or shared funding for health and social programs. The challenge confronting public health researchers and practitioners is to deepen the level of understanding of the link between health and social conditions. Social factors theoretically are recognized as important determinants of health , but they are generally considered outside the domain of public health practice. One consequence of our failure to make practical linkages between health and social conditions has been a fragmentation of related interventions, with programmatic efforts addressing different dimensions of the same problem viewed as competing rather than complimentary. In some cases, barriers to improved linkages are organizational as well as conceptual. For example, human service delivery systems that address poverty are organizationally independent of those that seek to prevent injury and illness. Also, service efforts are often organized by bureaucracies that are only modestly informed about the population groups they serve.

To achieve further gains in the health of minority women, public policies must reduce social inequalities and assure greater equity in access to resources that facilitate healthier environments and lifestyles. Minority communities in general, and minority women in particular, must be active participants in efforts that seek to improve their health and well-being. Public health initiatives should be community-based, that is, they should reflect a shared partnership that actively engages minority women in decision-making about their lives and is responsive to the *health* and *social* needs of minority women. Efforts that improve social conditions objectively provide opportunities for healthier lives and lifestyles. However, the need to continue to improve the quality of life of minority women should not overshadow the successes that have been made. The vast majority of Latina and African American women have survived the degrading experiences of second-class citizenship and are productive members of society. The gains achieved by minority women were, in large part, a consequence of public policies that reduced racial and gender-specific barriers to the economic opportunities available in this society. If we seek further progress, we should work to implement public policies that help overcome continuing discrimination and thus serve the goal of social equity and improved health status for all.

References

1. Hollingshead, A., and Redlich, F. *Social Class and Mental Illness*. John Wiley and Sons, New York, 1958.

2. Jackson, J.J. Black women in a racist society. In *Racism and Mental Health*. University of Pittsburgh, Pittsburgh, 1973.

3. Frazier, F. E. *The Negro Family in the United States*. University of Chicago Press, Chicago, 1939.

4. Clark, K. *Dark Ghetto*. Harper & Row, New York, 1965.

5. Texidor del Portillo, C. Poverty, self-concept, and health: Experience of Latinas. *Women Health* 12(3/4): 229–242, 1987.

6. Cooper, R., and David, R. The biological concept of race and its application to public health and epidemiology. *J. Health Polit. Policy Law* 11:97–115, 1986.

7. Krieger, N. Shades of difference: Theoretical underpinnings of the medical controversy on black/white differences in the United States,

1830–1870. *Int. J. Health Serv.* 17:259–278, 1987.

8. Zambrana, R.E. A research agenda on issues affecting poor and minority women: A model for understanding their health needs. *Women Health* 12(3/4):137–160, 1987.

9. Bennett, M.B. Afro-American women, poverty and mental health: A social essay. *Women Health* 12(3/4): 213–228, 1987.

10. Bassett, M.T., and Krieger, N. Social class and black-white differences in breast cancer survival. *Am. J. Public Health* 76: 1400–1403, 1986.

11. Dohrenwend, B.P., and Dohrenwend, B.S. *Social Status and Psychological Disorder: A Casual Inquiry*. Wiley Interscience, New York, 1969.

12. Neighbors, H. The distribution of psychiatric morbidity in black Americans: A review and suggestions for research. *Community Mental Health J.* 20(3):5–18, 1984.

13. Neff, J. Race differences in psychological distress: The effect of SES, urbanicity, and management strategy. *Am. J. Community Psychol.* 12(3):337-351, 1985.

14. U.S. Bureau of the Census. *Poverty in the United States: 1990*. Series P–60, No. 175. Washington, D.C., 1991.

15. U.S. Department of Health and Human Services. *Women's Health*. Report of the Public Health Service Task Force on Women's Health Issues, Vol. II. Washington, D.C., 1985.

16. Jaynes, G. D., and Williams, R. M., Jr. (eds.). *A Common Destiny: Blacks and American Society*. National Academy Press, Washington, D.C., 1989.

17. U.S. Bureau of the Census. *Statistical Abstract of the United States: 1991*, Ed. II. Washington, D.C., 1991.

18. U.S. Department of Health and Human Services. *Report of the Secretary's Task Force on Black and Minority Health*, 1: Executive Summary. Washington, D.C, 1985.

19. Trevino, F.M., and Moss, A.J. *Health Indicators for Hispanic, Black, and White Americans*. Vital and Health Statistics, Series 10, No. 148. DHHS Publication No. (PHS) 84–1576. National Center for Health Statistics, Washington, D.C., 1984.

20. Davis, K. et al. Health care for black Americans: The public sector role. In *Health Policies and Black Americans*, pp. 213-247. Transaction Publishers, New Jersey, 1989.

21. U.S. Department of Health and Human Services. *Health Status of Minorities and Low-Income Groups: Third Edition.* GPO:1991 271–848/40085. Washington, D.C., 1991.

22. U.S. Department of Health and Human Services. *Health, United States, 1990.* DHHS Publication No. (PHS) 91–1232. Washington, D.C, 1991.

23. Trevino, F.M. Falcon, A. P., and Stroup-Benham, C.A. (eds.). Hispanic Health and Nutrition Examination Survey, 1982–84: Findings on health status and health care needs. *Am. J. Public Health* 80 (Suppl.): 1–72, 1990.

24. Miller, W.J., and Cooper, R. Rising lung cancer death rates among black men: The importance of occupation and social class. *J. Natl. Med. Assoc.* 74: 253–258, 1982.

25. Muller, C.F. *Health Care and Gender.* Russell Sage Foundation, New York, 1990.

26. Navarro, V. Race or class or race and class? Growing mortality differentials in the United States. *Lancet* 336: 1238–1240, 1990.

27. Lerner, M., and Henderson, L.A. Income and race differentials in heart disease mortality in Baltimore City, 1979–81 to 1984–86. In *Health Status of Minorities and Low-Income Groups: Third Edition.* GPO: 1991 271–848/40085. U.S. DHHS, Washington, D.C., 1991.

28. Lerner, M., and Henderson, L.A. Cancer mortality among the disadvantaged in Baltimore City by income and race: Update from 1979–81 to 1984–86. In *Health Status of Minorities and Low-Income Groups: Third Edition.* GPO: 1991 271–848/40085. U.S. DHHS, Washington, D.C., 1991.

29. Otten, M.W., Jr. et al. The effect of known risk factors on the excess mortality of black adults in the United States. *JAMA* 263: 848–850, 1990.

30. Yergan, J. et al. Health status as a measure of need for medical care: A critique. *Med. Care* 19 (Suppl. 12): 57–68, 1981.

31. U.S. Department of Health and Human Services. *Current Estimates from the National Health Interview Survey, 1988.* Vital and Health Statistics, Series 10, No. 173, DHHS Publication No. (PHS) 89–1501. Washington, D.C., 1989.

32. Klag, M.J. et al. The association of skin color with blood pressure in U.S. blacks with low socioeconomic status. *JAMA* 265: 599–602, 1991.

33. Centers for Disease Control (National Center for Infectious Diseases, Division of HIV/AIDS). *HIV/AIDS Surveillance.* Atlanta, 1992.

34. Michaels, D. Occupational cancer in the black population: The health effects of job discrimination. *J. Natl. Med. Assoc.* 75: 1014–1017, 1983.

35. Robinson, J. Racial inequality and occupational health in the United States: The effects on white workers, *Int. J. Health Serv.* 15: 23–34, 1985.

36. Cromer, L. Plucking Cargill: The RWDSU in Georgia. *Labor Res. Rev.* 16: 15–23, 1991.

37. Lee, P.T. An overview: workers of color and the occupational health crisis. Labor Occupational health Program. U.C. Berkeley, California. In *The First National People of Color Environmental Leadership Summit*, pp. 76–79. Washington, D.C., October 1991.

38. Haynes, S. G., and Feinlieb, M. Women, work, and coronary heart disease. *Am. J. Public Health* 70: 133–141, 1980.

39. Rabinowitz, R. *Is Your Job Making You Sick?* Coalition of Labor Union Women, New York, 1991.

40. Commission for Racial Justice, united Church of Christ. *Toxic Wastes and Race in the United States.* Public Data Access, Inc., 1987.

41. Elson, J. Dumping on the poor. *Time Magazine,* August 1990, pp. 46–47.

42. Grossman, K. Environmental racism. *Crisis* 98(4): 14–17, 31–32, 1991.

43. Lee, C. The integrity of Justice: Evidence of environmental racism. *Sojourners,* 1990, pp. 23–25.

44. Bullard, R., and Wright, B.H. Environmentalism and the politics of equity: Emergent trends in the black community. *Mid-Am. Rev. Sociol.* 12: 21–38, 1987.

45. Blendon, R.J. et al. Access to medical care for black and white Americans: A matter of continuing concern. *JAMA* 261: 278–281, 1989.

46. Freeman, H.E. et al. Americans report on their access to health care. *Health Aff.* 6(1): 6–18, 1987.

47. Short, P.F., Cornelius, L.J., and Goldstone, D.E. Health insurance of minorities in the United States. *J. Health Care Poor Underserved* 1(1): 9–24, 1990.

48. Hahn, R., Mulinare, J., and Teutsch, S. Inconsistencies in coding of race and ethnicity between birth and death in U.S. infants: A new look at infant mortality, 1983 through 1985. *JAMA* 267(2): 259–263, 1992.

49.   Jones, C.P., LaVeist, T.A., and Lillie-Blanton, M. Race in the epidemiologic literature: An examination of the *American Journal of Epidemiology*, 1921–1990. *Am. J. Epidemiol.* 134: 1079–1084, 1991.

50.   National Institute on Drug Abuse. *Research Grants Program Catalog of Federal Domestic Assistance*, No. 93.279: Announcements and Guidelines. U.S. DHHS. Rockville, MD., 1990.

Notes

1.   Women of other racial groups (i.e., Asian and Pacific Islanders, Native Americans, etc.) were excluded from the analysis of the HIS data.

2.   The average poverty threshold for a family of four was $13,359 in 1990.

3.   The percentage of Latino and African American families headed by women increased by about 40 percent between 1970 and 1990, from 21.8 to 31.2 percent among African American families and from 13.3 to 18.8 percent among Latino American families (15).

4.   There was a twofold increase in the prison population during the 1980s, with young black males comprising almost half of that population in 1986 (15). Moreover, African American males aged 25 to 44 years have the highest mortality rates, 2.5 times the rate for white males in 1988 (10).

5.   These health problems were heart disease and stroke, cancer, cirrhosis, and other liver disease, diabetes, homicide and unintentional injuries, and infant mortality.

6.   Two notable exceptions are the Hispanic Health and Nutrition Examination Study (HHANES) and the Survey of American Indians and Alaskan Natives (SAIN)

Further Reading

AMA Council on Scientific Affairs. 1991. "Hispanic Health in the United States." *Journal of the American Medical Association* 265: 248–252.

C. P. Jones, Thomas A. LaVeist, Marsha Lillie-Blanton. 1991. "Race in the Epidemiologic literature: An Examination of the *American Journal of Epidemiology*, 1921–1990." *American Journal of Epidemiology* 134: 1079–1084.

U.S. Bureau of the Census. 1991. *Poverty in the United States: 1990.* Series P–60, No. 175. Washington, D.C.

Discussion Questions

1.   What are the most pressing issues facing minority women?

2.   How might examining the intersection of race, gender, and social class differently inform an analysis of health and illness? How might it inform policy?

3.   What directions do these findings suggest for changes in the health care system?

From *International Journal of Health Services*, Vol. 23 (3). Pp. 555-584. Copyright © 1993 by Baywood Publishing Company, Inc. Reprinted by permission. ✦

36

Impact of Marital Status on Outcomes in Hospitalized Patients

Howard S. Gordon
Gary E. Rosenthal

In this selection, Howard Gordon and Gary Rosenthal examine the relationship between marital status and various hospital outcomes. Health services researchers, like Gordon and Rosenthal, use indicators like hospital outcomes to determine the significant aspects of health, illness, and health care. Most clinical health services studies consider disease comorbidity; that is, when clinical researchers examine health outcomes of patients, they need to think about coexisting diseases that might contribute to a particular patient's health outcome. Outcomes frequently refer to the end result of care or treatment in health services research, but can also be used by clinical researchers to refer to the result of a specific kind of intervention or intentional change in a specific kind of service or treatment. Most clinical researchers are medical practitioners with training in public health, epidemiology, or a health related field like sociology or psychology.

Here, Gordon and Rosenthal examine the importance of the variable marital status, a social support variable, on hospital outcomes. In their examination, they hold constant severity of disease, age, and other factors that might result in different health outcomes for patients who differ on those characteristics. As you read

through this selection, think about the kinds of questions Gordon and Rosenthal ask about the influence of marital status on hospital outcomes. Think about the relevance of this selection to those you read on caregiving and caretaking. These authors argue that marital status is an important aspect of health and healing outcomes. Consider their discussion in relation to issues of social suppport and what you know about informal caregiving.

It is increasingly recognized that patient outcomes are dependent on a complex web of biological, psychological, and social factors. Although outcome studies have traditionally focused on biological parameters of disease,[1-4] an emerging body of evidence has demonstrated that non-biological factors can have a profound impact on patient outcomes. Identification of non-biological factors is important for several reasons. First, these factors may be important in prognostic stratifi-

Table 36-1
Characteristics in 40,820 Study Patients According to Marital Status*

| | Marital Status | |
	Unmarried[†] (N=21,219)	Married (N=19,529)
Mean (±SD)		
Age, y	55±22	58±16
Gender		
Male	7654 (36)	11,068 (57)
Female	13,637 (64)	8461 (43)
Race		
White	10,489 (49)	15,638 (80)
Nonwhite	10,802 (51)	3891 (20)
Clinical service		
Medical	13,214 (62)	9850 (50)
Surgical	8077 (38)	9679 (50)
Admission severity of illness group		
0	7269 (34)	8217 (42)
1	5432 (26)	5116 (26)
2	5356 (25)	3967 (20)
3	2949 (14)	2072 (11)
4	285 (1)	157 (1)

*The difference between unmarried and married admissions is significant, $P<.001$. Unless otherwise indicated, values indicate number (percent).

†Includes divorced, widowed, and never-married patients.

cation and in developing methods for severity and case-mix adjustment. Second, these factors may have impact on the effectiveness of medical interventions and may alter the relative costs and benefits of treatments in individual patients. Moreover, these factors may be useful in identifying patients at higher risk of adverse outcomes and for targeting costly interventions to specific patients. Finally, identification of nonbiological factors may provide important insight into the pathophysiology of disease and weaknesses in the organization and delivery of health care.

Recently, several studies have shown that patients with lower levels of social support had worse outcomes. These studies found, for example, that patients who were unmarried,[5,6] living alone,[7] or socially isolated[8,9] had shorter survival and were at higher risk for recurrent illness—providing empirical evi-

dence of the importance of social support on longer-term patient outcomes.

Although a substantial number of outcomes studies have examined shorter-term outcomes of hospitalized patients and although several studies have identified patient and provider characteristics associated with hospital outcomes, little attention has been given to the potential impact of social support on hospital outcomes. Therefore, we conducted this study to determine the relationships between an important aspect of social support—marital status—and several key hospital outcomes after adjusting for admission, severity of illness and other covariates.

Results

The mean age of the 40,820 study patients was 56±19 years; 46 percent of the patients

Table 36-2
Hospital Outcomes in 23,064 Medical and 17,756 Surgical Patients According to Marital Status

Outcome	Patient Group	Marital Status	
		Unmarried*	Married
In-hospital deaths, No. (%)	Medical	617(4.7)	489(5.0)
	Surgical[†]	297(3.7)	244(2.5)
Discharges to nursing home, No. (%)[‡]	Medical[†]	794(6.3)	220(2.4)
	Surgical[†]	465(6.0)	152(1.6)
Mean (±SD) length of stay, d	Medical[†]	6.2±7.0	5.7±6.8
	Medical[†]	6.1±6.8	5.4±6.3
	Surgical[‖]	9.7±13.0	8.9±10.9
	Surgical[§&]	9.2±12.3	8.5±10.2
Mean (±SD) charges, [#]	Medical[†]	5403±6928	5313±7758
	Medical[†]	5176±6450	4906±6563
	Surgical[§]	12,065±19,483	11,640±16,141
	Surgical[§]	10,979±16,956	10,848±14,050

*Includes divorced, widowed, and never-married patients.
† The difference between unmarried and married patients is significant, P<.001.
‡ Excluding in-hospital deaths and patients admitted from nursing homes (N=39,105).
§ Excluding in-hospital deaths (N=39,173).
‖ The difference between unmarried and married patients is significant, P<.01.
& The difference between unmarried and married patients is significant, P<.05.
# Hospital charges were standardized based on mean charges in a nationally representative database.[16]

were men and 64 percent were white. The study sample included 21,291 (52 percent) unmarried and 19,529 (48 percent) married patients. Compared with married patients, unmarried patients were younger ($P<.001$) and were less likely ($P<.001$) to be male, white, and to have undergone a surgical procedure (Table 36-1). Unmarried patients also had higher admission severity of illness; 40 percent of unmarried patients had moderate to high severity of illness (admission severity groups, 2 through 4) compared with 32 percent of married patients ($P<.001$).

In-hospital death occurred in 4 percent of the study sample. Rates of death among surgical patients were higher in unmarried than in married patients (3.7 percent vs 2.5 percent, $P<.001$), but were not significantly different ($P=.30$) in unmarried and married medical patients (Table 36-2). Rates of nursing home discharge, however, were more than two-fold higher in unmarried than in married patients among both medical and surgical patients. The

mean length of stay was roughly 9 percent higher in unmarried patients among both medical and surgical patients, although mean charges were higher only in unmarried medical patients. After excluding in-hospital deaths, the mean length of stay in unmarried patients was 12 percent and 8 percent higher in medical and surgical patients, respectively, and the mean charges were higher only in unmarried medical patients.

Independent Association Between Marital Status and In-Hospital Death

To determine the independent association between marital status and in-hospital death, a series of multiple logistic regression analyses were performed to control for severity of illness and other covariates, including diagnosis, age, gender, and race. Among all study patients, the relative risk of death (as estimated by the multivariable OR) in unmarried compared with married patients was 1.08 and was not significantly different from 1.0 (Table 36-3). However,

Table 36-3
*Relative Risk of Death for Unmarried Patients Compared With Married Patients as Determined by Multiple Logistic Regression Analysis Controlling for Diagnosis, Age, Gender, Race, and Admission Severity of Illness**

Patient Group	No. of Patients/ No. Of Deaths	Multivariable Odds Ratio	95 % CI†	P
All	40,820/1647	1.08	0.96-1.22	.23
Medical				
All	23,064/1106	0.98	0.84-1.15	.82
Female	12,838/582	0.90	0.73-1.12	.36
Male	10,226/524	1.00	0.80-1.25	.99
Nonwhite	10,251/457	0.98	0.76-1.26	.88
White	12,813/649	1.00	0.82-1.21	.99
Age, y				
18-64	13,597/455	0.99	0.78-1.26	.96
≥65	9467/651	0.97	0.78-1.20	.78
Surgical				
All	17,756/541	1.30	1.06-1.58	.01
Female	9260/265	1.30	0.97-1.75	.08
Male	8496/276	1.27	0.95-1.68	.11
Nonwhite	4442/169	1.06	0.73-1.54	.77
White	13,314/372	1.38	1.09-1.75	.008
Age, y				
18-64	10,815/228	0.87	0.64-1.20	.41
≥65	6941/313	1.55	1.17-2.06	.003

* The risk of death is estimated by the multivariable odds ratio.
† CI indicates confidence interval.

in stratified analyses, the relative risk of death in unmarried patients was significantly higher among surgical patients (OR, 1.30; 95 percent confidence interval, 1.06 to 1.58). In further stratified analyses of surgical patients, the increased risk of death in unmarried patients was similar among men (OR, 1.27; 95 percent CI, 0.95 to 1.68) and women (OR, 1.30; 95 percent CI, 0.97 to 1.75) but differed according to age and race, being more than 1.0 ($P<.0l$) only among patients who were aged 65 years and older and among patients who were white. Among medical patients, the risk of death was similar in unmarried and married patients across all subgroups examined.

Further analyses (not shown) found that, among all subgroups, the relative risk of death was higher in never-married patients (OR, 1.16; 95 percent CI, 1.01 to 1.35) compared with married patients but was similar in divorced (OR, 1.05; 95 percent CI, 0.71 to 1.56) and widowed (OR, 1.04; 95 percent CI, 0.89 to 1.22) patients. As would be expected the increased risk of death in never-married patients was higher among surgical patients (OR, 1.33; 95 percent CI, 1.04 to 1.70) than among medical patients (OR, 1.09; 95 percent CI, 0.91 to 1.31).

Independent Associations Between Marital Status and Nursing Home Discharge

To determine the independent associations between marital status and nursing home discharge, a series of multiple logistic regression analyses were performed, again controlling for severity of illness and other covariates. Among all patients, the relative risk of nursing home discharge (as estimated by the multivariable OR) was 2.67 times higher ($P<.001$) for unmarried compared with married patients (Table 36-4). In stratified analyses, the relative risks of nursing home discharge for unmarried compared with married patients

Table 36-4
*Relative Risk of Nursing Home (NH) Discharge for Unmarried Patients Compared With Married Patients as Determined by Multiple Logistic Regression Analysis Controlling for Diagnosis, Age, Gender, Race, and Admission Severity of Illness**

Patient Group	No. Of Patients†/ No. of NH Discharges	Multivariable Odds Ratio	95 percent CI‡	P
All	39,105/1631	2.67	2.33-3.06	.001
Medical				
All	21,920/1014	2.45	2.07-2.92	.001
Female	12,224/705	2.11	1.68-2.66	.001
Male	9696/309	2.81	2.17-3.63	.001
Nonwhite	9788/417	2.16	1.60-2.91	.001
White	12,132/597	2.56	2.07-3.16	.001
Age, y				
18-64	13,138/141	4.29	2.72-6.78	.001
≥65	8782/873	2.02	1.67-2.45	.001
Surgical				
All	17,185/617	3.04	2.43-3.80	.001
Female	8974/449	2.36	1.77-3.15	.001
Male	8211/168	3.73	2.62-5.29	.001
Nonwhite	4263/134	1.71	1.04-2.81	.04
White	12,922/483	3.49	2.72-4.48	.001
Age, y				
18-64	10,577/78	5.24	3.03-9.07	.001
≥65	6608/539	2.32	1.80-3.00	.001

* The risk of nursing home discharge is estimated by the multivariable odds ratio.
† Excluding deaths and patients admitted from a nursing home.
‡ CI indicates confidence interval.

were 2.45 and 3.04 times higher (*P*<.001) among medical and surgical patients, respectively. In further stratified analyses, these relative risks remained significantly higher for unmarried patients among all subgroups (age, gender, and race) of medical and surgical patients examined (Table 36-4). Additionally the risk of nursing home discharge was significantly higher for divorced (OR, 1.89; 95 percent CI, 1.20 to 2.99), widowed (OR, 1.73; 95 percent CI, 1.50 to 2.00), and never-married (OR, 3.28; 95 percent CI, 2.83 to 3.81) patients compared with married patients when these groups were examined separately.

Independent Associations Between Marital Status and Length of Stay and Charges

To determine the independent associations between marital status and length of stay and total hospital charges, a series of multiple linear regression analyses were performed, again controlling for severity of illness, diagnosis, age, gender, and race. Among all study patients, multivariable models estimated that charges

and length of stay were 5 percent and 8 percent higher (*P*<.001), respectively, for unmarried compared with married patients (Table 36-5 and Table 36-6). Among medical patients, charges and length of stay were 6 percent and 9 percent higher (*P*<.001), respectively, for unmarried patients; these results were similar among men and women, white and nonwhite patients, and older and younger patients (Tables 36-5 and 36-6). Among surgical patients relative charges and length of stay were 4 percent and 7 percent higher (*P*<.001) for unmarried compared with married patients; results were similar in men, white and nonwhite patients, and younger patients (Tables 36-5 and 36-6). In additional multivariable analyses (not shown), exclusion of patients discharged to a nursing home (n=1679) did not change the relationship between marital status and charges or length of stay. For example, among all patients, after excluding discharges to a nursing home, charges and relative length of stay remained 5 percent and 7 percent higher (*P*<.001), respectively, for unmarried com-

Table 36-5
Relative Hospital Charges for Unmarried Patients Compared With Married Patients as Determined by Multiple Linear Regression Analysis Controlling for Diagnosis, Age. Gender, Race, and Admission Severity of Illness

Patient Group	Relative Charges	95 percent CI*	P
All	1.05	1.04–1.07	.001
Medical			
All	1.06	1.04–1.08	.001
Female	1.04	1.01–1.07	.004
Male	1.06	1.03–1.10	.001
Nonwhite	1.04	1.01–1.07	.02
White	1.07	1.05–1.10	.001
Age,y			
18–64	1.06	1.03–1.09	.001
≥65	1.05	1.02–1.08	.002
Surgical			
All	1.04	1.03–1.07	.001
Female	1.02	1.00–1.05	.10
Male	1.07	1.04–1.10	.001
Nonwhite	1.07	1.03–1.12	.002
White	1.03	1.01–1.06	.002
Age, y			
18–64	1.06	1.03–1.08	.001
≥65	1.03	1.00–1.07	.05

* CI indicates confidence interval.

Table 36-6
Relative Length of Stay for Unmarried Patients Compared With Married Patients as Determined by Multiple Linear Regression Analysis Controlling for Diagnosis, Age, Gender, Race, and Admission Severity of Illness

Patient Group	Relative Length of Stay	95 percent CI*	P
All	1.08	1.06–1.10	.001
Medical			
All	1.09	1.07–1.l1	.001
Female	1.06	1.03–1.10	.001
Male	1.10	1.06–1.14	.001
Nonwhite	1.06	1.02–1.09	.001
White	1.11	1.08–1.14	.001
Age, y			
18–64	1.09	1.05–1.12	.001
≥65	1.08	1.04–1.11	.001
Surgical			
All	1.07	1.05–1.10	.001
Female	l.04	1.01–1.07	.01
Male	1.11	1.07–1.15	.001
Nonwhite	1.11	1.05–1.17	.001
White	1.06	1.03–1.08	.001
Age, y			
18–64	1.07	1.04–1.11	.001
≥65	1.06	1.02–1.11	.001

* CI indicates confidence interval.

pared with married patients. Finally, in analyses examining specific subgroups of unmarried patients, charges and length of stay were 4 percent and 7 percent higher (*P*<.001), respectively, for widowed patients and 5 percent and 7 percent higher (*P*<.001), respectively, for never-married patients, but were not significantly different for divorced patients.

Comment

Social support has been increasingly recognized as an important determinant of patient outcomes in several longitudinal studies.[6,8] However, the impact of social support on outcomes in hospitalized patients has been poorly studied. Therefore we studied 40,820 discharges from an academic medical center from 1988 through 1991 to examine the relationships between marital status and several hospital outcomes. We emphasize five findings. First, compared with married patients unmarried patients tended to have higher admission severity of illness, using a validated and widely used commercial method. Second, unmarried patients were more than 2.5 times more likely to be discharged to nursing homes. Third, unmarried patients had an 8 percent higher mean length of stay and 5 percent higher mean charges. Fourth, unmarried patients who underwent surgical procedures had a 30 percent higher risk of in-hospital death, after adjusting for age, severity of illness, and other potential covariates. Finally, these differences tended to be greatest among patients who were never married.

While marital status alone does not fully measure the entire spectrum of social support, marital status is commonly recorded among hospitalized patients and has been used in prior studies as a proxy measure of social support.[5,7,18] Moreover, it is likely that married patients have more complex social networks than unmarried patients. Thus, we suspect our findings are, in large measure, related to several aspects of social support. First, married patients may be more likely to have a caregiving spouse or child, which may allow for earlier discharge home and/or obviate the need for nursing home entry. Second, married patients may have higher levels of advocacy, which may lead to better access to medical care, encouragement to seek medical care earlier in the course of illness, better communication to medical staff of present and prior medical history, and improved compliance with treatment. Third, married patients are likely to have higher socioeconomic support that may lead to more timely and effective medical care. Finally, spousal support may modify or alleviate emotional stress that may produce physiologic benefit by unknown neural and/or neurohumoral pathways, as recently reviewed by Bucher.[19]

Alternatively, our findings may reflect differences in the quality or aggressiveness of care received by married and unmarried patients. Physicians and nurses may make different treatment decisions for married and unmarried patients, as a direct result of differences in spousal or family support. Our findings may also reflect differences in unmeasured severity of illness or comorbidity between married and unmarried patients, independent of differences in treatment or social support. We suggest that to understand the differences in outcomes between married and unmarried patients observed in this study, future studies of hospital patients directly measure specific aspects of social support, as well as potential differences in patient management and/or quality of care.

Notes

1. Brewster, A. C., Karlin, B. G., Hyde, L. A., Jacobs, C. M., Bradbury, R. C., and Chae, Y.M. MedisGroups: a clinically based approach to classifying hospital patients at admission. *Inquiry*. 1985;22:377–387.

2. Iezzoni, L. I. and Moskowitz, M. A. A clinical assessment of MedisGroups. JAMA. 1988;260:3159–3163.

3. Knaus, W. A., Wagner, D. P., Draper, E. A. et al. The Apache III prognostic system: risk prediction of hospital mortality for critically ill hospitalized adults. *Chest*. 1991;100:1619–1636.

4. Charlson, M. E., Pompei, P., Ales, K. L., and MacKennzie, C. R. A new method of classifying prognostic comorbidity in longitudinal studies: development and validation. *J Chronic Dis*. 1987;40:373–383.

5. Williams, R. B., Barefoot, J. C., Califf, R. M. et al. Prognostic importance of social and economic resources among medically treated patients with angiographically documented coronary artery disease. *JAMA*. 1992; 267:520–524.

6. Berkman, L. F. and Syme, S. L. Social networks, host resistance, and mortality: nine-year follow-up study of Alameda county residents. *Am J Epidemiol*. 1979;109:186–204.

7. Case, R. S., Moss, A. J., Case, N., McDermott, M., and Eberly, S. Living alone after myocardial infarction: impact on prognosis. *JAMA*. 1992;267:515–519.

8. Welin, L., Tibblin, G., Svardsudd, K. et al. Prospective study of social influences on mortality: the study of men born in 1913 and 1923. *Lancet*. 1985;1:915–918.

9. Ruberman, W., Weinblatt, E., Goldberg, J. D. and Chaudhary, B. S. Psychosocial influences on mortality after myocardial infarction. *N Engl J Med*. 1984;311:552–559.

10. Rosenthal, G. E., Landefeld, C. S. Do older Medicare patients cost hospitals more? Evidence from an academic medical center. *Arch Intern Med*. 1993;153:89–96.

11. Epstein, A. M., Stern, R. S., Weissman, J. S. Do the poor cost more? a multihospital study of patients' socioeconomic status and the use of hospital resources. *N Engl J Med*. 1990;322:1122–1128.

12. Rich, E. C., Gifford, G., Luxenberg, M., Dowd, B. The relationship of house staff experience to the cost and quality of inpatient care. *JAMA*. 1990;263:953–957.

13. Healthcare Knowledge Resources. *Hospital Inpatient Charges, 1990. Cost Containment Series*. Ann Arbor, Mich: Healthcare Knowledge Resources; 1992.

14. SAS Institute Inc. The logistic procedure. In: *SAS/STAT User's Guide, Version 6*. Cary, NC: SAS Institute Inc; 1989;1071–1126.

15. SAS Institute Inc. The GLM procedure. In: *SAS/STAT Users Guide. Version 6*. Cary, NC: SAS Institute Inc; 1989;891–996.

16. Jencks, S. F., Kay, T. Do frail, disabled, poor, and very old Medicare beneficiaries have higher hospital charges? *JAMA*. 1987;257:198–202.

17. Searle, S. R. *Linear Models*. New York, NY: John Wiley & Sons Inc; 1971.

18. Chandra, V., Szklo, M., Goldberg, R., Tonascia, J. The impact of marital status on survival after an acute myocardial infarction: a population-based study. *Am J Epidemiol*. 1983;117:320–325.

19. Bucher, J. C. Social support and prognosis following first myocardial infarction. *J Gen Intern Med*. 1994;9:409–417.

Further Reading

Colleen L. Johnson. 1985. "The Impact of Illness on Late-Life Marriages." *Journal of Marriage and the Family* 47: 165–172.

Leonard Pearlin and Carmi Schooler. 1978. "The Structure of Coping." *Journal of Health and Social Behavior* 19: 2–21.

Peggy Thoits. 1986. "Multiple Identities: Examining Gender and Marital Status Differences in Distress." *American Sociological Review* 51: 259–272.

Discussion Questions

1. What do Gordon and Rosenthal suggest about the relationship between marital status and health outcomes?

2. What do Gordon's and Rosenthal's findings suggest about marital status and informal caregiving?

3. What differences do you see in the way these health services researchers examine social support and in the discussions in the previous section by Emily Abel and Karen Lyman?

Organizing Systems of Health Care

37

Why the U.S. Health Care System Does Not Respond to People's Needs

Vicente Navarro

The idea that human beings are affected by environmental factors is an old one. The conception that environmental factors include characteristics like gender, race, class, and age is more contemporary. In this selection, Vicente Navarro examines the link between social class and health care. He underscores the significance of social class interests at every level of health care— at the level of individual status, health care provision, health care decision-making, and in the composition of governing bodies. Navarro locates experiences of illness and health in the contemporary fabric of United States society, making relevant comparisons with other countries. His Marxist emphasis on social class establishes a perspective for considering the differential distribution of disease by class within the United States.

Current debates about the accessibility of health care in the United States suggest that

health care is now more accessible than ever before; still, Navarro's discussion challenges this notion of accessibility with critical analysis of the U.S. class system. He raises questions about inequities in illness and health structured into the provision of health services in the United States. Consider how Navarro's data on lack of health insurance are correlated with reports of illness and poor health outcomes in United States society described in previous selections.

Health care in the United States is in a state of profound crisis. In 1992 the United States spent $838 billion ($3,010 per person) on health services. No other country in the world spent such a large amount, which came to 14 percent of the Gross National Product, or GNP, almost double the average for capitalist countries with similar levels of economic development. Yet despite this high level of expenditure, 38 million Americans—17 percent of the population—have *no* health benefits, another 50 million have major gaps in their benefits, and the overwhelming majority do not have comprehensive coverage (see Figure 37-1). The average annual cost for long-term care is $27,243, far more than a family earning the median income ($30,000) can afford. Not surprisingly, the inability to pay for health care is the primary cause of personal bankruptcy in this country. People are constantly denied care because they cannot pay their medical bills, or their health benefits are dropped because they cannot pay their health premiums or because they cost their employers or insurers too much. David Himmelstein and Steffie Woolhandler of Harvard University estimate that 100,000 people in the

Figure 37-1
Who Are the Uninsured?

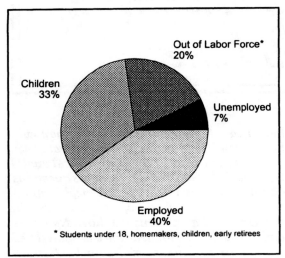

United States die each year from lack of care—three times as many as die from AIDS.

High costs and insufficient coverage are the key characteristics of the U.S. health care non-system, the most inefficient and inhuman of any health care system in any developed capitalist country. The United States and South Africa are the only major countries whose governments do not provide a national health program that guarantees access to health care in time of need. Health care in the United States is not a right; it is a privilege. At a time when the U.S. government declares that it is the great defender of human rights around the world, it continues to ignore this basic right at home. Forty years after the United Nations passed the Declaration of Human Rights, which includes—among other things—the right to access to health care, the U.S. government does not guarantee a right that is guaranteed in most other developed countries. Why?

In order to understand this situation, we must look not only at the practice of medicine but at the society of which this practice is a component. In other words, in order to understand the tree—the health sector—we must study the forest—the society we live in. We therefore have to start our analysis by focusing on the social, economic, and political forces that shape our society and that also

shape its health care, including its organization and its funding. This point cannot be overemphasized.

How can we go about understanding this context? This is a good question, and it has a complex answer.

First we need to understand power and how it is distributed. Power is very unevenly distributed. Most of us recognize, for example, that blacks, Hispanics, and other minorities in the United States have less power than whites, and that women have less power than men. Race and gender are categories of power, and much has been written about how racism and sexism continue to operate in the society at large, as well as in its health care system.

But the United States is divided not only by race and gender, but also by *class*. Class is the most important category of power for understanding U.S. society and its system of medicine. Yet class is rarely discussed in either the scientific literature or the mainstream media. It is considered an almost "un-American" category. Yet in other countries, class is considered an extremely important category for understanding how people live, work, dress, vote, enjoy themselves, get sick, and die. In the United States, however, the category of class disappears: the majority of the population is supposed to be in the middle. It is accepted that there are extremes—the rich and the poor—but most Americans are believed to belong to the middle class.

But the United States does have classes. How people live, get sick, and die, as well as the type of health care that they receive, depends not only on their race and gender but primarily on the class to which they belong.

Understanding the class structure of the United States and how it is reproduced over time is of enormous importance if we are to understand U.S. society and its health sector.

The U.S. Class Structure

At the top is a very small group (not more than 1.3 percent of the population) that has enormous power. This is what we can call the corporate class, and it includes individuals whose incomes come primarily from property rather than work. This class is predominantly white and its leaders are predominantly male.

The next group is the middle class. Contrary to popular belief, the middle class does not constitute the majority of Americans, although it is much larger than the corporate class. It includes professionals, small business people, self-employed shopkeepers, artisans, and so on.

The largest group is the working class, which includes almost 75 percent of the population. This is a class whose occupational structure and race and gender composition have changed over the past fifty years. The blue-collar sector of the working class—those working in heavy manufacturing—has declined, while the service sector has grown dramatically. The health sector is the fastest growing sector in the economy, and the health care industry is now the largest employer in the country. The total number of jobs in this sector increased by 639,000 from May 1990 through May 1992, while the total number of jobs *fell* by almost 1.8 million.

At the same time there has been a change from a predominantly white male working class to one in which women and minorities represent more than half of all wage earners. Changes in the labor force in the health care industry reflect the changes in the racial and gender make up of the working class as a whole. Today, most workers in the health sector are women, and 28 percent are minorities.

In the analysis of the U.S. class structure, we can see two striking phenomena that typify our society. One is the enormous concentration of wealth at the top. To cite just one statistic, the top one percent of the population, members of the corporate or capitalist class, owns 40 percent of all the property in this country, including stocks, bonds, and private land.

The other key characteristic of the U.S. class structure is the concentration of income at the top. Nobel Prize winner Paul Samuelson, in his book *Economics*, wrote that "If we made today an income pyramid out of a child's blocks, with each layer portraying $1,000 of income, the peak would be far higher than the Eiffel Tower, but almost all of us would be within a yard of the ground."[1]

The social class structure is different in each of the three major sectors of the economy—the monopolistic sector, the competitive sector, and the state sector.

Of the three sectors, the monopolistic sector is the most influential. It includes the large financial and manufacturing companies and is the world of "corporate America"—the fortune 500 companies and other large employers. This sector employs approximately 25 percent of the labor force. A few companies control each specific area of production or services. A key industry in this sector is the insurance industry, which plays, as we shall see, a very important role in the financing of health services.

The second sector, the market or competitive sector, used to be the largest of the three sectors in terms of both employment and economic activity, but it has declined over the past thirty years. This sector is generally labor intensive and local or regional in scope. The labor force is scattered in small units and seldom unionized. Examples are small businesses, restaurants, drugstores, and, in the medical sector, fee-for-service solo or group practices.

The third major sector is the state (or government) sector, which is in turn divided into two subsectors. In the public service subsector, the government both funds and provides services—an example is the Public Health Service. It does this at all levels of government, federal, state, and local. The other subsector—the contractual subsector—includes those activities that the government funds but that are delivered by the private sector under contract. For the most part, the government contracts with the monopolistic sector—the defense industry is a prime example. The United States, unlike most developed capitalist countries, does not have a nationalized defense industry that produces armaments; instead the government contracts with large corporations for their manufacture. Two other examples of this type of contractual arrangement between the government and the private sector are Medicare (the federal program that funds health care for the elderly) and Medicaid (the federal program for the medically indigent). These, along with other federal and state health pro-

Table 37-1
Major Manufacturing and Service Companies Operating in the Health Care Industry

Company	Fortune 500 Rank (1984)	Sales (billions $)	Major Areas of Production	Medical Production
IBM	6	45.0	Controls 60 percent U.S. computer, business typewriter, office equipment market	No. 1 in hospital computer market
General Electric	9	27.0	Consumer, industrial, military, technical systems; no. 6 contractor to Pentagon ($4.5 billion in sales); no. 2 producer of nuclear reactors	Diagnostic-imaging equipment; CAT scanners, X-ray, ultrasound, MRI
McDonnell-Douglas	34	9.5	Military and commercial aircraft; F-4 Phantom and F-15 Eagle: DC-9 and DC-10; no. 1 Pentagon defense contractor ($7.7 billion)	Health Services Division, formerly McAuto, fiscal intermediary for NYC Medicaid; acquired Science Dynamics Corp., renamed McDonnell-Douglas Physicians Systems, specializing in medical data bases and electronic claims-processing capabilities
Honeywell	56	6.0	Computer, information, and data systems in aerospace and defense; spacecraft; military and commercial aircraft; 10 percent of business with Pentagon	Controls 5 percent of hospital patient monitoring market; 1981 joint venture with NV Philips, manufacturing medical electronic systems
Siemens AG*	—	14.5	Germany's leading technology firm; world's third largest in telecommunications; supplying Brazil with 4 nuclear reactors	World's largest supplier of X-ray equipment and other diagnostic-imaging machinery
Avon Products	127	3.0	World's largest direct-selling business; cosmetics, toiletries, fragrances	Purchased Malinckrodt in 1982, producer of radiopharmaceuticals, X-ray contrast

*German-based multinational

grams, make up 42 percent of all expenditures in the health sector. The government contracts with private service providers or with health insurance companies for the delivery of health care to the private sector. Most hospitals and physicians are private, and many of the facilities, equipment, drugs, and other commodities used in the health services are also produced and provided by private companies. As Table 37-1 shows, most of the major suppliers to the health sector are also major suppliers to the defense industry.

These corporations are major components of both the military-industrial and medical-industrial complexes. Other components of the medical-industrial complex, besides the medical and hospital equipment industries, are the insurance companies, the drug companies, the hospitals, and the medical professional associations. These are the dominant power holders in the health sector.

The Insurance Industry in the Health Sector

Insurance companies (such as Prudential and John Hancock) write more than 50 percent of the health insurance premiums in this country. They are referred to in the health sector as the *commercial health insurance companies* to distinguish them from the *voluntary health insurance companies*, or the Blues, which until the 1960s controlled most of the premiums. The Blues' share of the private health insurance market dropped from

45 percent in 1965 to 33 percent in 1986, and it continues to decline.

The Blues were established during the Depression of the 1930s by the hospitals (which established Blue Cross) and the American Medical Association (which established Blue Shield) in order to ensure that hospitals and physicians would not run out of patients. For an annual payment—called a premium—these two groups promised to cover many, although not all, of the health care needs of those they insured. Working people could afford to pay a fixed (and at that time, small) amount of money for premiums but could not afford to pay doctors' fees for every service they needed. Later on, after the Depression, the price of premiums increased considerably, but the system of prepayment remained. Blue Cross has continued to be the insurance instrument of the hospital industry and Blue Shield of the medical profession.

Blue Cross pays the hospitals for their "reasonable" costs, leaving the hospitals to define what is reasonable. Blue Shield pays physicians according to "usual and customary" fees; if these are not too far from the fees of other physicians in the area, Blue Shield will pay. Such a generous physician reimbursement policy does not exist anywhere else in the world.

The Blues were given tax exempt status in return for their agreement to offer coverage based on an average premium for the community in which they operated, rather than requiring sicker people to pay higher premiums and healthy people to pay lower premiums. But once the commercial insurance companies began to enter the health premium market, the Blues were forced to compete for customers. This forced them to choose only customers who would be "good risks"—healthy people who would not need expensive care. Before long both the Blues and the commercial insurers were avoiding the sick and vulnerable and favoring the young and healthy. In 1986, Congress, recognizing this development, withdrew the Blues' tax exemption.

There is a great deal of competition between the Blues and the commercial insurance companies over control of the premium market. The commercials have been winning the battle, since the insurance companies have far more economic and political influence than the Blues. The large commercial insurance companies are not just health insurers—health is but one piece of their business. Their assets are enormous: Prudential has $116 billion in assets; Metropolitan Life, $94 billion; Aetna, $49 billion; Connecticut General, $31 billion; Travellers, $30 billion; and so on. The boards of directors of the insurance companies are filled with the world's wealthiest people. To take only one example, James Lynn, chief executive officer of Aetna, earned an astounding $23 million in 1990. In 1992, President Clinton's candidate for attorney general, Zoë Baird, made $1.5 million as a vice-president of Aetna.

The dominance of the insurance companies in the health care sector has meant that they, rather than the providers of care, are the ones who have a commanding voice in that sector. As a result, it is frequently not physicians and other health professionals who decide what their patients need; it is the insurance companies. What many people do not realize is that any procedures a physician recommends must be approved by the patient's insurance company. A physician can spend up to an hour a day seeking permission to do what he or she considers best for the patient. The insurance companies base their decision on their own criteria of cost-effectiveness, which are not disclosed to either the patient or the physician. This degree of intrusion into the physician-patient relationship by a third party—the insurance company—is unheard of in other countries.

The Power of the Insurance Industry

Table 37-2 shows PAC contributions from the health industry during 1992 elections. The insurance companies—the commercials and the Blues—as well as the other components of the medical-industrial complex, such as the medical-provider lobbies, the hospital lobbies, the equipment and pharmaceutical lobbies, among others, are the main forces responsible for the fact that the United States is the only major capitalist country without a national health program that guarantees universal and comprehensive health benefits to our population. The overwhelming majority of the population is dissatisfied with health care in this country, and 82 percent wants major and profound changes in the system of funding health care.[2] By a majority or large plurality, Americans since 1952—when the Gallup polls first asked this question—have wanted the federal government to finance health care. But they still do not have it. Back in the 1970s, the labor unions and their allies in Congress—Senator Edward Kennedy and Congresswoman Martha Griffiths—put forward a proposal for a national health program that would cover everyone and would be financed by the federal government, which would then contract directly with the providers of health services (as is done in Canada). The government would be the *single payer for health services*, eliminating the insurance companies. Need-

less to say, the insurance lobbies and their close friends in Congress mobilized to stop that proposal.

We saw the enormous political influence of the insurance companies during the 1992 election campaign. Even though the majority of Americans would prefer a health system like the Canadian one, not one of the candidates dared to propose it, afraid of antagonizing the insurance industry and the medical-industrial complex. Even Tom Harkin, considered one of the most liberal members of the Senate, remained silent about the need to establish a national health program, emphasizing instead—as a cop-out—the need to improve our "preventive services." Harkin received $270,404 from the medical-insurance PACs, which may explain his deafening silence on one of the major topics of the campaign. Similarly, the directors of the health

Table 37-2
Major PAC Contributors

Political action committees that contributed the most money to candidates in the 1992 election

National Association of Realtors	$2,950,138
National Medical Association	2,936,086
International Brotherhood of Teamsters	2,442,552
Association of Trial Lawyers of America	2,336,135
National Education Association	2,323,122

Political action committees in the health industry that contributed the most money to candidates in the 1992 election

American Medical Association	$2,936,086
American Dental Association	1,420,958
American Academy of Ophthalmology	801,527
American Chiropractic Association	641,746
American Hospital Association	505,888
American Podiatry Association	401,000
American Optometric Association	398,366
American Health Care Association	382,019
American College of Emergency Physicians	330,725
American Nurses Association	306,519
Association for the Advancement of Psychology	273,743
American Physical Therapy Association	198,941
Eli Lilly & Company	195,530
Pfizer Inc.	188,100
Schering-Plough Corporation	186,050

components of both the Bush and Clinton campaigns were Washington lobbyists for the insurance companies. The Republican's chief health advisor was Deborah Steelman, a lobbyist representing the Pharmaceutical Manufacturers Association, Aetna Life and Casualty, and others. The Democrat's chief health advisor was Bruce Fried, also a lobbyist for the major health insurance companies.

The corrupting influence of corporate America over the political process is encouraged by the "revolving door"—the movement of former politicians and the staff of the major health-related congressional committees to jobs in the medical industrial complex. The majority of Washington lobbyists for the medical-industrial complex once worked in the Congress and have retained close contacts there.

Former President Ronald Reagan used to work for the American Medical Association and opposed the establishment of Medicare. In a phonograph record sent by the AMA to doctors' wives, Reagan warned: "If you and I don't stop Medicare we will spend our sunset years telling our children and children's children what it was like in America when men were free."[3] Both former President Bush and former Vice-President Dan Quayle used to work for the pharmaceutical industry.

The U.S. Constitution starts with that splendid sentence, "We, the People. . ." To be accurate, we should add a footnote that would read "and the medical-industrial complex." The latter has a far greater voice than the people in deciding what can and cannot be done in the health sector.

Class Control of the Health Care Institutions

The corporate class's control over the health care sector does not begin and end with its control of funding; it continues with control over the health care institutions themselves and over the political institutions that influence how these work. Money, the energy that moves the system, passes through institutional channels that are controlled, or heavily influenced, by groups that are similar, although not identical, to those

that have dominant influence in the funding of those institutions.

Who controls the health care institutions, such as the medical research foundations, teaching hospitals, voluntary hospitals, and others? The question is difficult to answer. There are many groups that shape these institutions, but one that has enormous power is the board of directors (or trustees, or executive board) of each institution. These boards not only set policy, but generally appoint the executive officers and many members of upper level management in these institutions. Listen to Abraham Flexner, author of the famous *Flexner Report*, which established medical education in the United States as we know it today. Flexner wrote that "the influence of the board of trustees of the university determines in the social and economic realms an atmosphere of timidity, which is not without effect on critical appointments and promotions."[4] Feminists have long been aware of this point and have rightly called for a change in the gender composition of the boards of directors of our health institutions. Blacks, Hispanics, and other minorities have been equally aware of the problems of having all-white boards and have demanded a change in their racial and ethnic composition so that they will better reflect the diversity of the communities they serve.

But the issue of the class composition of these boards is seldom raised. Figure 37-2 compares the class composition of the United States as a whole with the class composition of the boards of trustees of the top ten medical research foundations, the private medical teaching institutions, the state medical teaching institutions, and the voluntary hospitals.

The figure shows vividly the enormous overrepresentation of the corporate and upper middle classes and the dramatic underrepresentation of the majority of the population—members of the lower middle and working classes. Further, the small changes in the gender and racial/ethnic composition of these boards have not had much effect on their class composition. Only in the case of the voluntary not-for-profit hospitals do members of the working class appear on

Figure 37-2
Social Class and Gender Compositions of U.S. Labor Force, Health Labor Force, and Boards of Trustees in the Health Sector

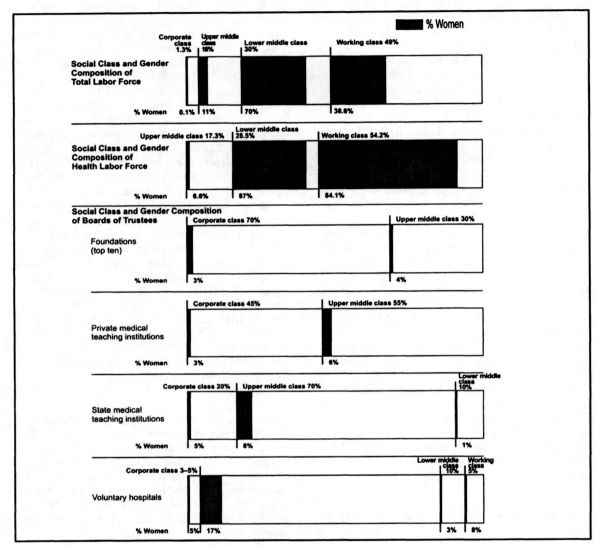

these boards. As R.M. MacIver has written, "The typical board member is associated with large-scale business, a banker, a manufacturer, business executive or prominent lawyer."[5]

You could say—and it has often been said—that there is a justifiable explanation for the class control of these institutions: members of the corporate class are needed to raise funds for the institution. But while that may have been the case in the past, it is not anymore.

Most of the funding of the leading private teaching institutions is overwhelmingly public—in other words, the funds come from the majority of the American people, ordinary folks who are not represented on the boards of directors.

This class discrimination is not only the least recognized type of discrimination in the United States, but it is the most persistent and continuous form of discrimination.

There has been an improvement in the representation of women and African-Americans in the medical student body. Although these changes are too timid, at least something is being done to correct this discrimination. The strongest, most persistent, and unchangeable form of discrimination is class discrimination. In 1920, only 12 percent of all medical students came from families at or below the median family income—that is, in the lower economic half of the population. This percentage remained the same in 1992, seventy years later. This is a discrimination that very few people talk about.

Class Power And The State in the Health Sector

Having described the patterns of class dominance over the financing of health care and the administration of health care institutions, let me now touch on a third component of what is going on in the health care sector. This is the class influence on the government, including its executive, legislative, and judicial branches. According to official rhetoric, the U.S. government represents the voice of the people. As one widely used textbook put it, "In our nation, political power reflects the will of all people, not the will of a few at the top."[6]

The reality, however, is otherwise. The overwhelming majority of senators are members of the corporate and upper middle classes. The same applies to the cabinet. Business was the largest single occupational group in cabinet positions from 1989 to 1990: of all the cabinet members during this period, more than 80 percent had been in business of one sort or another. This situation persists in President Clinton's cabinet. In spite of Clinton's populist message, sustained throughout his presidential campaign, seven of his cabinet members are lawyers with close ties to corporate America. All seven made more than $1 million before being appointed.

The same pattern of class domination holds for the House. A total of 102 congresspeople held stock and well-paying executive positions in banks or other financial institutions, and 81 received regular income from law firms that generally represented big business. Sixty-three percent got income from

stock in the top defense contractors; 45 percent from the giant (and federally regulated) oil and gas industries; 22 percent from radio and television companies; 11 percent from commercial airlines and 9 percent from railroads. Ninety-eight congresspeople were involved in numerous capital gains transactions.

It is important to note that while much has been written about the limited representation of women, and of blacks and other minorities, in top political positions, almost nothing has been written about the very limited class representation in these same bodies.

Some might argue that while there is indeed a pattern of class domination in our major political institutions, they are still representative because these politicians were elected by the majority of citizens, who are, as we saw earlier, mostly working class. The problem with this argument is that the majority of the working class does not vote. People are fully aware of the enormous power that corporate America has over their political institutions: 72 percent, according to a recent *New York Times* poll, believe that the Congress represents powerful economic interests rather than ordinary people.[7] In fact, barely half of the population of voting age goes to the polls in presidential-year Congressional elections (52 percent in 1988 and 54 percent in 1992) and less than half in non-presidential-year Congressional elections (38 percent in 1990). Since the half that votes is predominantly the upper economic half, we can conclude that the lower half, which includes the majority of the working class, does not vote.

Diversity Within the Dominant Classes and the Health Policy Debate

There is, however, a diversity of interests within the dominant classes, a diversity that is evident in the proposals for reforming the health care system put forward by different groups. For example, large financial capital (such as the major insurance companies) has different interests than manufacturing companies or medical practitioners (as represented by the AMA). These differences cause conflict. It is these conflicts between different corporate interest groups that are at the center of the de-

432 Section 5 ◆ *Social and Cultural Structures of Care*

bate on health care reform. The large insurance companies support the "managed competition" model, a solution first put forward by Alain Enthoven (former deputy director of defense under Robert McNamara when he was directing the Vietnam war and later health advisor to Prime Minister Margaret Thatcher on her plan to privatize the National Health Service in Great Britain). According to the managed competition proposal, which is supported by the insurance companies, the AMA, the *New York Times*, and the Clinton-Gore administration, employees would have to enroll in insurance-operated health care plans chosen for them by their employers. The employees could expect to see their choice of providers, and their benefits, dramatically reduced.

A few corporate leaders, however, including those in such industries as automobile manufacturing, want the government to play a direct role in controlling the costs because these have become so high. For instance, employee health benefits are a larger component of the cost of a car than the steel it is built from: $700 of the cost of a car now goes to pay for health benefits, compared to only $200 in Canada or Japan. Further, large employers have come to realize that the growing cost of health insurance is cutting into company profits, at least in the short term. In the long term, of course, they can pass these costs on to workers by cutting wages. In fact, the growth in the cost of health benefits is the primary reason wages in the United States have remained constant since 1972. As noted by the Congressional Budget Office, "Since 1973, the increased costs for health care and other benefits have absorbed most of the gains in inflation-adjusted compensation, leaving little room for wages and salaries."[8]

Conflicts between workers and employers over health benefits were the primary cause of strikes in 1991 and 1992. This situation led large employers to provide their own health insurance rather than contracting out to the insurance companies. Today 60 percent of all employers self-insure their employees. This means that they have health insurance departments that administer health care benefits in order to control costs directly—rather than indirectly through the insurance companies. These employers were primarily re-sponsible for the ERISA law, which allows an employer to curtail, reduce, or even eliminate health benefits for any employee who, because of a chronic condition such as AIDS, has health care costs that the employer considers too excessive for it to sustain. What this means is that an employee whose employer is self-insured has no medical security. This situation, recognized as legal by the Supreme Court, faces millions of workers who think that they have benefits until the moment they really need them—at which point they are dropped from their employers' health plan. Capitalism in the United States is a rough, cruel capitalism, a capitalism without gloves. You can see that there is a diversity of interests within the dominant classes in which insurance companies have different interests from large employers, which, in turn, have different interests from the medical trade and professional associations.

Despite the diversity of proposals for health care reform, there is a bias in the system that explains why some proposals have a far better chance than others, depending on whether or not they conflict with the structure of power that sustains the interests of the various groups. As one perceptive observer has written, the "flaw in the pluralist heaven is that the heavenly chorus sings with a very special accent . . . the system is askew, loaded and unbalanced in favor of a fraction of a minority."[9] The political debate that reflects this pluralism takes place within the framework of a common understanding and acceptance of certain premises and assumptions that consistently benefit some classes rather than others.

Even though a large plurality or a majority of people have, since 1952, wanted a health care system in which the health services are allocated according to need rather than ability to pay, none of the proposals put forward by the White House or by the congressional leadership has even come close to suggesting such a system. This is a clear sign of class dominance.

The Origins of Employment-based Health Coverage

Understanding class dominance is of paramount importance not only for understanding why the United States does not have a national health plan, but also for understanding why health benefits are provided through the workplace. In 1989, for instance, 56.9 percent of workers received health benefits through their jobs. Why? To answer this question, we must go back to the late 1940s and early 1950s, the period after World War II. The U.S. working class made enormous sacrifices during World War II. It was a war against fascism and nazism, a war for a better future for working people and their children. Not surprisingly, then, at the end of the war people's expectations were high: they believed that their sacrifices had to have served a purpose. Powerful groups were asking for a redistribution of wealth, for the nationalization of banking, and for the establishment of a national health program run by the government. Working people were pushing for these demands, demands that threatened the capitalist and upper middle classes. In response to this threat, these classes developed an aggressive anti-working-class campaign. Congress, where the dominant classes had enormous influence, led the fight. The targets included progressive individuals in all areas of political, social, and academic life. That campaign—called McCarthyism—was brutal.

In 1947, Congress passed the Taft-Hartley Act, which—among other things—outlawed sympathy strikes: for instance, coal miners could not go out on strike in support of steel workers. In other words, class pressure was outlawed. In no other Western developed capitalist country do workers face such restrictions. Indeed, it is not unusual to see a whole city—or even a whole country—in Europe paralyzed by a general strike, in which *all* the workers go on strike in support of demands that would benefit the majority of workers and their families. In the United States, a general strike is forbidden.

The Taft-Hartley Act also mandated that workers and their unions obtain health benefits from their employers through the collective bargaining process rather than, as in Europe, through the state. In other words, the unions had to negotiate the employers' payment of health insurance premiums for the workers and their families. This has meant that workers and their unions have to pressure their employers to get or to extend health benefits. Needless to say, wherever unions are strong, health benefits are extensive; where they are weak—as they are in most sectors of the economy—health benefits are limited.

The United States is therefore the only country in the developed world where workers and their families lose their health benefits when they lose their jobs. Relating health benefits to employment is an enormously effective way to discipline labor. Even changing jobs may mean changing the level of health benefits. According to a *New York Times*/CBS poll conducted in August 1991, 32 percent of working people stayed in jobs they did not like for fear of losing their health benefits.[10] The current shift from high-wage to low-wage, from union to non-union, and from full-time to part-time jobs has also meant a shift from good health benefits (in high-wage, unionized, and full-time jobs) to poor or nonexistent coverage (in low-wage, non-unionized, and part-time jobs). This shift was particularly large in the 1980s, during the Reagan/Bush years, when class aggression against the working class intensified. In 1979, 14.6 percent of the population (or 28.4 million people) did not have *any* form of health benefits. By 1985, this number had grown to 17.5 percent (36.8 million people). The majority were workers and their children. Thirteen percent of all full-time workers are uninsured. Most work for small employers who do not want, or cannot afford, to pay health benefits for their employees. Only 39 percent of small firms (those with twenty-five or less employees) offer health insurance to their workers, compared with 99 percent of firms with one hundred or more employees.

The same *New York Times*/CBS poll showed that 44.7 percent of those who change jobs or whose employment is for some reason interrupted did not have any form of health benefits for up to twenty-eight months. This percentage was even higher for blacks and Hispanics, who tend to be concentrated in low-wage nonunion jobs. Twenty percent of African-Americans and 33 percent of Hispanics are uninsured. Millions of people have loved ones who are sick and are not able to do anything about it because they cannot afford medical care.

But the problem does not end there. Compounding this inhuman situation is the huge reduction in benefits for working people that occurred during the 1980s. There was an almost 50 percent reduction in the hourly benefits (in dollar amounts) paid by employers for health insurance from 1980 to 1989 (from $1.63 per hour in 1980 to $0.85 in 1989), which led to a significant reduction in health care benefits for the majority of working people. In other words, during the 1980s, workers were not only growing more afraid of losing their jobs, and thus their health coverage, but even those who kept their jobs saw their benefits significantly reduced. This was the direct result of linking health care benefits to employment, and it is the situation that is favored by large employers.

All these realities are the result of class power—the power of the dominant class—which is a power unparalleled in any other major capitalist country. Let me give you an example of how unparalleled that power is. We recently saw how Prime Minister Margaret Thatcher had to resign because of her growing unpopularity, which was largely due to the imposition of what the British call a poll tax. According to Thatcher's proposal, local services were to be financed by a flat tax on each household, so that rich households and working-class households would both pay the same amount. The Labour Party loudly denounced the poll tax and mobilized so much opposition that Thatcher was forced out of office.

Yet in this country most of us are forced to pay for health care according to a system that is not unlike the poll tax: every employee in a particular business or industry pays the same amount (we call it a premium rather than a poll tax) for their health benefits, regardless of income. Thus the chairman of Bethlehem Steel, whose annual salary is $1.2 million, pays approximately the same premium for himself and his family as does the unskilled black or white steelworker in one of his mills, in spite of the fact that his income is forty times larger. And it is the Democratic Party that is leading the way in expanding rather than changing this profoundly regressive way of funding health care.

In the United Kingdom, as well as in all the other developed capitalist countries, workers have fought to divorce health benefits from the job and to make the funding of benefits progressive. This is why the overwhelming majority of the labor movements in the Western world made access to health care a universal entitlement, with the government guaranteeing that such a human right is implemented. Part of this human right is the funding of benefits through progressive taxation. In the United States, both the Republican and the Democratic parties have been proponents of the regressive funding of health services.

Notes

1. Paul Samuelson, *Economics* (8th ed.; New York: McGraw-Hill, 1972), p. 110.
2. Vicente Navarro, *The Politics of the Welfare State*.
3. Vicki Kemper and Viveca Novak, "What's Blocking Health Care Reform?" *Common Cause Magazine* 18, no. 1 (January/February/March 1992): 8-13, 25.
4. Abraham Flexner, *Universities: American, English, German* (rev. ed., New York: Oxford University Press, 1930), p. 180.
5. R.M. MacIver, *Academic Freedom in Our Time* (New York: Goodwin Press, 1967), p. 78.
6. William H. Hartley and William S. Vincent, *American Civics* (Orlando, FL: Harcourt Brace Jovanovich, 1987), p. 434.
7. *New York Times*, 24 September 1992.
8. U.S. Congress, Office of the Budget, *Economic Implications of Rising Health Care Costs*, October 1992, p. 37.
9. E.E. Schattschneider, *The Sovereign People: A Realistic View of Democracy in America* (New York: Holt, Rinehart, & Winston, 1960), p. 31.
10. New York Times/CBS Poll, August 1991.

Further Reading

Common Cause. 1992. "Why the United States Does Not Have a National Health Program." *International Journal of Health Services* 22: 619-644.

Jonathan S. Feinstein. 1993. "The Relationships Between Socioeconomic Status and Health: A Review of the Literature." *Milbank Quarterly* 71: 279-322.

Vicente Navarro. 1993. *Dangerous to Your Health*. New York: Cornerstone Books.

Discussion Questions

1. Give some examples of your own experiences or those of others that reflect Navarro's claims about U.S. health care and social class. How are Navarro's points illustrated by other authors in this section?

2. How might new health policies or changes in the organization of health care affect the situation Navarro describes?

3. What specific actions will prompt the U.S. health care system to respond to people's needs?

38

The Canadian System

David U. Himmelstein
Steffie Woolhandler

One concern about adopting a single player system of health care like Canada's in the United States is the belief that it will not allow expensive or life saving services. Single payer systems involve universal health insurance coverage under one plan, administered through federal or state governments. Himmelstein and Woolhandler explain that Canada's single payer health service system does not compromise care. Instead, the Canadian system manages health services and care differently from that in the United States. Take a look at the three graphs related to transplantation, breast cancer, and research that follow. Compare the variation between these graphs of the U.S. and Canadian health care services. Does

this evidence suggest a single payer system would be detrimental to American health?

Opponents of a single payer system have asserted that high technology care is unavailable in Canada. In fact, compared to Americans, Canadians have comparable rates of heart and/or lung, liver, bone marrow transplants, and kidney transplants (Figure 38-1).

Canada has regionalized most of these services. A relatively small number of centers each perform a large number of procedures. Such regionalization improves the quality of care since high volume centers are better able to maintain competence, and minimizes cost by avoiding the unnecessary duplication of expensive facilities.

Figure 38-2
Breast Cancer Care: Less Delays in British Columbia Than in Washington State

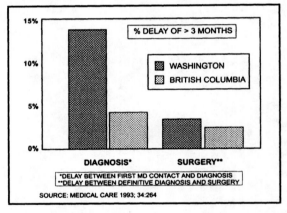

The U.S. media has prominently reported anecdotes of waits for care in Canada. However, this systematic study of waits in breast cancer care found that Canadians received more timely care. Fewer Canadian women waited more than three months between their first contact with a physician for breast symptoms and a definitive diagnosis of their breast cancer. Canadian women were also slightly less likely to experience a prolonged delay between the time of diagnosis and surgery (Figure 38-2).

Opponents of a National Health Program often argue that such reform would compromise innovation in U.S. health care. There is

Figure 38-1
Transplants: U.S. and Canada, 1990

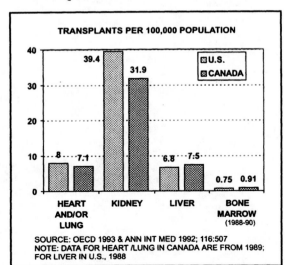

Figure 38-3
Medical Articles Published per Million Population

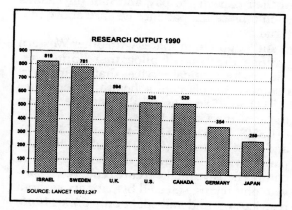

RESEARCH OUTPUT 1990

SOURCE: LANCET 1993;i:247

no evidence to support this argument. The overwhelming majority of basic bio-medical research is supported by grants from government or non-profit foundations. Often, as in the case of the HIV drug AZT, the results of government funded basic research are turned over to drug firms who do minimal additional scientific work, but reap rich rewards. Drug and equipment firms spend more for marketing than for research, and may label as "research" some marketing activities. Moreover, much drug industry research focuses on developing so-called me-too drugs that offer no clinical advantage over existing medications, but yield a chemically distinct, and hence patentable, version of an older drug.

We are unaware of systematic international comparisons of research productivity. However, the limited data reproduced on this chart (Figure 38-3) does not support the view that the U.S. research establishment is more productive than researchers in nations with national health programs.

Further Reading

Jennifer Brundin. 1993. "How the U.S. Press Covers the Canadian Health Care System." *International Journal of Health Services* 23: 275-77.

John K. Iglehart. 1986. "Canada's Health Care System." *New England Journal of Medicine* 315: 202-208.

Leslie L. Roos, Elliot S. Fisher, Ruth Brazauskas, Sandra M. Sharp, and Evelyn Shapiro. 1992. "Health and Surgical Outcomes in Canada and the United States." *Health Affairs* 11:56-72.

Discussion Questions:

1. How are U.S. systems of paying for health care structured? How does a single payer system differ from U.S. payment systems?

2. Why might Americans believe that a system like the Canadian system would compromise their health care?

3. Do you believe that the Canadian system of care would compromise health care? Why or why not?

39

Japan's Medical Care System

John K. Iglehart

John Iglehart notes that the Japanese system of care is based on three objectives: "ready access, high quality, and reasonable cost." Keep these objectives in mind as you read Iglehart's discussion of the Japanese health care system. We see in the Japanese health care system that physicians are administrators of health care institutions and the principal care providers in Japan. This stands in contrast to specifically trained administrators and the layers of care providers—nurse practitioners, clinical pharmacists, physicians' assistants—found in the United States. Consider what this means for physicians' status in Japan.

The elaborately organized system of insurance ensures all Japanese citizens access to care under employee insurance or community health insurance, still, Japanese citizens, like United States citizens, bear the rising cost of out-of-pocket expenses for medical care. Unlike in the United States, however, Japanese insurance plans protect patients from financial ruin from a long term or serious illness. Would this type of insurance system be effective in the United States? What kinds of social structural and cultural differences between Japan and the United States would need to be considered to introduce this type of system in the United States?

Japan's medical care system, like those of most Western industrialized nations, is based on three essential objectives: ready access, high quality, and reasonable cost. Within that framework, however, every culture influences the provision of medical care in countless ways. For example, Japan's medical system reflects in some respects the entrepreneurial, market-driven nature of its economy, yet it also expresses a policy that hospitals should be organized on a nonprofit basis, that all citizens should have access to care regardless of their capacity to pay, and that physicians should place the patient's welfare above material gain.

Although Japan shares with other Western nations the task of allocating limited resources for medical services that are in heavy demand, its per-capita health expenditure ($831) in 1986 was significantly less than those of the United States ($1,926), Canada ($1,370), Sweden ($1,195), France ($1,039), and West Germany ($1,031). Indeed, how Japan provided its citizens universal access to comprehensive medical care rendered by private physicians, selected by patients without restrictions, and still spent only 6.7% (1986) of the country's Gross Domestic Product (GDP) in doing so, is one of the most fascinating questions about the system. The estimate was calculated by the Organization for Economic Cooperation and Development on the basis of data provided by Japan's Ministry of International Trade and Industry.[1] Japan's Ministry of Health and Welfare estimates that spending totaled only 6.4% of the country's GDP in 1986. The difference is one of definition. Although this percent is low by comparison with that of other nations, the real annual rate of growth in health expenditures per capita (9.1%) during the period 1960 to 1984 was more rapid in Japan than in any other Western country, according to the Organization for Economic Cooperation and Development.

Japan's ability to finance a substantial increase in its per-capita expenditures for medical care during the 1970s without major political or public complaint derived from the rapid growth of its economy. In more recent years, the government, as the chief overseer of Japan's largely privately financed health insurance plans, has grown restive over the increasing portion of the GDP that is allocated to medical care, particularly for the elderly. Persons 65 years and older constituted 10.3% (12.5 million) of Japan's population in 1985. By the year 2010, it is expected that the number will more than double, to 27.1 million or 20%. Over the same period, the ratio of active to retired workers will drop from 5.9:1 to an estimated 2.8:1. By the year 2020, Japan's population will be among the oldest in the world.

This report will discuss the current status of Japanese medical care, a fee-for-service system cherished by its citizens because they believe steadfastly in the medical model and the physicians who symbolize it and because they place a high value on their personal health. I collected the information on which this essay and a subsequent report are based during two recent two-week trips to Japan, in which I interviewed a variety of physicians, government officials, and other persons with a stake in Japanese medical care. I also searched the English-language literature on the system.[2-10]

The Evolution of Japanese Medical Care

Japan's health care system has evolved over centuries to serve its 122 million citizens, who live on four major islands (and 3900 adjacent smaller islands) that stretch over an area of 377, 435 km^2—slightly smaller than the state of California. Japan's capital, Tokyo, a vast metropolis with a population in 1985 of 8.4 million, lies almost at the latitudinal center of the Northern Hemisphere. More than two-thirds of Japan's land mass is covered by mountains and forests and is thus uninhabitable. As a consequence, most of its people live on only a tiny fraction of the land, making Japan (behind Bangladesh and South Korea) the third most densely populated country in the world, with 318 people per square kilometer in 1984. The comparable world average is 35 people, and the United States' average is 25.

Situated on the border of East and West, Japan has demonstrated a capacity over the centuries to learn foreign cultures and ideas and then adapt them to its own milieu. Within this context, two major paradigmatic shifts marked the evolution of Japanese medical care. The first was the introduction of traditional Chinese medicine in the sixth century A.D., a period in Japanese history when acupuncture and herbal medications were the favored treatments for a wide variety of ailments. Almost a thousand years

later, Western medicine was introduced into Japan, largely through the influence of Portuguese Catholic missionaries. Later, between 1600 and 1867, a policy of isolationism dominated the country. Foreigners were forbidden to enter the country, with the exception of Dutch and Chinese traders, who were allowed to enter at only one location—the Nagasaki harbor. But through this entry point, Dutch medicine made its way into Japan, with notable influence on the provision of care.

Western influence on Japanese medical care accelerated after the Meiji Restoration, a reform era that followed a civil war in 1867. The war pitted an alliance of powerful landowners, young samurai, and mercantile capitalists in a successful struggle against the existing feudal system. The Meiji era (1868 to 1912) represents one of the more remarkable chapters in Japanese history.[11] Again, Japan's new leaders sought to replicate the institutions and practices of other countries that seemed best suited to the modernization of their own. For example, Japan adopted the methods of the British Navy and Merchant Marine, the Prussian Army, American business (in part), and German medicine, which at the time was considered the most advanced in Europe. The embrace of biomedicine by Meiji leaders was bolstered in large part by their attraction to Western technology in general.[12]

Although the present structure of social insurance is based largely on the Health Insurance Law of 1922, public and private actions dealing with citizens' welfare and the protection of workers date to the late 1800s. In imitation of the German experience, large corporations created mutual aid associations in the early 1900s, which financed care for some employees, and communities supported private clinics at which salaried physicians saw patients. The Relief Regulations of 1874, regarded as the forerunner of the modern Japanese social security system, were followed by other laws—the Factory Law of 1911, the Popular Life Insurance Law of 1916, and the Military Relief Law of 1917. The history is too rich to relate here, but suffice it to say that the Health Insurance Law of 1922 was not a radical departure in social policy, but rather a continuation and extension of existing programs in response to the needs of the times.[7]

More than 100 national laws govern health and medical affairs in Japan today. The Ministry of Health and Welfare is responsible for implementing most of these laws. Its activities span the range of public and environmental health, social welfare, medical care financing, pharmaceutical regulations, and pensions. Japan's 47 prefectures (jurisdictions similar to the states of the United States) and its local governments also have roles in the financing, administration, and delivery of public health and social services.

The government has never wavered in its view that physicians trained in biomedical science should be the dominant providers of medical care in Japan. This conviction is reflected in laws that make other health care workers subservient and a requirement that hospital administrators must be physicians, regardless of who owns the institutions. One reflection of the continued, if slight, influence of Chinese medicine is that health insurance schemes cover selected herbal medicines and that some pharmaceutical companies sell them to physicians. But herbal medicines represent only 1% to 2% of all drugs prescribed by physicians.

Health Status

Obviously, factors other than medical care and its availability enter into the complex equation that determines any society's health status.[13] For example, Japan's low-fat diet is considered a prominent ingredient in maintaining the health of its people. And certainly, the high rate at which Japanese men use tobacco products (63% smoke) places their well-being at greater risk. Other cultural factors that influence Japan's health status include its strong commitment to cleanliness and a resistance to invasive medical procedures. Whenever possible, Japanese people prefer bed rest and prescription drugs than any other Western nation, but its surgical rates are lower than those in the United States.

These cultural characteristics and a variety of other factors combine to make the Japanese population, according to several important indicators, the healthiest in the world. To appreciate the magnitude of this achievement fully, one must contrast it with the dire conditions that prevailed in Japan four decades ago, after World War II. In 1947, the estimated life expectancy at birth for Japanese male infants was 50 years and for female infants 53.9 years; in 1950, it was 59.6 years and 63 years, respectively, for male and female infants. One account of the conditions prevailing in Japan after the war was rendered by officials of the Section of Public Health and Welfare of the General Headquarters, Supreme Commander for the Allied Powers.

> During the war increased industrialization and urbanization on the four main islands of Japan, plus the dominance of military aims over all social welfare activities, had a pronounced influence on public health and welfare administration. Pressure of militarism brought greater emphasis on such emergency requirements as a rapid turnout of medical students, nurses and dentists. It also resulted in the cessation of many public health activities of benefit to the civilian population. The conversion of many factories, engaged in the manufacture of medical and sanitary supplies and equipment, to war material production, plus the lack of adequate professional people to serve the civilian population, resulted in a complete breakdown of all public health and welfare functions.[14]

The Section of Public Health and Welfare of the Allied Powers, headed by Dr. Crawford F. Sams, ordered immediate measures to control the epidemic of infectious diseases, but it also sought to institute Western-style reforms dealing with medical education, public health administration, and health information systems. After Japan recovered its autonomy in 1952, many of these reforms, based on Western values, were eventually abandoned, such as the medical internship system, which students had strongly resisted. One of the reforms, the development of a vital-statistics system, became an important permanent fixture of Japans's medical care system.[15]

By 1986 the life expectancy at birth of the average Japanese was 75.2 years for men and

80.9 years for women—the highest in the world. In 1987 Japan's infant mortality rate was the lowest among all countries—5.2 deaths per 1000 births. By comparison, life expectancy in the United States last year was 71 years for men and 78.1 years for women, and the U.S. infant mortality rate in 1986 was 10.6 per 1000 live births. Factors that influence Japan's low infant mortality rate include universal access to medical care, a literate society eager for medical advice, the availability of a handbook on maternal and child health that has been issued routinely to every pregnant woman since world War II, and one of the world's highest registered abortion rates (23.9 per 1000 women of childbearing age). The relation between Japan's abortion rate and its low infant mortality rate is not entirely clear, because almost all the induced abortions are sought for economic reasons rather than to eliminate high-risk pregnancies, according to the Ministry of Health and Welfare.

The country's intense drive to industrialize has led to dramatic improvements in living standards, but its narrow concentration on economic growth and material prosperity has also generated new social, cultural, and mental strains.[16] Japan's current rate of suicide is about twice that of the United States. Pollution and drug-induced disorders have been major problems since the 1960s, and lack of proper housing, inadequate sewage and garbage disposal systems, and increased traffic congestion and accidents have also exacted a toll on Japan's health status. Industrialization has led to a range of occupational hazards much like those faced by workers in Europe and North America[17] and a changing pattern of disease in Japan.

Although Japan's life expectancy and infant mortality rates continue to improve, its citizens report more sickness every year, perhaps as a consequence of the ready availability of medical care financed largely by third parties, the average citizen's close attention to his or her health, and the country's aging population. In 1985, 145.2 of every 1000 persons—1 in 7—reported in a national survey that they were sick. A similar increase in morbidity among Americans was reported recently in the *NEJM*.[18] The morbidity rates from the annual survey by the Japanese Ministry of Health and Welfare were based on responses to questions about whether the respondent was experiencing any "abnormality in physical or mental condition" at the time of the survey.

Physician's Services

One of Japan's responses to its rapid urbanization and other social phenomena has been the embrace of sophisticated, high technology medical services delivered by physicians. Japan has more CAT scanners per capita than the United States. On average, a Japanese citizen visits his or her physician 15 times a year, as compared with about 5 times in the United States. Physicians are revered figures in Japanese society, although their stature has eroded a bit in recent years. Patients' waiting times are long (patients are generally seen without an appointment on a first-come-first-served basis, and waiting one hour or more seems to be the norm), and the average encounter itself is very short, but physicians do not seem to be disparaged for this practice. Emiko Ohnuki-Tierney, a professor anthropology at the University of Wisconsin who studied elements of her native country's medical care system, has discussed the physician-patient encounter.[19]

> At most private offices, clinics and hospitals, doctors see large numbers of patients. For example, at hospital X [described as a 226-bed, private hospital in suburban Kobe] during three morning hours on May 19, 1979, two doctors at the internal medicine clinic saw 100 outpatients who were there for the first time, in addition to 102 patients who had been seen there at least once before. During the same period, the one doctor on duty at the eye clinic saw 48 patients. The obstetric-gynecology clinic, where I conducted most of my fieldwork, usually had one doctor on duty who was occasionally joined by a resident, and the average number of patients each morning was between 40 and 50. . . . Many Japanese blame the insurance system for people making frequent but virtually free visits to doctors and for doctors accommodating and often encouraging these visits. There is, however, another factor that is

responsible for the phenomenon—the relative readiness with which the Japanese both recognize departures from health and consult doctors about them.

The part played by private practitioners has always been important in Japanese medicine. Private doctors have remained the focal point of the system even though Japan's network of health insurance plans has led to a form of socialization of medial care. Care is rendered for the most part in two settings—private clinics and hospitals. There are some 9,400 hospitals in Japan and about 27,000 clinics with fewer than 19 beds. Any facility with 200 or more beds is considered a hospital. Most hospitals are owned by physicians, and virtually all the clinics are physician-owned and operated.

Japanese Health Insurance

The vast bulk of medical care in Japan is financed through a health insurance system that currently accounts for more than 90% of total medical expenditures when patients' cost-sharing amounts are included. The insurance system has evolved incrementally since 1922, resulting in a gradual expansion of coverage, which became universal in 1961. The Japanese Constitution, adopted in 1947, buttressed the importance attached to personal well-being by guaranteeing all citizens "the right to maintain the minimum standards of wholesome and cultured living." Article 25 declares: "In all spheres of life, the state shall use its endeavors for the promotion and extension of social welfare and security, and of public health."

The health financing programs that implement Japan's commitment to universal access to care can be divided into two broad categories: employee health insurance, under which 75 million people (employees of private corporations and of national and local governments and their dependents) are covered, and community health insurance (alternatively referred to as national health insurance), which extends financial protection to 45 million additional citizens. The latter fall into a variety of categories: all unemployed adults (including the elderly), employees of small businesses, the self-employed, and

farmers. As a rule, people covered under community-based plans are at higher medical risk and have fewer financial resources than those protected by employee health insurance. All employers must sponsor and partially finance a plan or contribute financially to a scheme that is publicly administered. The government pays the administrative expenses of all of Japan's health insurance plans, none of which are organized on a for-profit basis.

Employee plans are further divided into programs managed by private health insurance societies (large corporations) and those managed by the government (primarily plans for employees of medium and small businesses). In this role, government performs an administrative function as a fiscal intermediary. It does not underwrite the coverage, the cost of which is shared by employers and employees. As a rule, a health insurance society is the fiscal intermediary for a single company (generally, a firm with 700 or more employees). The health insurance societies, or KENPO-KUMIAI, as they are called, that perform the intermediary function for large corporations are regulated by Japan's Ministry of Health and Welfare. But their place in Japanese corporate life extends well beyond the intermediary function, as Wolfson and Levin have explained.[20]

> One of the mottos of Japanese companies—*kigyo wa hito nati*, or the company is people—recongnizes the value of each employee as a company asset. A healthy, well-informed employee is seen as the most important investment a company can have. The kenpos are the principal social and economic vehicles for helping to make this happen. At the end of fiscal 1984, there were 1711 kenpos providing coverage to about 28 million people. Of these, 12 million were employees and more than 16 million were dependents.

In addition, under the category of employee health insurance, there is seamen's insurance and mutual aid associations, whose beneficiaries include seamen, civil servants employed by the national and local governments, and teachers. The variety of categories reflects the evolutionary nature of Japan's health insurance system. Because the plans emerged incrementally, patients' cost-sharing arrangements and benefits are not all the same, producing some problems of equity among them.

Employee health insurance plans are financed by premiums based on earnings and cost sharing by patients. Under society-managed health insurance and mutual-aid-association insurance, premium rates range from 6 to 9.6% (of the monthly remuneration of the insured person, divided between employer and employee); each entity has the discretion to establish the contribution rate within this range. On average, the employer pays 4.6% and the employee 3.5%. An employee's contribution is deducted from his or her paycheck. The contribution rate of government-managed health insurance is 8.9% (of the monthly remuneration of the insured person, equally divided between employer and employee).

Under all the employee health insurance plans, an insured person must, in addition to contributing to the cost of the premium, pay 10% of the cost of the medical care he or she uses, with a limit of 54,000 yen ($400) per month. An employee's dependents face a cost-sharing requirement of 20% for inpatient care and 30% for outpatient care. These cost-sharing amounts are usually paid in cash by a patient before he or she leaves the physician's clinic or hospital. Although there are few or no available data, these cost-sharing requirements (combined with Japan's rising standard of living) have done little to diminish the average citizen's proclivity to visit the physician often.

Medical care benefits covered under employee health insurance include virtually every treatment a physician might render in both the inpatient and out-patient setting. The score of covered medical benefits is established by law. Exceptions to the liberal coverage offered include preventive examinations (similar to physical examinations in the United States) and the normal delivery of a baby. Because giving birth is not an expense prompted by the onset of disease, health insurance plans do not pay for deliveries, but if complications lead, for example, to a cesarean section, that procedure is covered. Like many other surgical operations, ce-sarean sections are performed far less frequently in Japan than in the United States.[21]

The standard hospital accommodation that employee health insurance covers is a semiprivate room with four to six beds. Wards of 8 to 12 hospital beds are not uncommon in Japan, particularly in older facilities. In one Tokyo facility that I visited, Shitaya Hospital, a private room with bath, telephone, and television set cost 16,000 yen extra a day. As a rule, the Japanese attach less importance to privacy in the hospital and physician's office than do Americans. As Ohnuki-Tierney explained in her book,

> In a private practitioner's office, the examination room is barely separated from the waiting room. Furthermore, while the examination goes on, nurses and other personnel may pass by, and the patient's family members often stay throughout the examination. In contrast to this open atmosphere, the examination process in the United States clearly expresses the cherished cultural values of privacy and the sacredness of the body. During an American examination, the doctor and the patient are alone in a room behind a closed door, with a thick wall guaranteeing absolute privacy.[19]

Beyond coverage of medical expenses, employee health insurance plans offer additional benefits not required by statute. These include cash benefits to cover normal deliveries and injury and sickness allowances, maternity allowances during absence from work, a nursing allowance (when an insured woman nurses her children, she receives 2,000 yen per child in a lump sum), and partial coverage of patient cost-sharing requirements. Some employee health insurance plans are no more generous than others in covering these items.

Community health insurance, a conglomeration of plans administered by cities, towns, villages, and private bodies representing specific trades or professions, provides coverage to an additional 45 million people. The medical benefits covered are essentially the same as those provided by employee health insurance, but additional cash benefits for sickness, injury, maternity, and the death of the insured person are considerably less generous under community-sponsored schemes. Community health insurance is financed by premiums paid by covered persons (the maximum per year in a household is 370,000 yen [$2,740]), a patient cost-sharing requirement of 30%, which can be lower depending on individual economic circumstances, and government subsidies. The premiums are calculated on the basis of a person's income and the actuarial value of the benefit. In addition to the premiums and patient cost-sharing amounts, which cover less than half the average cost of care to a patient, financing derives from national and local government support.

Although Japan's various health insurance plans impose different levels of cost-sharing on their beneficiaries, raising questions of equity that have long concerned the government but that remain nevertheless, all the plans protect their beneficiaries against the prospect of financial devastation by a serious illness. All plans include a ceiling (54,000 yen a month per illness, or $400) on the amount of out-of-pocket expenditures a patient can incur before all additional expenses are covered. For example, if an employee covered under employee health insurance incurred a hospital bill of 600,000 yen, 90% would be covered by the plan. Of the remaining 60,000 yen owned, the beneficiary would be required to cover 54,000 yen; the insured would be reimbursed by the health insurance plan for the remaining 6,000 yen.

Medical care for the elderly (defined as persons over 70 years of age and bedridden people between the ages of 65 and 70 years) is also a component of Japan's universal network of health insurance. Medical benefits for the elderly are financed through national government contributions (20%), local government bodies (10%, divided between prefectural and city, town, or village governments), and contributions from employee health insurance and community health insurance plans. Before the Health and Medical Services for the Aged law was enacted in August 1982, the national government was responsible for financing more of the medical care of the elderly. Because older people consume a great deal of care, community-based plans that paid for the bulk of their care were plagued with financial problems, often requiring assistance from the national government.

The 1982 law placed more of the burden of new medical spending for the elderly on employee health insurance plans paid by employers. Its enactment also demonstrated that Japan is more willing than the United States to impose policies on employers that are deemed to reflect their legitimate social obligation—in Japan's case, requiring employers and employees to shoulder a greater proportion of the cost of care for the elderly. The financial impact of the 1982 law is apparent in trends in the growth of Japan's medical care expenditures between 1983 and 1986. During that period, national government expenditures for medical care (and the percent of total expenditures they represented) rose only slightly, from 4.45 trillion yet (30.6%) to 4.46 trillion yen (26.1%), while employers' payments for their employee health insurance increased from 7.64 trillion yen (52.5%) to 9.32 trillion yen (54.6%). Employees' contributions represent the bulk of the remaining costs.

The 1982 law also imposed small cost-sharing requirements on the elderly—a controversial policy step designed to curb that population's increasing use of medical care. For every day in the hospital, an elderly patient must pay 400 yen ($3). The cost-sharing requirement for outpatient care is 800 yen a month ($6). Many elderly people who are taking a drug for an ailment visit a physician weekly to have their prescriptions refilled. The 1982 law also sought to reduce hospitals' current economic incentive for keeping elderly patients in the hospital for months (and sometimes years because of a very limited number of nursing home beds) by reimbursing facilities on a diminishing scale—the longer the stay, the lower the rate—and sought to encourage the use of more home care for the elderly to avoid hospital stays.

Despite the government's efforts to moderate the growth of medical care spending on behalf of the elderly, such spending has continued to rise more rapidly than that for the nonelderly, mostly because the rates at which the elderly use services have increased more sharply. In 1986, health-care expenditures on behalf of the elderly reached 30.1% (523,300 yen per capita versus 140,300 yen per capita for the population as a whole), although the elderly represent only 10.3% of the total population.

That they have comprehensive insurance is not the only reason that the elderly are using more medical care. Perhaps equally important is a cultural change taking place in Japanese society. The reverence in which Japan holds its elderly seems to be diminishing in the face of their increasing numbers, lack of space to care for elderly family members at home, and the increasing employment of women, the traditional care givers, outside the home. One consequence of these multiple developments is that elderly people are paying more visits to their physicians. Ohnuki-Tierney discussed this phenomenon:

> Because of rapid changes in attitude toward the aged and changed in family structure, which now emphasizes the nuclear family, these older people often feel lonely and uncomfortable, even when they are living with their offspring. Some of the waiting rooms at neighborhood doctors' offices have become local gathering places for the elderly. Some older people prefer to be hospitalized, even when their illnesses are not grave, and are unwilling to be discharged after recovery. Some doctors accommodate this behavior, either in their waiting rooms or in the hospitals, since their services to the elderly are reimbursed by the government. Others discourage the practice, pointing out that clinics and hospitals are not homes for the elderly.[19]

Japan's medical care system offers all its citizens an impressive array of services for a moderate price. Nevertheless, the government and providers of care are currently discussing many economic incentive issues. Some of these include the long hospital stays in Japan (the average for all patients, including both short-term and long-term care, is 39 days), the heavy use of pharmaceutical products, and the number of new physicians being trained in the country's medical schools. . . .

References

1. Schieber, G.J., and J.P. Poullier. 1988. International health spending and utilization trends. *Health Affairs* (Millwood) 7(4):105-12.

2. Ikegami, N. 1988. Health technology development in Japan. *International Journal of Technology Assessment* 4:239-54.

3. Fujii, M., and M.R. Reich. 1988. Rising medical costs and the reform of Japan's health insurance system. *Health Policy* 9:9-24.

4. Levin, P.J., Wolfson, J., and H. Akiyama. 1987. The role of management in Japanese hospitals. *Hospital and Health Services Administration* 32:249-61.

5. Gelb, A. 1985. Lessons from the Japanese. *American Journal of Gastroenterology* 80:738-42.

6. Abe, M.A. 1985. Hospital reimbursement schemes: Japan's point system and the United States' diagnostic-related groups. *Medical Care* 23:1055-66.

7. Steslicke, W.E. 1982. Development of health insurance policy in Japan. *Journal of Health, Politics, Policy and Law* 7:197-226.

8. Medical care in Japan: the political context. *Journal of Ambulatory Care Management* 5(4):65-77.

9. Lock, M.M. 1980. East Asian medicine in urban Japan; varieties of medical experience. Berkeley: University of California Press.

10. Steslicke, W.E. 1973. *Doctors in politics: the political life of the Japan medical association.* New York: Praeger.

11. Hashimoto, M. 1984. Health services in Japan. In *Comparative health systems: descriptive analyses of fourteen national health systems*, ed. M.W. Raffel. University Park, PA: Pennsylvania State University Press, 335-70.

12. Long, S.O. 1987. Health care providers: technology, policy and professional dominance. In *Health, illness, and medical care in Japan: cultural and social dimensions*, ed. E. Norbeck and M. Lock. Honolulu: University of Hawaii Press, 66-88.

13. Payer, L. 1988. *Medicine and culture: varieties of treatment in the United States, England, West Germany, and France.* New York: Henry Holt.

14. Steslicke, W.E. 1987. The Japanese state of health: a political-economic perspective. In *Health, illness, and medical care in Japan: cultural and social dimensions*, ed. E. Norbeck and M. Lock. Honolulu: University of Hawaii Press, 24-65.

15. Marui, E. Japan's experience with public health reform in the early occupation days: foreigner's plans and indigenous systems. In *International cooperation for health: problems, prospects, priorities*, ed.

M.R. Reich and E. Marui. Dover, MA: Auburn House Publishing.

16. Sonodo, K. 1988. *Health and illness in changing Japanese society*. Tokyo: University of Tokyo Press.

17. Reich, M.R., and H. Frumkin. An overview of Japanese occupational health. *American Journal of Public Health* 78:809-16.

18. Barsky, A.J. 1988. The paradox of health. *New England Journal of Medicine* 318:414-18.

19. Ohnuki-Tierney, E. 1984. *Illness and culture in contemporary Japan: an anthropological view*. New York: Cambridge University Press.

20. Wolfson, J., and P.J. Levin. Health insurance, Japanese style. *Business and Health* 3(6):38-40.

21. Notzon, F.C, Placek, P.J., and S.M. Taffel. 1987. Comparisons of national cesarean section rates. *New England Journal of Medicine* 316:386-89.

Further Reading

John K. Iglehart. 1988. "Health Policy Report: Japan's Medical Care System—Part Two." *New England Journal of Medicine* 319: 1166-1172.

Emiko Ohnuki-Tierney. 1984. *Illness and Culture in Contemporary Japan: An Anthropological View*. Cambridge: Cambridge University Press.

Noriko Yamamoto and Margaret I. Wallhagen. 1997. "The Continuation of Family Caregiving in Japan." *Journal of Health and Social Behavior* 38(2): 164-176.

Discussion Questions

1. What are some of the basic differences between the Japanese health care system and the U.S. system?

2. How does the Japanese system meet the three objectives Iglehart defines? How does it fall short?

40

Twenty Years of Care in Japan

Sakuji Uehara, as told to Hiroko Akiyama by Toshiomi Asahi

This interesting account merges the personal perspectives of caregiver, Mrs. Uehara, and caretaker, Dr. Asahi, in a description of one man's experience of the Japanese health care system. Hiroko Akiyama assembles these accounts and places them within the structural context of the Japanese health care system and culture. This selection highlights some of the crucial aspects of health insurance coverage in Japan—resources it makes available, and those it cannot. As you read this selection, think about your own experiences with the U.S. health care system or other systems of care. Reflect on the similarities and differences in health care organization, care provision, and resource availability.

Medical History

Mr. Uehara's story begins in the summer of 1971. While at work on July 26, Mr. Uehara began to have stomach pains. Not wanting to leave work on account of a stomach ache, Mr. Uehara rested at work and then had a friend follow him home to be sure he got home safely. At home he went on with life as usual, drinking his usual two decanters of "sake" and going to sleep.[1] He never told his wife of his stomach pains, and her only clue to things being not quite normal was his insistence that the "sake" tasted like water. In the morning his stomach still hurt so he decided to stop by the neighborhood clinic on the way to work. Without checking either his pulse or blood pressure, the doctor gave Mr. Uehara some pain killers and an injection. Mr. Uehara lost consciousness.

Mrs. Uehara was called to the clinic and told that her husband had lost consciousness after receiving an injection for his stomach pain. He had suffered a stroke, perhaps as a result of the treatment. When Mr. Uehara awoke, he complained of paralysis in his right arm. At this point, Mrs. Uehara decided that it would be best to seek treatment for her husband at the Police Hospital. She had the clinic call her a taxi and took her husband directly from the clinic to the hospital.

At the Police Hospital Mr. Uehara was put into an oxygen tent. Mr. Uehara again lost consciousness and remained unconscious for two weeks. The doctor at the Police Hospital told Mrs. Uehara to call the family together and inform them of Mr. Uehara's condition.

Mr. Uehara remained hospitalized from July 27, 1971, to April of the following year. After his discharge from the Police Hospital, the Ueharas returned to their home in Suginami (a section of Tokyo). Once back in Suginami, Mrs. Uehara concentrated on helping her husband regain his strength. He was able to return to work.

Until 1984, Mr. Uehara was under the care of a neighborhood doctor. In October 1984, Mr. Uehara began to be troubled by muscle convulsions in the right side of his body and, as a result, began to consult Dr. Asahi. As the convulsions became more serious it became necessary for Mr. Uehara to be hospitalized for the second time. On November 15, 1984, Mr. Uehara entered the hospital. He remained hospitalized until December 24 of the same year.

Prior to his second hospitalization, Mr. Uehara had been bedridden for four to five years. His second hospitalization introduced rehabilitation and physical therapy into Mr. Uehara's treatment. With the help of his wife, Mr. Uehara was able to attend at least one physical therapy session a week. After much hard work on both his and his wife's part, Mr. Uehara regained his ability to walk short distances.

Mr. Uehara was hospitalized for the third time on May 28, 1987, due to an inflammation of his liver. He remained hospitalized until December 27 of the same year. After his release he resumed his once-a-week rehabilitation sessions and was soon able to go out on short walks.

In June of 1988, Mr. Uehara was hospitalized for the fourth time with an occlusion of the right common iliac artery, which caused him pain in his right leg. Bypass surgery was performed on July 5, 1988. After his surgery, Mr. Uehara again resumed his physical therapy sessions. This time, however, he did not regain his ability to walk. He was released from the hospital on March 3, 1989.

The Ueharas are currently participants in a home health care program. Mrs. Uehara takes care of her husband's daily needs with the help of a health nurse and a physical therapist, who both visit once a week, and by helpers provided by the city, who visit once every two weeks. Mr. Uehara also sees Dr. Asahi once a month.

Even with physical therapy, Mr. Uehara has not regained enough strength to be able to get up on his own. Without the help of either his wife or his doctor, Mr. Uehara remains confined to his wheelchair. Although his wife could help lift him, both felt it would be best not to put undue stress on her back. To get exercise Mr. Uehara does take his wheelchair out in the evening for a stroll around the neighborhood, occasionally even giving his wife a ride on the chair with him.

In Japan, wheelchairs more often than not become mere decorations in the house. This is in part due to the "tatami" matting and raised entrances found in many Japanese homes.[2] "Tatami" mats inhibit the use of wheelchairs in that wheelchairs can damage the expensive mats. The raised entrances make it difficult for individuals in wheelchairs to get in and out of the home. While ramps are not unheard of, neither are they common. The Ueharas improvised, using a board to make it easier to get Mr. Uehara in and out of the house. Mr. Uehara's level of activity is somewhat unusual compared to other Japanese in similar situations. The doctor suggests that his history as a police officer and his wife's help with his rehabilitation exercises accounts for his level of activity.

Prior to his stroke, Mr. Uehara had given very little information to his wife that would have led her to believe that her husband was in poor health. She knew that he occasionally had high blood pressure and that a physical examination had revealed signs of heart trouble. Her husband had told her that if he should ever collapse, it would most likely have something to do with his heart. The fact that he had passed his physicals as a police officer and that he monitored his blood pressure regularly led her to believe that there wasn't much to worry about. It was only after her husband had his first stroke that she learned from a friend of his that he had been suffering from stomach discomfort severe enough to make him lie down at work.

According to Dr. Asahi, an embolism was the most likely cause of Mr. Uehara's original stroke (at the same time he does not discount the possibility of thrombosis playing a part in the original attack). Mr. Uehara is presently troubled by liver dysfunction, atrial fibrillation, and hip and knee problems. The occlusion of his right common iliac artery has also left him unable to walk.

Mrs. Uehara on Hospitals

When she first checked her husband into the Police Hospital, she was immediately told by the doctors that they would like the family to stay with Mr. Uehara. Their eldest daughter had just recently graduated from college and taken a job. The youngest was still just a sophomore in college. Not being able to either pay someone or rely on her children to help her care for her husband, Mrs. Uehara had to stay with her husband and care for him entirely on her own. This had the advantage of giving the patient the comfort of being taken care of by his own family. Mrs. Uehara moved into the hospital with her husband and stayed the entire time he was hospitalized.

Mr. Uehara and his wife initially had a room that they shared with one other patient. Mrs. Uehara ate and slept in the same room as her husband at the hospital. After Mr. Uehara's health improved and he regained consciousness, they moved him into a larger room that he shared with five other patients. The closeness of their quarters made privacy and sleeping difficult at first. Two of the biggest problems were when one of the other patients would either talk or snore too loudly. Room assignments had to be changed occasionally when roommates didn't get along. Mrs. Uehara occasionally even got into arguments with the hospital staff over such things as the setting on an air conditioner.

Meals were not provided at the Police Hospital. Mrs. Uehara had to either prepare the meals herself, or go out to buy the meals. Having to provide meals herself made it more difficult to take care of her husband. In Mr. Uehara's later hospitalizations breakfast was not served, but lunch and dinner were. This lightened Mrs. Uehara's workload and made it easier to take care of her husband.

While doctors consult the family on planned operations and the dangers of such operations, leaving medical decisions up to the doctor is characteristic of Japanese patient-doctor relations. The Ueharas were no exception. After talking to the doctors, Mrs. Uehara would talk matters over with her husband and his family. She would then report back to the doctors. It was Mrs. Uehara's responsibility as the "Yome" (wife) to report back to his family.

A Japanese patient's relationship with the hospital or with a doctor is different than it is in the United States. In Japan, patients rarely ask for second opinions. The doctor looks at a second opinion as a questioning of his/her competence. Interhospital relations are also more complicated. Hospitals like to treat patients that see their doctors rather than those referred to them by outside doctors. A hospital will usually respond that they are full rather than take in patients from other doctors. When Mr. Uehara underwent surgery on the occlusion of his common right iliac artery, he was referred to a hospital by Dr. Asahi. Dr. Asahi lent Mr. Uehara's file and X-rays to the other hospital, sat in on the pre-operation meetings, and expressed his desire not to have Mr. Uehara's leg amputated. This was unusual and does not often occur in the Japanese health care system. According to Dr. Asahi, interhospital relations are more often bad than good.

On Caring for Mr. Uehara at Home

At the time of the interview, Mrs. Uehara had been taking care of her husband for 18 years. The strain of caring for both her husband and family led to poor health and at one point resulted in her own hospitalization. Mrs. Uehara is presently aided by her now married daughter and by her grandchildren who have moved into her home. Everybody helps with the household chores, especially dinner. One of the most difficult chores is getting Mr. Uehara into the bathtub in the evening. To do this, Mrs. Uehara enlists the help of her daughter and grandchildren.

When asked by the interviewer if having a sick grandfather ever posed problems in the intergeneration household, the answer was no. The grandchildren have grown up with their grandfather in a wheelchair and realize that he has special needs that they as a family must work together to meet. For example, there are certain foods that Mr. Uehara isn't allowed to eat; dinner is always prepared with this in mind. The whole family also takes part in helping Mr. Uehara with his rehabilitation sessions. Mrs. Uehara states that one of the biggest problems was control over the television set at evening meals. She had worried that when the children became older they would complain that they were never able to watch the show they wanted. The children, however, are used to their grandfather's needs and will thus go upstairs to watch their television programs.

Mrs. Uehara was asked by the interviewer if she would ever consider a form of short-term day-care for Mr. Uehara so that the family could go on outings and trips together. Mrs. Uehara's response was that she couldn't and wouldn't consider handing her husband's care over to someone else. She would worry about her husband and wouldn't be able to enjoy either an outing or a trip without him. When her husband's health had looked the worst, her response had been "I will make him better!" Eighteen years of caring for her husband has made her feel that in a sense she is personally responsible for her husband's recovery.

The Ueharas are helped by a public health care nurse and a rehabilitation nurse, who visit the Uehara's home once a week. The public health nurse checks such things as Mr. Uehara's pulse, blood pressure, and temperature. The nurse also reminds Mrs. Uehara to keep Mr. Uehara from catching cold.

The rehabilitation nurse works with Mr. Uehara for 5 to 20 minutes each visit. The rest of the time is spent training the family to help Mr. Uehara with his exercises. Altogether, the rehabilitation nurse stays for a little over 30 minutes each visit.

At Dr. Asahi's hospital the types of services available to the patients are discussed with the patients before they are discharged from the hospital. A social worker comes to the hospital and talks over both the benefits and costs of each program. According to Dr. Asahi, such programs as are available today were not available even five years ago. Insufficient staffing resulted in public health and rehabilitation nurses being able to visit their patients only twice a month. An increase in staff has meant better care for patients. Ideally, Dr. Asahi would like to make further improvements, such as providing accessible vans or buses to make it easier for his wheelchair-bound patients to get to their rehabilitation sessions at the hospital. He also talks of developing a program through which the families of those receiving treatment could meet others in similar situations.

On Health Insurance

When Mr. Uehara collapsed he was 50 years old. Since he had not worked all the way up to his retirement age, his pension is small and making ends meet can be difficult. Most of the Uehara's health care expenses are covered by the Japanese national health insurance. For those over 65 years of age, visits to the doctor's office are generally free. However, for those under 65 there are some costs that the family must meet on their own. The biggest expenses are those small things, such as bandage costs, that are not covered by the national health insurance. These are sold to the patients at cost but can still become more of an economic burden than the original stay at the hospital. The public health care nurse and the helpers are covered partially by the city, but the patients must also pay a small fee for each visit. A visit from the public health care nurse costs 800 yen (about U.S. $6), and the helpers 1,200 yen (about $8). The rehabilitation nurse is free to the patient. The Ue-

haras are special participants in a health care program and have never been asked to pay for the services they have received from the city.

Closing Comments

According to Mrs. Uehara, they have been lucky and have received good health care. Dr. Asahi states that it was with a family willing to help that he and the hospital were able to provide the kind of health care that they did. He states that the Uehara case is somewhat different than that of the norm and that the interview focused mostly on the good points of the treatment he has received.

Notes

1. Sake is the word for Japanese rice wine, which usually contains about 14% alcohol.
2. Tatami mats are woven straw mats that take the place of carpet and could be found in most older homes.

Further Reading

Arnold S. Relman. 1992. "Reforming Our Health Care System: A Physician's Perspective." *The Key Reporter* Autumn: 1-5.

Marilynn M. Rosenthal and Marcel Frenkel, eds. 1992. *Health Care Systems and Their Patients: An International Perspective*. San Francisco: Westview Press.

Discussion Questions:

1. How does Dr. Asahi's account of Mr. Uehara's experience of health care in Japan differ from your own experiences of health care in the United States or other countries?

2. Can you imagine contexts of care in the United States that might be like those described by Dr. Asahi or Mrs. Uehara? Why or why not?

3. What kinds of structural differences in health care systems account for some of the differences you described above?

Section 6

The Social Construction of Illness: The Case of AIDS

This section is devoted to AIDS because of its incidence, ambiguity, and seriousness, and because its social construction underscores issues and arguments presented throughout this anthology. Protagonists do not always agree about what AIDS is, what it means, who contracts it, how it should be treated, which medical services should be given, and when, how, and to what extent these services should be given. A sometimes vocal scientific minority reject the generally accepted cause of AIDS—Human Immunodeficiency disease (HIV) (Fumento 1992). Wonder drugs flame hope and fuel the pharmaceutical industry. Today's costly regimen may cause tomorrow's deadly side effects. Definitions of AIDS and what to do about it lead to social policies, practices, and specific kinds of medical treatment. In turn, social policies and practices define, reaffirm, and perpetuate certain characterizations of AIDS. Questions arise about who has the power to define AIDS, its treatment, and services, who benefits from those definitions, who is disadvantaged by them, and when, why, and how benefits and disadvantages accrue.

The social significance of a pathological condition depends in part on its incidence in a population. Incidence reports rely on compiled statistics. The ways morbidity and mortality statistics are gathered and processed affect the assumed incidence of AIDS and the dispersion of resources to populations with HIV and AIDS. Gena Corea deftly raises questions about AIDS statistics. She argues that methods of classifying HIV infection can hide actual modes of transmission. A focus on risk groups rather than on behaviors leads to undetected cases and underestimated reporting. Social class differences, for example, can obscure reported numbers of cases. Overrepresented numbers of poor people and an underestimated count of affluent individuals result when only poor people use health services where AIDS and HIV are counted. As Corea suggests, knowledge is political. It is neither neutral nor acontextual.

Institutional reporting practices, as well as sophisticated epidemiological methods of data gathering, shape national and international knowledge of AIDS. An attempt to reduce the stigma of AIDS for patients and families can lead to emphasis on contributing conditions. A final and recorded cause of death may be an acute infection turned deadly because AIDS has depleted the person's immune system. AIDS sometimes appears in conjunction with other diseases. HIV may be underreported in some countries where it accompanies tuberculosis. It may be overreported in areas where grants and careers depend on increasing incidence. How, why, and where officials record the presence or absence of disease contributes to the social construction of AIDS and the treatment of HIV and AIDS. This has been especially true when it comes to reporting the incidence of AIDS in heterosexual women (Wortley and Fleming 1997).

Perceptions of risk, as Charles Bosk and Joel Frader imply, uphold the meanings and practices of hospital staff. Fear spawns stigma and separation from patients. In turn, separation generates professional justifications that mask ethical dilemmas about treatment decisions (Fox, Aiken, and Messikomer 1990). Some ethicists argue that the profession of medicine should oblige its practitioners differently than other professions: practitioners *should* attend to people with HIV and AIDS (Emanuel 1988; Pellegrino 1987). Attempts to change public behavior also spur a discourse on whose confidences will be kept, as questions of individual responsibilities and mandatory testing arise against the backdrop of the fear of AIDS (Alpert 1993; Bayer 1986).

Perhaps no disease has brought discussions of individual responsibility into the public arena more powerfully than AIDS. Yet these discussions may seem abstract and distant to their intended audiences. Moral tensions between personal gratification and individual responsibility lose abstractness and become immediate when people are infected with HIV and AIDS. Several of Miriam Cameron's interviewees are torn between seeking sexual pleasure without precautions or disclosure to partners and revising their sexual selves and activities.

Because AIDS is weighted with moral judgments, individuals with AIDS often search inward to find meaning in their experience of it and to explain why they might have it. In this case, the social understandings of AIDS merge with a reconstruction of self. The stigma and uncertainty of AIDS impose heavy burdens on people with HIV. Reconstruction of self also means coping with these burdens and their consequences. Rose Weitz tells poignant stories of

people with AIDS trying to come to terms with stigma, prospects of suffering, and uncertainty. Stigma, suffering, and uncertainty may arise from the diagnosis of AIDS alone before any severe physical distress begins. Maggie Callanan and Patricia Kelley's story of Brad tells of his being fired for having AIDS. Losing health insurance, much less losing a livelihood, causes many middle-class people to plummet into poverty at a time when they are physically and psychologically vulnerable (Light 1994). Like other serious illnesses, AIDS often turns productive people into isolated paupers. Brad was more fortunate than most in his final days. Poor people with hourly wages cannot take long leaves of absence to nurture a dying relative, as Brad's father did (Levine 1990).

The emergence of service communities, as Kent Sandstrom describes, partly eases the social, economic, and psychological distress that people with AIDS endure. These communities become sources of collective action, advocacy, and potential power. Their members become players in political and policy arenas. On an immediate basis, these communities offer individuals with AIDS psychological and social support as well as physical assistance. Community groups can mobilize resources and draw attention to AIDS-related concerns. Some observers believe the "epidemic" label for the AIDS crisis derived, in part, from the mobilization strategies of gay activists (Kayal 1993).

Labeling AIDS as an epidemic elicits images of crisis and fosters policies of immediate funding and intervention. Labels become taken as facts, and their implications are played out in programs and daily practices. Robert Broadhead and Douglas Heckathorn point out that AIDS transmission among intravenous drug users (IVDUs) became defined as a research problem. This definition resulted in funding multiple research centers with peer outreach workers to distribute informational material about the disease. Projects like these, however, may reflect political decisions to make a symbolic gesture to do something, but not much, about burgeoning numbers of AIDS cases among IVDUs (Charmaz and Olesen 1997). Piecemeal prevention and patchwork care to appease public concern and to ease political pressure have long been a part of the American health care scene (Navarro 1993).

New treatments extend the lives of many AIDS patients and keep them tied to expensive medication regimens. AIDS is becoming reconstructed as a serious chronic illness rather than terminal illness in countries where treatment is available. As AIDS holds less of the drama of death and more of the debilitating drain of chronic illness, will public sympathy diminish? Will it diminish more if the incidence of AIDS tumults further down the American social class structure and most affects low-income people of color and IVDUs and their partners? If a vaccine is developed, will AIDS become a syndrome of impoverished societies where few citizens have access to health care? Such questions point to how new reconstructions of the social meaning of AIDS could occur.

What we know of AIDS and how we know it reflects political choices, economic arrangements, and cultural beliefs. Macro–social policies and micro–ethical dilemmas flow from the social constructions of AIDS. The epidemiology of AIDS shapes crucial social images of it and beliefs about it. The relative effectiveness of prevention and treatment procedures defines those images. Both the epidemiology and relative efficacy of solutions affect ethical issues and dilemmas specific to AIDS. AIDS causes profound suffering—not simply of the body, but also of the spirit. It taxes social bonds and twists images of self. Earlier taken-for-granted assumptions about self erode. Yet despite loss and devastation, the resilience of the human spirit shines through. By becoming part of a larger community, people with AIDS may discover new meaning in life and realize theretofore hidden potentials of self. Thus, we come full circle back to the transformation of self that can occur through experiencing serious illness. Yet that transformation for people with AIDS may be more of a collective, rather than an individual process. If they have shared a community, people with AIDS may become transformed through the collective spirit infusing their existence and through the inspiring daily acts of exemplars.

References:

Sheri Alpert. 1993. "Smart Cards, Smarter Policy: Medical Records, Privacy, and Health Care Reform." *Hastings Center Report* 23(6):13-23.

Ronald Bayer. 1986. "AIDS, Power, and Reason." *The Milbank Quarterly* 64:168-182.

Kathy Charmaz and Virginia Olesen. 1997. "Ethnographic Research in Medical Sociology: Its Foci and Distinctive Contributions." *Sociological Methods of Research* 25:452-494.

Ezekiel Emanuel. 1988. "Do Physicians Have an Obligation to Treat Patients with AIDS?" *New England Journal of Medicine* 318:1686-1690.

Renee C. Fox, Linda H. Aiken, and Carla Messikomer. 1990. "The Culture of Caring: AIDS and the Nursing Profession." *The Milbank Quarterly* 67:226-258.

Michael Fumento. 1992. "Do You Believe in Magic?" *The American Spectator*, February. Pp. 16-21.

Philip Kayal. 1993. *Bearing Witness: Gay Men's Health Crisis and the Politics of AIDS*. San Francisco: Westview Press.

Carol Levine. 1990. "AIDS and Changing Concepts of Family." *The Milbank Quarterly* 68:33-58.

Donald W. Light. 1994. "Excluding More, Covering Less: The Health Insurance Industry in the United States." In *Beyond Crisis: Confronting Health Care in the United States*, Nancy F. McKenzie, ed. New York: Penguin, pp. 310-320.

Vicente Navarro. 1993. *Dangerous to Your Health: Capitalism in Health Care*. New York: Monthly Review Press.

Edmund D. Pellegrino. 1987. "Altruism, Self-Interest, and Medical Ethics." *Journal of the American Medical Association* 258:1939-1940.

Pascale M. Wortley and Patricia L. Fleming. 1997. "AIDS in Women in the United States," *Journal of the American Medical Association* 278:911-916. ✦

41

Brad

Maggie Callanan
Patricia Kelley

Brad's story echoes countless poignant scenarios among young people who have AIDS: youth and promise cut short by relentless disease. A secret identity as an AIDS patient masks an even greater secret and more fundamental identity—Brad's homosexuality. His story reflects profound losses in job, income, insurance, privacy. Nonetheless, Brad's story is also woven with bright threads. His parents' shock and sorrow turned into a loving and lasting commitment to care. His partner remained with him. The hospice nurses supplied technical assistance and emotional support to all. Though Brad's life may have been short, his dying allowed his family to give to him and to honor him, and his death had meaning.

Bright, handsome, kind and gentle by nature, Brad was an accomplished writer for a large advertising agency. Only thirty, he was far too young to die of anything, but especially of a tragic and ravaging illness. Suffering with the sudden and unpredictable ailments that come with AIDS, Brad in many ways personified the early days of the epidemic.

Brad and Adam, his partner of six years, shared a small, beautifully decorated townhouse in a city thousands of miles away from Brad's family home in Canada. Although Brad had pulled up stakes ten years before, he remained in close touch with his parents and brother, Lee, a commercial artist in Quebec. He called home every week and returned home each Christmas, always careful to conceal his sexual orientation and the degree of his closeness to Adam.

"They had no idea about our relationship or how sick Brad was," Adam told me. "He

struggled for years with how and when to tell his family he was gay. They're really wonderful, caring people, but he anguished about it; he was afraid the truth would break their hearts."

When Brad first began to come down with the opportunistic infections often associated with AIDS, he minimized them to his parents during their weekly phone calls. But they became increasingly more concerned with each problem Brad reported.

"It seemed strange to me that he was sick so often," his father said later. "He'd always been such a strapping, healthy young man."

When his boss realized that Brad had AIDS he fired him, claiming it was a necessary reduction in the staff. The firing cost Brad his income and his health-insurance coverage.

"Can you imagine that?" Adam said, with growing anger. "Brad had been one of their best employees for eight years. How's that for loyalty? Of course they denied any discrimination against him because of his illness or sexual orientation. We thought about hiring a lawyer to see what could be done, but frankly we didn't have the money and Brad was getting too sick to deal with it. We didn't want the notoriety anyway."

Adam, a respected sports reporter for one of the city newspapers, wasn't able to add Brad as a dependent on his health insurance or even use sick leave to care for him. All he could do was work as much overtime as possible to help pay the bills—amid the daily grind of changing soiled sheets, bathing Brad, and giving his medicines.

"His medical bills are unbelievable," Adam said. "The cost of just one of his medicines—AZT—is staggering! I begged him to level with his folks and seek their help, but he refused."

When Christmas came and pneumonia kept Brad from returning home, the matter was taken out of his hands. Missing their younger son and concerned about his health, Brad's parents decided to surprise him with a visit. They drove from Canada and knocked on Brad's door, only to receive a double-barreled shock.

"When they heard the word 'AIDS' there was a stunned silence for what seemed like an eternity," Adam said. "Finally Brad's father stood up and said to his wife, 'I need some fresh air. Will you join me?' They left together.

"My heart was aching for Brad *and* his parents," he said. "It must have been awful for them, and I knew Brad was afraid they would never come back. But two hours later they returned, faces puffy from crying. It was so sad. They hugged us and said, 'We'd like to stay and help if that's okay with both of you.' I can't tell you how relieved I was. Brad's eyes filled with tears."

The next few days were spent rearranging the den to make room for Brad's parents. His father called his business associate, explaining he'd be taking an indefinite leave of absence. His mother arranged for neighbors in Canada to watch their house and forward their mail. When Lee learned of his parents' plans, he offered to drive down the following weekend to bring additional clothing for his folks and some of his artwork for Brad's bedroom walls.

But sometimes love and family support aren't enough. Brad's condition was changing rapidly; he no longer could manage the trip to his doctor's office. His physician encouraged Adam and Brad's parents to consider hospice home care, as Brad needed regular monitoring by professionals. They agreed.

"Brad's so sick now that he can't be left alone at all," Adam said on my first visit. "I don't know what we would have done if his parents hadn't offered to stay. But we all need help and suggestions about taking care of him."

Brad quickly became bedridden and couldn't care for himself at all. The AIDS virus was affecting his brain. Confused, unable to speak, and possibly deaf, he'd fix his big brown eyes intently on whoever was near him, and follow that person with a look of urgency—as though he had something important he wanted to say.

We always spoke to him, explaining everything we were doing, assuming he could hear and understand. He rarely reacted, but we had a strong sense that he was aware of everything and everyone around him.

As the weeks and months passed, my admiration for Brad's parents grew. They never questioned or showed anger at his tragedy. They simply loved their son while gently and tirelessly providing for his every need. A mutual respect and love grew between them and Adam, as they worked together caring for Brad.

Becoming more debilitated, he stopped being able to swallow, but was receiving some fluids intravenously. We became concerned that these extra fluids might be prolonging his suffering and dying, rather than improving the quality of his life.

The doctor explained to Brad's parents that the IV fluids might delay his death by a few days, but that he was no longer really benefitting from them. He said the extra fluid might strain Brad's failing circulatory system, and recommended they be discontinued. This was a very upsetting and difficult change for Adam and Brad's parents to consider.

Our need to nurture is intense. We survive, thrive, and grow; we comfort, celebrate, and reward ourselves—and the people we care about—with food and drink. For parents, this need is profound, regardless of the child's age. Providing nourishment for our children is a essential part of a parent's role. Withholding it feels like denying love and nurturing—the very core issues of parenting. So, despite the inability of dying people to tolerate or benefit from fluids and nourishment, families and friends agonize over the question of ending them.

Brad's parents didn't want to stop the IV's. Adam and the doctor supported their decision. "This is difficult enough for them," the doctor said. "Continuing the IV's at a minimal rate won't make much difference to Brad, but if that helps his parents, then so be it."

When I visited, a few days later, Brad wouldn't look at me at all. Despite numerous attempts, I could not get his attention. His eyes were fixed, glaring at the IV bag hanging on the pole above his bed.

"Brad, I know this is hard for you," I said, holding his hand. "I bet you're really sick of it all and would like it to be over. You look like you're angry at the IV's, but we have them running as slowly as possible, so as not to drag this out. But your parents don't want to stop the fluids, because they love you so much. It's a decision that's too painful for them."

As I finished speaking, Brad shifted his gaze from the IV bag to the wall opposite his bed, where Lee had hung a charcoal sketch several months before. He stared intently at that picture. I hadn't paid much attention to it before, but on this day its symbolism was striking.

Lee had drawn a study in shadows and light, showing an old stone bridge, arched over a long dark mountain tunnel, at the far end of which a brilliant white light gleamed.

Many people report going through a passageway toward a wonderful bright light during Near Death Experiences; people who are dying slowly often have such occurrences, as well. I returned to Brad's side and took his hand again, stroking it.

"Brad, if you're ready to go, it's okay," I said. "I'll explain to Adam and your parents what I think you're trying to tell us."

We gathered around his bed as I explained my interpretation of Brad's behavior. By looking at the picture—with its image of passage—I thought perhaps he was attempting to tell us the time had come for his journey. Tearfully they hugged and kissed him, giving him permission to go.

"We love you and we'll miss you, Brad," Adam said. "But you've fought long enough and we're ready for you to go whenever you need to." Brad closed his eyes and relaxed.

During the next two days, Brad alternated between deep sleep and periods of being "glassy-eyed," seeming to look through us at something we could not see. Lee was called to come.

Everyone was restless, wandering in and out of Brad's room, taking turns napping and sitting with him. Touching and stroking him, they murmured soft reassurances. From deep sleep he drifted into a brief coma, barely noticed. He then quietly died with the people he loved around him.

At Brad's funeral, Lee said, "We were so close growing up we could almost read each other's minds. So it means a lot to me that he told us he was ready to die through my picture. It feels like I helped talk for him when he couldn't talk for himself anymore."

Unable to speak, Brad still could communicate his awareness that death was near. And, with help, his caregivers were able to understand his nonverbal message, giving him the permission he needed to go, and themselves the opportunity to prepare for his death. . . .

Further Reading

Harold Brodsky. 1996. *This Wild Darkness: The Story of My Death*. New York: Henry Holt.

Paul Monette. 1988. *Borrowed Time: An AIDS Memoir*. San Diego: Harcourt, Brace, Jovanovich.

Stephen O. Murray. 1996. *American Gay*. Chicago: University of Chicago Press.

Discussion Questions

1. How might Brad's earlier life have shaped his dying?

2. What kinds of social policies would foster quality care of AIDS patients?

3. What do you see as the main advantages and disadvantages of early disclosure of AIDS to family, friends, and co-workers for men and women in Brad's position?

42

Update: Trends in AIDS Incidence, Deaths, and Prevalence— United States, 1996

Centers for Disease Control

As research changes our understandings of HIV and AIDS, surveillance of human immunodeficiency virus (HIV) and acquired immunodeficiency syndrome (AIDS) has taken various forms. Programs to prevent HIV infection and to alleviate the opportunistic infections resulting from AIDS can only target populations and problems that we already comprehend. This report updates our understandings of the incidence and prevalence of HIV and AIDS. Note the changes in populations affected by the virus from 1981 to the present. Note the increases and decreases in this phenomenon for subsets of the population. Using other readings in this section as a guide, see if you can outline the changes in the definition and social context of HIV and AIDS that have altered the national incidence and prevalence of the disease. Consider whether future trends in HIV and AIDS related deaths are the best predictors of successful health education programs.

The national acquired immunodeficiency syndrome (AIDS) surveillance system is used to describe the impact of HIV-related morbidity and death in the United States. This report presents trends in AIDS incidence during 1996 and describes recent declines in deaths among persons reported with AIDS

(AIDS deaths) and increases in AIDS prevalence.

Cumulative AIDS cases among persons aged≥13 years reported to CDC based on the 1993 expanded surveillance case definition from the 50 states, the District of Columbia, Puerto Rico, and the U.S. territories were analyzed by year of report, race/ethnicity, and mode of risk/exposure.[1] Estimates of AIDS incidence and deaths were adjusted for the effects of delays in reporting. For analyses by mode of risk/exposure, estimates were adjusted for the anticipated reclassification of cases initially reported without an HIV risk/exposure.[1] To adjust for the expansion of the reporting criteria in 1993, estimates of the incidence of AIDS-opportunistic illnesses (OIs) were calculated from the sum of cases diagnosed with an AIDS-OI and the estimated dates of an AIDS-OI diagnosis for cases reported based on immunologic criteria.[1] AIDS-OI incidence was estimated quarterly through June 1996, the most recent period for which reliable estimates were available. Estimates of AIDS-OI incidence rates per 100,000 population were based on 1995 population estimates from the Bureau of the Census. Deaths among persons with AIDS were identified by review of medical records and death certificates and include both deaths from AIDS and from other causes. AIDS prevalence was estimated from cumulative AIDS incidence minus cumulative deaths.

Reported AIDS Cases

From 1981 through 1996, a total of 573,800 persons aged≥13 years with AIDS were reported to CDC by state and local health departments (Table 42-1). The expansion of the AIDS surveillance case definition in 1993 resulted in a large increase in reported cases during 1993 followed by declines in numbers of AIDS cases reported each year from 1994 through 1996. The 68,473 AIDS cases reported during 1996 was substantially higher (47%) than the number reported during 1992.

From 1992 through 1996, non-Hispanic blacks, Hispanics, and women accounted for increasing proportions of persons reported

Table 42-1

*Number and percentage of persons aged≥13 years reported with AIDS,
by sex and race/ethnicity — United States, 1981–1996*

Year of Report Characteristic	1992 No.	1992 %	1993* No.	1993* %	1994 No.	1994 %	1995 No.	1995 %	1996 No.	1996 %	1981–1996 No.	1981–1996 %
Sex												
Male	40.330	(86)	87,945	(84)	64,730	(82)	59,285	(81)	54,653	(80)	488,300	(85)
Female	6,307	(14)	16,671	(16)	13,830	(18)	13,682	(19)	13,820	(20)	85,500	(15)
Race/Ethnicity												
White, non-Hispanic	22,320	(48)	47,468	(45)	32,677	(42)	29,402	(40)	26,229	(38)	267,487	(47)
Black, non-Hispanic	15,576	(33)	37,523	(36)	30,373	(39)	28,729	(39)	28,346	(41)	198,780	(35)
Hispanic	8,223	(18)	18,410	(18)	14,612	(19)	13,961	(19)	12,966	(19)	101,253	(18)
Asian/Pacific Islander	334	(<1)	761	(<1)	573	(<1)	558	(<1)	561	(<1)	4,090	(<1)
American Indian/ Alaskan Native	121	(<1)	369	(<1)	246	(<1)	237	(<1)	207	(<1)	1,544	(<1)
Total†	46,637	(100)	104,616	(100)	78,560	(100)	72,967	(100)	68,473	(100)	573,800	(100)

* Year the expanded AIDS surveillance case definition was implemented.
† Totals include persons with unknown or missing race/ethnicity.

with AIDS. In 1996, non-Hispanic blacks accounted for 41% of adults reported with AIDS, exceeding for the first time the proportion who were non-Hispanic white, and women accounted for an all-time high of 20% of adults reported with AIDS.

AIDS-OI Incidence

In 1995, AIDS-OIs were diagnosed in an estimated 62,200 persons, an increase of 2% over the estimate for 1994 (61,200) (Figure 42-1). From January 1994 through June 1996, the quarterly incidence of AIDS-OIs was stable (mean: 15,200 cases per quarter).

During 1995, estimated AIDS-OI incidence rates per 100,000 population were approximately sevenfold higher among non-Hispanic blacks (99) and three than among non-Hispanic whites (15). Estimated rates were lowest among American Indians/Alaskan Natives (14) and Asians/Pacific Islanders (6) and were nearly five fold greater among men (48) than among women (10).

From 1994 through 1995, estimated AIDS-OI incidence was approximately constant (a decrease of 2%) among men who have sex with men (MSM) (Figure 42-2) and among heterosexual injecting-drug users (IDUS) (an increase of 2%) (Figure 42-3), but increased substantially among persons infected through heterosexual contact (17%) (Figure 42-4).

Of the 30,100 persons in whom AIDS-OIs were diagnosed during January-June 1996, 46% were MSM, 29% were IDUS, and 17% were infected through heterosexual contact.

Figure 42-1

*Estimated AIDS-opportunistic illness (OI)
incidence and estimated deaths among
persons with AIDS (AIDS deaths),
adjusted for delays in reporting, by quarter
year of diagnosis/death — United States,
1984–June 1996*

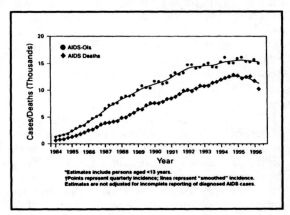

Figure 42-2
Estimated AIDS-opportunistic illness (OI) incidence and estimated deaths among persons aged ≥ 13 years with AIDS (AIDS deaths), by exposure category (men who have sex with men), adjusted for delays in reporting, by quarter year of diagnosis/death — United States, 1984–June 1996

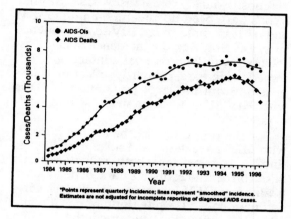

Figure 42-3
Estimated AIDS-opportunistic illness (OI) incidence and estimated deaths among persons aged ≥ 13 years with AIDS (AIDS deaths), by exposure category (injecting-drug use), adjusted for delays in reporting, by quarter year of diagnosis/death — United States, 1984–June 1996

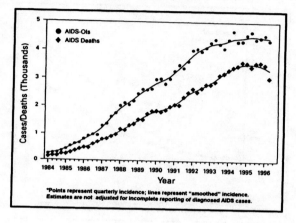

Deaths Among Persons Reported With AIDS

The estimated number of deaths among persons reported with AIDS increased steadily through 1994 (approximately 49,600 deaths among persons with AIDS during 1994) (Figure 42-1) but increased only slightly in 1995 (approximately 50,000 deaths). During January–June 1996, the estimated number of AIDS deaths (22,000) was 13% less than that estimated during January-June 1995 (24,900), and the number of deaths declined in each of the four regions of the United States (Northeast [15%], South [8%], Midwest [11%], and West [16%1]). The number of AIDS deaths also declined among all racial/ethnic groups (non-Hispanic whites [21%], non-Hispanic blacks [2%], Hispanics [10%], Asians/Pacific Islanders [6%], and American Indians/Alaskan Natives [32%]) and among men (15%) but increased 3% among women. By risk/exposure category, deaths declined 18% among MSM (Figure 42-2) and 6% among IDUs (Figure 42-3) but increased 3% among persons infected through heterosexual contact (Figure 42-4),

the only risk/exposure group with large increases in AIDS-OI incidence during 1995.

AIDS Prevalence

As of June 1996, the estimated prevalence of AIDS was 223,000 U.S. residents aged ≥ 13 years (Figure 42-5), representing increases of 10% and 65% since mid-1995 and January 1993, respectively. Of prevalent cases of AIDS, 82% were among men; 43%, non-Hispanic whites; 38%, non-Hispanic blacks; and 19%, Hispanics. By risk/exposure category, MSM accounted for the largest number of prevalent cases of AIDS (44%), followed by IDUs (26%) and persons infected through heterosexual contact (12%); all other risk/exposure groups combined accounted for 18% of prevalent cases of AIDS. The largest proportionate increase in AIDS prevalence from June 1995 through June 1996 occurred among persons infected through heterosexual contact (19%) while the largest absolute increase occurred among MSM (5100).

Reported by: State and local health depts. Div of HIV/AIDS Prevention—Surveillance and Epidemiology, National Center for HIV, STD, and TB Prevention, CDC.

Figure 42-4

Estimated AIDS-opportunistic illness (OI) incidence and estimated deaths among persons aged ≥ 13 years with AIDS (AIDS deaths), by exposure category (HIV infection acquired through heterosexual contact), adjusted for delays in reporting, by quarter year of diagnosis/death—United States, 1984–June 1996

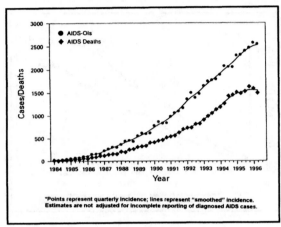

Points represent quarterly incidence; lines represent "smoothed" incidence. Estimates are not adjusted for incomplete reporting of diagnosed AIDS cases.

Figure 42-5

Number of prevalent AIDS cases among persons aged ≥ 13 years, adjusted for delays in reporting, by quarter year— United States, 1988–June 1996

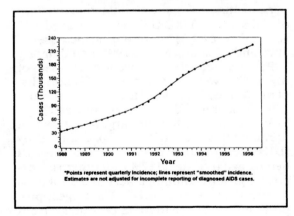

Points represent quarterly incidence; lines represent "smoothed" incidence. Estimates are not adjusted for incomplete reporting of diagnosed AIDS cases.

Editorial Note: The findings in this report document a substantial increase in AIDS prevalence in the United States. Prevalence is a function of both the rate of new infections and the duration of illness. The increase in AIDS prevalence reflects declines in AIDS deaths and stable AIDS incidence. The increased prevalence of AIDS indicates the need for medical and other services for persons with HIV infection and for prevention programs to reduce the number of persons becoming infected with HIV.

The leveling of AIDS-OI incidence nationally in 1995 was preceded by a gradual deceleration in the rate of increase of new AIDS diagnoses during previous years.[1] Similar trends have been documented among MSM and IDUs in clinic-based HIV-seroprevalence surveys.[2] However, the incidence of cases associated with heterosexual contact has continued to increase, primarily reflecting transmission from the large population of IDUs with HIV/AIDS to their heterosexual partners.

For the first time, deaths among persons with AIDS have decreased substantially. This finding is consistent with recent reports, based on death-certificate data, of declines in deaths from HIV infection in New York City[3] and nationally.[4] Despite these trends, during 1995 HIV infection remained the leading cause of death among persons aged 25–44 years (Figure 42-6), accounting for 19% of deaths from all causes in this age group.

The decrease in AIDS deaths reflects both the leveling of AIDS-OI incidence and improved survival among persons with AIDS. Increased survival reflects recent improvements in medical care, of therapy with antiretroviral agents, and increasing use of prophylactic drugs to prevent secondary AIDS-OIs.[5] In addition, the widespread availability of protease inhibitors, approved by the Food and Drug Administration in 1996, may further improve survival.[6]

The higher AIDS-OI incidence rates among non-Hispanic blacks and Hispanics than among non-Hispanic whites may reflect reduced access to health care associated with disadvantaged socioeconomic status, cultural or language barriers that may limit access to prevention information, and differences in HIV risk behaviors.[7] The number of AIDS deaths did not decrease among women or persons infected through heterosexual contact, reflecting, in part, continued increases in AIDS incidence and differences in access to treatment, which may vary by sex,

Figure 42-6
Death rates* for leading causes of death among persons aged 25–44 years, by year — United States, 1982–1995†

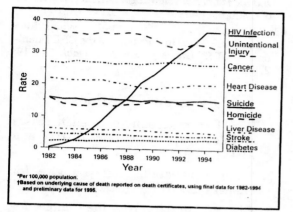

*Per 100,000 population.
†Based on underlying cause of death reported on death certificates, using final data for 1982–1994 and preliminary data for 1995.

region, race/ethnicity, and risk/exposure. To assist prevention efforts and treatment services, surveillance systems are being developed to access to counseling, testing, and care.

Monitoring AIDS prevalence will help direct resources to persons most in need of treatment for severe HIV disease. However, because the clinical status of most HIV-infected persons has not yet progressed to AIDS,[8] AIDS prevalence underestimates the total number of HIV-infected persons in need of related services. Advances in treatment and improved survival also will affect efforts to monitor the HIV epidemic based on the current AIDS surveillance definition and, therefore, will require surveillance systems that are less sensitive to changes in the progression of HIV disease. Among the 26 states that conducted surveillance for cases of both HIV infection and AIDS in 1996, prevalence of HIV and AIDS among reported cases (126,491) was 2.5-fold higher than the prevalence of AIDS (51,217).[1] However, this represents a minimum estimate of HIV prevalence in these states because not all HIV-infected persons seek testing and some persons are tested anonymously.

The Council of State and Territorial Epidemiologists has recommended that all states consider implementing surveillance for HIV infection and AIDS.[9] Population-based surveillance for both HIV and AIDS provides a more complete measure of the number of HIV-infected persons and a more timely measure to detect emerging patterns of HIV transmission than does AIDS surveillance alone. CDC provides technical assistance and funding to areas that conduct both HIV and AIDS case surveillance. CDC also supports research to develop optimal surveillance methods that meet the need for important behavioral, biomedical, and treatment data for persons with HIV and AIDS public health and community concerns about factors that may influence decision-making regarding testing or treatment.

Future trends in the HIV/AIDS epidemic in the United States will reflect the effectiveness of programs to prevent new HIV infections, to promote timely diagnosis, and to continue improving clinical management. CDC has established as a primary prevention strategy efforts to involve affected communities in planning and evaluating HIV-prevention programs.[10] To continue to provide data for planning, directing, and evaluating HIV prevention and care services at the federal, state, and local levels, HIV/AIDS surveillance systems must adapt to changes in the diagnosis and clinical management of HIV and AIDS.

References

1. CDC. *HIV/AIDS surveillance report.* Atlanta: U.S. Department of Health and Human Services, Public Health Service, 1996:3-4,20,30-3. (Vol 8, no. 1).

2. CDC. *National HIV serosurveillance summary: results through 1992.* Atlanta: U.S. Department of Health and Human Service, Public Health Service, CDC, November 1993.

3. Chiasson, M., L. Berenson, W. Li, S. Schwartz, B. Mojica, and M. Hamburg. "Declining AIDS mortality in New York City [Abstract]." In: *Program and abstracts of the IV Conference on Retroviruses and Opportunistic Infections, 1997.* Alexandria, Virginia: Infectious Diseases Society of America for Retrovirology and Human Health, 1997.

4. National Center for Health Statistics. "Births, marriages, divorces, and deaths for July 1996." Hyattsville, Maryland: U.S. Department of Health and Human Services, Public Health Service, CDC, 1997. (Monthly vital statistics report; vol. 45, no. 7, suppl.)

5. Jones, J.L., D.L. Hanson, J.W. Ward, J.E. Kaplan "Incidence trends in AIDS-related opportunistic illnesses in injecting drug users and men who have sex with men [Abstract]." Vancouver, British Columbia: XI International Conference on AIDS, 1996.

6. Carpenter, C.C.J., M.A. Fischi, S.M. Hammer et al. "Antiretroviral therapy for HIV infection in 1996: recommendations of an international panel." *JAMA*, 1996;276:146-54.

7. CDC. "AIDS among racial/ethnic minorities—United States, 1993." *MMWR*, 1994; 43:644-7, 653-5.

8. Karon, J.M., P.S. Rosenberg, G. McQuillan, M. Khare, M. Gwinn, and L. Petersen. "Prevalence of HIV infection in the United States, 1984 to 1992." *JAMA*, 1996; 276:126-31.

9. Council of State and Territorial Epidemiologists. "CSTE: position statement 2. Surveillance of HIV infection and disease." Atlanta: Council of State and Territorial Epidemiologists, 1991.

10. Valdiserri, R.O., T.V. Aultman, and J.W. Curran. "Community planning: a national strategy to improve HIV prevention programs." *J Community Health*, 1995; 20:87-100.

Further Reading

Allan Brandt. 1987. *No Magic Bullet: A Social History of Venereal Disease in the United States Since 1880.* New York: Oxford University Press.

Centers for Disease Control. *Medical and Mortality Weekly Report*. Boston: Massachusetts Medical Society.

Steven Epstein. 1996. *Impure Science: AIDS Activism and the Politics of Knowledge*. Berkeley: University of California Press.

Carol Levine and Gary Stein. 1991. "What's in a Name? The Policy Implications of the CDC Definition of AIDS." *Law, Medicine, and Health Care* 19: 278-90.

Discussion Questions

1. What factors account for rapid increases and decreases in the rates of HIV and AIDS?

2. What explanations can you give for changes in AIDS related death rates?

3. Given these data from the Centers for Disease Control, what sorts of trends might you expect to see in the incidence of HIV and AIDS in the next five years?

4. How might future trends in the incidence and prevalence of HIV and AIDS enable us to decipher the effectiveness of health education programs in the United States?

From Centers for Disease Control, 1997. ✦

43

The Invisible Epidemic: The Story of Women and AIDS

Gena Corea

A *rapid increase in HIV and AIDS infected women began in 1989. Before that time, women remained invisible victims. In this selection, Corea recounts the rapid increase in women's participation in programs for people with AIDS (PWAs) in the early 1990s. She documents clinics in the northeast where men receive the greater proportion of education and treatment in spite of rapidly increasing numbers of women with HIV and AIDS. Corea, like Lillie-Blanton and her coauthors, reports that the risk factors facing African-American and Latina women go unrecongnized in systems of classification and methods of identifying people at risk for HIV and AIDS. Consider some of the evidence Corea provides for this claim in her account of women at risk. Compare her accounts with those provided by Rose Weitz in the following selection. Think about the reasons why standard modes of classification and particular health education methods established by the Centers for Disease Control (CDC) do not prove effective in either categorizing or educating many of the women Corea discusses. Consider how attention to the problems and dilemmas conveyed here by Corea might alter the direction of trends reported in the previous data by the CDC.*

There was a dramatic switch in 1989 to a greater percentage of HIV transmission through heterosexual intercourse and to a greater percentage of infected women. This switch was reported in a number of places.

"When I first came on board in 1987," Evelyn Figarowa of the Woodfield Family Services in Bridgeport, Connecticut, said, "we didn't have one woman in the [HIV buddy] program. It was interesting to see our first woman [in 1989]. And then it was like, all of a sudden, all the new referrals that we got were all women. It seemed for a while there that most of the referrals came from women."

From July 1990 to June 30, 1991, there were fifty-eight PWAs in the buddy program—thirty-nine men and nineteen women. The program had no women at all in 1988; in such a short time to suddenly have a three-to-two ratio of men to women Figarowa found extraordinary.

In the Brown University AIDS program, where an estimated 95 percent of all the HIV-infected women with AIDS in Rhode Island were seen, before June 1989 almost all the HIV transmission—81 percent—was attributed to sharing of needles by IV drug users.

"Around June of 1989," Dr. Charles Carpenter of that program reported, "we began seeing a lot more heterosexual transmission. During the next nine months, the ratio of heterosexual transmission to IV drug use transmission was roughly fifty-fifty. During the nine-month period starting in March 1, 1990, the bulk of the transmission has been by the heterosexual route: roughly two-thirds. That's been a very striking change in the recent past. It's been statewide. Throughout this period, the ethnic backgrounds of the patients have remained roughly the same: 15 percent black, 15 percent Hispanic, and 70 percent Caucasian."

So, in a short period of time, the dominant mode of transmission in women in Rhode Island switched from IV drug use to heterosexual transmission.

In the women infected through sexual contact, the median number of sexual partners the women had had throughout their lives was small, Carpenter reported. Only three. Though a standard AIDS prevention message to women is "Reduce risk by lowering the number of sexual partners," some American women are learning what had long been the case for African women: with even one or two lifetime partners, you can get AIDS.

In New Jersey, Dr. Patricia Kloster, chief of the only women's HIV clinic in New Jersey, reported that in the mid-1980s, the HIV infected women she saw at University Hospital in Newark were about 80 percent IV drug users. The remaining 20 percent of patients had been infected through heterosexual intercourse or by unknown means. But by 1989, 48 percent of the women had been infected through sex.

Dr. Carmen Zorilla, who has been working with HIV patients in Puerto Rico since 1986, reported that in 1987, 28 percent of the women with AIDS acquired it through sexual contact. By 1990, this had increased to 43 percent.

"We can observe a clear pattern of increasing prominence of cases attributed to sexual transmission," she said. "Without sophisticated mathematical analysis, we can predict that within the next two years, heterosexual transmission will be the principal cause of AIDS in women in Puerto Rico. Most of our patients—82 percent—acquired infection through the sexual route."

Dr. Janet Mitchell, chief of perinatology at Harlem Hospital Center in New York, and colleagues looked at former IV drug users at a methadone program in New York City, a third of whose clients were women. These seven hundred women had a higher rate of HIV infection—61 percent—than the men in the clinic—on the order of 56 percent. This, she pointed out, was probably because the women were doubly exposed to HIV—through shared needles and sexual contact.

"So you don't know how they got it," she said. "You don't know which came first—the chicken or the egg. . .".

The CDC's method of classifying the way in which a person became infected with HIV could be hiding even more cases of heterosexual transmission in women. The transmission categories are set up hierarchically. That means that the first risk behavior a person admits to is the one her case is classified in. So a woman who admits to IV drug use and has HIV would be counted as having acquired the disease through dirty needles. But most often that woman is also sexually active

and may actually have been infected through sexual intercourse.

Women with AIDS are twice as likely as men with AIDS to be reported without an established risk factor, Dr. Ruth Berkelman, chief of the CDC's surveillance branch, reported. (According to Dr. Judith Cohen, director of the Association for Women's AIDS Research and Education [AWARE] in San Francisco, this is partly because some women die so soon after they are diagnosed that there is no time to schedule an interview with them to determine what their risk factor may have been.)

Many of these cases in which the risk factor had not been pin-pointed may actually be due to heterosexual transmission, the CDC's Berkelman noted. She reported that between 1988 and 1989, there was a 33 percent increase in AIDS cases attributed to heterosexual transmission in the United States.

"AIDS cases attributed to heterosexual transmission are rising among both men and women, but more cases are occurring among women than men," she stated.

The dramatic change in the AIDS epidemic was also happening in the predominantly white, middle-class suburbs of Long Island, New York. In fact, Long Island has more people with AIDS than any other American suburban region. A full 28 percent of the clients served by the Long Island Association for AIDS Care (LIAAC) are women.

In the next few years, many women living in suburbs who feel perfectly safe, who have no idea they are at risk, will get AIDS, LIAAC director Gail Barouh predicted. By 1994, she calculated, 42 to 45 percent of LIAAC's cases would be women.

Because the AIDS message had focused on categories of *people* at risk rather than on *behaviors*, women who did not belong to those categories—*they* were monogamous and nondrug-addicted—felt unjustifiably safe. But maybe their husband, identifying himself as a heterosexual, sometimes had sex with men.

Jeri Woodhouse, assistant to Manhattan Borough president Ruth Messinger on special projects including AIDS, worried about this.

People working with street youths in the city talked with her about the men who drive in from the suburbs, pay the street youth—boys and girls—for sex, and then drive home to the suburbs where their wives have no idea that their husbands have a secret sex life.

It's hard for women who've been married for a long time to know how to discuss this openly with their husbands, Woodhouse said. Suburban women tell her, "If I want to bring up that issue, he assumes I'm accusing him of cheating on me so I can't speak to him about it." Or, "I married him thirty years ago. How do I now say, 'Let's use condoms?' when we've not used them all these years?" Or the women fear their husbands will get angry and turn it around on them: "If you're thinking of this, you must be fooling around."

Among white, single women on Long Island, Gail Barouh now saw blanket denial that there was any problem, a chanting of charms that made them feel safe: "He doesn't look gay." "He hasn't gone out with a lot of different people; he was in steady relationships." "He looks safe so we don't need condoms." "He's into bodybuilding so he wouldn't be using drugs." "We used condoms at the beginning but we've been going out six months now so we don't do that anymore."

In the support groups LIAAC ran were women whose sisters had died of AIDS. Yet they themselves were sleeping with men without condom protection.

Thus a number of experts believe the current scale of the problem among married women in the suburbs may be somewhat underestimated to the extent that HIV infection in women is not being identified or counted.

"These [HIV-infected] women are going to their gynecologists," Figarowa of Woodfield Family Services in Connecticut says. "They're getting frequent infections, and it's attributed to anything else [other than HIV]. The doctor would never ask—and the wife would never have any idea. Unless they're tested or their husband comes down with the illness." She could as well have been speaking of Patricia Daugherty in rural Maine.

In Brooklyn, Marie-Lucie Brutus of WARN believed the false sense of safety middle-class white women felt about AIDS was due not only to the CDC's use of risk groups rather than risk behaviors but to the politics of knowledge. Poor women of color will be the ones mostly counted in official statistics on AIDS, she said, because they go to the places where counting is done: hospital clinics and social agencies.

"But the ones who do not go to the places where you can count—you don't know about them."

It was true that women in poor communities were being hard hit by the AIDS epidemic, she emphasized.

Food, shelter, clothes to cover us in winter—those are primary needs and these women don't have it! Let alone education. If they don't have it, of course they are going to be the group that will be most likely to be infected with a virus that is transmitted sexually. Because the drugs are already there. The alcohol is already there. The misfunction of the families is already there. All the social ills that are a breeding ground for any problem are already there.

But because white middle-class women tend not to go to agencies where the counting is done, we don't know where the disease may be spreading, undetected, Brutus pointed out.

"That's why I keep telling people not to be complacent," Brutus said.

Within the next three to five years, Barouh predicted, AIDS would be as much a woman's problem as a man's problem. At least on Long Island. What was happening on Long Island would happen in other areas, she feared. In many ways, Long Island was a suburban trend-setter.

Barouh could sum up Long Island's response to the AIDS crisis in two words: denial and apathy. Politicians were quiet about AIDS. County executives did not speak on it publicly or consider it their long-range planning. Long Island had done little to deal with its current AIDS problem or to prepare for the more massive AIDS epidemic that was coming.

Barouh was worried because many of the prevention strategies for women had not worked. Obviously. She and her colleagues at LIAAC thought training HIV-infected women to educate women in the community on AIDS prevention would be effective. But that was difficult because the HIV-infected women felt they needed to hide to protect themselves. They had to consider the consequences of their openness to their families. Would their children be thrown out of school and the whole family out of their housing? Would they lose their jobs? It was a big risk. Early in the year, when a woman who lived in Huntington, Long Island, revealed that she worked for an AIDS organization, a swastika was painted on her fence, Woodhouse reported.

> The women who are infected in the suburbs tend to believe that they are isolated cases, alone and stigmatized, so they are not going to tell anybody around them about it.

The women most directly affected by AIDS in the suburbs weren't talking. When the numbers of women infected got real bad, then something would be done. But government agencies were keeping the numbers low through a narrow definition of AIDS. Those artificial numbers were going to explode. Soon more and more people would know people with AIDS. It would be harder to keep the problem under wraps. Then maybe something would be done. When it was a colossal disaster. . . .

Further Reading

Michael Fumento. 1989. *The Myth of Heterosexual AIDS*. New York: Basic Books.

Lewis H. Kuller and Lawrence A. Kingsley. 1986. "The Epidemic of AIDS: A Failure of Public Policy." *Milbank Quarterly* 64: 56-78.

June Osborne. 1989. "Public Health and the Politics of AIDS Prevention." *Daedalus* 118(3): 123-144.

Randy Shilts. 1987. *And the Band Played On: Politics, People, and the AIDS Epidemic*. New York: St. Martin's Press.

Discussion Questions

1. According to Corea, what makes African-American and Latina women at greater risk than men or other groups of women for HIV and AIDS?

2. What sorts of issues need to be addressed in the identification of groups at risk for HIV and AIDS?

3. Why would a focus on behaviors rather than on particular social strata be a more effective method for identifying people at risk?

44

Becoming a Person with HIV Disease

Rose Weitz

How do people learn that they have a disease? In this chapter, Rose Weitz demonstrates the difference between biological process and social meaning. Reflect upon how official labels such as diagnoses affect thoughts, feelings and actions. Until people know and acknowledge being HIV infected, they are unlikely to alter their view of themselves. The path to discovering a diagnosis may neither be smooth nor clear. Think about how Weitz' interviewees learned of their conditions. Compare them with the personal accounts and studies you read in Section Two. False negatives and false positive test results render a person's status ambiguous. What people suspect about their health depends upon their situations.

Like other diseases, AIDS may have an insidious onset with amorphous, but explainable, symptoms. To the extent that people can downplay or explain symptoms, they will forego seeking treatment. Then when they receive a diagnosis, they may attribute varied meanings to it. Look for the range of meanings held by these research respondents. Weitz found that some of them assumed they could emerge victorious over AIDS while others crumbled in defeat to a death sentence. Certainly societal definitions of a disease and immediate support or its absence for one's view of it sustain or negate this view. However people define themselves in relation to HIV disease, once they acknowledge infection, they seek to explain how and why they have it. They place it within their biographies and imbue it with meaning. Such reflection leads to thoughts of the future with revised plans and, sometimes, dashed hopes. An uncertain future, an ambiguous course of illness, and unpredictable treatment place heavy burdens on individuals to find ways to reduce uncertainty.*

Interpreting Symptoms and Seeking Diagnoses

The initial symptoms of HIV disease can take many forms, including rashes, fevers, night sweats, weight loss, diarrhea, tiredness, difficulty breathing, and swollen lymph nodes. Once symptoms begin to appear, individuals must decide how to interpret them and how to respond.

The problems involved in making these decisions differ depending on whether or not individuals know they are or might be infected with HIV. Those who know have readily available explanations for any symptoms that appear. Yet they still must wonder if these symptoms are a result of HIV disease or of some unrelated health problems. Carol, for example, even though asymptomatic, was tested for HIV once she learned that the one person she occasionally shared needles with had been diagnosed with HIV disease. Her ambiguous health status causes her constant stress:

> That's the things that are aggravating to me about living with the HIV and just wondering day to day when is it going to progress to the next stage. Every time I have a headache, every time I can't remember something quite right, I wonder is it the stress and all the bullshit that's going on [in my life] or, my God, is this going into the second stage? And then how quick will it go into AIDS after it's gone into the second stage? That's something you live with day to day. Every little thing. I'll get a sore throat and think, "Oh, it's in my lymph nodes." You know and you start feeling around. It's just, it's scary. [It's] something that never goes away.

The appearance of symptoms presents a different set of problems for those who do not know they are infected with HIV. Because symptoms generally build gradually, persons with HIV disease at first can accommodate to them. As a result, they, like persons who develop other chronic illnesses, initially may explain their symptoms using preexisting cognitive frameworks that minimize the symptoms' importance.[1] Several blamed their night sweats and exhaustion on the Arizona heat. Others confused the symptoms of HIV disease with the side effects of drug use or drug withdrawal, both of which can cause weight loss, sweating, and diarrhea. Although these theories eventually proved wrong, in the interim they reduced uncertainty and hence stress by allowing individuals to feel they understood what was happening to them.

Although some individuals minimized their symptoms out of ignorance, most appeared consciously or unconsciously to downplay their symptoms because they preferred to maintain unrealistic theories about their health rather than to obtain accurate but depressing knowledge. Compared to the other people I interviewed, Kevin, a twenty-three-year-old sales clerk, seems far more overwhelmed by his illness, unable to cope either intellectually or emotionally with his situation. In the months before he was diagnosed, he had considerably more difficulty than most of those I interviewed in acknowledging that he might be infected with HIV. Although he had lost significant weight, experienced substantial pain, and seen his physical condition deteriorate, he had put off seeing a doctor as long as he could. As he explains, "I didn't want to find out I had AIDS. Even though I kind of figured I did, I didn't want to know. I wanted to live a normal life for as long as I could." Avoiding diagnosis and thus avoiding knowledge that was likely to be unpleasant had helped Kevin maintain his emotional health, despite his growing lack of control over his physical condition.

As Kevin's example demonstrates, those who downplay the importance of their symptoms, for whatever reason, may defer seeing a physician for some time. Of those who went for HIV testing only after they developed symptoms, almost every one did not seek medical care until they were sick enough to be diagnosed as having AIDS or ARC, rather than simply as HIV-infected. As the disease progresses, however, individuals eventually find that their health deteriorates to the point

where they can no longer maintain their everyday living patterns and thus can no longer maintain the fiction that nothing is wrong. As their former ideas about the meaning of their symptoms crumble, persons with HIV disease face an intolerably ambiguous situation. Once they reach this point, the incentive grows to seek diagnosis and treatment.

Because the test for HIV was developed for use by blood banks, many public health workers worried when the test first appeared that gay men might donate blood so that they could get tested for HIV. As a result, the federal government funds at least one public blood-testing facility in every state so that gay men can learn whether they are infected without donating blood. Individuals who recognize that they might have HIV disease and go to one of these facilities soon have an explanation for their illness. Those who go to private physicians, however, may find it considerably more difficult to obtain a diagnosis. Many physicians simply lack the knowledge needed to diagnose HIV disease.[2] Others may not consider such diagnoses unless they know that their clients are at risk, even if their clients' symptoms fit the classic patterns for HIV disease. Yet some clients do not realize that they are at risk and others will not tell their physicians that they are at risk for fear of the stigma attendant on drug use or homosexual activity. These problems are probably most acute for those who live in areas where HIV disease is still relatively rare and still not very salient for doctors.

For all these reasons, then, persons with HIV disease may not receive accurate diagnoses until several months after they seek care. In the interim, and at least initially, some individuals accept or even welcome the alternative diagnoses that their physicians propose. When symptoms continue, however, they find themselves in what Stewart and Sullivan have described (with regard to multiple sclerosis) as "an ambiguous and uncertain limbo," in which they suffer anxieties about the meaning of their symptoms and cannot function normally, but in which those around them may neither believe that they are sick nor relieve them of any responsibilities.[3] Consequently, they cannot indefinitely sustain their own belief in these diagnoses.

To cope with this situation, some individuals will go from doctor to doctor to obtain a more believable diagnosis. Others research their symptoms, diagnose themselves, and then press their physicians to test for HIV. Even then, they may have difficulty obtaining a diagnosis. Several persons I interviewed complained that their physicians neither tested them for nor diagnosed them with HIV disease, even though they had classic symptoms (such as night sweats, persistent diarrhea, and weight loss), stated that they were gay, and requested that their blood be tested for HIV. Caleb, a forty-five-year-old mechanic, describes how his physician refused his several requests for testing, even though the physician knew he was gay and that something was wrong with his immune system. He says, "I was concerned. The symptoms were there, and I was not getting any better, not feeling any better, still getting weaker and weaker, losing more weight, and I kept mentioning all these things, and I said 'Look, I've been reading more articles about AIDS.' And he said, 'Oh, people are just panic-stricken. You don't have AIDS. I'm not doing a test on you.'" Stories such as this suggest that even when physicians have the necessary information, they may consciously or unconsciously avoid diagnosing HIV disease.

Diagnosis with HIV Disease

The experience of receiving one's diagnosis and the immediate aftermath of this experience vary widely from individual to individual. One critical factor is the doctor's familiarity with HIV disease. Those who suspect that they have HIV disease and seek diagnosis either at HIV testing facilities or from doctors who specialize in this illness usually receive sympathetic, detailed, and accurate information about their condition and prognosis. So do those who do not suspect that they have HIV disease but whose primary practitioners specialize in gay populations and therefore have become educated about this illness. The rest are not always so lucky. Unlike doctors in places like California or New York, most doctors in other parts of the country, such as Arizona, have little experience with HIV disease. Consequently, although some doctors prove both sympathetic and knowledgeable, others make their ignorance and prejudice immediately known. They can do so by adopting unnecessary precautions against contagion such as donning gowns and masks, informing people who are infected with HIV but have yet to develop any opportunistic infections that they will die within a few months, speaking rudely or abruptly, and warning persons with HIV disease that they can infect their families if they hug them, cook their meals, or wash their clothes. Such stories were told to me by people diagnosed as recently as 1989.

The treatment Linda, Calvin, and Carrie received at diagnosis was considerably less humane than that received by the other people I interviewed, for these three had the misfortune to learn of their diagnosis while in "total institutions"—prison, a psychiatric hospital, and the military, respectively.[4] When prison authorities learned in 1986 that Linda had HIV disease, they transferred her from the minimum-security facility where she held a job outside the walls to isolation at a maximum-security prison. There she was served all her meals in her cell on Styrofoam plates and was segregated from other prisoners twenty-four hours a day. Similarly, that same year, when Calvin and his doctors at the county hospital psychiatric ward where he was receiving treatment following a suicide attempt learned that he had HIV disease, he was abruptly transferred to a maximum-security ward at the state mental hospital. According to Calvin:

> I was treated worse than a caged leopard. I was put in solitary confinement. I wasn't allowed to use the same bathroom as anybody else. I wasn't allowed to eat with the regular patients. All of my food came in disposable Styrofoam containers and they'd write on the container, "Calvin——, isolation, AIDS." And the staff were very abusive, [telling me] "Stay away from me. I don't want you near me. . . ." The first night. . .two of them threw their keys down and quit. They weren't about to work with a faggot with AIDS.

Three years later, in 1989, Carrie was tested for HIV by the military. When her superior officer learned that she was infected with HIV, he immediately and without explanation relieved her of her duties and cancelled her upcoming leave. A few days later, and still with no explanation, he sent her to a doctor who told her she was infected and should "prepare to die." The doctor also told her she had probably infected her children, "did not deserve" ever to have sexual contact again, and should consider herself a "murderer" if she did so.

The reactions of persons with HIV disease to their diagnosis vary as widely as their doctors' reactions. At least at first, some individuals, whether diagnosed simply as HIV-Infected or as having AIDS, assume that they can "beat" their illness. They thus refuse to take seriously any dire predictions about their future. Others cope with their situation by intellectually accepting that they have HIV disease but emotionally denying that fact. For example, two months after his diagnosis, Chris's doctor sent him to the hospital to test a culture the doctor had grown from a fungal infection on Chris's foot. Chris reports, "I'm reading this paper that he sent me over with and halfway down the paper it says, 'Caution: patient has AIDS,' and I almost turned around and walked back to him because I thought I had the wrong paper." Although this sort of denial cannot last long, it is comforting in the short run.

Conversely, other persons with HIV disease immediately consider their diagnosis "a death sentence"—again whether they are asymptomatic but infected or whether they have AIDS. Carol, for example, has yet to develop any health problems. Nevertheless, she considers her prospects bleak. She says:

> The most difficult part [of being infected with HIV] is knowing you have no control over it. I'm a person that likes to be in control of my situation of whatever comes along. [With HIV,] you have control to make it worse, but you have no control to make it better. It's not like a cold that you know you're going to get over in a week. Or whatever it is. Gonorrhea that you go and get a penicillin shot for. You have no control. It's there. And it's going to get you.

Five of the individuals I interviewed, including Carol, had attempted suicide shortly after their diagnosis, and several others had contemplated it often; other studies have conservatively estimated the rate of suicide among persons with AIDS to be from twenty-one to thirty-six times higher than that of the general population.[5] Others whom I interviewed had expressed their self-destructive feelings immediately following diagnosis in other ways, such as punching a hole in their living room wall or going on three-week drinking binges.

One reason Carol had tried to kill herself, and one reason she was among the most depressed and guilt-ridden individuals I interviewed, was that she had learned simultaneously that she was infected with HIV and that she had infected her newborn son. For two years before her diagnosis, Carol had been trying to get her husband to agree to a divorce. Consequently, when she accidentally became pregnant, she had difficulty truly acknowledging that fact. As a result, although during an earlier pregnancy she had stopped illegal drugs and had not even used aspirin, during this pregnancy she occasionally injected cocaine. She knew she could put her fetus at risk by doing so, but did not want to believe that she was really pregnant. Describing how she felt when she learned that her baby was infected, Carol says, "I was so devastated at first I didn't care. It made no difference if I was going to be dead in two weeks or twenty years. I was just floored. And so ashamed of myself that I had used drugs during my pregnancy and that I had done this to my child. I felt like I had put a gun to his head and was just waiting to pull the trigger." Carol's sense of guilt "never goes away" and has overwhelmed her abilities to cope emotionally with her illness.

Following diagnosis, then, persons with HIV disease may experience a gamut of emotions, including guilt, depression, and fear. They also face a gamut of responses from others, ranging from sympathy to hostility, as they begin learning how to live with this new moral, social, and biological status. In subsequent days they face a series of decisions regarding when and with whom they should hide or reveal their new status—to try, in

Goffman's terms, to remain "discreditable" rather than "discredited."[6]

The first such decision must be made before they leave their doctors' offices, for federal law requires doctors to report to the government the names of all persons with AIDS and Arizona law requires doctors to report all persons who are infected with HIV. Although laws supposedly protect the confidentiality of these reports, many physicians and patients fear that the information will leak out. As a result . . . to protect persons with HIV disease from possible legal, social, and financial repercussions, some doctors will bend the rules to avoid reporting. Similarly, individuals and their physician's may decide not to report diagnoses to insurance companies for fear the companies will terminate coverage or inform the individuals' employers. To further reduce the stigma, some persons with HIV disease will request insurance reimbursement only for treatments that will not trigger questions about the nature of their diagnosis. Thus, from the time of diagnosis, individuals have to begin developing ways of coping with potential or actual stigma.

After Diagnosis: Explaining Why HIV Disease Strikes

Diagnosis with HIV disease ends individuals' uncertainty about what is wrong with them. It raises new questions, however, about why this terrible thing happened. Only by answering these questions can individuals make their illness comprehensible.

The search for meaning is often a painful one, set as it is in the context of popular belief that HIV disease is punishment for sin. At least on the surface, the majority of the individuals I interviewed reject the idea that their illness is a divine judgment.

Instead, those who believe in God stress that God is the source of love and not of punishment. In addition, gay persons with HIV disease often argue that God would not have created gay people only to reject them as sinners. These individuals and others I interviewed emphasize that HIV disease results from the same biological forces that cause other illnesses. Consequently, they dismiss the idea that they or anyone else deserve this illness. As David, a thirty-nine-year-old floral designer, says "Nobody deserves it. I have friends that say 'well, hey, if we weren't gay, we wouldn't get this disease.' That's bullshit. I mean, I don't want to hear that from anybody. Because no germ has mercy on anybody, no matter who they are—gay, straight, babies, adults." Persons with HIV disease who agree with this philosophy may also bolster their argument by stressing that this illness originated with heterosexuals in Africa and thus could not be a punishment for homosexuality. They assert that it was simply bad luck that the first Americans infected with HIV were gay men or drug users.

These alternative explanations for their illnesses allow individuals to reject their rejecters as prejudiced or ignorant. Describing the Reverend Jerry Falwell's pronouncement that HIV disease is God's punishment for sin, Chris adds, "Somebody like that really ought to be put away. He's doing so much damage. It's pathetic and he doesn't know what he's talking about and that's real sad."

Yet in the same way that members of other oppressed groups sometimes feel they deserve their oppression, other statements by some of these same individuals suggest that at a less conscious level they do feel they are to blame for their illnesses.[7] For example, twenty-four-year-old Marshall denies that he deserves HIV disease, nevertheless suggests that his illness might be God's way of punishing him for being gay or "for not being a good person." He adds, "I should have helped people more, or not have yelled at somebody, or been better to my dad even though we have never gotten along. . . . Maybe if I had tried to get along better with him, maybe this wouldn't be happening."

Others maintain that they do not deserve HIV disease, but use language that suggests considerable ambivalence. Several, for example, attribute their illness not to their "nonmonogamy" or "multiple sexual partners" but rather to their "promiscuity." Chris, for example, believes he got HIV disease "probably because I was a royal whore for about four years." Others mention their "stupidity" or "carelessness." Their use of such morally loaded terms suggest that they are not simply describing their behavior objectively but rather are condemning it on moral grounds. Thus it seems they believe emotionally, if not intellectually, that they deserve punishment, although perhaps less severe punishment than HIV disease.

Still others have no doubt that they deserve HIV disease because of either their "immorality" or their lack of forethought in engaging in high-risk behaviors. For example, although at the time Daryl had convinced himself that HIV disease did not exist in Phoenix, in retrospect he blames himself for not taking more precautions. When asked how he felt when he learned his diagnosis, he replied, "Angry, I guess, at myself for allowing it to happen when I knew better. I mean, it's like, you deserve it. You knew what was going on and yet you slipped and this is the consequence." He reported feeling "disappointed in myself for allowing it to happen. It is something I brought on myself because I knew the possible consequences of what was going to happen."

Others explicitly state that they deserve HIV disease as punishment for activities they consider immoral. In these cases, diagnosis seems to unleash preexisting guilt about sexual activity or, to a much lesser extent, drug use. Such guilt seems particularly prevalent among gay men from fundamentalist Christian or Mormon families. Of the nine such persons I interviewed, five expressed regret about being gay and six at least partially believe that they deserve HIV disease. The most extreme reaction came from Brian, a thirty-five-year-old fundamentalist Christian. He says, "I reaped what I sowed. I sowed sin, I reaped death. I believe, biblically, I received AIDS as a result of my sexual sin practices." Such extreme feelings of self-blame are uncommon among the women, apparently because they never experienced such great conflicts about the behaviors that put them at risk.

The argument that HIV disease is a divine punishment can appear in inverse fashion among those who consider themselves innocent victims of this illness. Debbie, a middle-class mother and wife infected through a blood transfusion, says, "AIDS's a punishment from God. I just feel like he's telling the gay population to knock it off. And if they continue to do so, and infect each other knowingly, then they deserve what they get." She compared her own situation to that of the "innocent babies" whom the Bible says God killed to induce Pharaoh to release the Jews from Egypt: "There's always your innocent victims. We pay the price, but we're the ones that people stand up and look and get attention for, the innocent people and the babies."

None of the individuals I interviewed in 1986 or 1987 used Louise Hay's theory, which claims that illness is caused by individuals' lack of self-love, to explain their own illness (although one did use Hay's tapes for relaxation and inspiration). Of the twelve persons I interviewed in 1989, however, three are familiar with these ideas. Debbie's sister enrolled her in a seminar by Hay and added her name to Hay's mailing list. Although Debbie so far has resisted the pressures to adopt these theories, Sally and Sarah have concluded that they developed HIV disease because of their emotional conflicts over their sexual desires. Sally is a former call girl who wants to enter a legitimate occupation but misses the money and excitement of her former life, whereas Sarah believes that she was highly active sexually because she received little affection from her parents as a child. Belief in Hay's theory is probably more common on the two coasts, where it has gained the widest publicity, than in Arizona. Because so many gay magazines and newspapers have promoted Hay's view, it is also probably more common among gay men than among others at risk for HIV disease. Such ideas will become more common in the future, as they continue to spread from the two coasts to the interior and from gays to mainstream society. The local Phoenix newsletter for persons with HIV disease for example, seems to print an increasing number of articles on the topic with each passing year.

Not all persons with HIV disease, however, have found it necessary to attribute blame to themselves or others in an effort to explain their illness. Instead, and despite the price exacted by their illness, five of the thirty-seven men and women I interviewed define their illness in positive terms as a gift from God. Brent, a thirty-three-year-old computer operator and a staunch Catholic, considers his illness to be a divine gift rather than divine retribution. In the past, his disastrous choice of lovers had left him suicidal on several occasions. As a result, he regards his illness literally as an "answer to a prayer," because it provides the extra incentive he needs to avoid any further romantic entanglements. In slightly different fashion, Carrie, Grace, Sarah, and Jeremy have found benefits in their illness by adopting an altruistic perspective. Carrie, Grace, and Sarah are heterosexual women with firm religious convictions who have never injected illegal drugs. They believe that God has given them this illness to increase their compassion, sensitivity, and ability to work with those less fortunate than themselves and to enable them to champion the rights of all persons with HIV disease, including those who are far less likely to receive sympathy from the general public. Similarly, Jeremy, a twenty-six-year-old gay fundamentalist Christian, believes his illness has helped him pursue his lifelong goals of improving the position of gays and sharing his religious faith with others. As he explains:

> The only thing that I can actually think of, the only reason why I would get AIDS,. . . is the fact that I really feel that me getting AIDS has opened a lot of doors for me to share with people—either gay people who feel that God rejects them because they're gay, but even more so to the "Christian" community who refuse to accept homosexuals as being Christian. That's the only reason I can think of, is because I know I'm a Christian, and I can share this with certain people. I've got to share the things that have happened. Since I've got AIDS, I've been able to share the fact that you can be a homosexual and still go to heaven with people up in [rural towns] and all over. Just unbelievable.

All four individuals are working to improve the position of persons with HIV disease, and all have spoken publicly about their situations. In addition, Carrie is planning on filing an antidiscrimination suit against her employer, the military.

Regardless of how an individual explains why he or she got HIV disease, simply having an explanation makes it easier to tolerate the illness. For this reason, those who believe that others deserve to contract this illness, but that they themselves do not, appear the most distressed. They rage at the unfairness of their situation. Jeanne, for example, feels that HIV disease is fitting punishment for gays, but not for drug users like herself, while Marshall says, "I get real angry. I don't know how to explain why I got it and somebody else didn't because I don't consider myself that I was that promiscuous. When I go out, I see other guys out in the bars and they're hopping around, two and three guys a night basically. And it's like why aren't they getting it? Why is it me?" Individuals who engage in such downward social comparison increase the anxiety caused by uncertainty about why this has happened to them, but decrease their feelings of stigma by labeling others more immoral or deviant than themselves.[8]

Having HIV disease is also particularly distressful for those who believe they could not have avoided contracting the illness. Those who believe they were born gay consider it unfair that their innate sexual orientation put them at risk for HIV disease, whereas those who had quit using drugs before becoming ill feel that they are being punished unfairly for past sins. Such persons must cope with both the physical trauma of illness and the emotional trauma of losing their faith that this is a just world. Calvin vividly describes what this feels like:

> I often put myself in the situation of standing in a courtroom and trying to justify what I did and why I did it, but the judge and jury have decided, and the courtroom is empty and nobody is there but me. They've already sentenced me, and I'm standing there saying, "Hey, yoo hoo. Wait a minute. I've got something to say! Wait! You don't understand. There's a reason I did what I did!" And all you get is a hollowing echo, and there's nobody home, nobody listening. You just stand there with no one to turn to and you say, "So be it, I understand." And you go on with what's left.

Envisioning the Future

Diagnosis with HIV disease forces individuals to begin reconstructing their image of what their futures will be like. Because this illness can affect the body in so many ways, it is difficult to know what to expect. Some will become blind because of infection with cytomegalovirus, some will become disabled because of tuberculosis, and some will live for months or even years with only minimal health problems. Consequently, individuals face tremendous uncertainty about the nature of their remaining days.

Fear of death is minimal compared to fear of what one's life may become. In particular, individuals fear that they will be among the approximately 40 percent who suffer mild neurological impairment, the 10 percent who suffer true dementia, or the 10 percent who become disfigured by the lesions of Kaposi's sarcoma.[9] In addition, they especially fear esoteric illnesses whose effects they cannot predict. As Jeremy says, "I'm not [as] afraid of getting infections from people as I am from inanimate objects, like fruits and moldy tile. . . . I know what a cold is like. . . . [It's] something that I have experienced. I've never experienced a mold infection."

Persons with HIV disease have little control over whether they will develop such infections. To cope with this lack of control, some try to maintain unrealistic images of their futures by avoiding learning about their illness. Kevin, who had put off diagnosis as long as he could, also put off learning about HIV disease. He echoes the sentiments of several others when he explains that he has not joined a support group for persons with this illness because he does not "want to see what other people look like." Such feelings are especially common among persons at earlier stages of HIV disease and among those at later stages who, like Kevin, seem especially distraught over their situations. These individuals fear that gaining knowledge will lead to depression and therefore conclude that they can better cope with uncertainty about the future by maintaining ignorance.

Other individuals cope with uncertainty and lack of control by developing realistic predictions about their futures. To learn about the consequences and treatments of various infections (and to obtain emotional support), individuals may attend support groups offered by community organizations that deal with HIV disease. They can also research their illnesses on their own, and in some cases they develop extensive libraries on the subject. The knowledge that they gain allows them to feel that they can respond appropriately should some problem arise, and thus can exert some control over their situations.

This strategy, however, is really only available to those who live in major cities. In smaller cities and towns, libraries and bookstores are often too small to help, and support groups may not exist. In Arizona, only Tucson and Phoenix have support groups. Persons who live in other cities may not even know that these groups exist. Debbie, for example, who lives in an outlying city of about fifty thousand people, only learned of the community organizations that deal with HIV disease through our interview, even though she was diagnosed three years earlier and receives most of her major care in Arizona treatment center for HIV disease. Moreover, if she had wanted to attend a group, she would have had to travel more than two hundred miles each way to do so.

Even if they live in major cities, heterosexuals with HIV disease may have trouble getting the information they need. The medical literature on HIV disease largely relies on studies conducted on gay men or, less commonly, men who use intravenous drugs. Given the highly variable course of HIV disease, that literature is not necessarily applicable to any women or to men who contract this illness in other ways. Similarly, support groups and community organizations for persons with HIV disease cannot answer all the questions heterosexuals have because they, too, rely primarily on the shared experiences of gay men for their knowledge. In addition, even if support groups can provide useful information, heterosexuals may not attend because they consider the groups to be essentially gay social events, feel angry at gay men who they believe caused the epidemic, or, like many Americans, are uncomfortable interacting with gay people. To date, all attempts in Arizona to start a support group solely for women have failed. Attempts to start a group for drug users have been only partially successful, with the single resultant group meeting intermittently.

Questions about the future are difficult to answer for those who initially receive diagnoses of ARC or chronic HIV infection rather than AIDS, and even more difficult for those who learn while still asymptomatic that they are infected with HIV. Faced with conflicting estimates of when and whether they will develop AIDS, such persons experience enormous stress. Interviewed after her first negative ELISA test, Grace, the woman whose HIV status remains undetermined, said, "I'm not excited. I'm not relieved. I'm puzzled. And I'm not going to accept it at face value. . . . I don't feel that just this one negative ELISA is enough to make me go out and open a bottle of champagne and celebrate." Instead, she has concluded that it is emotionally safer to assume that she is infected with HIV than to assume that she is not and risk having her hopes dashed. She stated that she would rather know that she was positive than continue not knowing, "Because for me, personally, in all areas of my life, not knowing is harder for me. I can take the truth and deal with it. Not knowing, I have a harder time dealing with it." Brent echoes her feeling in describing how his emotional state changed when his diagnosis changed from ARC (at the time of the first interview) to AIDS (at the time of the six-month follow-up interview). He says, "The worst feeling was when I was ARC, waiting for a bomb to explode. Not knowing when or if ever it would do it. There was always that tentative in my life that it may or may not. Beware! Now that the diagnosis has come in, it's like 'Okay. I can relax now. The worst is over.'" As these quotes suggest, for many individuals, even the most devastating knowledge is preferable to living with uncertainty.

Conclusions

The process of becoming a person with HIV disease centers around coming to terms with uncertainty. Although uncertainty is a central concern for all seriously ill persons, it seems to have an especially great impact on those who have HIV disease. First, persons with this illness are more likely than most ill persons to know prior to diagnosis that they are at risk. As a result, they experience difficulties other ill persons do not, for uncertainty and anxiety often sap their emotional energy and physical resources months or even years before they become ill. Second, persons with HIV disease are more likely to feel guilt about the behaviors that led to their illness and, consequently, to believe that they deserve their illness. Moreover, these individuals are far more likely to find that their friends, families, and the general public also believe that they caused and deserve their illness. As a result, these others often reinforce the guilt that persons with HIV disease feel. Third, persons with HIV disease are more likely to face difficulties in obtaining an accurate diagnosis. Like other illnesses, HIV disease can be difficult to diagnose because it is rare and causes multiple symptoms. These problems are exacerbated when physicians deliberately (if unconsciously) avoid questions or actions that would lead to diagnosis. Fourth, persons with HIV disease face greater uncertainty than other ill persons in predicting how their illness will affect their lives, for HIV disease causes more extensive and less predictable physical and mental damage than most other illnesses. Finally, because HIV disease is such a new disease, infected individuals are more likely than other ill persons to lack answers to their questions about treatment and prognosis. Moreover, because physicians' understanding of HIV disease is rapidly developing and constantly changing, persons who have this illness often are reluctant to trust the answers they do receive.

Uncertainty seems particularly troubling for persons with HIV disease who are not gay men. These individuals face additional problems in obtaining diagnoses because they may not know they are at risk. Some women, for example, do not know that their male partners are bisexual. Other men and women believe that only gays are at risk. Moreover, their physicians may be less alert for and knowledgeable about HIV disease than the physicians of gay men, who in many instances specialize in gay health care. Following diagnosis with HIV disease, individuals who are not gay, and especially women, also experience more difficulty in predicting their futures because most studies have only investigated how HIV disease affects gay men. In addition, they are far less likely to have networks of fellow sufferers to turn to for advice and information. Some live on the margins of society and lack either access to or knowledge of community resources. Others are either unwilling because of their own homophobia to accept help from groups dominated by gay men or are unable to get help because their problems are too different from those of gay men. Finally, heterosexuals with HIV disease may suffer greater uncertainty about whether they might transmit HIV to others. Although most gay men with HIV disease also worry about infecting sexual partners, they function in social circles where everyone is presumed to be at risk. Consequently, their fear of infecting others generally does not have the same overwhelming quality as that experienced by heterosexuals who believe that they are the sole potential source of infection for their loved ones.

Despite all the difficulties persons with HIV disease face because of uncertainty, however, they are not helpless against it. Rather, they can find ways to reduce or, if necessary, to live with uncertainty. These data highlight the role that control plays in making uncertainty tolerable. Persons with HIV disease cope with uncertainty by developing normative frameworks that make their situations comprehensible. Even when inaccurate, these frameworks help individuals choose (albeit from among limited options) how they will live their lives. They therefore help persons with HIV disease feel at least minimally in control. In the final analysis, it is this sense of control that enables these individuals to live with uncertainty.

Notes

1. See, for example, Michael Bury, "Chronic Illness as Biographical Disruption," *Sociology of Health and Illness* 4 (1982): 167-182; Bill Cowie, "Cardiac Patient's Perception of His Heart Attack," *Social Science and Medicine* 10 (1976): 87-96; Joseph W. Schneider and Peter Conrad, *Having Epilepsy: The Experience and Control of Illness* (Philadelphia: Temple University Press, 1983); and David C. Stewart and

Thomas J. Sullivan, "Illness Behavior and the Sick Role in Chronic Disease: The Case of Multiple Sclerosis," *Social Science and Medicine* 16 (1982): 1397-1404.

2. Charles E. Lewis, Howard E. Freeman, and Christopher R. Corey, "AIDS-related Competence of California's Primary Care Physicians," *American Journal of Public Health* 77 (1987): 795-800.

3. For similar findings with regard to other illnesses, see Bury, "Chronic Illness as Biographical Disruption," p. 172; Stewart and Sullivan, "Illness Behavior and the Sick Role"; Schneider and Conrad, *Having Epilepsy*.; and Charles Waddell, "The Process of Neutralisation and the Uncertainties of Cystic Fibrosis," *Sociology of Health and Illness* 4 (1982): 210-220.

4. Erving Goffman, *Asylums* (New York: Doubleday, 1961).

5. Peter M. Marzuk, Helen Tierney, and Kenneth Tardiff, "Suicide Rate of Men with AIDS," *Journal of the American Medical Association* 259 (1988): 1333-1337; and Kenneth W. Kizer, Martin Green, Carin I. Perkins, Gwendolyn Doebbert, and Michael J. Hughes, "AIDS and Suicide in California," *Journal of the American Medical Association* 260 (1988): 1881. These estimates are based on death certificates. Because both suicides and AIDS are underreported on death certificates, these estimates are very conservative.

6. Goffman, *Stigma: Notes on the Management of Spoiled Identity* (Englewood-Cliffs, N.J.: Prentice-Hall, 1963), pp. 41-42.

7. For a discussion of self-blame among other oppressed groups, see Barry Adam, *The Survival of Domination: Inferiorization and Everyday Life* (New York: Elsevier, 1978). For similar findings with regard to persons with HIV disease, see Moulton, "Adjustment to a Diagnosis of AIDS."

8. For a discussion of downward social comparison, see Frederick X. Gibbons, "Stigma and Interpersonal Relationships," in Stephen C. Ainlay, Gaylene Becker, and Lerita M. Coleman, eds., *The Dilemma of Difference: A Multidisciplinary View of Stigma* (New York: Plenum Press, 1986), pp. 123-144.

9. My thanks to Dr. James Allender for these statistics and for helping me understand the neurological implications of HIV disease.

Further Reading

Erving Goffman. 1963. *Stigma: Notes on the Management of Spoiled Identity*. Englewood Cliffs, NJ: Prentice-Hall.

Phillip Kayal. 1993. *Bearing Witness: Gay Men's Health Crisis and the Politics of AIDS*. San Francisco: Westview Press.

Susan Sontag. 1989. *AIDS and Its Metaphors*. New York: Farrar, Straus & Giroux.

Discussion Questions

1. How has uncertainty for AIDS patients changed since Weitz's study in 1991?

2. In which ways do these research respondents' explanations for their HIV status or AIDS draw upon American social values and culture?

3. What are the implications of Weitz's findings for her respondents' self-concepts?

45

Ethical Problems Involving Sexuality

Miriam E. Cameron

Moral dilemmas in handling an illness go far beyond medical professionals' conference tables. Rather, they reach into the most intimate areas of patients' daily lives. Neither medical professionals nor social scientists have fully apprehended nor appreciated patients' continual ethical challenges, ones that can undermine the integrity of self and tear apart significant relationships. Perhaps nowhere are chronic and terminally ill people's moral dilemmas so stark as with ethical questions about the sexuality of people with AIDS and their partners.

The voices of people with AIDS come alive in their moral dilemmas about how to be sexual persons. Miriam Cameron's interviewees reveal raw honesty as they talk about what many other uninfected adults may think about and seldom discuss. Compare their statements about present and potential risks with discussions you have witnessed. These interviewees divulge that what they do is not necessarily what they believe they should do. Look for how the individualism in the wider culture rings through their statements as they ponder whether wishes or needs of self or other should take priority. Most of Cameron's interviewees state that changing their sex practices resulted in new views of sexuality and revised images of themselves as sexual beings. However, if sexuality defines the self and social life, some individuals prefer to risk infecting or being infected rather than risk rejection.

The most common ways to transmit HIV disease are through vaginal and anal sexual intercourse. Mucosal tissues of the vagina and rectum are rich in superficial blood vessels. If these tissues have small tears, white blood cells harboring the virus that come into contact with the tissues can enter the host's blood stream (Green 1987).

To reduce the possibility of HIV transmission, public health officials have advised people to take responsibility for their sexual behavior. They have suggested that HIV-infected persons abstain from sexual intercourse or engage in sex with fully informed adults who use precautions. For persons without HIV disease, public health officials have recommended abstinence or monogamous sex with a non-HIV-infected partner. If these options are not likely, non-HIV-infected individuals should use protection when engaging in sex, have few sexual partners, and talk openly with their sexual partners about AIDS (CDC 1992; Cline, Johnson, and Freeman 1992).

Although the fear of AIDS has prompted some individuals to alter their sexual behavior, other people have not seemed to change, even after being told about modes of HIV transmission. Research indicates that teenagers may be engaging in unsafe sex at nearly the same rate as before AIDS was first identified (Brooks-Gunn and Furstenberg 1990; CDC 1992). Women may want to use protection, but they may feel they have little personal power to demand that men use condoms (Bell 1989). The self-esteem of some men who have sex with men may be so low because of society's homophobia that they take part in abusive sex. Persons who are under the influence of alcohol and drugs may not be able to make responsible choices about their sexual activities (Crimp 1988; Eliason and Randall 1991).

All of the participants seemed knowledgeable about modes of HIV transmission. . . . Fourteen PWAs (4 women and 10 men) and three significant persons specifically described ethical problems involving sexuality: "Should I engage in protected sex or unprotected sex?" "Should I be concerned about my partner's sexuality or focus on my own sexual needs?" "Should I accept or reject that I am gay?" "Should I be sexual as a heterosexual person even though I may infect someone with HIV?"

"Should I Engage in Protected Sex or Unprotected Sex?"

Roxanne

Roxanne, who became HIV-infected from "heterosexual sex," described conflict about whether she should engage in protected or unprotected sex. "Should I care about transmitting HIV to someone else?" she asked. "A lot of people think somebody gave them AIDS, and they're going to give it to everybody. They fuck everybody and don't give a fart. They are getting venereal diseases, and it's killing them faster. I don't want that to happen to me."

Describing her resolution to her conflict, Roxanne said, "I use condoms and avoid becoming infected by someone else." She rationalized, "I can't afford to catch anything from anybody or be infected with the virus again because that breaks my system down twice as fast. I don't want to be the cause of somebody dying because life is precious." After blowing her nose, she said, "My tears are because people don't take life seriously. . . ."

Andy

Andy became HIV-infected from blood products to treat his hemophilia. "Should I use condoms with women that I date?" he asked. "Should I tell them about HIV? I'm afraid to. They might reject me. Should I use condoms with my present girlfriend? She found out about me being infected and got bent out of shape."

"When I was dating other women," Andy said of his resolution, "I told them about HIV. The ones that wanted a condom, didn't make a difference to me. I felt that we can do this to keep you safe. With my present girlfriend, sometimes we use condoms, and sometimes we don't, the emotion at the moment."

Andy reasoned, "If I didn't have HIV, I wouldn't want nobody giving it to me. You might be taking a life, and that's wrong. I am a good person and don't want to hurt nobody. Before sexual encounters, it's best to let women know what they're up against so they can decide if it matters. I wish I could have made a decision about getting HIV."

Shari

Shari, a significant person and Andy's girlfriend, described conflict about whether to use protection when engaging in sex. "For the first 6 months we were together," she said, "I didn't know he's infected, and we didn't use condoms. I found out by overhearing him on the phone, and I cried. In my mind, he was saying he didn't care if he got me infected. We talked, but he refuses to use condoms, and I'm afraid I will become infected. I don't want to get AIDS because I have children. One is disabled. He's more comfortable without condoms. All men are like that."

"If it's only me and him," Shari continued, "I'm not afraid of AIDS. I found him with another female. He said it was his friend's girlfriend. I hope he don't be like all men and most females and want to share himself with someone else. I'm respecting him as a human being, not a diseased person, and he can respect me as a female. I have needs, being in the relationship one-on-one."

Shari described her resolution. "We don't use condoms," she said. "I go to the doctor to make sure I haven't gotten HIV. He's not planning to be with a girl no more than a night or couple of days, but I take it one step at a time."

Explaining her rationale for her resolution, Shari said, "Men or females with HIV should tell their partner in an adult way. AIDS shouldn't be spread to anyone else. Since I'm risking my life by having sex with him without condoms, I want him to be faithful. If I wanted to use condoms, he'd be willing, but I don't want nothing to be uncomfortable for him. I think more of him than myself. It doesn't bother me that we don't use condoms, because I go to the doctor regularly. If you're going to get AIDS, you're going to get AIDS. We all got to go some day."

'Should I Be Concerned About My Partner's Sexuality or Focus on My Own Sexual Needs?'

Diana

When Diana was in jail, she tested positive for HIV disease. She had not engaged in sex with her boyfriend, who injected drugs, for 2

1/2 months because "I don't feel good enough," and she questioned whether to be concerned about his sexuality or focus on her own. "I'm worried about my boyfriend passing HIV to somebody," Diana said. "He gave HIV to me, I wasn't messing around. AIDS is deadly, and I wouldn't want it to happen to someone else."

Diana said about her resolution, "I told him, 'I'm too sick to have sex with you, and if you go elsewhere, you'd better use a rubber, and make sure it's safe for the other person.' He promised he'd keep rubbers on him. I ask him, 'Have you had sex with anybody?' I told him, 'Rubbers not safe, they break.'"

"My boyfriend is a man," Diana reasoned, "and I can't expect him not to have sex because I don't have sex. I'm too scared to have sex with anyone but my boyfriend because I don't want to pass HIV on. That would be too much to keep having sex and passing HIV on."

Margo

"I don't know how I got it," Margo said about HIV disease. "My husband doesn't know how he got it, either." She described conflict similar to Diana's conflict.

"My husband has a high sex drive," Margo said. "He got to have sex, if it's four times a day, seven days a week. When a man is not satisfied, he's going to go somewhere else and get it. Both of us having AIDS has slowed him down, but I'm worried that he could spread the illness to someone else."

"I told him, 'Sex is there whenever you want it,'" Margo said, describing her resolution. "You have to be cautious to avoid HIV to be spread more. My sexual needs is, if I get it, fine. If I don't, it don't bother me. My husband is generous. He has never said, 'You can't have any,' or make an excuse. What we're doing about sex seems to be working. We have sex, but we use condoms. We don't have sex as much as we used to. It's monogamous, so we don't pass it on or bring something back."

"I rather him stay here and get sex," Margo rationalized. "That help me with my own sexual needs. A wife is for her husband alone. A husband is for a wife alone. It's not to be shared. It's breaking a commitment. I am serious about my marriage vows and my relationship with my husband."

Chris

Chris, a significant person, explained that his wife had become HIV-infected from a blood transfusion during surgery, which took place before blood was tested for HIV disease. He described conflict about whether to be concerned about his wife's sexuality or concentrate on his own sexual needs.

"I want to be sexually satisfied," Chris began, "but HIV makes me scared of sex with my wife, and protection limits my sexual satisfaction. I am concerned that I will lose an erection because of the condom. Sometimes I am tired or stressed. That's when the darn condom is a headache and helps to make me a failure, which is rare. Then she feels bad for me. Do I look elsewhere for sexual satisfaction? I am pulled between my love for her and desire to remain monogamous and my wish to be sexually fulfilled."

"My heart goes out to her, and her heart goes out to me," Chris said about his resolution. "We made a game of finding the best condom. Some were sloppy, messy, smelly. We found a thin, sensitive one that is more satisfactory. Now we always use condoms and jelly, and we've never broken one yet. She tries to compensate for their limitations. We are careful about washing. Our living is close to normal. We avoid having sex when we are overly tired or stressed. HIV hasn't diminished our sex life."

Chris explained his rationale, saying, "While condoms are not as satisfying as regular intercourse, they're better than nothing. Sex is only one part of the relationship. The right thing to do is be monogamous and live in harmony with our values. Having an affair or picking up a prostitute would be shallow. Why us? There isn't an answer. It's happenstance. You take the good with the bad, and accept what you can't change. Struggling with adversity is part of growing."

"Should I Accept or Reject That I Am Gay?"

Theo

When I asked Theo, a PWA, how he became HIV-infected, he said, "Ninety-nine percent chance gay sex and 1 percent needles." He explained that he and his life partner, who was not HIV-infected, used protection during sex. Eager to talk, he said, "I don't have anything to fear from people knowing." As we sat in his kitchen, he questioned whether to accept being gay.

"I lived most of my life feeling bad about being different," said Theo. "Like other gay boys and lesbian girls, I grew up in a heterosexual environment that is biased against homosexuality. We develop a strong gay or lesbian sexual identity in spite of rejection. I tried to change so people would love me, but I couldn't change being gay. Should I be honest about who I am?"

Theo described his resolution. "When I realized there was a name—gay—for what I was, that I could be proud of, I liked myself better," he said. "Hating myself didn't get me anywhere. I decided to love myself and be honest. Now I embrace my differences. I told my family that I was gay, and they didn't reject me. I am open with other people about being gay."

"I can't be the person everybody wants me to be," rationalized Theo. "I have to be me. Differences aren't bad, they are wonderful. Being gay doesn't make me a bad person. Most people like me even though they know I am gay. If it's too big of an issue for them, they make their choice."

Lewis

Lewis become HIV-infected from "gay sex." He had not had sex for "one year" but would engage in "safe sex." Unlike Theo, he was concerned about confidentiality, and we met secretly. "The conflict is that I've been gay all my life," Lewis said. "But if I wasn't gay, would I have gotten AIDS? Before I became educated, I morally thought that AIDS was punishment from God. I fight that issue. People have said to me, 'You chose this lifestyle, and AIDS is what you have to live with.' Society has put a stigma on gay people."

"When the voice inside says, 'If you hadn't been gay, you wouldn't have AIDS,' I answer with hope, strength, God," Lewis said about his resolution. "I say, 'I didn't choose to be gay. This is who I am.' I fight harder to stay alive and be healthy. I go with the flow and deal with it the best I know how."

Explaining his rationale, Lewis said, "People feel that if you weren't gay, AIDS wouldn't have happened. And that's sad. It makes a difference to me that AIDS can happen to anyone, and I'm not alone with AIDS. I'm a spiritual person. I was raised in church. God is an important part of my life, which gives me strength and hope. God knows all, and I don't think that AIDS is God's fault. AIDS isn't a punishment."

'Should I Be Sexual as a Gay Man Even Though I May Infect Someone With HIV?'

Jacob

Jacob, who became HIV-infected from "gay sex," described conflict about whether he should be sexual as a gay man. "As an Afro-American man growing up," he began, "it's important to experiment with sex. In the homosexual lifestyle, at least in the past, we tend to have more than one partner, which is like sleeping with a community of people. A lot of us are careless with sex. We say, 'They didn't look out for me, so why should I look out for them?' Should I be sexually involved with someone else and take the chance of infecting that person?"

"I want to be more aware, responsible, cautious about sex," Jacob resolved. "Unfortunately, I haven't been involved with someone because of AIDS. I like to keep my relationships to a minimum. To be fair, I want to be involved with someone who's also infected so I don't infect anyone else. An infected person will know what AIDS is like."

"I care about whether people get HIV because someone didn't care about me," Jacob reasoned. "If I had considered myself, I wouldn't have AIDS. It's important to care about other people and yourself. If you're a sexually responsible person, you protect yourself and the other person. By taking a few minutes, you won't get AIDS. You can be responsible regardless of your age or color. . . ."

Bruce

Bruce became HIV-infected from "gay sex, good sex!" Although celibate for four years, he questioned whether to be sexual even though he could infect someone with HIV disease.

"When I was diagnosed," Bruce began, "I wanted to share HIV with everybody. 'Fuck the doctors.' I had unsafe, casual sex. As an Asian Pacific gay man, I didn't love myself and wanted to use sex to validate myself. Having sex was a cultural sharing with my sub, subculture, being Pacific Islander and gay. I don't do that now, but I wonder, should I have a sexual relationship with my friends? Should I be honest with my parents about my sexuality and AIDS? I'm the oldest son and heir to what my parents built. I don't want them to suffer."

"How should I deal with the unfairness of AIDS and its effect on my sexuality?" he asked. "Death is coming soon for me. I am at the peak of my career. I have a lot to give, smiles for people, lovely things to say to clerks who work in stores on days when they should be off. I want better. That's a lot to ask."

"After my lover died," Bruce said about his resolution, "I was hospitalized, and they told me I was going to die. I woke up, and my room was bathed in an eerie, orange glow. A Filipino woman was wiping night sweat from my body and saying, 'God loves you.' God was talking to me, and the simple message was, if God loves me, I can love myself enough to take care of myself and not engage in this emotional, spiritual, physical self-flagellation, and not endanger others. When I got out of the hospital, I went back and asked to speak to the Filipino nurse. There was no Filipino nurse on duty that night."

"I decided to stop engaging in casual, unprotected sex," said Bruce. "I became celibate and an AIDS activist. I had to get a grip on myself, accept responsibilities taught to me as a child. I said, 'Bubba, stop this bullshit. It's stupid. Doesn't help. Makes the situation worse. Do the best you can. See your doctor every month. Take the medications.' I talked to my mother, and put all my cards on the table."

Bruce reasoned, "Engaging in self-flagellation isn't the cure for AIDS because AIDS is still here. I don't want to make somebody sick. I am not a destroyer of life. I became celibate because no matter how many con-

doms you use, the virus can get through. . . . My friends and I don't know who infected who, a sorrowful situation. Many of them have died, and I have grief issues about them."

"The gay community denies discrimination toward Asian Pacific Islanders," Bruce continued, "Rice queens, white men who are into Asian Pacific men, brought the virus into our culture. Generally they are aggressive or top and easily pass the infection to the passive or bottom. The Centers for Disease Control say that only a few Asian Pacific Islanders are infected, so we don't get money to fight AIDS. But almost all of us are infected. Death certificates don't say AIDS. They say pneumonia or heart insufficiency. I became an activist because no Asian Pacific Islander was saying a word about AIDS. So I am going to make a difference if I can."

"Should I Be Sexual as a Heterosexual Person Even Though I May Infect Someone With HIV?"

Marilyn

Marilyn, who became HIV-infected from "heterosexual sex," described conflict about being sexual. "I long for a companion to love me, AIDS and all," she said. "You can enjoy sex, laugh. You're a person. But do you want to tell that person about AIDS? That could be tough. I might never see him again. He may reject me if I insist on condoms. One man, I insisted on condoms. He said it didn't matter to him, he wasn't afraid of HIV. I said it did matter to me. So he didn't want to have sex with me."

"I'm young," Marilyn resolved, "but I'm refraining from sex now. I am looking for a long-term companion. If I find him, I will tell him about HIV and use protection when we have sex."

Explaining her rationale, Marilyn said, "You have to tell him about AIDS to give you peace inside. A person have a right to know. Keeping a secret is not telling who you are. It's like being pregnant with another man's baby, and you meet this guy, and you not showing. A relationship need to be based on honesty, not a lie. I would use protection because I don't want to destroy nobody, or I couldn't live with myself. Because of AIDS, I may have to live without a companion.

Tonio

Tonio became HIV-infected from a blood transfusion to treat his hemophilia before blood products were tested for HIV. "I take precautions to not infect my wife," he began, "but I'm concerned that they will not work. Sexual intercourse dropped after my diagnosis with HIV and even more with AIDS. I have a psychological blockage because there's chance of transmission. Condoms are a pain because your brain has to be working so you don't get carried away, and it says, 'Should you be doing this?'"

Tonio described his resolution to his conflict. "We use protected sex," he said, "and wait until we want to have sex rather than force it. My physician said my blockage was probably psychological. Rationalization took over, and for a while we were able to do it. Now it's infrequent again, but it's not true impotence any more. I don't perform like I did when we were first married. That falls off normally in a married couple."

"My psychological blockage may not be due entirely to AIDS," Tonio said, explaining his rationale, "because the males in my family were never oversexed. Sex is important, and we don't want to give it up, but it isn't the most important part of our relationship. Having sex less often hasn't affected our relationship. If anything it's firmer than before AIDS. . . ."

Vance

Vance, who became HIV-infected from a blood transfusion to treat his hemophilia, said that he was unmarried but in a long-time relationship with his girlfriend. "What is the right way to meet my sexual needs?" he asked. "For a young male, sex is way up there on the list of priorities, especially after a couple of drinks. Should I have a sexual relationship with my girlfriend? Protected sex is still dangerous, and I don't want to infect her. Should I be monogamous with her, or have a primary relationship with her while having relationships with other women? I want to be honest with her, but I don't want her to know

about my relationships with other women, or she might leave me. I want to keep my present girlfriend, yet I am attracted to other women."

"Before having sex with another woman, should I tell her that I have AIDS?" Vance asked. "I don't want to ruin my chances with her. Should I do what is ethically right or what brings me immediate physical gratification? How can I meet my sexual needs without hurting her? Is it right to pursue a sexual relationship knowing the risk that she is taking?"

"Usually, I use condoms when I have sex with my girlfriend, but they break or fall off," Vance said about his resolution to his conflict. "I engaged in unprotected sex with my former girlfriend before and after I found out that I was HIV-positive. Since she hadn't become infected previously, I figured she wouldn't become infected by having sex a few more times. When my buddy and I met a couple of women, I opted for immediate physical gratification. I had sexual relations with one of them without exactly telling her the situation, but I was careful."

"Since the relationship with my present girlfriend is improving, I have less desire for sex with other women, and I don't feel as much conflict," Vance rationalized. "It's important to use protected sex. I should tell a woman that I have AIDS before having sex with her. It is unethical to have sex, even if it is protected sex, without telling her that I have AIDS. It's not fair to her because she doesn't know that she is potentially risking her life."

Lisa

Lisa, a significant person and Vance's girlfriend, said that they did not consistently use condoms, and she questioned whether to be sexual with him even though she might become HIV-infected herself. Although she brought up the topic about sex, she seemed self-conscious to talk about it. She gave only a brief description before turning to another ethical problem.

"I love him and want a sexual relationship with him," explained Lisa, "but by having sex with him, I could get AIDS." Describing her resolution, she said, "I have a sexual relationship with him, and usually we use condoms." She reasoned, "I'm fine having a sexual relationship with him. I don't think about it. I'm not afraid of getting AIDS. I probably should be more worried, but what good will that do?"

Commentary

Given the danger of transmitting HIV disease, the participants asked if they should be sexual with other people at all. They craved involvement with individuals who would provide comfort and meaning for them and help to meet their sexual needs. As Marilyn put it, "I long for a companion to love me, AIDS and all. Because of AIDS, I may have to live without a companion."

However, the PWAs did not want to infect anyone, and the significant persons feared becoming infected themselves. Roxanne said, "I don't want to be the cause of somebody dying, because life is precious." They questioned whether using condoms would, in fact, prohibit HIV transmission. "I take precautions to not infect my wife," Tonio said, "but I'm concerned that they will not work." In asking whether they should be sexual, the participants expressed concern about AIDS taking away their sexuality. Bruce asked, "How should I deal with the unfairness of AIDS and its effect on my sexuality?"

Most participants resolved their conflict by being sexual. Jacob and Diana said that they only engaged in sex with other HIV-infected individuals. As Jacob put it, "To be fair, I want to be involved with someone who's also infected so I don't infect anyone else. An infected person will know what AIDS is like."

The PWAs who were sexual described a second conflict, whether to tell their potential sexual partners about having AIDS. On one hand, they said that HIV-infected persons should be honest about their diagnosis. As Vance explained, "It is unethical to have sex, even if it is protected sex, without telling her that I have AIDS."

On the other hand, the PWAs were reluctant to be honest with their sexual partners because they feared rejection. Also, they were angry about their diagnosis and being stigmatized by society. Roxanne said, "A lot of people think somebody gave them AIDS, and they're going to give it to everybody."

Many of the PWAs acknowledged that they had engaged in sex without disclosing their diagnosis or using protection, particularly right after being diagnosed with HIV infection. "When I was diagnosed," explained Bruce, "I wanted to share HIV with everybody. I had unsafe, casual sex."

The participants described a third conflict. Even if they decided to be sexual and talk openly about HIV disease, they questioned whether to use condoms. The women hesitated to ask their male sexual partners to use condoms. As Marilyn put it, "He may reject me if I insist on condoms." Shari said, "He refuses to use condoms, and I'm afraid I will become infected. He's more comfortable without condoms. All men are like that."

The women worried that if they did not sexually satisfy their partners, the men would be promiscuous or reject them and even transmit HIV disease to someone else. Diana, who felt too sick to have sex, said, "My boyfriend is a man and I can't expect him not to have sex because I don't have sex. I'm worried about my boyfriend passing HIV to somebody. He gave HIV to me." Margo explained about her husband who had AIDS, "My husband has a high sex drive. When a man is not satisfied, he's going to go somewhere else and get it. I rather him stay here and get sex."

The men explained that condoms reduced their sexual satisfaction and could lead to sexual impotence. Some male PWAs even said that if their sexual partners were willing, they did not use condoms. "The ones that wanted a condom," said Andy, "didn't make a difference to me. I felt that we can do this to keep you safe." However, he acknowledged, "With my present girlfriend, sometimes we use condoms, and sometimes we don't, the emotion at the moment." His girlfriend, Shari, said, "For the first 6 months we were together, I didn't know he's infected, and we didn't use condoms. I found out by overhearing him on the phone, and I cried. I don't want to get AIDS because I have children. One is disabled."

Even if the participants had engaged in unsafe sex in the past, most of them said that now they were taking steps to avoid HIV transmission, primarily through celibacy, being honest about AIDS, and using protection when engaging in sex. Jacob explained, "If you're a sexually responsible person, you protect yourself and the other person."

Some participants said that because of AIDS they were changing their views about sexuality. "I am a sexual person through nurturing, love, respect, and sharing," Eric said, describing his new perspective. "Sex doesn't need a nasty element to be fun. Sex isn't bad, it's a wonderful gift." Martin said, "From my relationship with my lover, I'm learning that sexuality and sexual intercourse aren't the same. I have to be myself, doing what feels good, safe, responsible."

Despite AIDS, some participants said that they were able to meet their sexual needs in caring relationships. "I am sexually active in my monogamous relationship," explained Eric. "I won't endanger my partner if I don't engage in activities that transmit HIV. HIV-infected persons build relationships that are loving with noninfected persons, and people start relationships with HIV-infected persons. They're having rich, full relationships."

The participants' stories support research findings indicating that HIV-infected persons frequently do not disclose their infection to their sexual partners (Marks, Richardson, and Maldonado 1991; McCusker, Stoddard, and McCarthy 1992; Schoeman 1991). Persons with HIV disease who have been honest about their diagnosis have been subject to discrimination and ruptured relationships (Winslade 1989). Individuals who knowingly expose other people to HIV disease may be reacting to their experience of discrimination, poverty, and alienation (Poku 1992).

Research has documented inequities in power between some women and men, as illustrated by the participants' stories. Traditionally, women have assumed responsibility for using protection when engaging in sex. Often, they feel that they have little personal power to demand that men use condoms, and even think that HIV infection is their due (Bell 1989).

Several studies have been reported about inconsistent use of condoms (Jemmott and Jemmott 1991; Smeltzer and Whipple 1991; Williams 1991). Additional research is needed to identify what should be done to encourage women to insist on protection when engaging in sex even though they risk losing their male partners. Also, research is needed about how to encourage men to value their female sexual partners over their own sexual satisfaction and take responsibility for using safer sex techniques.

Codependency is one explanation for why a non-HIV-infected individual would knowingly engage in unprotected sex with someone who has HIV disease. Lisa, who used condoms "sometimes," said, "I'm fine having a sexual relationship with him. I don't think about it. I'm not afraid of getting AIDS." Shari explained, "If I wanted to use condoms, he'd be willing, but I don't want nothing to be uncomfortable for him. I think more of him than myself. He's not planning to be with a girl no more than a night or couple of days, but I take it one step at a time." A few months later, the nurse who had arranged my interview with Shari told me that she had become HIV-infected.

Codependency is extreme involvement with another person or persons, which can be so pervasive that the codependent's self-esteem depends on the other person. The individual feels unable to survive without the significant other. Codependency places the individual at risk for emotional, physical, and social difficulties, including HIV disease (St. Onge 1992). Research is needed about effective ways to counteract codependency.

The participants' stories illustrate an important element that seems to be missing in current AIDS education. Being given information about AIDS does not appear to motivate some people to change their risky sexual behavior. Although all of the participants appeared to be knowledgeable about AIDS, some of them justified engaging in unsafe sexual practices. As Shari said, "It doesn't bother me that we don't use condoms because I go to the doctor regularly. If you're going to get AIDS, you're going to get AIDS. We all got to go some day."

The thinking of the participants who engaged in unsafe sex seemed to something like this: "Infecting another person or becoming infected is wrong, but being rejected is even worse. This one time I will engage in unprotected sex because the chance of the virus being transmitted is low." Research is needed to determine what kind of AIDS and ethics education are needed to overcome this type of reasoning so that people stop engaging in risky, unethical behavior while justifying their actions.

Gay PWAs described a fourth conflict involving sexuality. They questioned if they should hide being gay. As Tonio put it, "I lived most of my life feeling bad about being different. I tried to change so people would love me, but I couldn't change being gay. Should I be honest about who I am?"

Tonio's words illustrate the struggle of many gay women and men to accept their sexuality in a homophobic world. Homophobia permeates society and the health care system (Crimp 1988; Eliason and Randall 1991). Repressive measures have been used to eliminate homosexual behavior and persons. Hatred and misunderstanding have been heaped upon homosexual women and men by their families, communities, government, organized religion, and even the gay community itself (Murphy 1990, 1991).

Because of homophobia, gay men have actually been blamed for AIDS. As Lewis put it, "People feel that if you weren't gay, AIDS wouldn't have happened." Some people have claimed that AIDS is a just punishment for homosexual behavior (Murphy 1988).

Lewis and Theo described how they were dealing with homophobia. "When the voice inside says, 'If you hadn't been gay, you wouldn't have AIDS'," said Lewis, "I answer with hope, strength, God. I say, 'I didn't choose to be gay. This is who I am.'" Theo explained, "I decided to love myself and be honest. Now I embrace my differences." He joined Alcoholics Anonymous, participated in the gay community, and became an AIDS activist.

Like Lewis and Theo, many gay, HIV-infected persons are coming to terms with their sexuality and refusing to internalize society's homophobia. They are avoiding abusive behavior, such as unsafe sex. Rather than be angry and depressed, they are using their struggles concerning sexuality as an opportunity for personal growth (Barrows and Halgin 1988).

In summary, to deal effectively with AIDS, individuals need to take responsibility for their sexual behavior by not infecting anyone or becoming infected themselves. Society's responsibility is to fund research about sexuality, codependency, homophobia, and effective AIDS and ethics education and to provide education based on the findings.

References

Barrows, P.A., & Halgin, R.P. (1988). Current issues in psychotherapy with gay men. *Professional Psychology: Research and Practice, 19,* 395-402.

Bell, N.K. (1989). Women and AIDS: Too little, too late? *Hypatia, 4*(3), 3-22.

Brooks-Gunn, J., & Furstenberg, F.F., Jr. (1990). Coming of age in the era of AIDS. *The Milbank Quarterly, 68,* 59-84.

Centers for Disease Control. (1992). Selected behaviors that increase risk for HIV infection among high school students—United States, 1990. *Morbidity and Mortality Weekly Report, 41,* 231-240.

Cline, R.J.W., Johnson, S.J., & Freeman, K.E. (1992). Talk among sexual partners about AIDS: Interpersonal communication for risk reduction or risk enhancement? *Health Communication, 4*(1), 39-56.

Crimp, D. (Ed.). (1988). *AIDS: Cultural analysis/cultural activism.* Cambridge: MIT Press.

Eliason, M.J., & Randall, C.E. (1991). Lesbian phobia in nursing students. *Western Journal of Nursing Research, 13,* 363-374.

Green, R. (1987). The transmission of AIDS. In H.L. Dalton, S. Burris, & the Yale AIDS Law Project (Eds.), *AIDS and the law: A guide for the public* (pp. 28-36). New Haven, CT: Yale University Press.

Jemmott, L.S., & Jemmott, J.B., III. (1991). Applying the theory of reasoned action to AIDS risk behavior: Condom use among black women. *Nursing Research, 40,* 228-234.

Marks, G., Richardson, J.L., & Maldonado, N. (1991). Self-disclosure of HIV infection to sexual partners. *American Journal of Public Health, 81,* 1321-1323.

McCusker, J., Stoddard, A.M., & McCarthy, E. (1992). The validity of self-reported HIV antibody test results. *American Journal of Public Health, 82,* 567-569.

Murphy, T.F. (1988). Is AIDS a just punishment? *Journal of Medical Ethics, 14,* 154-160.

Murphy, T.F. (1990). Reproductive controls and sexual destiny. *Bioethics, 4,* 121-142.

Murphy, T.F. (1991). The ethics of conversion therapy. *Bioethics, 5,* 123-138.

Poku, K.A. (1992). Knowingly exposing others to HIV. *AIDS Patient Care, 6,* 5-10.

St. Onge, J.L. (1992). Codependence: Addictive relationships and HIV care. *AIDS Patient Care, 6,* 25-27.

Schoeman, F. (1991). AIDS and privacy. In F.G. Reamer (Ed.), *AIDS & ethics* (pp. 240-276). New York: Columbia University Press.

Smeltzer, S.C., & Whipple, B. (1991). Women and HIV infection. *Image: Journal of Nursing Scholarship, 23,* 249-256.

Williams, A.B. (1991). Women at risk: an AIDS educational needs assessment. *Image: Journal of Nursing Scholarship, 23,* 208-213.

Winslade, W.J. (1989). AIDS and the duty to inform others. In E.T. Juengst & B.A. Koenig (Eds.), *The meaning of AIDS: Implications for medical science, clinical practice, and public health policy* (pp. 108-116). New York: Praeger.

Further Reading

Kathy Charmaz. 1991. "Disclosing Illness." in *Good Days, Bad Days: The Self in Chronic Illness & Time.* New Brunswick, NJ: Rutgers University Press.

Timothy Murphy. 1994. *Ethics in an Epidemic: AIDS, Morality, and Culture.* Berkeley, CA: University of California Press.

Frederic Reamer (ed.). 1991. *AIDS & Ethics.* New York: Columbia University Press.

Discussion Questions

1. What parallels, if any, do you find in these accounts with concerns and priorities of sexually active adolescents and adults who are not HIV positive?

2. In which ways might these research participants' social worlds and world views influence their ethical beliefs and decisions?

3. Cameron portrays the moral dilemmas and ethical decisions faced by people with HIV disease and AIDS. How would you compare them with those faced by other people with chronic and terminal illnesses?

46

Confronting Deadly Disease: The Drama of Identity Construction Among Gay Men With AIDS

Kent L. Sandstrom

Kent Sandstrom's article lies squarely within the interpretive tradition of studies of health and illness. Find themes in it that are consistent with earlier chapters by Kathy Charmaz, Arthur Frank, and David Karp. In this short piece, Sandstrom shows how feelings shift and change as people who are identified as having HIV infections grapple with the knowledge of their new status and identity. The meaning of AIDS changes from an abstract category to imminent death. Unlike people with many other illnesses, a symbolic transformation occurs before the person experiences the direct effects of illness. Think about how wider social meanings of the threat and stigma of AIDS may result in transforming a newly diagnosed person's social and personal identities. Like people who have other serious illnesses, the foundations of this person's self becomes shaken. The web of social relations supporting the self may be torn apart. AIDS casts the person adrift in a sea of uncertainty and ambiguity. Loss after loss may follow.

The meaning of illness derives from the feelings the person holds about it. When gay men feel guilty about having contracted the virus or about being homosexual, Sandstrom finds that they believe they deserve the punishment of AIDS. Yet these men's uncertain lives and ambiguous statuses as persons with AIDS also allow them to reconstruct an empowered self. Their path to empowerment is fraught with interactional barriers and dilemmas. Support may be a sham; concealing one's diagnosis and illness may make sense. Isolation is risky; it may result in medical crises. Selective interaction and selective withdraw permitted identity management and prevented loss of control. But over time, Sandstrom found that these men's identity work resulted in their viewing AIDS as having transformed them.

The phenomenon of AIDS (acquired immuno-deficiency syndrome) has been attracting increased attention from sociologists. A number of observers leave examined the social meanings of the illness (Conrad 1986; Sontag 1989; Palmer 1989), the social influences and behavior involved in its onset and progression (Kaplan et al. 1987) and the larger social consequences of the AIDS epidemic (Ergas 1987). Others have studied the "psychosocial" issues faced by individuals who are either diagnosed with the illness (Nichols 1985; Baumgartner 1986; Weitz 1989) or closely involved with someone who has been diagnosed (Salisbury 1986; Geiss, Fuller and Rush 1986; Macklin 1988).

Despite this growing interest in the social and psychosocial dimensions of AIDS, little attention has been directed toward the processes of social and self-interaction (Denzin 1983) by which individuals acquire and personalize an AIDS-related identity. Further, given the stigmatizing implications of AIDS, there has been a surprising lack of research regarding the strategies of stigma management and identity construction utilized by persons with this illness.

This article presents an effort to address these issues. It examines the dynamics of identity construction and management which characterize the everyday lives of persons with AIDS (PWAs). In doing so, it highlights the socially ambiguous status of PWAs and considers (a) the processes through which they person-

alize the illness, (b) the dilemmas they encounter in their interpersonal relations, (c)
the strategies they employ to avoid or minimize potentially discrediting social attributions, and (d) the subcultural networks and
ideologies which they draw upon as they construct, avow and embrace AIDS-related identities. Finally, these themes are situated
within the unfolding career and lived experience of people with AIDS.

Method and Data

The following analysis is based on data
gathered in 56 in-depth interviews with nineteen men who had been diagnosed with HIV
(human immunodeficiency virus) infections.
On the average, each individual was interviewed on three separate occasions and each
of these sessions lasted from 1 to 3 hours. The
interviews, conducted between July 1987 and
February 1988, were guided by 60 open-
ended questions and were audiotaped. Most
interviews took place in the participants'
homes. However, a few participants were interviewed in a private university office because their living quarters were not condu-
cive to a confidential conversation. . . .

All respondents were gay males who lived
in a metropolitan area in the Midwest. They
varied in age, income, and the stage of their
illness. In age, they ranged from nineteen to
forty-six years, with the majority in the
twenty-eight to forty age bracket. Six persons were currently employed in professional
or white-collar occupations. The remaining
thirteen were living marginally on Social Security or disability benefits. Several members
of this latter group had previously been employed in either blue-collar or service occupations. Seven individuals were diagnosed
with AIDS, 10 were diagnosed with ARC
(AIDS-related complex), and 2 were diagnosed as HIV positive but both had more serious HIV-related health complications (e.g.,
tuberculosis).

On Becoming a PWA: The Realization of an AIDS Identity

For many of these men, the transformation
of physical symptoms into the personal and social reality of AIDS took place most dramatically when they received a validating diagnosis from a physician. The following account
reveals the impact of being officially diagnosed:

> She [the doctor] said, "Your biopsy did
> come out for Kaposi's sarcoma. I want
> you to go to the hospital tomorrow and to
> plan to spend most of the day there."
> While she is telling me this, the whole
> world is buzzing in my head because this
> is the first confirmation coming from
> outside as opposed to my own internal
> suspicions. I started to cry—it [AIDS] be-
> came very real . . . very real. . . .

> Anyway, everything started to roller
> coaster inside me and I was crying in the
> office there. The doctor said, "You knew
> this was the way it was going to come
> out, didn't you?" She seemed kind of
> shocked about why I was crying so much,
> not realizing that no matter how much
> you are internally aware of something, to
> hear it from someone else is what makes
> it real. For instance, the first time I really
> accepted being gay was when other peo-
> ple said "You are gay!". . . . It's a social
> thing— you're not real until you're real
> to someone else.

This quote illustrates the salience of social
processes for the validation and realization
of an identity—in this case, an AIDS-related
identity. Becoming a PWA is not simply a
matter of viral infection, it is contingent on
interpersonal interaction and definitions. As
depicted in the quote, a rather momentous
medical announcement facilitates a process
of identity construction which, in turn, entails both interpersonal and subjective transformation. Within the interpersonal realm,
the newly diagnosed "AIDS patient" is resitu-
ated as a social object and placed in a marginal or liminal status. He is thereby separated from many of his prior social moorings.
On the subjective level, this separation produces a crisis, or a disruption of the PWAs
routine activities and self-understanding.
The diagnosed individual is prompted to
"make sense" of the meaning of his newly acquired status and to feel its implications for
future conceptions and enactments of self.

Personalizing the Illness: Self-Feelings Evoked by AIDS

As he interprets and responds to the meaning of his condition, the diagnosed individual *personalizes* (Asher 1987) it, adjusting it to the distinctive features of his life (e.g., his work situation, family history, personal relationships, character traits, and access to resources). Certain self-feelings and psychic reactions are especially important in this personalizing process. For example, PWAs may feel anguished about the loss of their future, the loss of a highly valued job, or by a diminished sense of sexual desirability. They may also feel troubled by their loss of everyday skills or opportunities and their lack of involvement in normal interaction. The remarks shared by one interviewee are reflective of such sentiments:

Of course, I can't drive now and it is difficult to deal with that fact. That is a big loss, it really is . . . and also knowing that I can't go back to work. I'm getting used to not working but mentally it is a loss—your thinking is lessened. I don't have to give a quick answer anymore. When somebody would come up to me at work and ask a question, I would have the answer for them before they could even finish the question. Now that ability isn't there anymore. I had really enjoyed being able to do that.

These experiences of loss are typically accompanied by reactions of grief. Indeed, a few PWAs stressed that grief had become a predominant theme in their everyday lives. Most PWAs grieved about their loss of health, potential, and a normal life span. They also felt grief regarding the loss of previous sources of personal continuity and self-validation such as work, friendships, and sexual relationships.

Feelings of guilt can also be induced by an AIDS diagnosis. These feelings have several sources and dimensions. For instance, PWAs may feel guilty about the possibility that they infected their sexual partners. They may also feel guilty about the anguish, grief, or suffering that their diagnoses provoke among partners, friends, or family members. Furthermore, they may experience identification

guilt because they are members of groups which are stigmatized by cultural conceptions (Conrad 1986), media accounts (Seidman 1988) and conservative religious doctrines (Palmer 1989). These stigmatizing perspectives are sometimes internalized by PWAs and may lead them to (consciously or unconsciously) interpret their condition as a kind of punishment. Such a reaction is illustrated in the following remarks:

In the beginning, it [AIDS] triggered feelings that had to do with . . . well, I hesitate to say this but it was like I deserved this [illness]. This is exactly what I deserved! I've heard other gay men talk about the same thing like "God, we've tried to live such a decent life and we're being punished." We made that connection of somehow being punished . . . and even if we didn't come right out and say it was punishment or something, what we said or what I said was "Well, God's trying to tell us something here."

Finally, due to the fatality of this disease, being informed that one has AIDS can also elicit strong feelings of death anxiety:

After the doctor told me that I had Kaposi's sarcoma, I was really in bad shape. . . . I don't mean to be melodramatic but something inside me was saying "Holy shit, you're going to die! No you're not going to just die but you're going to die very soon!"

An AIDS diagnosis can evoke powerful images of death which may result in shock, denial, panic, and despair. These reactions inhibit the ability of newly diagnosed individuals to understand the immediate effects of their condition, to cope more effectively with the symptoms associated with the illness, and to deal with the demands of their everyday lives. Also, feelings of severe death anxiety make it more likely for PWAs to oscillate between phases of denial, anger, bargaining, depression, and acceptance as they grapple with the prospective implications of their diagnosis (Nichols 1985). . . .

The Liminal Situation of the PWA: Constraints and Opportunities

As an individual enters into and personalizes the status of being a PWA he finds his life characterized by ambiguity. The manifestations and consequences of his HIV infection are unclear and unpredictable. He is uncertain about what specific symptoms will be triggered by his illness, how he will feel from day to day, how much longer he can expect to live, and whether or not he will be able to live with dignity (Weitz 1989).

In the social realm, the experience of the PWA is especially ambiguous. Given the fear and mystery that surround AIDS, responses of others to his diagnosis can range from avoidance, hostility, and rejection to empathy and support. Regardless of the specific reactions of others, a shift or rupture occurs in the individual's social location. The PWA is not only separated from his previous social anchorages but he is not clearly linked to any new ones. Also, given the diverse and competing social definitions of AIDS, he is not provided with a precise indication of his current status. The newly diagnosed PWA thus becomes situated as *liminal persona*, that is, he is "neither here nor there; he is betwixt and between the positions assigned by law, custom, convention and ceremonial" (Turner 1969, 95).

Most important, recently diagnosed PWAs encounter both the constraints and opportunities that go along with their liminal social situation. On one hand, their liminal location can intensity problematic self-feelings and provoke a sense of confusion about the implications of their illness. Further, the ambiguous social meaning of their condition makes it more difficult for them to enact an AIDS-related identity. That is, although PWAs are provided with a medical designation, they are given a clear idea of what role or set of behavioral expectations correspond to this identity. They subsequently have few practical guidelines for constructing a meaningful course of action.

In a more positive light, the liminal situation of PWAs can elicit a sense of power and opportunity. Feelings of empowerment can be derived from the mystery and danger associated with liminality (Turner 1969). At the same time, a sense of opportunity can arise from the lack of conventions and guidelines applying to those with such a novel and ambiguous condition. In essence, since AIDS is a rather unique and vaguely understood phenomenon, PWAs are granted some room to improvise and maneuver when constructing a behavioral repertoire to go along with their medical identity. They are not simply constrained or captured by this identity. Instead, they are afforded a certain amount of power and opportunity to define what it means to be a PWA and to reshape the meaning of this identity in their social encounters. Nevertheless, in their ongoing efforts to construct and negotiate a viable identity, PWAs must grapple with a number of stigmatizing reactions and interpersonal dilemmas.

Interpersonal Dilemmas Encountered by PWAs

Stigmatization

Stigmatization is one of the most significant difficulties faced by people with AIDS as they attempt to fashion a personal and social meaning for their illness. The vast majority of our informants had already experienced some kind of stigma because of their gay identities. When they were diagnosed with AIDS, they usually encountered even stronger homophobic reactions and discreditation efforts. An especially painful form of stigmatization occurred when PWAs were rejected by friends and family members after revealing their diagnosis. Many respondents shared very emotional accounts of how they were ostracized by parents, siblings, or colleagues. Several noted that their parents and family members had even asked them to no longer return home for visits. However, rejections were not always so explicit. In many cases, intimate relationships were gradually and ambiguously phased out rather than abruptly or clearly ended.

A few PWAs shared stories of being stigmatized by gay friends or acquaintances. They described how some acquaintances subtly reprimanded them when seeing them at gay bars or repeatedly reminded them "to be careful" regarding any sexual involvements. Further, they mentioned that certain gay friends avoided associating with them after learning of their AIDS-related diagnoses. These PWAs thus experienced the problem of being "doubly stigmatized" (Kowalewski 1988), that is, they were devalued within an already stigmatized group, the gay community.

PWAs also felt the effects of stigmatization in other, more subtle ways. For example, curious and even sympathetic responses on the parts of others, especially strangers, could lead PWAs to feel discredited. One PWA, reflecting on his interactions with hospital staff, observed:

> When they become aware [of my diagnosis], it seemed like people kept looking . . . like they were looking for something. What it felt like was being analyzed, both physically and emotionally. It also felt like being a subject or guinea pig . . . like "here's another one." They gave me that certain kind of look. Kind of that look like pity or that said "what a poor wretch," not a judgmental look but rather a pitying one.

An experience of this nature can precipitate a crisis of identity for a person with AIDS. He finds himself publicly stigmatized and identified as a victim. Such an identifying moment can seriously challenge prior conceptions of self and serve as a turning point from which new self-images or identities are constructed (Charmaz 1980). That is, it can lead a PWA to internalize stigmatizing social attributes or it can incite him to search for involvements and ideologies which might enable him to construct a more desirable AIDS identity.

Counterfeit Nurturance

Given the physical and social implications of their illness, PWAs typically desire some kind of special nurturing from friends, partners, family members, or health practitioners. Yet displays of unusual concern or sympathy on the part of others can be threatening to self. People with AIDS may view such expressions of nurturance as counterfeit or harmful because they highlight their condition and hence confirm their sense of difference and vulnerability.

The following observation illustrates the sensitivity of PWAs to this problem:

> One thing that makes you feel kind of odd is when people come across supportive and want to be supportive but it doesn't really feel like they are supportive. There is another side to them that's like, well, they are being nice to you because they feel sorry for you, or because it makes them feel good about themselves to help someone with AIDS, not because they really care about you.

PWAs often find themselves caught in a paradox regarding gestures of exceptional help or support. They want special consideration at times, but if they accept support or concern which is primarily focused on their condition, they are likely to feel that a "victim identity" is being imposed on them. This exacerbates some of the negative self-feelings that have already been triggered by the illness. It also leads PWAs to be more wary of the motivations underlying others' expressions of nurturance.

Given these dynamics, PWAs may reach out to each other in an effort to find relationships that are more mutually or genuinely nurturing. This strategy is problematic, though, because even PWAs offer one another support which emphasizes their condition. They are also likely to remind each other of the anomalous status they share and the "spoiled" features (Goffman 1963) of their identities qua PWAs.

Ultimately, suspicions of counterfeit nurturance can lead those diagnosed with AIDS to feel mistreated by almost everyone, particularly by caregivers who are most directly involved in helping them. Correctly or incorrectly, PWAs tend to share some feelings of ambivalence and resentment towards friends, lovers, family members, and medical personnel.

Fears of Contagion and Death Anxiety

Fears of contagion present another serious dilemma for PWAs in their efforts to negotiate a functional social identity. These fears are generated not only by the fact that people with AIDS are the carriers of an epidemic illness but also because, like others with a death taint, they are symbolically associated with mass death and the contagion of the dead (Lifton 1967). The situation may even be further complicated by the contagion anxiety which homosexuality triggers for some people.

In general, others are tempted to withdraw from an individual with AIDS because of their fears of contracting the virus. Even close friends of a PWA are apt to feel more fearful or distant toward him, especially when first becoming aware of the diagnosis. They may feel anxious about the possibility of becoming infected with the virus through interactions routinely shared with him in the past (e.g. hugging and kissing). They may also wish to avoid the perils of being stigmatized themselves by friends or associates who fear that those close to a PWA are a potential source of contagion.

Another dimension of contagion anxiety is reflected in the tendency of significant others to avoid discussing issues with a PWA that might lead them to a deeper apprehension of the death-related implications of his diagnosis. As Lifton (1967) suggested, the essence of contagion anxiety is embodied in the fear that "if I come too close to a death tainted person, I will experience his death and his annihilation" (p. 518).

This death-related contagion anxiety often results in increased strain and distance in a PWA's interactions with friends or family members. It can also inhibit the level of openness and intimacy share among fellow PWAs when they gather together to address issues provoked by their diagnoses. Responses of grief, denial, and anxiety in the face of death make in-depth discussions of the illness experience keenly problematic. According to one respondent:

> Usually no one's ever able to talk about it [their disease and dying] without going to pieces. They might start but it only takes about two minutes to break into tears. They might say something like "I don't know what to do! I might not even be here next week!" Then you can just see the ripple effect it has on the others sitting back and listening. You have every possible expression from anger to denial to sadness and all these different emotions on people's faces. And mostly this feeling of "what can we do? Well. . . Nothing!"

Problems of Normalization

Like others who possess a stigmatizing attribute, people with AIDS come to regard many social situations with alarm (Goffman 1971) and uncertainty (Davis 1974). They soon discover that their medical condition is a salient aspect of all but their most fleeting social encounters. They also quickly learn that their diagnosis, once known to others, can acquire the character of a *master status* (Hughes 1945; Becker 1963) and thus become the focal point of interaction. It carries with it, "the potential for inundating the expressive boundaries of a situation" (Davis 1974, 166) and hence for creating significant strains or rupture in the ongoing flow of social intercourse.

In light of this, one might expect PWAs to prefer interaction contexts characterized by "closed" awareness (Glaser and Strauss 1968). Their health status would be unknown to others and they would presumably encounter fewer problems when interacting. However, when in these situations, they must remain keenly attuned to controlling information and concealing attributes relevant to their diagnosis. Ironically, this requirement to be dramaturgically "on" may give rise to even more feelings of anxiety and resentment.

The efforts of persons with AIDS to establish and maintain relationships within more "open" contexts are also fraught with complications. One of the major dilemmas they encounter is how to move interactions beyond an atmosphere of fictional acceptance (Davis 1974). A context of fictional acceptance is typified by responses on the part of others which deny, avoid, or minimize the reality of an individual's diagnosis. In attempting to grapple with the management of a spoiled identity, PWAs may seek to "break through" (Davis 1974) relations of this nature. In doing so, they often try to broaden the scope of interactional involvement and to normalize problematic elements of their social identity. That is, they attempt to project "images, attitudes and concepts of self which encourage the normal to identify with [them (i.e., 'take [their] role') in terms other than those associated with imputations of deviance" (Davis 1974, 168).

Yet even if a PWA attains success in "breaking through," it does not necessarily diminish his interactional difficulties. Instead, he can become caught in an ambiguous dilemma with respect to the requisites of awareness and normalization. Simply put, if others begin to disregard his diagnosis and treat him in a normal way, then he faces the problem of having to remind them of the limitations to normalcy imposed by this condition. The person with AIDS is thus required to perform an intricate balancing act between encouraging the normalization of his relationships and ensuring that others remain sensitized to the constraining effects of such a serious illness. These dynamics promote the construction of relationships which, at best, have a qualified sense of normalcy. They also heighten the PWAs sense that he is located in an ambiguous or liminal position.

Avoiding or Minimizing Dilemmas

In an attempt to avoid or defuse the problematic feelings, attributions, and ambiguities which arise in their ongoing interactions, PWAs engage in various forms of identity management. In doing so, they often use strategies which allow to minimize the social visibility of their diagnoses and to carefully control interactions with others. These strategies include *passing, covering, isolation,* and *insulation.*

The particular strategies employed vary according to the progression of their illness, the personal meanings they attach to it, the audiences serving as primary referents for self-presentations, and the dynamics of their immediate social situation.

Passing and Covering

As Goffman (1963) noted in his classic work on stigma, those with a spoiled identity may seek to pass as normal by carefully suppressing information and thereby precluding others' awareness of devalued personal attributes. The PWAs we interviewed mentioned that "passing" was a maneuver they had used regularly. It was easily employed in the early stages of the illness when more telltale physical signs had not yet become apparent and awareness of an individual's diagnosis was confirmed to a small social circle.

However, as the illness progresses, concealing the visibility of an AIDS-related diagnosis becomes more difficult. When a person with AIDS begins to miss work frequently, to lose weight noticeably, and to reduce his general level of activity, others become more curious or suspicious about what ailment is provoking such major changes. In the face of related questions, some PWAs elected to devise a "cover" for their diagnosis which disguised troubling symptoms as products of a less discrediting illness.

One informant decided to cover his AIDS diagnosis by telling co-workers that he was suffering from leukemia:

> There was coming a point, I wasn't feeling so hot. I was tired and the quality of my life was decreasing tremendously because all of my free time was spent resting or sleeping. I was still keeping up with work but I thought I'd better tell them something before I had to take more days off here and there to even out the quality of my life. I had already had this little plan to tell them I had leukemia . . . but I thought how am I going to tell them, what am I going to tell them, how am I going to convince them? What am I going to do if someone says, "You don't have leukemia, you have AIDS!"? This was all stuff clicking around in my mind. I thought, how could they possibly know? They only know as much as I tell them.

This quote reveals the heightened concern with information control that accompanies decisions to conceal one's condition. Regardless of the psychic costs, though, a number of our informants opted for this remedial strategy. A commonly used technique consisted of informing friends, parents, or co-workers that one had cancer or tuberculosis without mentioning that these were the presenting symptoms of one's AIDS diagnosis. Covering attempts of this kind were most often employed by PWAs when relating to others who were not aware of their gay identity. These relationships were less apt to be characterized by the suspicions or challenges offered by those who knew that an individual was both gay and seriously ill.

Isolation and Insulation

For those whose diagnosis was not readily visible, dramaturgical skills, such as passing and covering, could be quite useful. These techniques were not so feasible when physical cues, such as a pale complexion, emaciated appearance, or facial lesions made the nature of a PWAs condition more apparent. Under these circumstances, negotiations with others were more alarming and they were more likely to include conflicts engendered by fear, ambiguity, and expressions of social devaluation.

In turn, some PWAs came to view physical and social isolation as the best means available to them for escaping from both these interpersonal difficulties and their own feelings of ambivalence. By withdrawing from virtually all interaction, they sought to be spared the social struggles and psychic strains that could be triggered by others' recognition of their condition.

Nonetheless, this strategy was typically an unsuccessful one. Isolation and withdrawal often exacerbated the feelings of alienation that PWAs were striving to minimize in their social relationships. Moreover, their desire to be removed from the interactional matrix was frequently overcome by their need for extensive medical care and interpersonal support as they coped with the progressive effects of the illness.

Given the drawbacks of extreme isolation, a number of PWAs used a more selective withdrawal strategy. It consisted of efforts to disengage from many but not all social involvements and to interact regularly with only a handful of trusted associates (e.g., partners, friends, or family members). Emphasis was placed on minimizing contacts with those outside of this circle because they were likely to be less tolerant or predictable.

PWAs engaging in this type of selective interaction tried to develop a small network of intimate others who could insulate them from potentially threatening interactions. Ideally, they were able to form a reliable social circle within which they felt little need to conceal their diagnosis. They could thereby experience some relief from the burden of stigma management and information control.

Building and Embracing an AIDS Identity

Strategies such as passing, covering, isolation, and insulation are used by PWAs, especially in the earlier stages of their illness, to shield themselves from the stigma and uncertainty associated with AIDS. However, these strategies typically require a high level of personal vigilance, they evoke concerns about information control, and they are essentially defensive in nature. They do not provide PWAs with a way to reformulate the personal meaning of their diagnosis and to integrate it with valued definitions of self.

In light of this, most PWAs engage in more active types of *identity work* which allow them to "create, present and sustain personal identities which are congruent with and supportive of the[ir] self-concept[s]" (Snow and Anderson l987, 1348). Certain types of identity work are especially appealing because they help PWAs to gain a greater sense of mastery over their condition and to make better use of the behavioral possibilities arising from their liminal condition.

The most prominent type of identity work engaged in by the PWAs we interviewed was embracement. As Snow and Anderson (1987) argued, embracement refers to "verbal and expressive confirmation of one's acceptance of and attachment to the social identity associated with a general or specific role, a set of social relationships, or a particular ideology" (p. 1354). Among the PWAs involved in this study, embracement was promoted and reinforced through participation in local AIDS-related support groups.

Support Groups and Social Embracement

People facing an existential crisis often make use of new memberships and social forms in their efforts to construct a more viable sense of self (Kotarba 1984). The vast majority of respondents in this study became involved in PWA support groups in order to better address the crisis elicited by their illness and to find new forms of self-expression. They typically joined these groups within a few months of receiving their diagnosis and continued to attend meetings on a fairly regular basis.

By and large, support groups became the central focus of identity work and repair for PWAs. These groups were regarded as a valuable source of education and emotional support that helped individuals to cope better with the daily exigencies of their illness. At support group meetings, PWAs could exchange useful information, share feelings and troubles, and relate to others who could see beyond the negative connotations of AIDS.

Support groups also facilitated the formation of social ties and feelings of collective identification among PWAs. Within these circles, individuals learned to better nurture and support one another and to emphasize the shared nature of their problems. Feelings of guilt and isolation were transformed into a sense of group identification. This kind of *associational embracement* (Snow and Anderson 1987) was conveyed in the comments of one person who proclaimed:

> I spend almost all of my time with other PWAs. They're my best friends now and they're the people I feel most comfortable with. We support one another and we know that we can talk to each other any time, day or night.

For some PWAs, especially those with a troubled or marginal past, support group relationships provided an instant "buddy system" that was used to bolster feelings of security and self-worth. Recently formed support group friendships even took on primary importance in their daily lives. Perhaps because of the instability and isolation which characterized their life outside of support groups, a few of these PWAs tended to exaggerate the level of intimacy which existed in their newly found friendships. By stressing a romanticized version of these relationships, they were able to preserve a sense of being cared for even in the absence of more enduring social connections.

Identity Embracement and Affirmation

Most of the PWAs we interviewed had come to gradually affirm and embrace an AIDS-related identity. Participation in a support group exposed them to alternative definitions of the reality of AIDS and an ongoing system of identity construction. Hence, rather than accepting public imputations which cast them as "AIDS victims," PWAs learned to distance themselves from such designations and to avow more favorable AIDS-associated identities. In turn, the process of *identity embracement* was realized when individuals proudly announced that

they were PWAs who were "living and thriving with the illness."

Continued associations with other PWAs could also promote deepening involvement in activities organized around the identity of being a person with AIDS. A case in point is provided by a man who recounted his progression as a PWA:

> After a while, I aligned myself with other people with AIDS who shared my beliefs about taking the active role. I began writing and speaking about AIDS and I became involved in various projects. I helped to create and promote a workshop for people with AIDS. . . . I also got involved in organizing a support group for family members of PWAs.

As involvement in AIDS-related activities increases, embracement of an AIDS-centered identity is likely to become more encompassing. In some cases, diagnosed individuals found themselves organizing workshops on AIDS, coordinating a newsletter for PWAs, and delivering speeches regularly at schools and churches. Virtually all aspects of their lives became associated with their diagnosis. Being a PWA thus became both a master status and a valued career. This process was described by a person who had been diagnosed with ARC for two years:

> One interesting thing is that when you have AIDS or ARC and you're not working anymore, you tend to become a veteran professional on AIDS issues. You get calls regularly from people who want information or who want you to get involved in project, etc. You find yourself getting drawn to that kind of involvement. It becomes almost a second career!

This kind of identity embracement was particularly appealing for a few individuals involved in this study. Prior to contracting an AIDS-related infection, they had felt rejected or unrecognized in many of their social relationships (e.g. family, work, and friendships). Ironically, their stigmatized AIDS diagnosis provided them with an opportunity for social affirmation. It offered them a sense of uniqueness and expertise that was positively evaluated in certain social and community circles (e.g., public education and church forums). It could even serve as a springboard for a new and more meaningful biography.

Ideological Embracement: AIDS as a Transforming Experience

Support groups and related self-help networks are frequently bases for the production and transmission of subcultural perspectives which controvert mainstream social definitions of a stigma. As Becker (1963) argued, when people who share a deviant attribute have the opportunity to interact with one another, they are likely to develop a system of shared meanings emphasizing the differences between their definitions of who they are and the definitions held by other members of the society. "They develop perspectives on themselves and their deviant [attributes] and on their relations with other members of the society" (p. 81). These perspectives guide the stigmatized as they engage in processes of identity construction and embracement.

Subcultural perspectives contain ideologies which assure individuals that what they do on a continuing basis has moral validity (Lofland 1969). Among PWAs, these ideologies were grounded in metaphors of transformation which included an emphasis on *special mission* and *empowerment*.

One of the most prominent subcultural interpretations of AIDS highlighted the spiritual meaning of the illness. For PWAs embracing this viewpoint, AIDS was symbolically and experientially inverted from a "curse" to a "blessing" which promoted a liberating rather than a constricting form of identity transformation. The following remarks illustrate this perspective:

I now view AIDS as both a gift and a blessing. That sounds strange, I suppose, in a limited context. It sounds strange because we [most people] think it's so awful, but yet there are such radical changes that take place in your life from having this illness that's defined as terminal. You go through this amazing kind of *transformation*. You look at things for the first time, in a powerful new way that you've never looked at them before in your whole life.

A number of PWAs similarly stressed the beneficial personal and spiritual transitions experienced as a result of their diagnosis. They even regarded their illness as a motivating force that led them to grapple with important existential questions and to experience personal growth and change that otherwise would not have occurred.

For many PWAs, *ideological embracement* (Snow and Anderson 1987) entailed identity constructions based on a quasi-religious sense of "special mission." These individuals placed a premium on disseminating information about AIDS and promoting a level of public awareness which might inhibit the further transmission of this illness. Some felt that their diagnosis had provided them with a unique opportunity to help and educate others. They subsequently displayed a high level of personal sacrifice and commitment while seeking to spread the news about AIDS and to nurture those directly affected by this illness. Most crucially, their diagnosis provided them with a heightened sense of power and purpose:

Basically I feel that as a person with ARC I can do more for humanity in general than I could ever do before. I never before in my life felt like I belonged here. For the most part, I felt like I was stranded on a hostile planet—didn't know why. But now with the disease and what I've learned in my life, I feel like I really have something by which I can help other people. It gives me a special sense of purpose.

I feel like I've got a mission now and that's what this whole thing is about. AIDS is challenging me with a question and the question it asks is: If I'm not doing something to help others regarding this illness, then why continue to use up energy here on this earth?

The idea of a "special mission" is often a revitalizing formulation for those who carry a death taint (Lifton 1967). It helps to provide PWAs with a sense of mastery and self-worth by giving their condition a more positive or redemptive meaning. This notion also gives form and resolution to painful feelings of loss, grief, guilt and death anxiety. It enables individuals to make use of these emotions, while at the same time transcending them.

Moreover, the idea of special mission provides PWAs with a framework through which they can moralize their activities and continuing lives.

Beliefs stressing the empowering aspects of AIDS also served as an important focus of identity affirmation. These beliefs were frequently rooted in the sense of transformation provoked by the illness. Many of those interviewed viewed their diagnosis as empowering because it led them to have a concentrated experience of life, a stronger sense of purpose, a better understanding of their personal resources and a clearer notion of how to prioritize their daily concerns. They correspondingly felt less constrained by mundane aspects of the AIDS experience and related symptoms.

A sense of empowerment could additionally be derived from others' objectification of PWAs as sources of danger, pollution, or death. This was illustrated in the remarks of an informant who had Kaposi's sarcoma:

> People hand power to me on a silver platter because they are afraid. It's not fear of catching the virus or anything, I think it is just fear of identification with someone who is dying.

The interactional implications of such attributions of power also recognized by this same informant:

> Because I have AIDS, people leave me alone in my life in some respects if I want them to. I never used to be able to get people to back off and now I can. I'm not the one who is doing this, so to speak. They are giving me the power to do so.

Most PWAs realized their condition offered them an opportunity to experience both psychological and social power. They subsequently accentuated the empowering dimensions of their lived experience of AIDS and linked these to an encompassing metaphor of transformation.

Summary and Conclusions

People with AIDS face many obstacles in their efforts to construct and sustain a desirable social identity. In the early stages of their career, after receiving a validating diagnosis, they are confronted by painful self-feelings such as grief, guilt, and death anxiety. These feelings often diminish their desire and ability to participate in interactions which would allow them to sustain favorable images of self.

PWAs encounter additional difficulties as a result of being situated (at least initially) as liminal persons. That is, their liminal situation can heighten negative self-feelings and evoke a sense of confusion and uncertainty about the social implications of their illness. At the same time, however, it releases them from conventional roles, meanings, or expectations and provides them with a measure of power and maneuverability in the processes of identity construction.

In turn, as they construct and negotiate the meaning of an AIDS-related identity, PWAs must grapple with the effects of social reactions such as stigmatization, counterfeit nurturance, fears of contagion, and death anxiety. These reactions both elicit and reinforce a number of interactional ambiguities, dilemmas, and threats to self.

In responding to these challenges, PWAs engage in various types of identity management and construction. On one hand, they may seek to disguise their diagnoses or to restrict their social and interactional involvements. PWAs are most likely to use such strategies in the earlier phases of the illness. The disadvantage of these strategies is that they are primarily defensive. They provide PWAs with a way to avoid or adjust to the effects of problematic social reactions, but they do not offer a means for affirming more desirable AIDS-related identities.

On the other hand, as their illness progresses and they become more enmeshed in subcultural networks, most PWAs are prompted to engage in forms of identity embracement which enable them to actively reconstruct the meaning of their illness and to integrate it with valued conceptions of self. In essence, through their interactions with other PWAs, they learn to embrace affiliations and ideologies which accentuate the transformative and empowering possibilities arising from their condition. They also acquire the social and symbolic resources necessary to fashion revitalizing identities and to sustain a sense of dignity and self-worth.

Ultimately, through their ongoing participation in support networks, PWAs are able to build identities which are linked to their lived experience of AIDS. They are also encouraged to actively confront and transform the stigmatizing conceptions associated with this medical condition. Hence, rather than resigning themselves to the darker implications of AIDS, they learn to affirm themselves as "people with AIDS" who are "living and thriving with the illness."

References

Asher, R. 1987. "Ambivalence, moral career, and ideology: A sociological analysis of women married to alcoholics." Ph.D. diss., University of Minnesota.

Baumgartner, G. 1986. *AIDS: Psychosocial factors in the acquired immune deficiency syndrome.* Springfield, IL: Charles C. Thomas.

Becker, H. S. 1963. *Outsiders.* New York: Free Press.

Charmaz, K. 1980. "The social construction of pity in the chronically ill." *Studies in Symbolic Interaction* 3:123-45.

Conrad, P. 1986. "The social meaning of AIDS." *Social Policy*, 17:51-56.

Davis, F. 1974. "Deviance disavowal and the visibly handicapped." In *Deviance and liberty*, edited by L. Rainwater, 163-72. Chicago: Aldine.

Denzin, N. 1983. "A note on emotionality, self and interaction." *American Journal of Sociology* 89:402-9.

Ergas, Y. 1987. "The social consequences of the AIDS epidemic." *Social Science Research Council/Items* 41:33-39.

Geiss, S., R. Fuller, and J. Rush. 1986. "Lovers of AIDS victims: Psychosocial stresses and counseling needs." *Death Studies* 10: 43-53.

Goffman, E. 1963. *Stigma.* Englewood Cliffs, NJ: Prentice-Hall.

———. 1971. *Relations in public.* New York: Harper & Row.

Glaser, B. S., and A. L. Strauss. 1968. *Awareness of dying.* Chicago: Aldine.

Hughes, E. C. 1945. "Dilemmas and contradictions of status." *American Journal of Sociology* 50: 353-59.

Kaplan, H., R. Johnson, C. Bailey, and W. Simon. 1987. "The sociological study of AIDS: A critical review of the literature and suggested research agenda." *Journal of Health and Social Behavior* 28:140-57.

Kotarba, J. 1984. "A synthesis: The existential self in society." In *The existential self in society*, edited by J. Kotarba and A. Fontana, 222-33. Chicago: Aldine.

Kowalewski, M. 1988. "Double stigma and boundary maintenance: How gay men deal with AIDS." *Journal of Contemporary Ethnography* 7:211-28.

Lifton, R. J. 1967. *Death in life.* New York: Random House.

Lofland, J. 1969. *Deviance and identity.* Englewood Cliffs, NJ: Prentice Hall.

Macklin, E. 1988. "AIDS: Implications for families." *Family Relations* 37:141-49.

Nichols, S. 1985. "Psychosocial reactions of persons with AIDS." *Annals of Internal Medicine* 103:13-16.

Palmer, S. 1989. "AIDS as metaphor." *Society* 26:45-51.

Salisbury, D. 1986. "AIDS: Psychosocial implications." *Journal of Psychosocial Nursing* 24 (12): 13-16.

Seidman, S. 1988. "Transfiguring sexual identity: AIDS and the contemporary construction of homosexuality." *Social Text* 19/20:187-205.

Snow, D., and L. Anderson, 1987. "Identity work among the homeless: The verbal construction and avowal of personal identities." *American Journal of Sociology* 1336-71.

Sontag, S. 1989. *AIDS and its metaphors.* New York: Farrar, Straus, & Giroux.

Turner, V. 1969. *The ritual process.* Ithaca, NY: Cornell University Press.

Weitz, R. 1989. "Uncertainty and the lives of persons with AIDS." *Journal of Health and Social Behavior* 30:270-81.

Further Reading

Ronald Bayer. 1989. *Private Acts, Social Consequences: AIDS & the Politics of Public Health.* New York: Free Press.

Danielle Carricaburu and Janine Pierret. 1995. "From Biographical Disruption to Biographical Reinforcement: The Case of HIV-Positive Men." *Sociology of Health and Illness* 17: 65-88.

Joseph Kotarba and Darlene Hurt. 1995. "An Ethnography of an AIDS Hospice: Towards a Theory of Organizational Pastiche." *Symbolic Interaction* 18: 413-438.

Dorothy Nelkin (ed.). 1991. *A Disease of Society: Cultural and Institutional Responses to AIDS.* New York: Cambridge University Press.

Discussion Questions

1. What are the sources of experience for men with AIDS as compared with people who have other chronic or terminal illness?

2. Considering the analyses of Robert Murphy, Rose Weitz, and Kent Sandstrom,

outline what you have learned about stigma.

3. The course of AIDS is changing to a serious chronic illness for many patients.

How might this change affect identity construction?

From *Journal of Contemporary Ethnography*, Vol. 19 (3). Pp. 271-294. Copyright © 1990 by Sage Publications. Reprinted by permission. ✦

47

AIDS and Its Impact on Medical Work: The Culture and Politics of the Shop Floor

Charles L. Bosk
Joel E. Frader

In this selection, Charles Bosk and Joel Frader provide us a look at the micro-politics of medical work under changing definitions of health and risk of illness. Discovery of AIDS changed the practice of medical work. It forced medical personnel to reconstruct their ideas about risk and vulnerability. Bosk and Frader show that work with AIDS and people with HIV and AIDS did not follow the standard routine. As you read this selection, think about what practitioner vulerability means for medical work and its practice. Bosk and Frader speculate that AIDS even lessened the number of medical students intent on practicing primary care. In fact, the 1980s and early nineties show declines in students choosing primary care as an area of practice.

Other sociologists have demonstrated that most medical work is riddled with uncertainty: uncertain treatments and uncertain cures. Consider the ways AIDS challenged patient treatment and attention to work. In its introduction, workers unfamiliar with AIDS work touched patients less, used extreme protective measures, or passed an AIDS-related tasks to other workers more often than those who

worked with people with HIV and AIDS. Bosk and Frader speculate on how the uncertain risk of AIDS—resulting from incomplete scientific knowledge and limited personal knowledge—transformed the character of medical work on "the shop floor" of university teaching hospitals. As you read this selection, consider the consequences of HIV and AIDS for the current face of interactions between health practitioners and patients in the United States.

In 1979 when undergraduates applied in record numbers for admission to medical school, AIDS was not a clinical and diagnostic category. In 1990 when the applications to medical schools are plummeting, AIDS is unarguably with us, and not just as a clinical entity. . . .

This article is about the impact of AIDS on the shop floor of the academic urban hospital, an attempt to understand the impact of AIDS on everyday practices of doctors providing inpatient care. We wish to view AIDS as a total social phenomenon rather than as a mere disease. Procedurally, we shall concentrate on the house officer (someone who, after graduation from medical school, participates in medical specialty training) and the medical student to see how this new infectious disease changes the content of everyday work and the education of apprentice physicians learning how to doctor and to assume the social responsibilities of the role of the physician. We are going to look at professional and occupational culture as a set of shop-floor practices and beliefs about work.

At the close of this article we will make some generalizations about the impact of AIDS on medical training and reflect on how this affects the professional culture of physicians. This may distort the picture somewhat, as the urban teaching hospital is not representative of the whole world of medical practice. To the degree that AIDS patients are concentrated in them, any inferences drawn from large teaching hospitals overstate or exaggerate the impact of AIDS. At the very least, such sampling fails to catalogue the variety of strategies individual physicians may use to avoid patients with AIDS. It fails, as well, to capture the innovative approaches to AIDS of pioneering health professionals in nontraditional settings.

This sampling problem not withstanding, the urban academic teaching hospital is the arena of choice for studying the impact of AIDS on the medical profession. The concentration of cases in urban teaching hospitals means that students and house officers have high likelihood of treating patients with AIDS. They are the physicians on the clinical front lines, the ones with the heaviest day-to-day operational burdens.

Further, our attention to the house officers and students possesses a secondary benefit for this inquiry into shop-floor or work-place culture: namely, the natural state of the work place in its before-AIDS condition has been extensively documented. We use the terms shop-floor and work-place culture to invoke the sociological tradition for inquiries into work begun by Everett C. Hughes (1971) at the University of Chicago in the post-World War II years. This tradition emphasizes equivalencies between humble and proud occupations, the management of "dirty work," the procedures that surround routines and emergencies, and the handling of mistakes. Above all, the perspective invites us to reverse our "conventional sentimentality" (Becker 1967) about occupations. The idea of the hospital as shop floor is one rhetorical device for reminding us that house officers and students are workers in a very real and active sense.

. . .We can construct a before-AIDS shop-floor culture as a first step in assessing what difference AIDS makes in the occupational culture of physicians. Our picture of the after-AIDS shop floor arises from the pictures drawn in the medical literature, our teaching and consulting experience in large university health centers, and 30 interviews with medical personnel caring for AIDS patients. These interviews were conducted with individuals at all levels of training and provide admittedly impressionistic data which need more systematic verification. The interviews averaged an hour in length and explored both how workers treated AIDS patients and how they felt about the patients.

Shop-floor Culture before AIDS: Exploitation and Powerlessness

The pre-AIDS shop floor in academic medical centers is not a particularly happy place, as depicted in the first-hand accounts of medical education. . . . The set of everyday annoyances extends considerably beyond the long hours of work, although these alone are burdensome. Beyond that there is the fact that much of the work is without any profit for the house officer; it is "scut" work, essential drudgery whose completion appears to add little to the worker's overall sense of mastery and competence. (Becker et al. 1961 first commented that medical students, like their more senior trainees, disliked tasks that neither allowed them to exercise medical responsibility nor increased their clinical knowledge.) Consider here a resident's reaction to a day in the operating room, assisting on a major surgery:

> I urinated, wrote all the preoperative orders, changed my clothes, and had some dinner, in that order. As I walked across to the dining room, I felt as if I'd been run over by a herd of wild elephants in heat. I was exhausted and, much worse, deeply frustrated. I'd been assisting in surgery for nine hours. Eight of them had been the most important in Mrs. Takura's [a patient] life; yet I felt no sense of accomplishment. I had simply endured, and I was probably the one person they could have done without. Sure, they needed retraction, but a catatonic schizophrenic would have sufficed. Interns are eager to work hard, even if to sacrifice —above all, to be useful and to display their special talents—in order to learn. I felt none of these satisfactions, only an empty bitterness and exhaustion (Cook 1972, 74).

The complaint is not atypical.

In all accounts, house officers and students complain about the ways their energies are wasted because they are inundated with scut work of various types. If procedures are to be done on time, house officers have to act as a back-up transport service. If test results are to be interpreted and patients diagnosed, then house officers have to track down the results; they are their own messenger service.

In many hospitals house officers and students do the routine venipunctures and are responsible for maintaining the intravenous lines of patients requiring them. Routine bloodwork comprises a large amount of the physician-in-training's everyday scut work.

Their inability to control either their own or their patient's lives, their fundamental powerlessness, and the exploitation of their labors by the "greedy" institution (Coser 1979) that is the modern academic hospital are all at the center of physician's accounts of their training.

Clinical Coups and Defeats

The juxtaposition of labors that are both Herculean and pointless account for the major narrative themes in accounts of patient care. First, there are stories of "clinical coups." These are dramatic instances where the house officer's labors were not pointless, where a tricky diagnostic problem was solved and a timely and decisive intervention to save a life was initiated. Such stories are rare but all the house officer accounts, even the most bitter, tell at least one. These tales reinforce—even in the face of the contradictory details of the rest of the narrative—that the house officer's efforts make a difference, however small; that the pain and suffering of both doctors and patients are not invariably pointless; and that professional heroism may still yield a positive result, even if only rarely.

More numerous by far in the narratives are accounts of "clinical defeats." A few of these tales concern the apprentice physician's inability to come to the right decision quickly enough; these are personal defeats. The bulk of these tales, however, concern defeat (indexed by death) even though all the right things were done medically. Narratives of clinical defeats generally emphasize the tension in the conflict between care and cure, between quantity and quality of life, between acting as a medical scientist and acting as a human being.

The repeated accounts of clinical defeats reinforce at one level the general pointlessness of much of the house officers' effort. They recount situations in which house officers either are too overwhelmed to provide clinical care or in which the best available care does not insure a favorable outcome. But the stories of defeat tell another tale as well. Here, house officers describe how they learn that despite the failings of their technical interventions they can make a difference, that care is often more important than cure, and that the human rewards of their medical role are great. Each of the first-hand accounts of medical training features a tale of defeat that had a transformative effect on the physician in training. Each tale of defeat encodes a lesson about the psychological growth of the human being shrouded in the white coat of scientific authority. . . .

Psychological Detachment and Adolescent Invulnerability

The shop-floor culture of house officers and students is largely a peer culture. The senior authority of faculty appears absent, at best, or disruptive and intrusive, at worst, in the first-hand narratives of clinical training. That is to say, the clinical wisdom of faculty is unavailable when house officers need it; when clinical faculty are present, they "pimp" (humiliate by questioning) house officers during rounds with questions on obscure details or order them to perform mindless tasks easily performed by those (nurses, technicians) far less educated about the pathophysiology of disease. . . . "The patient is the one with the disease." The reverse, of course, is that the doctor does not have a problem. He or she is invulnerable. In the first-hand accounts of training, physicians' feelings of invulnerability appear and reappear. The doctors treat disease but they are rarely touched by it (save for the occasional exemplary patient with whom physicians make a psychological connection). To these young apprentice physicians, disease is rarely, if ever, personally threatening and rarely, if ever, presented as something that could happen to the physician. . . . Moreover, given that hospitals (outside of pediatrics and before AIDS) housed a high proportion of patients substantially older than house officers, patterns of mortality and morbidity themselves reinforced the sense of invulnerability. It is the rare patient close in age to the author who provokes distress and introspection about doctoring on the part of writers of first-hand narratives.

The fantasy of invulnerability takes on an adolescent quality when one notes the cavalier tone used to describe some of life's most awful problems and the oppositional stance taken toward patients and attending faculty. There may be something structural in this; just as adolescence is betwixt and between childhood and adulthood, the physician-in-training is likewise liminal, betwixt studenthood professional independence.

The Coming of AIDS to the Shop Floor: Risk and the Loss of Invulnerability

Before AIDS entered the shop floor, physicians in training had many objections to work-place conditions. Not only that, AIDS entered a shop floor that was in the process of transformation from major political, social, organizational, and economic policy changes regarding health care. These changes have been elaborated in detail elsewhere (Light 1980; Starr 1982; Relman 1980; Mechanic 1986) and need only brief mention here. Acute illnesses, especially infectious diseases, have given way to chronic disorders. The patient population has aged greatly. There has been a relatively new public emphasis on individual responsibility for one's medical problems—diet, smoking, nontherapeutic drug use, "excessive" alcohol use, exercise, etc. (Fox 1986).

Of great importance has been the redefinition of medical care as a service *like any other* in the economy with individual medical decisions subject to the kind of fiscal scrutiny applied to the purchase of automobiles or dry cleaning. Achieving reduced costs through shorter hospitalizations and other measures, however, has created more intensive scheduling for those caring for patients on the hospital's wards—even if the hospital's capacity shrinks in the name of efficiency. Fewer patients get admitted to the hospital and they stay for shorter periods of time, yet more things are done to and for them, increasing the house officers' clerical, physical, and in-

tellectual work while decreasing the opportunity for trainees to get to know their patients (Rabkin 1982; Steiner et al. 1987). The beds simply fill up with comparatively sicker, less communicative patients who need more intensive care.

All the shifts in the medical care system have changed the reality of hospital practice in ways that may not conform to the expectations of those entering the medical profession. In addition to the usual disillusionment occurring in training, the contemporary urban teaching hospital brings fewer opportunities for hope (Glick 1988). To the extent that AIDS contributes to the population of more desperately ill hospitalized patients, it exacerbates house officers' feelings of exploitation and, because of its fatal outcome, AIDS adds to their sense of powerlessness. We must assess the impact of AIDS against this background of old resentments and new burdens.

AIDS has certainly not improved the work climate of the medical shop floor. The most apparent phenomenon related to AIDS in the contemporary urban teaching hospital is risk or, more precisely, the *perception* of risk. The orthodox medical literature proclaims, over and over, that the AIDS virus does not pass readily from patient to care giver (Lifson et al. 1986; Gerberding et al. 1987). But some medical writing dwells on risks (Gerbert et al. 1988; Becker, Cone, and Gerberding 1989) and observations of behavior make clear that fear on the wards is rampant. Workers of all types, including doctors, have at times sheathed themselves in inappropriate armor or simply refused to approach the patients at all. Klass (1987, 185) put it quite starkly: "We have to face the fact that we are going through these little rituals of sanitary precaution partly because we are terrified of this disease and are not willing to listen to anything our own dear medical profession may tell us about how it actually is or is not transmitted."

Perceptions of risk can and do change with time and experience. Our interviewees and commentators in the literature indicate that as individuals and institutions have more patients with AIDS they begin to shed some of their protective garb. In one hospital we were told that the practice of donning gown, gloves, and masks became less frequent as doctors, nurses, housekeepers, and dietary workers "saw" that they did not get AIDS from their patients. This, of course, raises another interesting question: In what sense did personnel come to this conclusion? After all, the diseases associated with HIV infection typically have long latencies, up to several years, before symptoms develop. None of the institutions where our informants worked conducted routine surveillance to assess development of HIV antibody among personnel. Thus, staff could not really know if they had "gotten" HIV infection. Moreover, reports of individual physicians anxiously awaiting the results of HIV tests after needle sticks have now become a staple of the oral culture of academic medical centers.

On AIDS wards all personnel are far less likely to place barriers between themselves and patients for activities where blood or other body fluids might be transmitted. Beyond subspecialty units, however, medical, nursing, and support staff are far more fearful and employ many more nonrational techniques to prevent contamination. . . . One informant told us that HIV-infected hemophilia patients in one hospital often refuse hospitalization if it means getting a room on certain floors or nursing units. The patients prefer to delay needed treatment until a bed becomes available on a unit where they feel more humanely treated.

Several other curious phenomena have emerged regarding risks and AIDS in the medical work place. While in some locations lack of experience has led to classic reactions of fear and avoidance, in other places the paucity of experience permits denial to dominate. The comments of house staff in a hospital with only an occasional AIDS patient indicates that few residents followed Centers for Disease Control or similar guidelines for "universal precautions." Various explanations were offered, including the conviction that starting intravenous infusions, blood drawing, or similar procedures is more difficult when wearing gloves. When asked how surgeons accomplish complex manual tasks while wearing one or two pairs of gloves, residents usually replied that they had not learned to do things "that way." Here, one

kind of inexperience (with gloves) reinforces another (with AIDS), bolstering the feeling of invulnerability that was widespread before AIDS.

Some medical students and physicians have dealt with the problem of risk globally. They want to avoid encountering patients with AIDS altogether. In one medical school where we teach, there is a policy prohibiting students from refusing to care for HIV-infected patients. The policy infuriates many students, a fact we learned in medical-ethics discussion groups which met to discuss an AIDS case. They cited several reasons. The rules, some felt, were changed midstream. Had they known about the policy, they might have chosen another school. They felt they had no role in the formation of the policy and that the tremendous economic investment they made in the institution, in the form of tuition, entitles them to some decision-making authority. They objected to the rule's existence. They said such rules have no place in medicine. Doctors, they believe, should have as much freedom as lawyers, accountants, executives, or others to accept or reject "clients" or "customers." When presented with the notion of a professional obligation or duty, based upon generally acknowledged moral precepts, they balked. At other institutions we know there has been more controversy among medical students, with some making impassioned statements about the physician's obligation to treat. In this debate we see AIDS as a total social phenomenon acting as a vehicle for debating and defining standards of professional conduct.

Another aspect of medical risk avoidance may be revealed through the changing patterns of residency selection. For some time there has been a shift away from primary care specialties like internal medicine, family practice, and pediatrics, toward specialties such as orthopedics, ophthalmology, otolaryngology, and radiology (McCarty 1987). The reasons for this phenomena are not entirely clear, but include the technical, rather than personal, orientation of the medical training system and the higher compensation available in the latter group of specialties, sought, in part, because of staggering educational debts. In the past few years, the trend may have accelerated, with internal medicine (whose house staff and practitioners provide the bulk of the care for AIDS patients) training programs failing to find sufficient qualified applicants (Graettinger 1989; Davidoff 1989). This crisis has been most marked in the cities with large numbers of HIV-infected patients. A similar trend toward avoiding residencies in AIDS endemic areas may be emerging in pediatrics, according to faculty rumors; a substantial proportion of pediatric house officers, like those in internal medicine, would not care for AIDS patients if given the choice, according to one survey (Link et al. 1988). . . .

Surgical Risk and Historical Precedent

Even more remarkable in the AIDS-risk reaction has been the appearance in prestigious medical journals of complaints, whines, and pleas for understanding from doctors worried about contamination and ruination (Guy 1987; Ponsford 1987; Dudley and Sim 1988; Carey 1988; Guido 1988). These pieces offer various estimates of risk to person, career, family, future patients deprived of the skills of the author or his or her esteemed colleagues, and other justifications for not treating HIV-infected persons. . . . It is important to note that the medical literature on AIDS is not entirely negative; complaints can be matched against calls to duty (Gillon 1987; Zuger and Miles 1987; Pellegrino 1987; Kim and Perfect 1988; Friedland 1988; Emanuel 1988; Sharp 1988; Peterson 1989). On the shop floor and in the literature, AIDS as a total social phenomenon has become the lens for focusing on the obligations of members of the medical profession.

Surgeons have been particularly outspoken about the extent to which they are threatened, and there *is* reason for their special concerns (Hagen, Meyer, and Pauker 1988; Peterson 1989). After all, these doctors have a high likelihood of contact with the blood of patients. This involves not just working in blood-perfused tissues, but also a risk of having gloves and skin punctured by the instruments of their craft or having blood splash onto other vulnerable areas of the body (mucous membranes in professional parlance). Surgeons, by the very nature of their work, do more of this than many other doctors. But other physicians do find themselves in similar circumstances, depending on their activities. Intensive care specialists, invasive cardiologists, emergency physicians, pulmonary and gastrointestinal specialists, and others have frequent and/or sustained contact with the blood or other body fluids of patients who may be infected with HIV. House staff, as the foot soldiers doing comprehensive examinations, drawers of blood specimens, inserters of intravenous catheters or other tubes in other places, cleaners of wounds, or simply as those first on the scene of bloody disasters, are particularly likely to be splashed, splattered, or otherwise coated with patients blood, secretions, or excretions.

We do not have data on the extent to which fears have or have not been translated into changes in behavior in operating and/or procedure rooms. In some communities there may now be fewer operations and these procedures may take longer as extra time is taken to reduce bleeding and avoid punctures. This may not turn out to be as good as it might at first seem. To the extent that high-risk patients have operations delayed or denied or must undergo longer anesthetics and have wounds open longer, patient care may be compromised.

It is interesting to compare the current outcry with what happened when medical science discovered the nature of hepatitis and recognized the medical risks to personnel of serum hepatitis, now known as hepatitis B. As long ago as 1949 (Liebowitz et al. 1949), the medical literature acknowledged that medical personnel coming in contact with blood stood at risk from hepatitis. A debate continued through the 1950s, 1960s, and early 1970s about whether surgeons were especially vulnerable because of their use of sharp instruments, the frequency of accidental puncture of the skin during surgical procedures, and the likelihood of inoculation of the virus into the bloodstream of the wounded party. The risks were felt to be clearly documented in an article (Rosenberg et al. 1973) in the *Journal of the American Medical Association* that commented: "This study demonstrates the distinct occupational hazard to surgeons when they operate on patients who are capable of transmitting hepatitis virus. . . . We believe that serious attempts should be made to prevent future epidemics. . . . Education and constant vigilance in surgical technique are central to any preventive program." Nowhere does the article suggest surgeons should consider not operating on patients at risk for hepatitis.

Of course, hepatitis B is not associated with a fatal prognosis in a large proportion of cases and is not entirely comparable to AIDS. Nonetheless, the epidemiologic evidence gathered in the 1970s suggested that hepatitis B was very prevalent among physicians, especially surgeons (Denes et al. 1978), and that medical personnel seemed especially vulnerable to having severe courses of the disease (Garibaldi et al. 1973). A portion become chronic carriers of the virus, with the added risk later of liver cancer and liver failure from cirrhosis. Moreover, secondary spread from infected medical workers can occur to patients (through small cuts and sores on the workers' skin) and sexual partners (through exchange of bodily fluids). Despite all this, major medical journals did not carry discussions of whether doctors at risk might be excused from professional activities. It may be that our society's general risk aversiveness (Fairlie 1989) and tolerance of self-centeredness have escalated sufficiently to make public renunciation of professional responsibility more acceptable. More likely, the general medical professional ethic has changed to one closer to that of the entrepreneur, as was true for our students. But perhaps something else is going on that, being synergistic with the perceived loss of invulnerability brought on by AIDS, makes the AIDS era distinctive.

AIDS as a Total Social Phenomenon

The reaction to AIDS on the shop floor must be examined in light of the perceptions of risk, the epidemiology of AIDS, and moral judgments some make about activities that lead to acquiring the disease. Most AIDS patients have come from identifiable populations: the gay community, intravenous drug

users and their partners, and those who have gotten the disease from medical use of blood and blood products. While hepatitis B infections were prevalent in these populations and also entailed risks to medical personnel, hepatitis in such patients did not cause doctors to deny their professional responsibility to provide treatment. We are arguing that the unique combination of factors associated with AIDS prompts the negative reactions among doctors: changing tolerances of risk, the shift to an occupation bounded by entrepreneurial rules rather than professional duties, a specific fear of the terrible outcome should one acquire AIDS from a patient, objections to some of the specific behaviors which lead to AIDS, and class and racial bias. Below, we discuss some of the social characteristics of AIDS patients which affect the negativity of the professionals.

The demographics of AIDS is striking and flies rudely in the face of the last several decades of medical progress. Most AIDS patients are young adults. This is true of gays, drug users, and even the hemophiliacs, by and large. Most house officers, however naive and unprepared they are too confront devastating illness and death, at least have a general cultural and social expectation of, if not experience with, the death of old people. With AIDS, many of the sickest patients filling teaching hospital wards in high-prevalence cities are in their prime years, similar in age to the house staff providing the frontline care (Glick 1988). People so young are not supposed to die. These deaths challenge the ideology of the coming-if-not-quite-arrived triumph of modern medical science implicitly provided young doctors in medical education. (Two former house officers have written about the effects of AIDS on medical training: Wachter 1986; Zuger 1987.)

We do not want to paint with too broad a brush here. There are some important differences among the groups of AIDS patients, which influence the reactions of resident physicians. Our informants describe three nonexhaustive groups of patients to whom young doctors and students react: hemophiliacs and others who acquired AIDS through transfusion, young gay men, and drug users and their partners. (We have insufficient information to comment on the reaction to the rapidly growing infant AIDS population.)

In many ways, the patients who develop AIDS from blood products constitute a simple set. These patients are clearly seen as innocents, true victims of unfortunate but in inevitable delay between recognition of a technical problem—blood-borne transmission of a serious disease—and its reliable and practical prevention—cleaning up of the blood supply. A chief resident commented that her house officers talk differently about patients with AIDS caused by transfusions from the way they speak about other AIDS patients. "The residents see these cases [with blood-product-related disease] as more tragic; their hearts go out to them more." Hemophiliacs have an air of double tragedy about them: an often crippling, always inconvenient genetic disorder made worse as a direct consequence of their medical treatment.

Hemophiliac patients with AIDS in one of the hospitals where we made inquiries went out of their way to make the origins of their disease or other emblems of their identity known. These patients "display" wives and children to differentiate themselves from homosexual patients. One hemophiliac, reflecting on his desire to have others know that his HIV-positive status preceded his drug abuse, commented that this public knowledge was important because there is "always a pecking order" in who gets scarce nursing care. Even though few people hold these patients in any way responsible for their disease, behavior on the wards toward HIV-positive hemophiliacs clearly differs from attention given non-AIDS or non-HIV-infected patients. As mentioned earlier, their hospital rooms are not as clean as the rooms of hemophiliac patients not infected with HIV; the staff does not touch them as often as they once did. (Many of these patients were frequently hospitalized before the HIV epidemic; in effect, they have served as their own controls in a cruel experiment of nature.) Their care is compromised in small but painful ways.

Gay patients with AIDS occupy an intermediate position in the hierarchy. The social characteristics of many of these patients, in the eyes of our informants, were positive ones: the patients were well educated, well groomed, took an active interest in their treatments, had supportive family and/or networks that relieved some of the burdens from their care providers, and the like. Of course, not all medical personnel appreciate all of these features. Interest in care has emerged into social activism about treatment, which some physicians resent. For example, one patient who had developed severe difficulty swallowing, and was starving as a consequence, requested insertion of a feeding tube through his abdominal wall into his intestinal tract. His primary physicians tried to put him off, apparently believing he would succumb soon, no matter what was done. When he persisted, a surgical consultant was called. The surgeon initially treated the request as a joke, finally agreed after an attempt to dissuade the patient ("So, you really want to do this?"), and then provided no follow-up care. This is but one case, but our general impression is that the "turfing" (transferring) that Shem (1978) described as a major feature of shop-floor culture before AIDS has intensified. Physicians want to shift the burdens and responsibilities of care to others.

From the resident's point of view, there may also be a down side to the extensive support systems many gay patients enjoy. In the final stages of AIDS, little more can be done for patients beyond providing comfort. For the interested and compassionate resident, titration of pain medication and less technical interaction, i.e., talking with the patient, can be therapeutic for both. If the patient has become invested in alternative treatments for discomfort, from herbal medicine to meditation to imaging, and if the patient is surrounded by loving family and community, the house officer may feel she or he has nothing whatsoever to contribute. The helplessness amplifies the despair and the pointlessness of whatever scut work must be done. Here, there can be no transforming, heroic intervention, no redemption arising from clinical defeat.

The IV-drug-using HIV-infected patients represent the fastest growing and most problematic set of patients. Teaching hospitals have always had more than their share of patients who are "guilty" victims of disease, i.e., patients whose medical problems are seen as direct consequences of their behavior. Many of our prestigious teaching hospitals have been municipal or county facilities filled with substance-abusing patients with a wide spectrum of problems from which house staff have learned. Our informants suggested that the coming of AIDS to this population had subtly altered the way these patients are regarded. Now, drug users cannot be regarded with mere contempt or simple disrespect: there is fear among doctors who are afraid of acquiring AIDS from the patients. Whereas frustration and anger in some cases (especially when drug users were manipulative or physically threatening) and indifference in others used to constitute much of the response to drug-using patients, fear of AIDS has added a difficult dimension.

One might argue that before HIV, this underclass population had a set of positive social roles to play. Their very presence reminded doctors and nurses, perhaps even other patients, that things might not be as bad as they seemed. The intern might be miserable after staying up an entire weekend, but she/he could look to a better life ahead and know that she/he did not have to face homelessness and desperate poverty when finally leaving the hospital to rest. Moreover, the underclass patients provided chances to learn and practice that private patients could not offer. . . . But AIDS seems to have changed the balance for many who might have tolerated or welcomed the opportunities to care for the undeserved. For a medical student contemplating a residency, what was previously a chance to gain relative autonomy quickly in an institution with many substance-abusing patients may have become predominantly unwelcome exposure to a dreadful illness. If this is so, AIDS will trigger, in yet another way, a dreadful decline in the availability and quality of care for America's medical underclass.

Conclusion

The full impact of AIDS on the modern system of medical care will not be clear for many years. Nevertheless, the disease has already affected the culture of American medicine in a pivotal place: the urban teaching center. Al-

ready a scene beset with anger, pain, sadness, and high technology employed soullessly against disease, AIDS has added to the troubles. We cannot know for certain whether this new plague has contributed to the decline in interest in medicine as a career or to the flight from primary care. There is certainly no evidence that AIDS has prompted many to seek out a life of selfless dedication to tending the hopelessly ill.

For those who have chosen to train in hospitals with large numbers of AIDS patients, the disease has added to the burdens of the shop floor. The perception of risk of acquiring AIDS has undermined one of the best-established defenses house officers have relied on: the maintenance of an air of invulnerability. Some doctors are so scared they are abandoning their traditional duty and no longer seem able or willing to try to bring off the heroic coup against daunting clinical odds. To be sure, this fear is fed by other factors on the social scene: the economic changes in medicine, transforming the profession into the province of the entrepreneur; the youth and other characteristics of many AIDS patients; and the willingness of the entire society to turn away from the underclass, especially from those who are seen as self-destructive.

Nothing here suggests that AIDS will spark a turn to a kinder, gentler medical care system. Those in the educational system inclined to seek models providing compassionate medical care will likely find few attractive mentors. Instead, they will meet burned-out martyrs, steely-eyed technicians, and teachers filled with fear. Tomorrow's first-hand accounts of medical education and fictionalized autobiographies may, as a result, be even grimmer than yesterday's.

There is the possibility that this conclusion is too stark, too depressing. For those desperate for a more hopeful scenario, at least one other alternative suggests itself. As the numbers of medical students dwindle, perhaps those that enter will be more committed to ideals of professional service and, among those, some will enter with a missionary zeal for caring for AIDS patients. There is little to suggest this other than the portraits of the few heroic physicians one finds in Shilts's

(1987) account of the early years of the AIDS epidemic. If these physicians inspire a new generation of medical professionals, then the tone of future first-hand accounts will be more in line with the highest ideals of the medical profession.

References

Becker, H. 1967. Whose Side Are We On? *Social Problems* 14:239-47.

Becker, C.E., J.E. Cone and J. Gerberding. 1989. Occupational Infection with Human Immunodeficiency Virus (HIV): Risks and Risk Reduction. *Annals of Internal Medicine* 110:653-56.

Becker, H., B. Geer, E.C. Hughes, and A. Strauss. 1961. *Boys in White: Student Culture in Medical School.* Chicago: University of Chicago Press.

Carey, J.S. 1988. Routine Preoperative Screening for HIV (Letter to the Editor). *Journal of the American Medical Association* 260:179.

Cook, R. 1972. *The Year of the Intern.* New York: Harcourt Brace Jovanovich.

Coser, R.L. 1979. *Training in Ambiguity: Learning through Doing in a Mental Hospital.* New York: Free Press.

Davidoff, F. 1989. Medical Residencies: Quantity or Quality? *Annals of Internal Medicine* 110:757-58.

Denes, A.E., J.L. Smith, J.E. Maynard, I.L. Doto, K.R. Berquist, and A.J. Finkel. 1978. Hepatitis B Infection in Physicians: Results of a Nationwide Seroepidemiologic Survey. *Journal of the American Medical Association* 239:210-12.

Dudley, H.A.F., and A. Sim. 1988. AIDS: A Bill of Rights for the Surgical Team? *British Medical Journal* 296:1449-50.

Emanuel, E.J. 1988. Do Physicians Have an Obligation to Treat Patients with AIDS? *New England Journal of Medicine* 318:1686-90.

Fairlie, H. 1989. Fear of Living: America's Morbid Aversion to Risk. *New Republic* January 23:14-19.

Fox, D. 1986. AIDS and the American Health Polity: The History and Prospects of a Crisis of Authority. *Milbank Quarterly* 64 (suppl.) 1:7-33.

Friedland, G. 1988. AIDS and Compassion. *Journal of the American Medical Association* 259:2898-99.

Garibaldi, R.A., J.N. Forrest, J.A. Bryan, B.F. Hanson, and W.E. Dismukes. 1973. Hemodialysis-Associated Hepatitis. *Journal of the American Medical Association* 225:384-89.

Gerberding, J.L., C.E. Bryant-Le Blanc, K. Nelson, A.R. Moss, D. Osmond, H.F. Chambers, J.R. Carlson, W.L. Drew, J.A. Levy, and M.A. Sande. 1987. Risk of Transmitting the Human Immunodeficiency Virus Cytomegalovirus, and Hepatitis B Virus to Health Care Workers Exposed to Patients with AIDS and Aids-related Conditions. *Journal of Infectious Diseases* 156:1-8.

Gerbert, B., B. Maguire, V. Badner, D. Altman, and G. Stone. 1988. Why Fear Persists: Health Care Professionals and AIDS. *Journal of the American Medical Association* 260:3481-83.

Gillon, R. 1987. Refusal to Treat AIDS and HIV Positive Patients. *British Medical Journal* 294:1332-33.

Glick, S.M. 1988. The Impending Crisis in Internal Medicine Training Programs. *American Journal of Medicine* 84:929-32.

Graettinger, J.S. 1989. Internal Medicine in the National Resident Patching Program 1978-1989. *Annals of Internal Medicine* 110:682.

Guido, L.J. 1988. Routine Preoperative Screening for HIV (Letter to the Editor). *Journal of the American Medical Association* 260: 180.

Guy, P.J. 1987. AIDS: A Doctor's Duty. *British Medical Journal* 294-445.

Hagen, M.D., K.B. Meyer, and S.G. Pauker. 1988. Routine Preoperative Screening for HIV: Does the Risk to Surgeon Outweigh the Risk to the Patient? *Journal of the American Medical Association* 259:1357-59.

Hughes. E.C. 1971. *The Sociological Eye: Selected Papers on Work, Self, and Society.* Chicago: Aldine-Atherton.

Kim, J.H., and J.R. Perfect. 1988. To Help the Sick: An Historical and Ethical Essay Concerning the Refusal to Care for Patients with AIDS. *American Journal of Medicine* 84:135-38.

Klass, P. 1987. *A Not Entirely Benign Procedure: Four Years as a Medical Student.* New York: Putnam.

Liebowitz S., L. Greenwald, I. Cohen, and J. Litwins. 1949. Serum Hepatitis in a Blood Bank Worker. *American Medical Association* 140(17):1331-33.

Lifson, A.R.. K.G. Castro, E. McCray, and H.W. Jaffe. 1986. National Surveillance of AIDS in Health Care Workers. *Journal of the American Medical Association* 265:3231-34.

Light D. 1980. *Becoming Psychiatrists: The Professional Transformation of Self.* New York: W. W. Notton.

Link, R.N., A.R. Feingold, M.H. Charap. K. Freeman, and S.P., Shelov. 1988. Concerns of Medical and Pediatric House Officers about Acquiring AIDS from Their Patients. *American Journal of Public Health* 78:455-59.

McCarty, D. J. 1987. Why Are Today's Medical Students Choosing High-technology Specialties over Internal Medicine? *New England Journal of Medicine* 317:567-69.

Mechanic, D. 1986. *From Advocacy to Allocation: The Evolving American Health Care System.* New York: Free Press.

Pellegrino, E.D. 1987. Altruism, Self-interest, and Medical Ethics. *Journal of the American Medical Association* 258:1939-40.

Peterson, L.M. 1989. AIDS: The Ethical Dilemma for Surgeons. *Law, Medicine, and Health Care* 17(Summer): 139-44.

Ponsford, G. 1987. AIDS in the OR: A Surgeon's View. *Canadian Medical Association Journal* 137:1036-39.

Rabkin, M. 1982. The SAG Index. *New England Journal of Medicine* 307:1350-51.

Relman, A.S. 1980. The New Medical-Industrial Complex. *New England Journal of Medicine* 303:963-70.

Rosenberg, J.L., D.P. Jones, L.R. Lipitz, and J.B. Kirsner. 1973. Viral Hepatitis: An Occupational Hazard to Surgeons. *Journal of the American Medical Association* 223:395-400.

Sharp, S.C. 1988. The Physician's Obligation to Treat AIDS Patients. *Southern Medical Journal* 81:1282-85.

Shem, S. 1978. *The House of God.* New York: Richard Marek.

Shilts, R. *And the Band Played On.* New York: St. Martins.

Starr, P. 1982. *The Social Transformation of American Medicine.* New York: Basic Books.

Steiner, J.F., L.E. Feinberg, A.M. Kramer, and R.L. Byyny. 1987. Changing Patterns of Disease on an Inpatient Medical Service: 1961-62 to 1981-82. *American Journal of Medicine* 83:331-35.

Wachter, R.M. 1986. The Impact of the Acquired Immunodeficiency Syndrome on Medical Residency Training. *New England Journal of Medicine* 314:177-80.

Zuger, A. 1987. AIDS on the Wards: A Residency in Medical Ethics. *Hastings Center Report* 17(3):16-20.

Zuger, A., and S.H. Miles. 1987. Physicians, AIDS, and Occupational Risk: Historical Traditions and Ethical Obligations. *Journal of the American Medical Association* 258:1924-28.

Further Reading

Charles Bosk. 1979. *Forgive and Remember: Managing Medical Failure.* Chicago: University of Chicago Press.

Ezekiel Emmanuel. 1988. "Do Physicians Have an Obligation to Treat Patients with AIDS?" *New England Journal of Medicine* 318: 1686-90.

H. Fairlie. 1989. "Fear of Living: America's Morbid Aversion to Risk" *New Republic* January 23: 14-19.

Abigail Zuger. 1987. "AIDS on the Wards: A Residency in Medical Ethics" *Hastings Center Report* 17(3): 16-20.

Discussion Questions

1. How might perception of risk affect a practitioner's willingness to care for HIV and AIDS patients?

2. Where does uncertainty in working with AIDS patients come from? Cite specific examples from the selection that point to health professionals' uncertainty in working with AIDS patients.

3. Explain how perception of risk and uncertainty might characterize the nature of medical care for illnesses other than AIDS.

From *The Milbank Quarterly*, Vol. 68:2. Pp. 257-277. Copyright © 1990 by Blackwell Publishers. Reprinted by permission. ✦

48

AIDS Prevention Outreach Among Injection Drug Users: Agency Problems and New Approaches

Robert S. Broadhead
Douglas D. Heckathorn

Previous readings in this section define AIDS as a personal and public health issue. AIDS is also a social policy issue. Policy analysts show that combatting HIV and AIDS requires organized community decision making and action. Within the past few years, community outreach programs have constituted part of the plan to fight transmission of AIDS. These programs generally target specific segments of the population at risk for HIV and AIDS. Among these programs are interventions for intravenous drug users (IDUs). Robert Broadhead and Douglas Heckathorn report on one type of intervention and outreach program for IDUs.

The authors of this selection discover that micro-political contexts of peer networks provide successful avenues for community intervention. As you read this discussion, consider the organizational goals of community outreach programs more generally. Think through some of the goals that may be specific to IDU outreach programs. As with any organizations, problems arise when outreach workers are not invested in the dissemination of information to their peers. Consider some of the issues that arise for IDU outreach workers. In spite of many problems, Broadhead and Heckathorn show us that peer networks are relevant parts of the healing process. Both healthy and ill individuals rely on other individuals for support. And as we have seen in previous readings, friends and family can assist in self definition or in fulfilling daily tasks and obligations severely hindered by the illness. Likewise, organized community peer groups offer social support and, with some motivation, can serve as reliable vehicles for AIDS prevention and public health promotion.

Introduction

In June 1981, the first cases of gay men suffering from acquired immune deficiency syndrome (AIDS) were identified, a disease caused by human immunodeficiency virus (HIV) (Shilts 1987). The existence of HIV and its routes of transmission were established in 1983, but the official response to help high-risk groups, such as gays and injection drug users, protect themselves remained stalled for a number of years (National Commission on AIDS 1991). This response by political and public health officials during the early 1980s has been severely criticized by those who feel the opportunity was lost to limit the epidemic (Kuller and Kingsley 1986; Altman 1987; Perrow and Guillen 1990). Yet it is also clear that the AIDS epidemic presented, and continues to present, a challenge of unprecedented proportions. Understanding the obstacles to effective control of the AIDS epidemic has consequences not only for understanding the early history of the AIDS epidemic; it also reveals the constraints under which contemporary efforts to control AIDS must operate.

In this selection, we focus on the control of AIDS among injection drug users (IDUs). We base our analysis on theories of collective action (Olson 1965; Coleman 1990) and agency theory (Jensen and Meckling 1976). Drawing on recent theoretic developments in the understanding of collective action (Heckathorn 1990, 1993), and on original field research, we conclude that the organizational barriers to controlling AIDS among IDUs are significant but not insurmountable. We argue that more effective control of AIDS among IDUs may require a new approach that builds on the success of, but goes substantially beyond, the traditional outreach prevention efforts that have been used nationwide. We describe new forms of AIDS prevention that build on the experience of outreach interventions by relying on an active collaboration between IDUs and service providers. . . .

Controlling AIDS as a Collective Action Problem

. . . AIDS prevention is a collective action problem because it results from a conflict between individuals' behavior (in this case, sexual and drug use activities that individuals find rewarding), and the frequently unarticulated and unacknowledged common interests of the communities they belong to (in this case, collective enforcement of prevention norms requiring changes in individuals' risk practices). AIDS prevention constitutes a public good because the suffering resulting from HIV infection spills over from all affected individuals to their family members and friends. It also spills over to the community at large, because of the financial costs of treating HIV infections and diseases.

At the beginning of the AIDS epidemic, the large size of high-risk groups, and their lack of organization around public health issues, virtually guaranteed that levels of collective action to combat AIDS would be extremely low. In addition, the rewards of unsafe sex and drug use were powerful and immediate counter inducements; the efficacy of safer practices in preventing HIV infection was uncertain; and the risk from any single act appeared to be small and long delayed—all of which made changing individual behavior more difficult (Lawlor 1990). High-risk groups, therefore, tended to remain latent. Collective action could be expected to arise first in the more organized high-risk groups, such as gays. It might never arise in far less organized groups, such as IDUs.

Thus, at the beginning of the epidemic, high-risk groups were ill equipped to act quickly. In contrast, many low-risk politically or religiously-based groups were already organized around moral agenda related to sexuality and drug use. Such groups, drawn from both white and minority communities, were well situated to redeploy their organizational resources to hinder public health initiatives to combat AIDS (Quimby and Friedman 1989).

In sum, obstacles to containing the AIDS epidemic included the difficulty of mobilizing latent high-risk groups, and overcoming the high level of mobilization exerted by low-risk groups whose moral/political agenda conflicted with effective AIDS prevention measures. These conflicts continue to afflict AIDS prevention efforts. As the epidemic has matured, some high-risk groups have significantly increased their levels of organization. However other groups, in particular IDUs, remain nearly totally atomized in the United States. In addition, the influence of highly organized groups with moralistic agenda remains substantial.

These obstacles could be overcome in large measure if means were found to catalyze or facilitate the process by which high-risk groups mobilize for collective action. Such means would speed the process by which latent groups, such as IDUs, were able to identify common interests and create and enforce AIDS prevention norms consistent with them. . . .

Community-Based AIDS Outreach

By 1986, HIV seroprevalence rates among IDUs in New York City and northern New Jersey had climbed to 60 percent, compared to 12 percent in San Francisco (Haverkos 1988). Faced with a rapidly spreading AIDS epidemic, the federal government began seeking ways to reduce high-risk behavior among IDUs beyond the punitive measures that had long been part of the War on Drugs (Wisotsky 1991; Government Accounting Office [GAO] 1992). The new policy addressed the transmission of HIV among IDUs as a *research problem* and assigned it to the authority of the National Institute on Drug Abuse (NIDA 1991a). In 1987, NIDA (1987:1) funded six research demonstration projects intended to study "[t]he use of indigenous outreach workers [OWs] to identify, reach and communicate with I.V. drug abusers and associates in their natural communities" about the risks of HIV, and what steps IDUs could take to protect themselves. OWs were given three fundamental tasks: to recruit IDUs for HIV testing and counseling; to educate them on their own turf regarding AIDS risks; and to distribute prevention materials to IDUs, such as condoms and small bottles of bleach for cleaning needles. NIDA increased the program in 1988 by funding 41 outreach research projects in more than 60 targeted inner-cities with large numbers of IDUs, all part of the National AIDS Demonstration Research (NADR) Project (NIDA 1991a; Brown and Beschner 1993).

Research on the impact of outreach projects confirms the view of IDUs as a latent group, that is, a group with awareness of a common interest but a limited capacity for its individual members to act collectively based upon that interest. Even so, the finding that IDUs are capable of recognizing and, within limited domains, acting upon their interests was something of a revelation. Before the NADR program, it was often believed that IDUs did not care about their health and were unable to regulate their own and others' behavior (Friedman et al. 1987). This claim resulted from the *position* researchers, clinicians, and public health officials traditionally took toward IDUs. It rested on the following assumptions: if people shoot drugs, they do not care about their health; and, if people continue to shoot drugs, they will not change (Rivera-Beckman 1992a). With the advent of outreach projects working directly with IDUs on their own turf, it became apparent that these assumptions had blocked a recognition of both the very real concerns IDUs have about their health, and the changes IDUs are willing to make to protect it, short of "just saying no" to drugs or sex. This has included actions wholly independent of externally organized AIDS prevention programs. For example, Des Jarlais et al. (1985) found in 1983 that, even before outreach projects were initiated, some IDUs in New York City began reacting on their own to reports about the risk of AIDS by reducing needle sharing and increasing the demand for clean syringes. By 1984, IDUs' demand for clean needles was so great that it spawned a new market ripe for exploitation: dealers began repackaging used

needles and selling them as new (Des Jarlais, Friedman, and Hopkins 1985; Friedman et al. 1987).

Given IDUs' responses to the arrival of AIDS, it is not surprising that their reaction to outreach programs was positive. Many IDUs began to disinfect their needles with bleach, and to reduce needle sharing. IDUs also increased their use of condoms, though less successfully. For example, in San Francisco during the winter/spring of 1986, *before* outreach distribution of bleach and condoms began, only 3 percent of the city's estimated 15,000 IDUs reported that they regularly disinfected their syringes. OWs began distributing bleach in the streets in July 1986. One year later,

> 55.4% interviewed reported using bleach . . . [and analysis of] needle-sharing partners in the past year showed significant shrinkage in the reported size of needle-sharing circles and increased numbers of persons who reported not sharing needles (Watters et al. 1990a:592-93).

Similarly, in 1986, 9.8 percent of IDUs reported not sharing needles, which increased to 21 percent one year later. During that same year, only 4.3 percent of the respondents reported using condoms at least half the time they had sex. By 1987, 32.7 percent reported using condoms in general and "18.6 percent reported using them at least half of the time" (Watters et al. 1990a:593). Watters et al. (1990b:3-4) report that from the baseline measures taken in the winter/spring of 1986, "there was a near doubling of HIV seroprevalence [to] early 1987, from 7% to 13%. After this point the curve is relatively flat" through late 1989. Watters et al. (1990b:4) emphasize that "major behavior change occurred immediately following the implementation of outreach and bleach distribution."

Risk reductions by IDUs in response to outreach efforts in other cities were similarly' significant, as NADR researchers reported in New York City, Miami, Chicago, Denver, Baltimore, Cleveland, Hartford, and other sites (NIDA 1991b; Brown and Beschner 1993; Booth and Wiebel 1992; Chitwood et al. 1991; Neaigus et al. 1990; Stephens, Feucht, and Roman 1991; Weeks et al. 1990; Wiebel and

Lampinen 1991). Such changes occurred so rapidly following the implementation of outreach projects that secular trends, such as growing awareness of how HIV is transmitted, do not appear to be able to account for them. . . .

However, in examining the organizational dynamics of outreach projects nationwide, it has become clear that IDUs responded impressively to very unimpressive and uneven outreach efforts that drifted toward inertia, and that suffered from high levels of mal-and non-performance of OWs. These findings, reported below, suggest that a new approach to AIDS prevention among IDUs may be feasible, one that relies on a more active and direct collaboration between IDUs and service providers.

Agency Problems in Outreach Projects

Ethnographic research has accumulated on the inner workings of outreach projects, including how OWs have performed in the community in reaching IDUs (NIDA 1991a; Longshore 1992). Our analysis draws on this literature. Our analysis is also based on an ethnographic study of the San Francisco outreach project conducted by the first author. The ethnography consists of a year and a half of participant observation, beginning in June 1988, during which time the first author and two full-time associate ethnographers were trained as OWs and deployed as members of various outreach teams in targeted areas of San Francisco. It also includes interviews with 24 of the 33 OWs employed by the San Francisco project between July 1988 and January 1990.[2] All quotes that lack citation come from these interviews. In addition, in October 1989, the first author and an associate spent two weeks on the streets with the NADR outreach project in New York City at two different sites, Brooklyn and Queens. The observations of San Francisco and New York, and the literature on outreach in other cities, reveal a high degree of commonality in the manner in which outreach projects functioned across the country.

If collective action always succeeded, individuals at risk of contracting HIV would act collectively to neutralize that threat. However, in reality, collective action frequently fails, hence the need for AIDS prevention projects. Agency theory (Jensen and Meckling 1976; Eisenhardt 1985; White 1985) provides a useful conceptual framework for understanding the inner workings and problems of these projects. The theory focuses on *informational asymmetries* between individuals who contract for a service (principals), and those who enlist or are hired to provide that service (agents). For example, in the relationship between patients (principals) and physicians (agents), the latter's vastly greater access to specialized medical knowledge creates opportunities to control the patient through evasion, dissimulation, mystification and many other deceptive practices (Waitzkin 1991). Similarly, in the relationship between clients (principals) and lawyers (agents), the latter's use of specialized legal knowledge can mislead clients to act against their own interests (Bok 1978). More generally, any bureaucracy can be seen as a chain of principal-agent relationships that link principals ("superordinates") to agents ("subordinates") charged with fulfilling their delegated responsibilities. However subordinates' differential control over information frequently enhances their power and provides the opportunity to manipulate their superordinates.

Outreach projects could be analyzed at any of several levels, including that of NIDA officials as principals and research investigators as agents; or research investigators as principals and outreach supervisors as agents; and supervisors as principals and outreach workers as agents. In this selection, we limit our analysis to the latter relationship, because it is the closest to the street-level at which outreach interactions occur with IDUs, and because analyzing higher-level agency problems would exceed the scope of this selection. However, it is important to note that the problems identified in the performance of OWs may derive from agency problems higher in the organization (e.g., see Broadhead and Margolis 1993).

Outreach and the Problem of Adverse Selection

According to agency theory, two fundamental types of problems inevitably arise when the agent's interests fail to coincide with those of the principal. The first problem occurs *ex ante*, before the agent's services are retained. It is termed *adverse selection*, because the agents with the strongest incentives to offer their services to the principal tend to be those who are least qualified or motivated. For example, when advertising for a job, the applicants who respond do not come from a random sample of all people who are qualified for the job, because most such people are satisfied with their current unemployment. Instead, most responses come from people who are unemployed or are in the process of losing their current jobs. This group contains a larger proportion of workers with problems in competence or reliability than does the working population at large. Identifying the true suitability of candidates for a job is especially difficult, because applicants who are least qualified have the greatest incentive to withhold information that reveals their deficiencies.

. . . The ethnographic field research revealed problems of adverse selection. The most frequent and simplest problem occurred during employment interviews when applicants expressed a heartfelt desire to help drug addicts protect their health. After being hired, it became apparent, sometimes slowly, sometimes immediately, that their heart was never in the job. Thus, for example, "going into the field" came to include visiting the mall and shopping, goofing off with clients, chasing around, hanging out in bars, drinking beer, playing pool, and getting high. As one outreach supervisor noted, "All the problems that we deal with on the street, we have in our very own agency." . . .

As one OW observed while working a neighborhood in San Francisco: "This job would be the perfect cover if you wanted to run a scam." Later he was discharged by the project after he was discovered fencing stolen merchandise on the job. Another OW was confronted several times by the project director over rumors he was orchestrating the sale of drugs while distributing bleach and condoms. But such schemes were difficult to prove. In this case, the OW was also a team supervisor and, in observance of the strong street ethic never to "snitch," the OWs under him refused to tell what they knew to the project directors. In encouraging OWs to use constantly their street-based experience, outreach projects provided opportunities to tap into a complex and lucrative black market that offered goods and services in high demand. If OWs chose to take advantage of the opportunities they cultivated, as some did, they were in a good position to dabble and make a quick return on an investment, or to get more intensely involved.

Yet, it must be emphasized that there were many OWs who remained committed to their jobs and wished to perform like professionals. Studies of outreach projects throughout the country have revealed that many OWs worked hard at accessing IDUs and at promoting risk reduction (see Johnson 1988; Margolis 1990; Rivera-Beckman 1992b; Broadhead and Fox 1990). For those OWs, however, *the* most deflating and demoralizing experience was having to tolerate the shirking and con jobs of their colleagues. Such demoralization was a major occupational risk for those OWs who were well-meaning and highly motivated (Broadhead and Fox 1993). Thus, a very sincere OW who was able to stay with the San Francisco project for only a few months explained:

> When I worked with a volunteer agency, the volunteers worked harder and longer than we did. . . . So here is an agency where everyone is paid, but so little is happening, at least with the team I was with. Eventually I just felt like I was wasting my time. I even started to schedule personal things into my own work time, which I didn't think was right.

In contrast, an OW who constantly had to deal with his partner's large-scale con job eventually quit in desperation:

> I hate Sam, man, I just want to kill that dude! I'm just ready to say "Screw this job!". . . And Sam, he's still dealin' on the job! He's got four guys that I know of workin' for him. And they [clients] ask me if I "use," and I tell them, "No man, I don't anymore". . . The reason it bothers

me is that it makes me look like a fool. I'm out there trying to do something about this epidemic. So what does Sam do? He tells the guys on the street not to say anything to me.

Outreach and the Problem of Moral Hazard

A second type of agency problem occurs *ex post*, after an agent's services have been retained. If a principal lacks the means effectively to monitor an agent's performance, the latter may act in ways that serve his or her interest at the principal's expense. This risk stems from postcontractual opportunism and is termed "moral hazard," though it need not entail behavior that is either immoral or illegal.[3]

. . . First, OWs enjoyed considerable autonomy in the field for long periods of time, largely free of supervision or colleague control. Such autonomy is a generic feature of occupations at the "street-level" (Lipsky 1980), and many OWs regarded it as a major prerequisite of their job. Once in the field, OWs had many opportunities to shirk. Consequently, OWs frequently organized their days to accommodate personal matters, such as educational programs, artistic pursuits, avocations, and even part-time jobs. Some OWs kept "banker's hours," as a director of the San Francisco project acknowledged.

A second factor that impedes monitoring of OWs derives from local norms. In conforming to the ethics of the street, OWs were loath to "snitch" on one another, which made project monitoring even more difficult. For example, in joining an outreach team, one OW was given the following advice by her new teammates: "I was told, whatever happens *in* the team, *stays* in the team. Don't bring problems out in the staff meetings that are our business. We keep our own problems to ourselves."

Given the lack of effective monitoring, OWs had extensive opportunities to act in ways that conflicted with the official aims of outreach projects. These divergent actions resulted from (1) political conflicts, (2) conflicts between local culture and the goals of outreach, (3) the status needs of OWs, and (4) OWs' reactions to the occupational risks of outreach.

Political Conflict. Political conflicts between OWs and outreach projects aversely affected AIDS prevention efforts. Minority communities in the United States have been for some time disproportionately at risk of contracting HIV (National Commission on AIDS 1991). In addition, minority communities, especially African-American and Hispanic, tend "to see AIDS in the context of broader problems of poverty, drug addiction, inadequate education and employment" (Quimby and Friedman 1989:405). As such, in 1990, at nearly the same time that the Centers for Disease Control was announcing the success of outreach services, members of the Black Leadership Commission on AIDS in New York City were holding their own press conference to announce the opposite: from their perspective, the national AIDS outreach effort was a cop-out by the federal government that reflected a failure to deal with the pervasive problems afflicting minority communities (Broadhead 1991). As reported in the *New York Times* (1990:N14), the Black Leadership Commission "criticized public health officials in New York City for the bleach distribution, saying they were giving the poor a sop rather than real help;": and, "[b]leach distribution amounts to endorsing inexpensive ways to stop AIDS from spreading among users but failing to come up with the millions of dollars needed to help users get off drugs."

OWs who shared this position with their communities, and brought it to their job, had difficulty remaining committed to their work. Thus, for example, a young Latino OW felt compelled to quit after struggling for approximately six months, during which time he resumed a cocaine habit:

I just couldn't handle it anymore. There was something kinda weird about going up to old dope fiends and saying, "Hey man, want some bleach?" when it's like, "Well, you won't die from AIDS but, man, you might OD in two weeks." The project didn't even address that! It's like, "Oh, sure, we want to help you, so here, take some free bleach," you know (pointing his finger to his temple indicating that this is crazy). . . What about the real problems? It doesn't address the problem that all these kids in our community are dying from crack and from violence about drugs. . . .

Conflicts Between Local Culture and Outreach. Some OWs' indigenous identities in the community undermined their prevention efforts. Two examples from the San Francisco project suggest the complexity of the problem. One OW, who acknowledged having been a prostitute and hustler years earlier, joined the outreach project after becoming a born-again Christian. Her identity conflicts with the project were twofold. In being asked to work with prostitutes, her job as an OW constantly drew attention to a former identity she wanted to forget. In addition, by requiring OWs to be nonjudgmental in working with IDUs, she was prohibited from spreading the religious message closest to her heart, for which she wore a large, glittering pin that said "THINK JESUS." Her tenure with the project ended after several weeks of erratic performance. . . .

In general, OWs worked best with clients who were most like themselves. This meant that, for any OW, there were many types of clients with whom they were *unprepared* to work. Specifically, OWs' indigenous ingroup/outgroup alignments often reflected the same narrow attitudes and prejudices current among their peers. Thus, for example, a straight Latino OW, perhaps a former heroin addict, may feel confident about accessing and relating to people like himself. But he may be at a loss in having to work with Latina IDUs, or gay Latino or transvestite cocaine injectors, speed-using male or female prostitutes, black crack addicts, nondrug-using Latina or black sexual partners of IDUs, and white, runaway drug-using youth. Outreach projects specifically hired indigenous members of targeted communities to work as OWs, but much of what OWs brought to the job compromised their performance on the job.

Status Needs of OWs. In successfully establishing themselves in specific communities, OWs found that they enjoyed a kind of popularity and kinship with user populations; being well known and admired was a powerful reward. Yet becoming established created inertia. OWs found the prospects of having to break into new drug networks stressful. OWs found their work more satisfying if they stayed with clients who knew and respected them, instead of going into situations as strangers to face IDUs' deep-seated distrust. Thus, OWs tended to restrict their work to areas in which they were well known and felt comfortable, at the expense of breaking into new territories. So, their outreach efforts bogged down.

Status conflicts also arose between the clients of outreach and OWs. Outreach projects asked OWs to maintain a nonjudgmental attitude toward their clients' lifestyles and practices. Yet, some OWs were resocialized by drug treatment programs to attitudes that were highly negative toward drug use and addicts, especially in New York City. As reported by Rivera-Beckman (1991), almost all of the 23 OWs who staffed the AIDS outreach project she studied in New York identified themselves as recovering addicts and members of Narcotics Anonymous (NA). In turn, the philosophy of NA toward active users was highly disparaging: drug use *per se* was a repudiated activity that must be tolerated; users were denigrated; recovering addicts in NA who "slipped" were denounced by other members and stripped of rights and entitlements that could only be earned back through humiliating submission to the strictures and control of NA. As a result, given their local membership in NA, most OWs in New York had an *aversion* to working with IDUs and, as reported by Rivera-Beckman (1991), they refused even to place bleach in IDUs' hands. Instead, IDUs had to approach OWs, whose *modus operandi* was to stand behind portable tables set up on the street.

. . . Due to the OWs' perspective in New York as members of NA, during a ten-month period from June 1990 through April 1991, only 1.02 bleach bottles per OW were distributed on average per day (Rivera-Beckman 1991).

Reactions to the Occupational Risks of Outreach. OWs entered communities and worked directly with IDUs, which generally entailed walking the streets of blighted, crime-ridden neighborhoods. Individuals were hired as OWs, in part, because of their personal knowledge of the areas in which they would be working. Yet, as several OWs noted, they sometimes avoided those very areas in the past *because* of what they knew about them. As one OW reported, "when they said I was going to work down there as an OW I said, 'Oh no, that is *not* where I want to be!' "

Most inner-city areas containing large concentrations of IDUs have high predatory crime rates, and many OWs initially felt anxious about being assaulted while working in them. On a day-to-day basis, it was not uncommon to see people involved in confrontations and shouting matches; or undercover police running people down, hassling and rousting people in various locations, and making arrests. In such areas, the threat of physical violence was palpable and ever-present. Besides physical assault, the risk of being psychologically and emotionally assaulted was also high. OWs' clients lived in extremely deprived circumstances, the vast majority were homeless, addicted, unhealthy and impoverished. OWs spoke often, and with considerable emotion, of the psychological and emotional assaults they experienced in witnessing their clients' suffering and deprivation (Broadhead, Fox, and Espada 1990; Margolis 1990).

However, OWs' adjustments to their work situation went far beyond merely protecting their physical safety. To reduce their exposure to disturbing situations, OWs tended to restrict themselves to open, public spaces. Thus, for example, an OW reported in a staff meeting, "This week we went into the City Hotel and I want to tell you, I've never seen five floors of such absolute filth in my life like we saw there." The staff agreed that OWs were better off staying out of such places and positioning themselves to hand out prevention materials to clients as they came and went. OWs typically positioned themselves where they hoped community members would know where to find them (Johnson, Williams, and Kotarba 1990).

. . . In addition, OWs learned that in working to be accepted and trusted by IDUs, it was streetwise to copy IDUs' street demeanor. Members of drug using scenes try to avoid drawing attention to themselves and their activities. . . . Being low profile and cool helped OWs allay IDUs' suspicions and forge trusting relationships with them (Broadhead and Fox 1990). But the style worked against aggressive and widespread distribution of AIDS prevention materials.

The Role of IDUs in Outreach Efforts

The general picture of outreach that emerges from the research literature is that OWs adapted rationally to a risky and stressful work environment in ways that reduced both the number and diversity of IDUs they served. OWs' adjustments were also the result of working in projects that were bureaucratically organized, but that operated under conditions which allow hierarchy and supervision to break down easily, resulting in organizational drift and inertia. Yet, as documented earlier, IDUs made significant community-wide risk reductions in response to the outreach services they received. Indeed, this is only half the story: IDUs' responsiveness went beyond risk reduction changes *per se*. Specifically, in outreach projects throughout the country, OWs found, and ethnographers documented, that IDUs volunteered and helped OWs carry out AIDS prevention efforts in many ways (Broadhead and Fox 1990; Rivera-Beckman 1992b; Johnson, Williams, and Kotarba 1990).

IDUs frequently introduced OWs to other users, and vouched for OWs in new communities. IDUs commonly helped OWs fill and prepare bleach bottles, and helped OWs distribute bleach, condoms, and prevention information. It was also common for IDUs to aid OWs in locating users to be interviewed, or to find users who needed to return for follow-up interviews. As the directors of the San Francisco outreach project reported:

> In short, the IV drug users became deeply involved in helping us gather health information regarding AIDS and its means of transmission. They generally looked favorably on such efforts to involve them voluntarily and encouraged their friends to cooperate in a similar fashion (Feldman and Biernacki 1988:31-32).

. . . In sum, while it appears that outreach projects in many areas sparked risk-reduction changes, IDUs and other drug-scene members clearly augmented those projects substantially. In the course of doing so, IDUs further disseminated and reinforced the strength of prevention norms within the larger IDU community. What is now known about both the limitations of traditional outreach and the unexpected responsiveness of IDUs, suggests the potential for a new approach to AIDS prevention that relies on, and works to strengthen, the capabilities of drug users to promote risk reduction among their peers. . . .

Efforts to Promote Self-Organization Among IDUs

The responsiveness of IDUs to outreach efforts has encouraged many AIDS researchers to call for future prevention efforts that are based on active *collaborations* between drug users and prevention workers (Carlson and Needle 1991; Chitwood et al. 1990; Des Jarlais and Friedman 1990; Feldman and Biernacki 1988; Wiebel 1988). However, only one such program has been both implemented and assessed in the professional literature. In the Williamsburg section of New York City in 1988, Friedman et al. (1991) encouraged ex-users to recruit active users into self-help groups. Using a storefront, the organizers initiated weekly meetings of female IDUs for several months with an attendance of 6 to 20, and later, weekly meetings of male IDUs with between 3 and 18 participants. This experiment encountered agency problems similar to those found in traditional outreach projects. For example, the staff of ex-users often sought to prevent active users from encroaching on their authority, and even acted to discourage active users from becoming engaged in the program. Similarly, the staff sought to deny active users any overt recognition for the program's achievements. So, the program fell prey to the status needs of staff. Because of such problems, the experiment was unable to cultivate a durable user-organization. . . Given its success in motivating user self-help, the preliminary results were nonetheless encouraging. Des Jarlais and Friedman (1990:143) conclude that, "Public health officials should address the immediate need to reduce the spread of HIV, including advocating prevention programs that involve collaborative efforts with current members of drug use subcultures."

As the above example illustrates, the problem of designing a system to harness the potential contributions of IDUs is challenging. The special demands of IDUs' lifestyle, a product in large part of the War on Drugs (Goode 1993; Drug Policy Foundation 1992), frequently reduce IDUs' ability to perform satisfactorily in traditional organizational roles. In addition, it would not suffice merely to hire IDUs to replace OWs because the same agency problems that hampered OWs' efforts would also afflict IDUs. More creative organizational arrangements are required. . . .

The first task of outreach is recruiting IDUs into prevention programs. As in traditional outreach programs, the nexus of a "peer-driven intervention," or PDI, is a facility, such as a storefront, that provides HIV testing and counseling, risk reduction education, and prevention materials. In a PDI, IDUs are motivated to recruit other users for the above services via a coupon system: for each IDU recruited bearing a coupon, the user who recruited him or her receives a modest monetary reward. Only modest rewards are required, because the cost involved in exercising influence over peers is usually small, and there now exists widespread concern about AIDS and its threat to the welfare of peers.

Each recruit, in turn, is also given a limited number of coupons to recruit still other IDUs within their network. Thus, the mechanism coopts user networks to serve as a medium to recruit further IDUs. If adequate incentives are employed, with the number of coupons strictly limited per IDU so that no one single member can monopolize recruiting, the expanding system of chain-referrals may be robust enough to saturate the IDU population. In addition, all members of the IDU community are provided an equal opportunity to participate in the intervention, and to be rewarded. This approach has several advantages. First, it puts the burden of identifying recruits on those with the best current information: active users. Of course, users vary in community, so they can be expected to vary in the success of their recruitment efforts. However, as the network research on the "small-world problem" demonstrates (Killworth and Bernard 1978/79), only a handful of linkages are required to connect even highly disparate positions in real-world social networks. The implication is that peer-re-cruitment mechanisms can operate virtually irrespective of network structure.

Second, the pay-for-performance design of a PDI rewards the most productive recruit-ers, thereby reducing problems of moral haz-ard. As a result, subjects are paid in direct proportion to the success of their recruit-ment efforts, and those who recruit no one receive nothing.

Third, a PDI offers a built-in accommoda-tion to the cultural diversity in the user popu-lation: with IDUs accessing their peers, the recruitment effort is couched in terms appro-priate to each user subgroup. Thus, a PDI has built into it a performance-based monitoring system that effectively avoids the agency problems commonly afflicting bureaucratic organization.

Another central task of outreach is distrib-uting AIDS prevention information. Tradi-tional programs educate IDUs both in the field, and through education modules on HIV, STDs, safer injection practices, and so on at a storefront, van, or similar space. In a PDI, IDUs are given incentives to educate their peers in the community. The extent to which IDUs pass on information to those they recruit can be measured through ques-tions added to standard interview schedules, and the reward to the recruiter depends on the knowledge of the recruit. This approach has several advantages. First, it puts the re-sponsibility for educating IDUs on those who are most likely to be influential: their peers. One of the most effective ways of motivating students to invest in a body of knowledge is to have them teach one another (Juzang 1992). Second, it entails considerable repeti-tion. Subjects are first educated by their peer-recruiter, then by project staff, and finally subjects rehearse what they have learned when educating and recruiting their peers. Third, its pay-for-performance design re-wards the most effective educators, thereby reducing problems of moral hazard. Fourth, it gives the outreach effort ongoing feedback for assessing the comprehension of preven-tion messages by users of different cultural and ethnic groups.

The final essential task of outreach is dis-tribution of AIDS prevention materials such as bleach, condoms, and (if legally and ad-ministratively permissible) syringes. In a PDI, secondary incentives also can be used to motivate IDUs to distribute materials to their peers in the community. Thus, IDUs can look forward to receiving rewards that they have *earned* by referring their peers for education and testing, and for distributing AIDS pre-vention materials and information.

The most durable interventions are those that change community norms. Strictly indi-vidualized incentives, which affect only incli-nations, tend to have results that are tran-sient and erratic (Andenaes 1974). In con-trast, alteration of regulatory interests has more durable effects because it creates a sys-tem of supportive norms. When recruiting and educating their peers, individuals draw upon whatever reserves of social influence they may possess. If such norms are consis-tent with previously existing regulatory inter-ests within the group, they can, so to speak, take on a life of their own (Heckathorn 1988). In relatively cohesive groups, norms can per-sist long after the external sanctions upon which they are based have withered or been withdrawn. In more atomized groups, the in-tragroup control resources that are available, however weak, can be harnessed on behalf of the norms. Consequently, changes in norms have the potential to produce more abiding alterations in group behavior.

Financial constraints add urgency to the task of seeking more efficient means to de-liver human services to IDUs. Most outreach projects nationwide have been funded by the federal government as demonstration pro-jects for only three to five years. Many are now losing federal funding and are too ex-pensive for many state and local govern-ments to continue. Thus, the San Francisco outreach project was defunded at the end of 1990. When the first author returned to San Francisco in May 1991 to a neighborhood he had served as an OW, some of the IDUs com-plained that no one was giving out bleach anymore on the streets. The result was, as one IDU noted, "People back doin' some bad shit, 'homes'."

The defunding of outreach projects has caused considerable alarm at the federal con-gressional level (Weiss 1990). Despite OWs' success at reducing the spread of HIV, outreach projects are now being abandoned in many parts of the country. Other programs have lost funding because of agency problems like those described above (Hartford Courant 1992). Given a PDI's greatly reduced reliance on paid staff, such an intervention would be far less expensive than traditional outreach, by nearly an order of magnitude, and avoid many organizational problems found to afflict such projects. . . .

References

Altman, Dennis. 1987. *AIDS in the Mind of America*. Garden City, New York: Anchor Books.

Andenaes, Johannes. 1974. *Punishment and Deterrence*. Ann Arbor: University of Michigan Press.

Bok, Sissela. 1978. *Lying: Moral Choice in Public and Private Life*. New York: Random House.

Booth, Robert, and W. Wayne Wiebel. 1992. "Effectiveness of reducing needle-related risks for HIV through indigenous outreach to injection drug users." *American Journal on Addictions*, 1:277-287.

Broadhead, Robert S. 1991. "Social constructions of bleach in combating AIDS among injection drug users." *Journal of Drug Issues*, 21:713-37.

Broadhead, Robert S., and Kathryn J. Fox. 1990. "Takin' it to the streets: AIDS outreach as ethnography." *Journal of Contemporary Ethnography*, 19:322-48.

———. 1993. "Occupational health risks of harm reduction work: Combating AIDS among injection drug users," in *Advances in Medical Sociology, Vol. III: The Social and Behavioral Aspects of AIDS*, eds. Gary L. Albrecht and Rick Zimmerman, 123-142. Greenwich, Conn.: JAI Press.

Broadhead, Robert S., Kathryn J. Fox, and Frank Espada. 1990. "AIDS outreach workers." *Society*, 27:66-70.

Broadhead, Robert S., and Eric Margolis. 1993. "Drug policy in the time of AIDS: The development of outreach in San Francisco." *Sociological Quarterly*, 34:497-522.

Brown, Barry, and George M. Beschner. 1993. *Handbook on Risk of AIDS: Injection Drug Users and Sexual Partners*. Westport, Conn.: Greenwood Press.

Carlson, Gregory, and Richard Needle. 1991. "Sponsering Addict Self-organization (Addicts Against AIDS): A Case Study." In Community-based AIDS Prevention: Studies of Intravenous Drug Users and Their Sexual Partners: Proceedings of the First AnnualNADR National Meeting, ed. The National Institute on Drug Abuse (DHH's Pub. No.

80M-91-1752), 342-49 Washington, D.C.: U.S. Government Printing Office.

Chitwood, Dale D., Clyde B. McCoy, James A. Inciardi, Duane C. McBride, Mary Comerford, Edward Trapido, H. Virginia McCoy, J. Bryan Page, James Griffin, Mary Ann Fletcher, and Margarita A. Ashman. 1990. "HIV seropositivity of needles from shooting galleries in south Florida." *American Journal of Public Health*, 80:150-52.

Chitwood, Dale D., Mary Comerford, Elizabeth L. Khoury, and Judith A. Vogel. 1991. "Behavior changes of intravenous drug users after an intervention program," in *Community-Based AIDS Prevention: Studies of intravenous Drug Users and Their Sexual Partners: Proceedings of the First Annual NADR National Meeting*, ed. National Institute on Drug Abuse (DHHS Pub. No. 8OM-91-1752), 449-455. Washington, D.C.: U.S. Government Printing Office.

Coleman, James S. 1990. *Foundations of Social Theory*. Cambridge: Belknap Press.

Des Jarlais, Don C., Samuel R. Friedman, and William Hopkins. 1985. "Risk reduction for AIDS among intravenous drug users." *Annals of Internal Medicine*, 103:755-759.

Des Jarlais, Don C., and Samuel R. Friedman. 1990. "Shooting galleries and AIDS: Infection probabilities and 'tough' policies." *American Journal of Public Health*, 80:142-45.

Drug Policy Foundation. 1992. *National Drug Reform Strategy*. Washington, D.C.: The Drug Policy Foundation.

Eisenhardt, K. 1985. "Control: Organizational and Economic Approaches." *Management Science*, 31:134-49.

Feldman, Harvey W. and Patrick Biernacki. 1988. "The ethnography of needle sharing among intravenous drug users and implications for public policies and intervention strategies," in *Needle Sharing Among Intravenous Drug Abuse: National and International Perspectives*, eds. R.J. Battjes and R.W. Pickens, 28-40. National Institute on Drug Abuse Research Monograph No. 80. Washington, D.C.: U.S. Government Printing Office.

Friedman, Samuel R., Don C. Des Jarlais, Jo L. Sotheran, Jonathan Garber, Henry Cohen, and Donald Smith. 1987. "AIDS and self-organization among intravenous drug users." *The international Journal of the Addictions*, 22:201-19.

Friedman, Samuel R., Meryl Sufian, Richard Curtis, Alan Neaigus, and Don C. Des Jarlais. 1991. "AIDS-related organizing of intravenous drug users from the outside," in *Culture and Social Relations in the AIDS Crisis*, eds. E. Schneider and J. Huber, 115-130. Newbury Park, Calif.: Sage.

Goode, Eric. 1993. *Drugs In American Society.* New York: McGraw-Hill.

Government Accounting Office. 1992. Drug Abuse Research: Federal Funding and Future Needs. (GAO/PEMD-92-5).Washington, D.C.: Government Account Office.

Hartford Courant. 1992. "Hartford agency loses AIDS grant." October 6:Al.

Haverkos, Harry W. 1988. "Overview: HIV infection among intravenous drug abusers in the United States and Europe," in *Needle Sharing Among intravenous Drug Abuse: National and International Perspectives,* eds. R. J. Battjes and R. W. Pickens, 7-15. National Institute on Drug Abuse Research Monograph No. 80. Washington, D.C.: U.S. Government Printing Office.

Heckathorn, Douglas D. 1988. "Collective sanctions and the emergence of prisoner's dilemma norms." *American Journal of Sociology,* 94:535-62.

———. 1990. "Collective sanctions and compliance norms: A formal theory of group-mediated social control." *American Sociological Review,* 55:366-84.

———. 1993 "Collective action and group heterogeneity: Voluntary provision versus selective incentives." *American Sociological Review,* 58:329-350.

Jensen, Michael C., and William H. Meckling. 1976 "Theory of the firm: Managerial behavior, agency costs, and ownership structures." *Journal of Financial Economics,* 3:305-60.

Johnson, Jay. 1988. "Community health outreach workers and AIDS intervention: An ethnographic analysis." Master's thesis, Department of Sociology, University of Houston. Unpublished manuscript.

Johnson, Jay, Mark L. Williams, and Joseph A. Kotarba. 1990. "Proactive and reactive strategies for delivering community-based HIV prevention services: An ethnographic analysis." *AIDS Education and Prevention,* 2:191-200.

Juzang, Ivan. 1992. *Reaching The Hip-Hop Generation.* MEE Productions, Philadelphia: Unpublished manuscript.

Killworth, Peter D., and H. Russell Bernard. 1978-79. "The Reversal Small-World Experiment." *Social Networks,* 1:159-192.

Kuller, Lewis H., and Lawrence A. Kingsley. 1986. "The epidemic of AIDS: A failure of public policy." *Millbank Quarterly,* 64:56-78.

Lawlor, Edward J. 1990. "When a possible job becomes impossible: Politics, public health, and the management of the AIDS epidemic," in *Impossible Jobs in Public Management,* eds. Erwin C. Hargrove and John C. Glidewell, 152-176. University Press of Kansas.

Lipsky, Michael. 1980. *Street-Level Bureaucracy: Dilemmas of the Individual in Public Services.* New York: Russell Sage.

Longshore, Douglas. 1992. "AIDS education for drug users: Existing research and new directions." *Journal of Drug Issues,* 22:1-16.

Margolis, Eric. 1990. "Visual ethnography: Tools for mapping the AIDS epidemic." *Journal of Contemporary Ethnography,* 19:370-91.

National Commission on AIDS. 1991. *The Twin Epidemics of Substance Use and HIV. Report No. 4.* Washington, D.C.: U.S. Government Printing Office.

National Institute on Drug Abuse. 1987. "AIDS Community Outreach Demonstration Project." *Grant announcement DA-87-13, January.* Unpublished manuscript.

———. 1991a. *Community-Based AIDS Prevention: Studies of Intravenous Drug Users and Their Sexual Partners: Proceeding of the First Annual NADR National Meeting,* ed. National Institute on Drug Abuse (Pub No. 8OM-91-1752). Washington, D.C.: U.S. Government Printing Office.

———. 1991b. "NIDA's AIDS projects succeed in reaching drug addicts, changing high-risk behaviors." *NIDA NOTES 6,* (Summer/Fall):25-27.

Neaigus, Alan, Meryl Sufian, Samuel R. Friedman, Douglas S. Goldsmith, Bruce Stepherson, Patrice Mota, Jacqueline Pascal, and Don C. Des Jarlais. 1990. "Effects of outreach intervention on risk reduction among intravenous drug users." *AIDS Education and Prevention,* 2:253-271.

New York Times. 1990. "Black group attacks using bleach to slow spread of AIDS." June 17:NI4.

Olson, Mancur. 1965. *The Logic of Collective Action.* Cambridge, Mass.: Harvard University Press.

Perrow, Charles, and Mauro F. Guillen. 1990. *The AIDS Disaster: The Failure Of Organizations In New York and The Nation.* New Haven, Conn.: Yale University Press.

Quimby, Ernest, and Samuel R. Friedman. 1989. "Dynamics of black mobilization against AIDS in New York City." *Social Problems,* 4:403-15.

Rivera-Beckman, Joyce. 1991. "Process ethnography report on the AIDS Outreach and Prevention Program: A report to the New York Division of Substance Abuse Services." National Development Research Institutes, Inc. New York City. Unpublished manuscript.

———. 1992a. "Voices from an underground needle exchange." Paper presentation at the 3rd International Conference on Drug-Related Harm Reduction (March), Melbourne, Australia.

———. 1992b. "Community outreach in the time of AIDS: The San Francisco, Chicago and POCAAN Models: A report to the New York State Division of Substance Abuse Services." National Development Research Institute, Inc. New York City. Unpublished manuscript.

Schuster, Charles R. 1988. "Intravenous drug use and AIDS prevention." *Public Health Reports*, 103 (No. 3): 261-266.

Shilts, Randy. 1987. *And The Band Played On: Politics, People and the AIDS Epidemic*. New York: St. Martin's Press.

Stephens, Richard C., Thomas E. Feucht, and Shadi W. Roman. 1991. "Effects of an intervention program on AIDS-related drug and needle behavior among intravenous drug users." *American Journal of Public Health*, 81:568-71.

Stern, L. Synn. 1992. "Self-injection education for street level sexworkers," in *The Reduction of Drug-Related Harm*, eds. P.A. O'Hare, R. Newcombe, A. Matthews, E.C. Buning, and E. Drucker, 122-128. New York: Routledge.

Waitzkin, Howard. 1991. *The Politics of Medical Encounters*. New Haven: Yale University Press.

Watters, John K., Mohr Downing, Patricia Case, Jennifer Lorvick, Yu-Teh Cheng, and Bonnie Fergusson. 1990a "AIDS prevention for intravenous drug users in the community: Street-based education and risk behavior." *American Journal of Community Psychology*, 18:587-96.

Watters, John K., Yu-Teh Cheng, Mark Segal, Jennifer Lorvick, Patricia Case, Francis Taylor, and James R. Carlson. 1990b. "Epidemiology and prevention of HIV in heterosexual IV drug users in San Francisco, 1986-1989." Paper presentation at the Sixth International Conference on AIDS (June). San Francisco.

Weeks, Margaret R., Merril Singer, Jean J. Schensul, Zhongke Jia and Maryland Grier. 1990. "Project COPE: Preventing AIDS among injection drug users and their sexual partners comprehensive data report." Project COPE, Hartford, Conn. Unpublished manuscript.

Weiss, Ted. 1990. "Strategies to prevent transmission of HIV among intravenous drug users." Opening statement before the Human Resources and Intergovernmental Relations Subcommittee of the Committee on Government Operations, United States House of Representatives, September 18.

White, H. 1985. "Agency as control," in *Principals and Agents: The Structure of Business*, eds. J. Pratt and R. Zeckhauser, 187-214. Boston: Harvard Business School Press.

Wiebel, W. Wayne. 1988. "Combining ethnographic and epidemiologic methods in targeted AIDS interventions: The Chicago Model," in *Needle Sharing Among Intravenous Drug Abuse: National and International Perspectives*, eds. R.J. Battjes and R.W. Pickens, 137-50. National Institute on Drug Abuse Research Monograph No. 80. Washington, D.C.: U.S. Government Printing Office.

Wiebel, W. Wayne, and Thomas M, Lampinen. 1991. "Primary prevention of HIV/1 among intravenous drug users." Journal of Primary Prevention 12:35-48.

Wisotsky, Steven. 1991. "Beyond the War on Drugs," in *The Drug Legalization Debate*, ed. J.A. Inciardi, 103-29. Newbury Park, Calif.: Sage.

Notes

1. We thank Patrick Biernacki, in whose memory this paper is dedicated, for his enormous contributions as a sociologist to combating AIDS among injection drug users, and his thoughtful reactions to this analysis which builds on much of his work. We also thank Samuel R. Friedman, Gaye Tuchman, Joyce Rivera-Beckman, Noel Cazenive, Judith Levy, Susan LoBello, Steven Maser, Mark Abrahamson and Robert Antonio for their helpful comments and advice. Gayle N. Williams, and especially Kathryn J. Fox, helped in collecting the ethnographic data drawn upon in the analysis, for which we are grateful. We thank Denise Anthony, Steve Harvey and Kathleen Cahill for their assistance. We also thank the National Institute on Drug Abuse (ROI DA05517) for the research support given to Robert Broadhead, and the National Science Foundation (SES-9022926) for the support given to Douglas Heckathorn. We were also supported by a grant from the National Institute on Drug Abuse (ROI DA08014). An earlier version of this paper was presented at the VIII International Conference on AIDS, Amsterdam. The Netherlands, July 1992, and the American Sociological Association meetings, Miami, August 1993.

2. Some of the OWs were interviewed during and after their tenure with the San Francisco project. The names of project staff members appearing in the text are pseudonyms.

3. The problems of adverse selection and moral hazard are conceptually distinct. However, they are sometimes difficult to discriminate in particular cases because they become intertwined. For example, inadequate monitoring of agent performance can lead to postcolonial opportunism (moral hazards) such as running con jobs on the project. Subsequently, the prospect for con jobs can serve to attract re-

cruits who are on the lookout for opportunities to exploit thereby creating a problem of pre-contractual opportunism (adverse selection). In either case, agency theory locates the source of the problem in informational asymmetries.

Further Reading

Phillipe Bourgois, Mark Lettiere, and James Quesada. 1997. "Social Misery and the Sanctions of Substance Abuse: Confronting HIV Risk Among Homeless Heroin Addicts in San Francisco" *Social Problems, 44(2): 155-73.*

Robert Broadhead and Kathryn Fox. 1990. "Takin' it to the Streets: AIDS Outreach as Ethnography" *Journal of Contemporary Ethnography* 19: 322-48.

Robert Broadhead and Eric Margolis. 1993. "Drug Policy in the Time of AIDS: The Development of Outreach in San Francisco" *Sociological Quarterly* 34: 497-522.

Charles Perrow and Mauro Guillen. 1990. *The AIDS Disaster: The Failure of Organizations in New York and the Nation.* New Haven: Yale University Press.

Discussion Questions

1. List some of the strengths of community based outreach programs.

2. What are some of the organizational and agency issues that prohibit IDUs from being effective outreach workers?

3. What sorts of solutions might you propose to remedy some of the problems of community based intervention programs revealed in this selection?

4. In your opinion, can community-based programs of the kind described by Broadhead and Heckathorn be an effective instrument in public health education? Explain your position.

Section 7

The Future of Health, Illness, and Healing

Although growth in health care expenditures has slowed within the past five years, the United States spends more of its Gross Domestic Product (GDP) on health care expenditures than any other industrialized country. In 1995, the United States invested $988 billion—13.6 percent of the GDP—in health care expenditures (Prospective Payment Commission 1997). The decrease in national expenditures has been transferred to organizational and personal out-of-pocket costs. Still, U.S. health expenditures are projected to reach more than $2 trillion by 2003. The rising costs of health care are most often attributed to inflation and scientific and technological advances (Callahan 1990; Prospective Payment Commission 1997).

Quandaries about what services to provide, who will offer these services, and who will receive them plague government officials, policymakers, and administrators. During the early 1990s, national attempts to restructure health insurance and to introduce a plan for those without insurance failed. Speculations about why national plans have been unsuccessful in the United States range from perceived lack of feasibility for businesses to general distrust of presidential administrations. At present, the United States health care system is an illness care system in which costs keep rising and an increasing number of people are without basic care. Paradoxically, the United States has one of the best medical care systems in the world when we consider advanced technologies, medical specialty training, and dollars for research.

Despite large government expenditures, many Americans do not have health insurance, and the gap between "have" and "have-nots" is getting bigger. A number of Americans, insured through their worksites, accumulate greater out-of-pocket expenses for themselves and their dependents as administrators struggle to control organizational costs. Still, many men and women maintain employment but are uninsured or underinsured workers. Review the graph presented by Himmelstein and Woolhandler. Their illustrations depict the increasing number of weeks an average wage earner works to cover health care costs. Not surprisingly, the "working poor" now constitute the most rapidly growing segments of the population dependent on public assistance for health insurance (Seccombe and Amey 1995). Timothy Kenny's personal account depicts just what could happen to a worker unable to work due to chronic degenerative disease. Lack of insurance can shatter dreams and destroy taken-for-granted daily lives. Kenny tells of the struggles the chronically ill must face when confronting a debilitating illness without insurance.

Peter Conrad and Phil Brown explain the U.S. health insurance and care deficit as one way of rationing care. All societies ration medical care. In the United States, rationing depends on the ability to pay for treatment.

For individuals, the fact of unemployment, underemployment, or disability often restricts access to less-than-optimal care, if any. Nationally, restricted payments for specific Diagnostic Related Groups (DRGs) took form in the seventies to control the skyrocking government expenditures on Medicaid. Under DRG restrictions, hospitals and physicians are reimbursed fixed amounts for specific procedures and treatments rather than establishing their own payment schedules. At the organizational level, managed systems of care—like Health Maintenance Organizations (HMOs)—design methods of rationing based on cost, where organizational expenditures for treatment are spread over a group of people enrolled in a managed care plan. Alternatives for rationing care advise rationing by social group, allocating the greatest proportion of health care resources to the young and diminishing access to care for individuals over 65 years of age, for example.

Health care rationing is intimately related to economic systems. Capitalist societies, like the United States, ration health care by ability to pay for care. In Japan, decentralized governments offer care by occupation through worker- and government-based insurance. Socialized systems spread cost over the entire population, offering basic care to all citizens. Regardless of the form rationing assumes, national health care costs increase substantially as more people live longer and as technologies begin to take once unimaginable forms. And efforts to cut the costs of health care trickle from governments to hospitals and other organizations; in more recent years, they have affected physicians and individual citizens.

Rationing requires making judgments, and no decision about care is without moral character. Concern over tensions between cost and quality direct quests to measure and to compare quality of care in various organizations, assuming cost-cutting strategies to exchange quality of care for reduced expenditures. Currently, both government and organizational methods of standardizing and comparing quality of care are immature and of questionable validity. To date, few attempts have matched patients' individual experiences of care with organizational and world

health measures. No measurement scale could embody difficult individual and group decisions about treatment and quality of life.

The selection by David Hilfiker allows us to witness decisions physicians must make when treating terminally ill persons. Complicated treatment regimens translate into organizational cost. Hospital organizations spend a disproportionate amount of money and technological resources on the last months of life. Aggressive and intensive medical treatment do not ensure a life of quality. Coupled with issues of cost cutting that plague every hospital administration—issues more recently filtering to physicians as agents of health care organizations—the dilemmas Hilfiker presents are frightening.

Charles Bosk shows how distressing quality of life dilemmas are, bringing us inside an intensive care, pediatric consultation group. Bosk notes that no single individual wants to bear the burden of advancing futile treatment or carry responsibility for ending a potential life. More physicians claim that they do not have a treatment choice. Legally, physicians must save life where there is one, regardless of life quality and, as Bosk indicates, irrespective of parental decisions. Do Not Resuscitate (DNR) orders embody one way of translating patient, family, and physician decisions into health care treatment. Fearful, reluctant, and unwilling patients do not talk with their physicians about end-of-life treatment decisions. Robert Zussman's observations in an intensive care ward show us, however, that DNR orders serve principally as legal and organizational documentation. Rules for resuscitation are always up for negotiation. Advanced directives for care emerge as the tragedies of illness unfold (Kaplan 1988; Siminoff and Fetting 1991). Patients giving advanced directives for end-of-life care often change their minds about that care, becoming more favorable toward aggressive measures in advanced stages of illness. One thing is certain: no single person wants responsibility for terminating technological intervention or for prohibiting its initiation. Both Bosk and Zussman suggest that public and organizational records show only collective decision making about end-of-life decisions. Thus, the records implicate no single care provider for complicated judgments. Because medical judgments about life quality are moral judgments, ethics consultations in intensive care wards are not unusual. Ethicists grow in number in academic departments at schools of medicine and in hospitals as health care decisions become increasingly complex. Despite the involvement of ethicists, definitions about quality of life are not entirely separate from decisions about cost (Curtis and Rubenfeld 1997).

Levels of moral decision making also include political agendas and research opportunities. Shumaker and Smith underscore how women's involvement in the American health care agenda enhances medical innovations in health care. Women's increased participation in medical research agendas and their role as the subjects of clinical trials expands treatment definitions and possibilities for care. Innovations in scientific and medical research have increased the number of questions to be answered. Advancing technologies challenge the parameters of research possibilities and medical procedures and are at the forefront of ethical debates. The proliferating frontiers of science and medicine now force us to settle questions of what "ought to be" and to address possibilities for what "can be" with advances in reproductive technologies, organ transplantations, tissue regeneration, and genetic research (O'Neill 1994). How far will scientific research and medical technologies take us? At what economic and social costs?

Daniel Callahan explains that emphasis on acute illness and accommodation of individual care, coupled with rapid technological advancement, escalates personal demands for medical treatment. An "illusion of necessity" for treatment—because advanced technologies make the unimaginable possible—drives costs up in the United States and in Canada (Evans 1988). Focus on the personal needs and remedies for acute illnesses force immediate individual attention over consideration of long-term necessities and general public good. Rapid and complex care regimens prevail over global strategies for illness prevention and health promotion (Department of Health and Human Services 1997; Mechanic 1990). The acute model of care, still embedded in the American health care system, no longer serves patients or health care providers. Strauss and Corbin explain that chronic illness is normative rather than exceptional. They highlight how myopic attention to acute care and economic issues cannot help us to reform American health care.

Can attention to economic issues rescue us from the spiraling costs of care and individual demands? Will attention to social issues help redefine life quality? Do economic and social decisions assist in creating individually and institutionally relevant health care policies? The answers to these questions lie in future debates that recognize and respond to health and illness as the intersection of selves, social contexts, and societies.

References

Daniel Callahan. 1990. "Hopes, Vain Hopes: The Pursuit of Efficiency." *What Kind of Life: The Limits of Medical Progress.* Washington, D.C.: Georgetown University Press, pp. 69-102.

J. Randall Curtis and Gordon D. Rubenfeld. 1997. "Aggressive Medical Care at the End of Life." *Journal of the American Medical Association* 278(12):1025-1026.

Robert G. Evans. 1988. "'We'll Take Care of It for You'—Health Care in the Canadian Community." *Daedalus* 117 (Fall), p.185.

Kenneth Kaplan. 1988. "Assessing Judgment." *General Hospital Psychiatry* 9:202-208.

David Mechanic. 1990. "Promoting Health." *Society* 27: 16-22.

Terry ONeill. 1994. *Biomedical Ethics.* San Diego: Greenhaven Press, Inc.

Prospective Payment Commission. June 1997. *Medicare and the American Health Care System: Report to the Congress.* Washington, D.C.

Karen Seccombe and Cheryl Amey. 1995. "Playing by the Rules and Losing: Health Insurance and the Working Poor." *Journal of Health and Social Behavior*, pp.168-181.

L.A. Siminoff and J.H. Fetting. 1991. "Factors Affecting Treatment Decisions for a Life-Threatening Illness: The Case of Medical Treatment of Breast Cancer." *Social Science and Medicine* 32(7):813-818.

U.S. Department of Health and Human Services. 1997. *Healthy People 2000: National Health Promotion and Disease Prevention Objectives.* Washington, D.C. ✦

Bioethical Issues

49

Playing God

David Hilfiker

Physicians make life and death decisions every day they practice medicine. Some decisions are simple. Others are complicated. David Hilfiker shows us exactly how complicated some decisions are. Dr. Hilfiker provides insight into his own feelings and decisions for treating Elsa Toivonen, an elderly nursing home patient. Through his account, you will witness one physician's personal struggles with medical progress and intervention in the private lives of patients. Hilfiker indicates that medical expertise and social status may permit physicians absolute authority over technical treatment decisions. Medical decisions often have conflicting messages about the quality of human life; no heroic measures, do everything possible, keep her comfortable. Hilfiker's quandary about how to treat Mrs. Toivonen in her final stage of life raises several critical questions about the power of physicians and the quality of human life.

The phone rings, pulling me from that deepest sleep which comes during the first hours of the night. I can barely remember who I am, much less why the phone might be ringing. I manage to find the receiver next to the bed and pick it up.

"Hello?"

"Hello, Dr. Hilfiker? This is Ginger at the nursing home. Elsa has a fever."

In the silence my mind is immediately clear. Elsa Toivonen, eighty-three years old, confined to the nursing home ever since her stroke three years ago, bedridden, mute. In an instant I remember her as she was before the stroke: her dislike and distrust of doctors and hospitals, her staunch pride and independence despite the crippling back curvature of scoliosis, her wry grin every time I suggested hospitalization for some problem. I remember admitting her to the hospital after her stroke, incontinent, reduced to helplessness, one side completely paralyzed, speech gone; and I remember those first few days during which I aggressively treated the pneumonia that developed as a complication of the stroke, giving her intravenous antibiotics despite her apparent desire to die. "Depressed," I had thought. "She'll get over it. Besides, she may recover substantially in the next few weeks." She did, in fact, recover from the pneumonia, but she remained paralyzed and without speech. For the last three years she has remained curled in her nursing-home bed, my own grim reminder of the power of modern medicine.

"Dr. Hilfiker?" Ginger Moss's voice brings me back to my tired body.

"Oh . . . yeah," I say. My mind is focused; I just can't get my mouth to work. "Any other symptoms?"

"Well, you know Elsa. It's hard to tell. She hasn't been eating much the last few days, and she's had a little cough. Mary noticed her temperature on the evening shift, but she didn't want to bother you."

"So why are you bothering me now?" I want to say. Instead I ask, "What's her temperature?"

"One hundred three point five, rectally."

"Oh . . . all right," I say reluctantly. "I'll be right down."

Driving down the hill, I go through my usual jumble of irrational emotions. First I'm angry at Elsa for having her fever, then irritated with Mary for not having called me earlier in the evening, and finally I'm annoyed with Ginger for not waiting until morning. I'm glad I have this ride; otherwise I'd offend a lot of people. By the time I get to the nursing home, my irritation his subsided, and compassion for Mrs. Toivonen has begun to take over. Ginger is waiting for me in the dark hall just outside Mrs. Toivonen's room, chart in hand. "She looks pretty sick, David."

She does indeed! Wasted away to sixty-nine pounds, chronic bedsores on the bony protuberances of back and hip, she peers at me from behind her blank face. I'm used to all that from my regular monthly visits, but this morning there is no movement of her eyes, no resistance to my examination, nothing to indicate she's really there. Worse yet, there is little more to learn about the history of her fever than what Ginger has already told me over the phone. Mrs. Toivonen, of course, hasn't talked in three years, nor has she understood anything I've said as far as I call tell; so there is no hope of further information from her. My exam is brief as I look pointedly for the most common causes of fever in the elderly—upper respiratory infection, pneumonia, bladder infection, a viral illness. I realize I'm not being thorough, and feel briefly guilty as I recall an article I've read suggesting that nursing-home patients receive less thorough medical attention simply because they are old and feeble. It's true, of course. I know perfectly well that if this were a forty-seven-year-old schoolteacher in the emergency room with a fever, I would be spending an hour checking him out and talking with him. I try to assuage my guilt with the thought that I can't exhaust myself now, in the middle of the night, if I'm going to give decent care to all the other patients who need me in the morning. In my heart, though, I know it's a lousy excuse.

Listening to Mrs. Toivonen's chest, I hear the noises I expected, faint crackling pops indicating irritation in the lungs, probably pneumonia. I complete the rest of the exam without finding anything else and look up at Ginger. "I think she's got pneumonia," I say, and we both stare at Elsa's withered body I wonder to myself, "What am I going to do now?" Ginger's glance tells me the same question is going through her head. I ask her to call Mark out of bed for a chest x-ray, and I write orders for a urine culture in the morning just to make sure a bladder infection is not causing the fever. While waiting for the x-ray, Ginger and I sit at the nurse's station, writing our respective reports in the chart.

Ginger looks up. "Mabel Lundberg said she hoped there wouldn't be any heroics if Elsa got sick again."

"I know. She talked to me, too." What does she mean by "heroics," though? I suddenly feel irritated again, but I keep my mouth shut. Almost thirty years younger than Elsa, Mabel is the only friend Mrs. Toivonen has, her only visitor at the nursing home. Mabel was a neighbor and before Elsa's stroke she would help her with shopping, drive her to her clinic visits, run errands, and generally help out. She probably knows better than anyone what Elsa would really want, but Elsa's only relative, a niece I've never met who lives in another state, called some months ago asking that "everything possible" be done for her aunt. "Heroics"—"everything possible": each phrase refers to the same intervention but means something totally different. We all want "everything possible" done for our poor, bedridden aunt; but at the same time we all want to spare her those terrible medical "heroics" in which doctors "prolong needlessly the agony of the dying." It all depends on the words you choose.

Essentially alone in the middle of the night, foggy from tiredness, I'll make decisions that will probably mean life or death for this old woman. I think back to medical school and university hospital where a thousand dollars' worth of laboratory and x-ray studies would have been done to make sure she really did have pneumonia: several x-rays of the chest, urine cultures, blood cultures, microscopic examinations of her phlegm (which could only be obtained by putting a needle through the neck and into the trachea of this sixty-nine-pound, eighty-three-year-old lady), blood counts, a Mantoux test to make sure she doesn't have tuberculosis, possibly even lung scans to check for blood clots. The list is limited only by one's imagination, each test "reasonable" in its own way once you enter the labyrinth of medical thoroughness. I can almost hear the residents suggesting obscure possibilities to demonstrate their erudition. . . .

There in the middle of the night I consider doing "everything possible" for Mrs. Toivonen: transfer to the hospital, IVs for hydration, large doses of penicillin, thorough lab and x-ray evaluation, twice-daily rounds to be sure she is recovering, other more toxic antibiotics to cover the chance of an infection resistant to penicillin, even transfer to our regional hospital for specialist evaluation and care. None of it is unreasonable, and another night I might choose just such a course; but tonight my human sympathies lie with Mrs. Toivonen and what I perceive as her desire to die. Perhaps it is because Ginger is working, and I know how impatient she is with technological "heroics." Perhaps it is because I've been feeling a little depressed myself in the last few days and imagine I can better appreciate Mrs. Toivonen's perspective. Although who knows what thoughts are—or aren't—going on behind the impenetrable mask of that face? Perhaps, I think to myself, it is because I'm tired and lazy and don't want to bother.

In any event, I decide against the "heroics," but I can't just do nothing, either. Everything in my training and background pulls against that course, so there is no way I'm going to be able to be consistent and just go home. Instead, I compromise and write an order in the chart instructing the nursing staff to administer liquid penicillin by mouth, encourage fluid intake, and make an appointment with my office so I can reexamine Mrs. Toivonen in thirty-six hours. My orders make no real medical sense, of course. Such a debilitated lady's pneumonia will probably require the higher doses of penicillin possible only through an IV; Mrs. Toivonen is also likely to refuse the nurses' attempts to give her extra fluids. And my compromise makes even less ethical sense. Am I or am I not treating Mrs. Toivonen? Am I or am I not prolonging her life artificially?

On my way out of the dark hospital I talk with Mark, who looks sleepier than I feel, and we check the x-ray. I've known all along that the information it can offer me will be questionable at best. With her severe back curvature, Mrs. Toivonen is always difficult to x-

ray, and she has chronic changes in her lungs which make early pneumonia difficult to detect. I thank Mark for the x-ray, wondering why I ever ordered it. Driving up the hill, I wonder why the practice of medicine is so often dissatisfying.

As usual, it takes me an hour to get back to sleep.

Mrs. Toivonen survived her pneumonia, more because of her constitution than my treatment, but even my compromise treatment was an important ethical choice. I had decided that the quality of her life was not valuable enough to warrant aggressive medical treatment. Situations like Mrs. Toivonen's are common. In my practice and in those of other physicians I see around me, the old, chronically ill, debilitated, or mentally impaired do not receive the same level of medical evaluation and treatment as do the young, acutely ill, and mentally normal. Two physicians studied the response of nursing-home staff to fevers in the elderly residents and discovered that the older and more debilitated the patients were, the less likely they were to receive aggressive treatment.[1] The nursing aide was less likely to bring a fever to the attention of the supervising nurse, the nurse less likely to call the physician, the physician less likely to examine the patient personally, and the fever less likely to be treated with antibiotics. During my student years I was working with a particularly caring and competent doctor. When the nurses one day on hospital rounds reported that a debilitated elderly patient had a fever, I was shocked to watch my preceptor write an order for aspirin without even investigating the cause of the fever. Without further explanation he lamely apologized to me by explaining that it was "probably just a virus." Only years later did I understand that this physician had developed his own way of allowing certain patients to die by withholding all available care.

Some may believe I acted irresponsibly and unethically in not treating Mrs. Toivonen more aggressively. There has been a widespread perception in medical circles that all patients should receive the maximum possible care for any given medical problem. In medical schools, in conversations between physicians, and—until very recently—in the medical literature, there has been the tacit assumption that all patients (with the possible exception of the terminally ill) receive the maximum care. But it isn't so. We rarely discuss this reality or debate its ethics. Only recently has there been acknowledgment that this extraordinarily common, profoundly disturbing ethical deliberation is a daily part of our lives. Instead, the practicing physician has been left to fly by the seat of his pants.

Some might be tempted to dismiss the entire problem with the simple assertion that all patients deserve maximal care. Consider, however, the following situation. We have in our nursing-home a young woman who has been comatose for five years as a result of an accident. Although there is no reasonable chance that she will ever improve, she is not "brain dead" and is supported only by routine nursing care, consisting of tube feedings, regular turnings, urinary catheters, and good hygiene; she is on no respirator or other machine. If, on a routine yearly examination, her physician were somehow to discover that she was in danger of a life-threatening heart attack within the next few years, few persons, I think, would recommend full-scale evaluation for possibly corollary bypass surgery. The decision not to offer her maximal care might be justified in any one of several ways, but most often the question would simply not arise. It would seem obvious to the practicing physician that this particular patient should not receive such heroic treatment.

I think few would quarrel with the decision to withhold such evaluation and treatment. But once we have allowed that some persons should not receive some treatments that will prolong their lives, we must begin the thorny ethical process of "drawing lines": which patients? which treatments? If this comatose young woman should not get the bypass surgery, then what kinds of treatment might we offer her? How far should we go? Would we perform a major abdominal operation to repair a dangerous ballooning of the aorta, a major artery that would otherwise probably rupture and kill her within a matter of weeks? Would we perform routine surgery to cure appendicitis? Would we give her an IV to compensate for fluid loss if she had diarrhea? Would we give her medicines by mouth to treat an uncomplicated urinary-tract infection? Would we put in a new stomach tube so that she could be fed? Each person would draw the line differently, but once it is agreed that a certain heroic treatment will not be offered, that still doesn't tell us what to do. . . .

Notes

1. N.K. Brown and D.J. Thompson. Nontreatment of Fever in Extended Care Facilities. *New England Journal of Medicine* vol. 300 (1979): 246-250.

Further Reading

Daniel Callahan. 1990. *What Kind of Life: The Limits of Medical Progress*. Washington, D.C.: Georgetown University Press.

Marcia Millman. 1977. *The Unkindest Cut: Life in the Backrooms of Medicine*. New York: William Morrow.

Samuel Shem. 1978. *The House of God*. New York: Dell.

Discussion Questions

1. What sort of role should physicians play in treatment decisions concerning dying patients?

2. What kinds of criteria should physicians use for making end of life treatment decisions? What sorts of criteria do you think patients use? Where do family members fit in?

3. Should patients receive the maximum possible care for any given medical problem? Why or why not?

50

Baby Doe Before Regulations

Charles Bosk

Charles Bosk explores how shared understandings become translated into medical ethics. His perspective as a sociologist also forces him to ask what responsibility sociologists should assume for making sense of "what's going on." Bosk shows that, regardless of parental decisions, hospital personnel, however conflicted they might be, will not refuse treatment to an infant with severe congenital defects. In most instances, physicians try to avoid making any definitive decisions. Difficult questions, indicated in the previous selection by Hilfiker, become more complex as the number of persons responsible for the decision increases. As you read this selection, consider the personal and individual patient-related questions that Hilfiker raises. Bosk presents some of the same issues, this time, with regard to institutional and social group responsibilities for care and ranges of treatment. Consider the responsibilities of the sociologist, not merely as a researcher but as a member of the medical ethics team.

Medical decisions are multi-layered and require the participation of individual, institutional, and cultural actors. Who is legally liable? Who will accept moral responsibility? Private tragedies emerge as public discourse. Complicated ethical debates become obfuscated by legal quandaries. Personal conflict melds into group consensus. Consensus about treatment reduces individual lives and decisions to organizational outcomes and numbers. Ultimate accountability is not easy to pinpoint where medical ethics are concerned.

. . . In the NICUs (Neonatal Intensive Care Unit) of pediatric hospitals, the activist, indi-vidualistic ethos of American culture virtually enjoins the physician to act and the parents to wish for that action. The problem in intensive care then, is patterns of overzealous treatment, rather than neglect. What made the Baby Doe regulations such an intriguing development was that the entire drift of reports from intensive care units—whether they were autobiographical recountings of families, the reports of medical scientists in established journals, or sociological accounts of the dynamics of aggressive intervention in the NICU—indicated that the regulations, however they were modified, amended, understood, and applied, had the problem backwards (Guillemin and Holmstrom 1986; Stinson and Stinson 1979, 1983; Silverman 1981). . . .

Two Cases

The fact that genetic counselors were involved in each of the following cases meant that disagreements had spilled out of the private intensive care unit into the hospital and were a source of public trouble. Because both these cases became public hospital issues, previously unacknowledged differences became visible, and there was no simple way to disentangle participants, no way to smooth over ruffled feathers. These cases are separated in time by three years. Read that way, they are a simple illustration of how little progress had been made in one major American hospital in dealing with the kinds of questions and problems that arise when the shared understanding of physicians and parents of what is in the best interests of the child breaks down. Since the last case, "ethical consultation" has become available. How that changes situations when there is a conflict of intentions between parental and medical narratives for the child (Hunter 1991) is an important topic for future exploration. My intent in providing the detail I do in describing these cases is to give a sense of a "same-old, used-to-be" to describe the pediatrics hospital before "ethics" had a widespread presence at the bedside.

One last prefatory note: That the cases are separated by three years means that the depth of my access to data and my understanding of that data was different. When the first case arose, I was literally a few days in the field. It was my first attendance at rounds. I was unknown to many and trusted by few of the people in the setting. The second case became an issue at the end of my three years in the setting. By this time, more than a little trust had been built up. This case I was able to observe quite closely. I was quite literally dragged along into all negotiations by Palmer as "someone who could provide us some advice on what we are doing." The clear implication of this inclusion was that my advice was in the service, the thrall really, of Palmer's objectives. I was asked to be a witness, and also not to limit myself to witnessing alone. If I could provide some advice on how to avoid a disaster, in either human or public-relations terms, I should feel free to do so.

Case 1: The Baby

Case 1 is not so much a case as a discussion that occurred in clinical genetics rounds, the weekly meeting of pediatricians, social workers, nurses, and lab technicians who are involved in the ongoing work of the genetic counseling team. Dr. Bill Smith presented the case. He began by stating that for reasons "that would become clear," he neither wanted to bring the child down for the group (which numbered around thirty) to see, nor did he want the group to visit the bedside. That much said, he began to present the baby's history. He reported that he first saw the baby at ten hours of age. (Interestingly; in this case the baby was always referred to as *the baby* and never as *Baby Girl Smith* or even *the baby girl.*) The baby, he reported, had been born with multiple birth defects. The child was born without three limbs, without a jaw, with fusion of lip and palate, and with splenic-gonadal fusion. He continued his reporting: There was no known history of consanguinity in the family, nor was there any history of drug intake during pregnancy. Neurologically, the child was alert as a neonate should be. Given this clinical picture, he concluded that a diagnosis of one of the madibular syndromes with limb hypogenesis best fit the baby. These, he informed the group, were all mostly sporadic. At this point Dr. Smith had completed the normal presentation of a case

during genetic rounds: he had described the physical findings, identified the syndrome associated with those findings, and provided a recurrence risk.

At this point, the normal order of rounds would have been to discuss Dr. Smith's diagnosis—evaluate its adequacy—or if there were no questions, move on to the next case. But in this case, something else happened.[1] Dr. Smith continued his narrative. He said, "I don't know if this is the place to bring it up, but we've been agonizing over it for days now. The child has severe defects. The parents have asked for no surgical procedures. The surgeons are convinced this is a salvageable child, [who] has no life-threatening problems and will live with minor surgery. The parents plainly do not want any surgery."

Dr. Berger, chief of the genetics unit, was the first to speak after Smith had laid the doctors' dilemma on the table. He said, "We know how the Spartans felt about such babies. We are dealing here with a severely damaged child. It is hard to get the family to accept what is an impossible situation. We have to take a very hard, philosophical approach. This is a little like the thalidomide babies."

The baby's pediatrician, Dr. Abbott, refocused the discussion on the parents' rejection of the child and their resistance to surgical intervention: "The parents do not want this child treated. They do not want the child to go home. They have voiced this over and over again."

Berger here reminds the group that this is a statement which cannot be tolerated. "But obviously some future has to be faced. Not in one year. Not in two years. But now."

At this point, a physician whose name I had not yet learned, asked the question which until then had not been asked directly: "What if the family absolutely refuses surgery?"[2]

The question invited speculation. This baby, these parents. These times (the early years of the Carter administration). This surgeon. Those lawyers. This hospital administration. With so much variation, each new case has only weak precedents. Dr. Berger, official leader of the group, took a stab at answering the question: "Well, we leave to know what is the position of the hospital and what is the position of the parents in making this decision. In making these decisions, the courts have in the past made a plan for the child. Of course, it's also possible in the current climate that the courts would let the child die.[3] But such a course would be hard. I gather from the consultants that the plastic surgeons think they can do something for the child, and rehabilitation thinks they can do something for the child."

Realizing that the drift of this logic is into the surgical suite, Dr. Eggleston attacks a basic underlying premise of Berger's argument: the analogy to thalidomide babies. "Yes, but this is not like the thalidomide babies. Here we need an intervention. This is different. You have to make a positive decision to undertake surgery."

As far as Berger is concerned, *plus ça change, plus c'est la meme chose:* "But it is only minor surgery. A conservative approach would be to intervene, because this is a rehabilitable child."

At this point, Smith reenters the conversation with the observation that "socially, the parents want to abandon the child." Berger points out to him the distance between the desiring and the doing: "I don't know how easy it is for parents to abandon children."[4]

The questioner who opened up this whole sequence by asking, What if the parents absolutely refused? now complicates his own hypothetical question: "What would we do if the parents were Seventh-Day Adventists?" Smith, perhaps uneasy about all of this speculation, reports another item of the parents' behavior: "The parents have asked to have the child killed." This is a request that Berger takes at face value. "That's a shock reaction." The doctors' dilemma won't go away: What if they absolutely refuse? The original framer of this hypothetical question projects it into the future: "What if they took the child home and it died? What if we did nothing? Could they be prosecuted?"[5]

Smith fields this question with a discussion of what the drill is for today, not tomorrow: "This is all becoming a question of hospital policy." He then states his understanding of that policy: "We are not going to starve this child. If it arrests, we are not going to resuscitate." This is not a policy nor a plan that satisfies Berger. He grumbles: "That's

wishing away a bad situation, and it's not just going to go away. The child is not going to die."

Berger's remark seems to generate yet another hypothetical question: "If the state intervenes and if the child undergoes surgery, then who is financially responsible?" The normally pragmatic Berger fails to answer this question and responds with a Panglosian piety: "These are extreme situations which we are beginning to face everyday; whose financial problem is the child? This is such a rare situation. It's a chance event. Why should we victimize the parents and tell them to dedicate their lives because of a random event. If society decides that these children should be saved, then let society take care of them. And let us let the parents come to some moral and spiritual resolution of this situation themselves."

Berger has a certain sympathy for Smith's immediate problems. But he reminds him and the assembled group that the parents should not be crushed because the physicians found themselves squeezed between the rock of what a physician's sense of responsibility obligated him or her to do and the hard place of the society's lack of resources for dealing with the chronically handicapped: "Well we can't treat these parents like they are victims of the Inquisition. Who knows how any of us would react? We can't force people either to cope or not to cope with such extreme situations."

At this point, the physician who originally objected to the thalidomide analogy reinvokes it: "There's always the danger of brainwashing the parents. You're always citing the exceptions, the children, the thalidomide children who did well."

Berger agrees: "Yes, we also have this myelomeningocele, where two-thirds are retarded. Yet we are always talking about the one-third that does well. And now society is getting more and more into the act, which is very much different than saying, 'Here's your baby, go find a quiet cliff and deal with it.'"

Smith at this point adds an encouraging note: "Well, we are evolving solutions to these problems. But they [the parents] are trying to make the baby disappear. We're trying to keep it alive." At this point, Berger closed discussion of the case with the pronouncement: "Well, we can't make an ultimate projection of what the parents will do or how the baby will do in the long run."

Let me note that the case had the following resolution. Surgery was planned despite the parents' objections. However, as this was all happening, the infant developed a breathing problem and died. Berger was wrong; some bad situations do disappear. Three years later, the parents gave birth to a healthy infant.

Time Passes

It is three years later. All the contextual variables in which clinical decisions are made have changed. The field of applied human genetics has advanced technically. Changes are, of course, too numerous to detail here and still discuss the process of decision making when parents challenge physicians; nevertheless, some deserve mention. Operationally, the most important is that the status of amniocentesis has changed from that of a procedure that is assumed safe, but not definitely known to be so, to one whose safety has been documented by the Canadian, United States, and United Kingdom registry studies. Amniocentesis is now a clinical routine of obstetrics. Further advances in the technology of cytogenetics have made it possible to identify genetic abnormalities through increasingly subtle "markers." At the same time, technical progress in the field of neonatal intensive care has made it possible to salvage babies of lower and lower birth weights. The American Public has been kept aware of such advances and their downside risks through local television media, local newspapers, and a variety of national magazines, including *Consumer Reports, Atlantic,* and *Time.*

At a local level, both the genetic counseling group and the facilities for neonatal intensive care have evolved. Most obviously, its members, in Schutz's memorable phrase, "have grown older together" (1971, 220). Over three years, operating rules of thumb, tacit understandings, and informal norms for handling work have been in constant flux because of changes in membership.[6] Twice now, clinic coordinators have come and gone. A social worker or genetics associate, the clinic coordinator is a key figure in organizing the work of the genetics group. More significantly, Berger, the leader and academic patron of the younger physicians who are genetic counselors, has left. His replacement, Dr. Palmer, is an unknown quantity. His investment in the "special mission" of genetic counseling is suspect. However, as chair of the Pediatrics Department, his political authority in the hospital is firmly established. Careers are at stake in personnel changes such as this; it was a highly stressful time for the genetic counselors. Brooding about the future had become a very popular collective activity.

Things have not been all that calm in either the newborn nursery or the neonatal intensive care unit either. Nurses in the newborn nursery have taken issue on several occasions with physicians' decisions both to attempt or to refrain from attempting salvage of compromised neonates. After much wrangling, an official policy has been outlined detailing the broad criteria on which judgments are based.

Despite this effort, a lack of clarity still remains about the process of making judgments: who is involved, with what authority, and with what dispute-resolution mechanisms are all areas of continuing uncertainty. Meanwhile, intensive care has become one of the areas where the "action" is in pediatrics. The nurses view themselves as an elite corps with special skills, disposition, and courage. The field also has a charisma and ethos for physicians. . . . In the world of pediatric intensive care, physicians and nurses casually wear their "courage to fail" ethos on the sleeves of their scrub suits.

Moreover, what Berger referred to as the "current climate" when speculating about what actions the courts might take if the parents absolutely refused surgery has changed. First, a significant right-to-life group has moved politically from the fringe to the mainstream—to breakfast at prayer meetings with a newly elected president. These groups have grown more militant and aggressive in their protection of fetal and neonatal "rights." All of the physicians at the pediatric hospital were well aware of the potential politicization of any decision not to treat, and the attendant media spectacle that could result. How this constrained their thinking about cases is difficult to gauge precisely; that it did so is undeniable.

Finally, the fieldworker has changed as well. I took in the first case described here with the phenomenological wonder of a child. The second I took in with a sense of phenomenological fatigue, a weariness from seeing all too many of what the genetic counselors refer to as "God's mistakes." In fact at the time of the second case, I had officially withdrawn from the field, ostensibly to begin writing up my data. However, the impending birth of my first child made it unbearable to see, on a routine basis, so many parents whose desires for a "perfect" baby had been disappointed at the start. I was called back both by Smith and by Palmer, each of whom for reasons of their own wanted a sounding board to share their thoughts, feelings, and frustrations as the case unfolded. Smith and Palmer had been generous with themselves as informants; I owed them much, and I could not easily refuse their request to help out by observing a case that they described as "one I would be interested in."[7] I returned to the field, but I took notebook in hand with much reluctance.

To provide some comparability between the discussions of the two cases, I shall, as with the first case, report only on one conference, despite the fact that I was privy to much more. The conference was called after the contest over clinical autonomy was resolved, and its purpose was to review that resolution.

Case 2: Baby Boy Flannery

Boy Flannery had been born seven days previously with trisomy 21 and duodenal atresia (a stricture in the intestine that makes normal feeding impossible). At the time that the neonatologist explained the treatment options to the father, he included in his presentation the right to refuse surgery. The father of the child (the mother at this time was not yet informed of the child's problems) chose to exercise this option. This decision was unacceptable to the nursing staff of the newborn nursery—they refused to carry it out. For them, not treating in this instance was not a branch of the decision tree. Operation-

ally, the nurses on staff had the organized authority to call the question. As a group, they rejected not treating as an option. The neonatologists then negotiated an agreement late on a Friday afternoon to assume custody of the baby, arrange for its transfer to Nightingale which is affiliated with the newborn nursery, repair its stomach, and then place it up for adoption.

First thing Monday morning, Friday's agreement proved unworkable. No mechanisms existed, to the satisfaction of all parties for the parents quickly and definitively to relinquish custody, for the courts to authorize repair, for the surgeons to repair, and for the child to secure "an alternative parental environment."[8] Nightingale Children's Center refused to accept transfer of the child without a surgical consent. Tuesday passed trying to arrange transfer of the child to another hospital that would agree to nonrepair. No hospital could be found. By this time, a third party ready to press for the child's right to life in court had materialized. On Wednesday, the parents agreed to the transfer. On Thursday the surgery was done. Friday was conference day.

I was informed of the conference about two hours before it was to begin, by Bill Smith. I asked Smith what the hurry was. He told me that he had objected strongly to the conference: "It's appropriate to have a conference when the dust has settled, but not now, you know what I mean? Emotionally and scientifically, what good can it do now? People are too involved."[9] He pointed out that, as a rule, death and dying conferences were held two weeks after the event, and that gave people a little time to cool out. He said that he was "frightened" about what could come out of a conference. Smith told me that, "knowing no good" could come of this conference, he had tried to block the neonatology fellow from scheduling it. The fellow, whom he described as a stubborn type, dug in his heels and would not reschedule the conference. Smith went over his head and called one of the attendings in neonatology. From him he learned that the entire group of neonatologists wanted the conference and wanted it now. As a group, they had all supported offering the nontreatment option to the parents. They felt "sandbagged" by the administration. The group was "angry, very angry" and, "short of quitting," did not know what to do. The neonatologists felt that they were "being told how to practice medicine and that they had been blocked from a legitimate treatment option."

It's worth noting that at the time (1981), the neonatologists had every reason in the world to believe that they had indeed been sandbagged. It's also worth noting that times have changed. A new norm has emerged. Today the neonatologists are much less likely to support the parents. The parents, faced with in-hospital ethical help, are less likely to push the point. But consensus reached is not always consensus sustained. Scarce resources, the need to constrain medical cost, less collective generosity for the chromosomally different—all threaten the current ethical consensus. One never knows until cases make new problems. But back then, the physicians were sandbagged, and the nurses were right. Operationally, not treating was not part of the decision tree at Nightingale.

The conference, which was scheduled for 1:00 P.M., started a mere ten minutes later, a remarkable display of punctuality for such an ad hoc meeting. There were twenty-seven people in attendance: representatives of neonatology, genetics, surgery, and social services, as well as several "interested" members of the hospital community who had heard about the case. Dr. Mackrides—head of the Newborn Nursery—sat on the left front side of the table; Dr. Palmer, at the right. Whether ominously or innocently, no one took that place at the head of the table. Dr. Mackrides began the conference. She directed everybody's attention to a handout detailing what happened when, gave a brief oral summary of the case, announced the purpose of the meeting as being "to discuss what happened," and turned the floor over to Dr. Palmer.

Dr. Palmer began: "This is an instructive case, just as all cases should be instructive to physicians. The first thing we need to do is recognize the physician's responsibility in cases of this sort. The first responsibility of the physician is to give an expert explanation of Down's syndrome, trisomy 21, and its obvious association with the vomiting in this case. This was done right from the beginning,

since Dr. Smith had met with the family [the father] for three hours on Friday, the day the child was born. What is known in this case is that the child has a relatively easily correctable defect, that it is a viable child without heart disease but with mongolism. Rather than to inject our own values into the case, our responsibility is to present every reasonable treatment option. In this case we learned what our reasonable options are; we also learned what the nonviable options are. For twenty-four to forty-eight hours, we had all thought we would be able to assume custody of the child. The next time this happens—and the next time will probably be next week, since these things happen in twos and threes—well, we'll know that option is not present."[10]

There was then some discussion in which various members of the hospital staff involved with the case all expressed their surprise at finding out that the transfer of custody was legally complicated. One member of the audience was incredulous. He asked, "How does this case differ from guardianship? Hospitals assume guardianship all the time. How is this different from going to the courts and getting an order?"

Mackrides does not so much answer this question as frame all the hospital's actions as being guided by the goal of providing the parents' support. She says, "In our attempts to support the parents, we did not want to obtain a court order. We felt that would be violating the rights, the beliefs, the whatever-you-have, of the parents. We decided not to take the case to court, but to try and support them."

Dr. Palmer places this support in the larger context of alternative scenarios the physicians might have had to face in this case. "I want to back up and talk about the options. The first is to tell the parents what mongolism is and means, to say that the child has no heart lesion but, with gastrointestinal surgery, will be a normal Down's syndrome child, and then have the parents say, 'This is a child, this is our child, and this is one we want to take home. We want the child to be repaired.' Obviously this did not happen in this case. That brings us to option two. Here the parents say, 'We want the child to have normal surgery and care, and we will reserve the decision about the child's ultimate disposition. We will all work together to make long-run decisions in the future.' This option was also rejected in this case. The parents then have option three—they can say 'We have decided we do not want the child to live. We feel in our hearts that we cannot let this child come into our home. We cannot let this child live.' If the parents choose this option, as was the case here, then there are two branching options that have to be considered: Whether this will happen in this institution, or whether the child will go elsewhere. It is this hospital's policy not to carry out neglect both for legal reasons and because of the institution's philosophy. This leaves parents the option of taking the child home to die. Frankly, I would not have mentioned to the parents the option of refusing surgery. It confused the parents, and we all did not appreciate the legal aspects of taking the child home. The parents could be slapped with a neglect or a murder suit by the prosecutors. The way this case evolved, the parents—we all—had to be educated to their real options. At any time, the institution could have said, 'We'll go to the courts.' But we wanted to help the parents to come to the right decision, and a court order would have created more problems than it would have solved. At one time, the parents' lawyer and the hospital's lawyer went to the courts to gather information privately. Now I wasn't a party to those discussions, but the parents must have found they had no good option, because they decided to sign for surgery."

Dr. Farley, a pediatrician interested in medical ethics, felt Palmer's presentation narrowed the parents' options unreasonably. "I think the parents got bad advice if they were told that they didn't have the right to refuse treatment. The trend in this country in the courts so far has been to maximize the patient's right to refuse care. No state has gone against this trend. The most recent case which has a bearing here—the New Jersey Supreme Court ruling in the Quinlan case—sees this decision as a private matter between the family and the physicians. As one looks over twenty years of legal precedent, the right to maximize refusal seems to be fairly well

established. The option to refuse treatment is real in many states, including a neighboring one. As far as I am concerned the rights of the child and of the parents have been abrogated in this case."

Palmer responded, "Let's assume that what you say is correct—and I'm not willing to grant that—our institutional policy is not to support neglect. We will support parents in their decision making. I am familiar with a case where the parents took the child home, and it died later. The parents could go somewhere else. Either way if you go either way, you have to be certain in this state, in this country, of the legal ramifications—be sure you know what is going to happen to you. I am not a lawyer. I am not a judge. I am not God. Both the parents and I have to be sure no prosecutor is going to bring charges."

Dr. Mackrides here tried to move the discussion from hypothetical to empirical matters. "If the parents had refused, the hospital was determined, if it did not get permission within a certain time, to get a court order. This is not a personal theory; this was going to happen."

Farley here points out that there is a difference between trying to obtain a court order and actually having one. "But the court could have said no. This is a matter of privacy. It is between the families and physicians to agree on a course of action. In fact, it is hard to imagine the courts countermanding the parents' decision to refuse."

There is one weakness in Farley's hypothetical point; it is an empirical one, and Palmer is quick to point it out. "If that is the case," he wanted to know, "why did they go to court on Wednesday and come away signing for the operation."

Farley is undeterred. He maintains, with a correctness more fitting to law review articles than to everyday life, that "the trend in the law is to back away from such matters and call them private."

As this debate on legal theory wound down, Dr. Mackrides added a new piece of information. "I should mention here that a member of a child-advocate group called me to get information on the child in order to get an injunction to forbid the parents from signing the child out against medical advice. It was a matter of timing. If the parents had signed out AMA, an agency was going to get an injunction that would have tried to force the parents to consent to surgery." Palmer pointed out that this was an example of a point he had been trying to make, that the parents were bound to be put under lots of pressure.

Dr. Kraft, a neonatologist, asked, "What finally turned the parents around?"

Palmer answered, "I wish I knew."

Here the surgeon who performed the surgery added a pious homily: "May I suggest that the case was turned around because the parents realized that we were—that the doctors in this case realized that it was not just a child but a family that needed help—that we came *to* but not *at* the parents." He added that the family was now considering taking the child home.

Dr. Mackrides had some difficulty with this description. "That is a very idealistic picture. I think what happened was that they exhausted all other possibilities. My perception is that at one point they were asking what is worse, the publicity from signing or not signing. They repeatedly talked about the publicity, the newspapers, the intrusion on their private lives. It wasn't an idealistic move. Right now they are exploring adoption agencies."

At this point, someone asked, "What if they had refused?"

Palmer responded, "That is a reasonable question. I had decided if they wanted to sign out AMA, that we would allow them to do so. Any hospital has to allow this. I cannot answer what I would have done if they had signed out—if I had an obligation to report neglect, to seek an injunction, to file a CY 147 [a report of suspected child abuse]. I think personally I would not have sought an injunction, but as to whether the hospital would have, I do not know." For Palmer, who is chairman of pediatrics of the hospital, this distinction between what he would do and what the hospital would do is an extreme equivocation or an act of public discretion. What is interesting is what is not said: what the hospital would have done. And surely as the doer of hospital action, Palmer had at least a theory about that. His "personal" position is clear. His official, "public" policy is not articulated.[11]

Someone points out, "But there was a third party ready to seek an injunction."

Palmer answers, "There is always a third party in this kind of institution."

At this point, a short discussion of adoption policy and lots of side involvement mark the meeting. The discussion is put on course by a neonatology fellow who asks, "What about the charge that the parents were badgered, that they were in a grief reaction, and that they couldn't make up their minds. Why didn't we use hyperal solution to hydrate the baby until the parents got over the initial shock?"

Mackrides, Palmer, and the surgeon all assured the questioner that this was exactly what happened. Following this, Farley objected that all the effort in this case had been toward coercing consent and that nontreatment was never realistically considered. Palmer stated that no one in the hospital had threatened the parents with legal action, but that they themselves bowed before the legal threat nontreatment represented.

Mackrides added, "A major side of this case hasn't been discussed. When the parents first decided not to treat, prior to their attempts to relinquish custody, I had agreed with the parents' decision not to support it. I went to the nurses to say that this is the situation. Here is the baby, we are not going to support it. I had a nursing revolt on my hands. My young nurses looking at this healthy baby couldn't carry out this decision. They thought this was a place to maintain life. The same sentiment emerged among medical students, house officers, and fellows. The question I have is how to carry out a decision that involves such grief and pain to my staff."

Palmer said that he had been through this once or twice before and that "inevitably the surgery gets done. If the physicians agree to support the parents, the administration doesn't. If administration is supportive, then the nurses aren't. And if the nurses support the parents, and they inevitably do not, then there are outside threats. The best thing to do is to defuse the situation as quickly and quietly as possible."

One neonatologist stated, "Then one of the things we have learned is not doing anything is not an option."

Farley objected that it was important that it remain an option.

Palmer responded, "No, logically, it is not an option. Because here you are using duodenal atresia as a method of euthanasia. I want to sort that out. We can't use one condition as a reason for euthanasia because of another condition, mongolism."

This would have seemed to end the discussion, but someone asked if the parents had to be told before the surgery that the child had trisomy 21. A long discussion on truth-telling and its pros and cons followed. Once this discussion ended, Dr. Mackrides began to wrap up the conference. "No one can deny that it is a difficult problem. I have calculated that excluding today's conference, 386 man-hours have gone to resolving it. Perhaps Dr. Palmer would like to make a few concluding remarks."

Palmer states, "This case has been an important learning experience. What is important is that now we know what the real options are. What caused such problems here is that we held out to the parents an option that didn't exist. In the future, we must avoid this. We must judge each case on its own merits with respect for the dignity of the persons involved. We must recognize that there are at least three patients." But there is a contradiction here, for if all trisomy 21 children will be operated on, if that is the general rule, then there is no reason to look at each case on its merits.

This speech closed the conference. As I left the room, Palmer came over to me. He asked me what I thought. I shrugged my shoulders. He said, "if this is what goes on at Mecca, I would hate to see how these things are handled in the boondocks."

Time Stops

In this section, I turn to an analysis and interpretation of the situations, decisions, and presumptions that governed decision-making in the two Baby Doe analogues presented above.

Before doing so, let me add a gratuitous editorial comment or two, so that the reader can better gauge my own biases. First, although the parents' desire for nontreatment is similar in the two cases, each presents to the pediatricians involved very different questions. Had I been required to act rather than just observe, my response to each case would have been very different. In the first case, I would have had no problems with nontreatment. The magnitude of the child's problems, the potential quality of life, the parents' response—all of these made intervention appear less than noble to me. In addition, I never escaped the feeling that an overly optimistic picture of the child's future was being projected by the surgeons and the physicians in rehabilitation medicine—this feeling was confirmed by the child's demise. But there was no necessity to this. Save for a "breathing problem," a miracle might have been manufactured.

With the second case, like Palmer, like the parents as the situation unfolded, I am extremely uncomfortable using duodenal atresia as a pretext for euthanasia of children with trisomy 21. But, like Farley, I am troubled by the constriction of choices. The hospital's mode of resolving the problem unsettled me. I am not sure that the parents hadn't become the victims to the Inquisition that the recently departed Berger had warned about in the first case.

Collective vs. Individual Responsibility

For me, as a sociologist, the most striking feature of the way each of the two cases is defined is this: No single physician claims decision-making authority in either case. Health care in America is not yet socialized; yet it certainly seems that, at least in this hospital, responsibility for patients has been. This jointly held responsibility explains why conflicts over nontreatment were so difficult to resolve. In complex bureaucratic settings such as hospitals, with their delimited zones of formal authority, patients move in and out of different administrative classifications, confusing who is in charge. The discourse by the physicians does not stress individual responsibility. Rather it frames the question collectively: "What should *we* as a medical staff do?" This framing recognizes how often responsibility is transferred either temporarily to a colleague on call or, more permanently, to those outside the NICU. Collective rather than individual responsibility maximizes the opportunity for a group consensus to operate, but it maximizes as well the potential for disagreement and, absent mechanisms for resolving such discord, it maximizes the opportunities for decision-making paralysis.

There are, it should go without saying, some structural features related to the organization of care which reinforce this pattern of collective decision making. First, the patients are neonates. By definition, there is no long-standing relationship with a family on which to draw in evaluating treatment options. The therapeutic relationship here is among strangers.[12] Second, the staffing patterns of the NICU encourage collective responsibility. Attendings are on for a week, rotate off for two, and then are back on. When on, attendings have total responsibility; when off, only so much as they wish to assume. As a result, attendings know that they will have to live with a certain number of collegial decisions that they might have handled otherwise and vice versa.

In addition, most of the problematic cases fall outside the boundaries of what might be called normal intensive care. These are neonates with multisystem problems. Thus, to the team of intensive care physicians are added all the consultants that inhabit modern research centers. In cases of disagreement, these physicians not only have to consider the well-being of the individual patient, they need to consider their future work relations with one another. In cases where parents disagree with physicians, and physicians disagree with one another, a recurrent question is, "How are the claims of these parents whom I deal with but once matched against the claims of colleagues I need to work with day in and day out."

There are a number of dangers inherent in defining the clinical responsibility as collective. The first is, of course, that although decision making involves hordes of physicians,

it is not collective in any deeper sense which reflects a communal consensus, which echoes a shared normative order. Rather, it might just as well be the case that when all the physicians gather together in one room, colleagues bow to those physicians involved with the strongest feelings about what should be done. In the two cases presented above, the pediatric surgeon consulted was also a born-again Christian with very strong feelings about each child's right to life. Here the confluence of personal beliefs and professional capacity operates to nullify parental choice.

In a context that looks like open debate, something else operates. That something else is very close to the tendency to view clinical autonomy in *absolute* terms and to brand any infringement of it as anathema. From such a viewpoint, peer review of medical care, technology assessment, cost-benefit approaches to alternative therapeutic regimes, consulting with ethics committees, and so on are unacceptable and are therefore resisted. Absolute views of clinical freedom likewise discount patient wishes and quality-of-life arguments. The general point is that conceptions of collective responsibility with special structures and processes do not of themselves guarantee enlightened decision making. Especially when inside the collective forum, some believe that no limits may sensibly be placed on the physician's duty to save a life. In this ethos it is playing God to limit the physician, while aggressive treatment is a human thing to do. That the terms of the debate might be skewed is rarely, if ever, the focus of the debate.

So seen, collective responsibility in some ways reduces each decision maker's stake in the outcome. This allows those without some special interest to leave the field to those with ideological axes to grind. Collective rituals of decision sharing can become ways in which responsibility is abrogated as well as embraced. As a result, the genetic counselors, whatever their misgivings about their colleagues' actions, collude with those colleagues. They act less as mediators of conflict and more as facilitators for treatments that they do not necessarily approve. When parents do not dig in their heels, little conflict is generated. However, when parents resist, the kinds of tensions these cases illustrate proliferate. Genetic counselors, however, (in the language of the housestaff) are not "players" in resolving this trouble. Their position is clear; their value-neutrality and commitment to client autonomy lead them to support parents. Yet their actions do not reinforce their sentiments. Their deference to "green-suited claims to authority" renders them unable even to articulate these sentiments.

If others do not constrain aggressive NICU intervention, neither does the allocation of the costs of mistakes and misjudgments. None of the key medical decision makers have to live with any of the consequences of their decisions. There are no economic costs that fall upon providers from salvaging infants that are better left unsalvaged. Because in the American system there is no fixed sum allocated for health-care, there is no pressure on any individual physicians to consider the costs of a treatment, or the resource implications of salvaging a particular child, or even what it might mean to the emotional life of the family. This is not to say that individual physicians never consider these issues, but that there is very little incentive for them to do so. This reinforces whatever tendencies exist to divorce clinical action from individual responsibility. In the first case, had the child lived, the physicians involved were in a position to congratulate themselves, and they would have been shielded to a large degree from any of the negative features of the salvage. As much as the genetic counselors may have felt it was wrong "to victimize the parents and force the parents to dedicate their lives to a random event," they seemed, if not quite willing to allow that to happen, powerless to stop it. Moreover, had it happened, all of the actors debating what to do would have had limited long-term involvement with the family. This allows the freedom to intervene, whether it is individual or collective, to operate without a commensurate sense of responsibility for consequences.

Public vs. Private

The second layer of complexity in these cases rests on whether they are defined as public or private issues. In the first case we see in Berger's comments about the tendency of society to get involved the realization that old ways are changing. Three years later this change is complete, at least in the minds of medical personnel. A generalized fear of third parties dominates discussion of the second case. Only marginally does concern about what they should do guide the doctors' talk about the case. Rather, there is a preoccupation with what others will do if they pursue this or that course of action. Significantly, this concern is grounded in reality, the dubious direct interest of others in the case notwithstanding. For example, in Danville, Illinois, the aftermath of a "do not feed" order involving newborn Siamese twins illustrates just how decisive third parties can be (Robertson 1981). Nurses in the hospital disobeyed the order and secretly fed the twins. The Illinois Department of Children and Family Services was given an anonymous tip that the children were ordered to be starved to death. Armed with custody and transfer orders, the department and state's attorney moved to protect the lives of the twins. Charges of attempted murder (and thirteen other lesser offenses) were brought against the parents and physicians on the basis of complicity in the "do not feed" order.

In the more recently publicized Baby Jane Doe case, a Vermont lawyer and right-to-life advocate filed briefs to overturn a Long Island couple's refusal to consent to surgery for their severely damaged newborn.[13] What goes on in the doctor-patient relationship is clearly not private and confidential in any ordinary sense. There appears to exist a rather wide audience of interested bystanders ready to act if the clinical autonomy of doctor and/or patient strays too widely from some unspecified rule about what is just and moral. This problem is, of course, exacerbated in an American context where care is framed in a rhetoric of individual rights and entitlements rather than in a rhetoric of balancing collective needs.

Further, the difficulties of exercising autonomy in an intensive care setting are amplified by a design feature of the environment. As most are well aware, the typical intensive care unit is one of several large open rooms. Their design makes it possible to wheel in whatever supportive equipment is necessary to support life and to permit monitoring of patients from a single vantage point. All action is public: it takes place in the open in full view of the entire medical and nursing staff, as well as visitors to the unit. Ethics of the practice aside, it is physically impossible to leave infants to the side to die; there is no such place out of the view of others.

Although the treatment of neonates at the margin of viability is a public issue, it has a private dimension as well. As Guillemin and Holmstrom point out, "almost all American babies are hospital born, and, if critically ill, are transported to intensive care within a closed bureaucratic system managed by like-minded hospital personnel. The transfer of an infant from a community hospital to a central hospital, or from an obstetric division to the NICU in the same hospital, avoids critical outside judgment. The captive clientele nature of critically ill newborns referred to intensive care reduces the possibility of conflict about referral, and consequently, the chances of legal dispute" (1983, 94). Furthermore, intensive care is regionalized in the American system. As a result, transport often removes parents from an effective decision-making role. The complexity and immediacy of much of the decision making regarding critically ill newborns also makes such activity a private medical matter, further reducing the parents' involvement.

There are two sides to the public and private nature of decision making in intensive care. By and large, the majority of cases become private decisions of the medical staff. In those rare cases where parents object to medical action, or physicians and parents agree to salvage efforts, the public nature of the decision is likely to come into play. This issue is framed in terms of the infant's rights and the threat that non-treatment poses not just to this infant, but to the class of all such infants. In the American context, there are really quite limited opportunities for withholding treatment from infants. The pressure in the American context is for treatment. Needless to say, automatic treatment is hardly a careful balancing of interests. In this light, the two cases presented above are interesting for what they reveal about how physicians feel constrained by forces well outside their control.

Professional vs. Personal Considerations

The third and last aspect of the cases under discussion that warrants discussion is the types of rationales which support action. Here we find the greatest divergence between medical and lay decision makers. It is a sociological commonplace to claim that medical authority in particular and professional authority in general rests on mastery of a formal body of theoretic knowledge. Physicians in Nightingale's intensive care units see their patients in terms of malfunctioning systems and what is needed to correct them. Talk about patients at rounds is organized by a ten-point checklist, or systems review. Residents refer to the discussion of cases at rounds as "going down the numbers." There is no irony here; the talk about patients in rounds is almost entirely talk about numbers. Discussion of family variables is rare enough to prompt a request to return to the topic (Frader and Bosk 1981). Progress is thought of in numeric terms: Are today's numbers better than yesterday's? All of this technical talk may be necessary if sick neonates are to be cared for properly. It is the essence of professional mastery. It is also a radical decontextualization of the patient as a person.

Physicians as professionals think about patients in one other set of professional terms: Physicians have also come to speculate about the legal bearing of their actions. Both cases presented in this selection contain a great deal of hypothetical legal thinking. This is the most common form of ethical discourse that one finds in medical settings. In recent years, the development of internalized dispute-resolution mechanisms has only accelerated the translation of ethical questions into legal terms. This reduction of complicated ethical problems to legal matters no doubt makes sense. It has, as well, the unfortunate consequence of taking a complicated issue such as who decides the standard of care and translating it into a question of power and authority.

The point here is not that physicians make bad legal philosophers (some do, some do not); rather the point is that a great deal of the world's complexity is washed out when severely compromised neonates are viewed in either technical terms (Can we save this baby?) or legal ones (For what consequences am I liable if I treat or fail to treat, this infant whose life I have the capacity to save?). Entire cultural frames disappear.

Of these, perhaps the most significant is the biographical, familial frame in which parents tend to view their children. If physicians decontextualize infants into organ systems, parents recontextualize them as children in families. Children are beings for whom parents have wishes, dreams, desires, fears, and anxieties. Parents project onto children a role in a family system. Quite literally, parents and physicians talk about children in two different realms of discourse that offer few, if any, points of contact. What is so striking about the cases related above is how inattentive, almost deaf, the physicians are to the parents' concerns (Hunter 1991). Even when the parents are heard, their concerns are seen as human and understandable, but certainly not decisive. Generally, physicians as decision makers need not pay great attention to parental wishes and desires, which are seen as subjective and unreliable (Anspach 1988) or irrelevant (Frader and Bosk 1981).

This point only underscores one more persistent "rough edge" of medical practice: There are simply some fault lines where professional and lay criteria do not meet. Neonatologists measure their craft by their success at salvaging lower and lower birth-weight babies. Follow-up of those babies over the long haul has not been necessary for establishing professional authority. Parents are concerned for a child's healthiness and normality. They measure their fortune or misfortune by how close to the norm their child is. Between these two standards, there is much room for misunderstanding. Each position provides a different warrant for the exercise of decision-making authority. Given how different these warrants are, we might well wonder that there are not more times of open discord between treating physicians and resisting parents.

Public Myth and Private Fears

My task in this selection was to present two cases where parents sought (and failed) to withdraw treatment over physician objections. These cases illustrate the philosophical and ethical problems in making treatment and nontreatment decisions. What remains is to tie together the description and analysis and to anticipate some likely sources of criticism.

Let us begin with the last task first. The first objection I would raise concerns the narrative framework of the cases discussed. The presentation of the cases does some violence to reality. As the cases unfolded, the events did not emerge quite as neatly as the case presentation here makes it appear. This text is clearly a reconstructed, edited version. The meetings, as they happened, took longer and were less orderly than the narrative discussion implies. Speakers made false starts. Long digressions have been edited out. This editing is quite clearly a potential source of bias. I have turned two meetings in one hospital into stories. Sociologists analyze data; ethnographers do so by interpreting accounts of behavior that they themselves create. Why accept an account from an ethnographic witness?

How do we know they are true stories? The fact that when participants were shown the narrative it accorded with their sense of what happened is hardly comfort. This was how the actors remembered the events. But this is really a weak defense: their memory could be as self-serving as mine. A stronger defense is that narratives are an extraordinarily human way to recall the past. The way parts are arranged into a whole is what creates a tale of social conduct out of an account of mere behavior. The claim for my narrative descriptions is not that their are completely accurate renditions of what happened or the only possible ones. Palmer and Farley, not to mention Bill Smith, all tell very different stories. The claim is more modest: They are a plausible reconstruction, which makes confrontation of certain social dilemmas unavoidable. The goal of the narrative reconstruction is not a phenomenologically perfect snapshot, but an impressionistic sketch—all the better to evoke a response and reaction (Nisbet 1976; Van Maanen 1988).

Even if they are plausible narrative reconstructions, these two cases discuss rare events. Baby Doe situations where a decisive medical intervention will save a life and where the parents are opposed are rare. But underlying conflict between lay persons and professionals is not. Among physicians and patients, the most common cases involve no such disputes over dramatic intervention. Those that do are cases that unfold slowly over time, without a clear-cut decisive moment, and with distrust building slowly—a bricolage of missed signals and offhand remarks. These cases are unrepresentative of the complexity of nontreatment issues raised by aggressive treatment of the newborn. One sinks, rather than leaps, into disaster.

To this objection there is a good deal of truth, and the answer to it is not wholly satisfactory. That is to say, Baby Doe cases represent a public myth about the structure of medical care in the hospital context. Questions of empirical frequency aside, examining the myth serves to lay bare some of the underlying tensions that beset medical care. The resolution of Baby Doe regulations as a chapter in the bureaucratic regulation of medical practice does not, of course, fully resolve the tensions concerning who is a legitimate decision maker in a nontreatment decision when the patient is incompetent.

Such tensions have entered the public arena in other forms, their presence signaled by case names: Quinlan, Bouvia, Cruzan. That neither of the two cases described here reached such notoriety does not mean that they did not rehearse the same issues. Rather, it indicates that in neither case did the parents want to sacrifice their privacy to make in a public arena their claims of private sovereignty over their child's well being.

Notes

1. There is a little retrospective judgment here. I could not, at the time (this being of rounds), have known how this case was not typical or normal.

2. Remember this is my first day in this setting. I did not know who was who. I was phenomenologically overloaded. I had heard that physicians discussed such things, but I had never heard such a discussion. It was hard enough to grasp what was being said, let alone record who was saying what. Sometimes, the trickiest bit of ethnographic work is the first part: the getting straight of who said what to whom.

3. Berger's estimate of the current climate has only grown more accurate. At any rate, invocations of the "current climate" are extemporaneous judgment. There is a recurrent frustration in writing about the "current climate" in applied clinical genetics: the climate changes quickly; the publication process for any report on the current climate is much slower.

4. According to a considerable historical literature, it may not be so difficult for parents to abandon children as Berger suggests. Certainly, evidence of child abandonment is not absent in contemporary American society. To be fair, the normative response appears to be the opposite: parents assume responsibility for less-than-perfect newborns.

5. The questioner might have asked about his own legal liability here as well: Is silence consent? And if in all this there is a felony and felons, are there not also accessories? The boundaries in these matters, being set by prosecutorial creativity, are difficult to trace with precision.

6. Numerous as these changes are, flux is perhaps the normal standard of things in American teaching hospitals, what with regular rotations, academic leave, and the normal mobility that is part of a career.

7. Ethnographers have not, as a rule, spent enough time thinking about how our subjects produce data for us on the basis of their judgments of what we might find interesting; how they place us "on call" for the things they think we want to see.

8. The quotation marks here indicate not a naive usage at the time, but a relabeling years later by me of this last question, which was the place where understanding broke down.

9. Ethnographers often criticize documentary journalism for "putting into words" subjects' private thoughts. We ethnographers don't do that sort of thing, of course. But here I report a "snatch" from a private phone conversation. What kind of person behaves this way? Don't accurate reports from the backstage inevitably violate some sort of privacy? And, more gloom, still, doesn't the violation of privacy by

individual ethnographic actions weaken privacy as a collective ideal?

10. Palmer's reference here to things happening in cascades ("twos and threes") reflects a widespread folk-belief among physicians that rare events cluster in time in ways that defy mere statistical probability. Certainly, the general surgeons I have studied (Bosk 1979) shared this belief. I suppose it could be empirically tested. But if the belief was not verified, was shown to be mere "occupational superstition," it would not matter much. The workgroup in the hospital is not without its genuine need for some magical thinking.

11. Because Palmer speaks for himself, no one speaks for the hospital; a curious omission.

12. Rosenberg (1987) pointed out that relationships among strangers are a feature of hospitalized care more generally. In the ICU setting, the nature of being a stranger is amplified.

13. One outcome of the second Baby Doe case was to limit the judicial standing of such distant third parties.

References

Anspach, Renee R. 1988. "Notes on the Sociology of Medical Discourse: The Language of Case Presentation." *Journal of Health and Social Behavior* 29: 357-75.

Bosk, Charles L. 1979. *Forgive and Remember*. Chicago: Univ. of Chicago Press.

Frader, Joel, and Charles L. Bosk. 1981. "Parent Talk at Intensive Rounds." *Social Science and Medicine* 15E: 267-74.

Guillemin, Jean, and Eleanor Holmstrom. 1983. "Legal Cases, Government Regulations and Clinical Realities in Newborn Intensive Care." *American Journal of Perinatology* 1: 89-97.

Hunter, Kathryn. 1991. *Doctor's Stories: The Narrative Structure of Medical Knowledge*. Princeton, NJ: Princeton Univ. Press.

Nisbet, Robert. 1976. *Sociology as an Art Form*. New York: Oxford university Press.

Robertson, J. 1981. "Dilemma in Danville." *Hastings Center Report* 11, no. 5: 5-8.

Rosenberg, Charles. 1987. *The Care of Strangers: The Rise of America's Hospital System*. New York: Basic Books.

Schutz, Alfred. 1971. *Collected Papers 1: The Problem of Social Reality*. The Hague: Martinus Nyhoff, 207-59.

Silverman, William. 1981. "Mismatched Attitudes about Neonatal Death." *Hastings Center Report* 11: 12-17.

Stinson, Robert, and Peggy Stinson. 1979. "On the Death of a Baby." *Atlantic Monthly* 1979: 64-72.

———. 1983. *The Long Dying of Baby Andrew*. Boston and Toronto: Atlantic Monthly Press Book—Little Brown, 1983.

Van Maanen, John. 1988. *Tales from the Field*. 1988. Chicago: Univ. of Chicago Press.

Further Reading

Troy Duster. 1990. *Backdoor to Eugenics*. New York: Routledge.

Jean Guillemin and Eleanor Holmstrom. 1986. *Mixed Blessings: Intensive Care for Newborns*. New York: Oxford University Press.

Kathryn Hunter. 1991. *Doctor's Stories: The Narrative Structure of Medical Knowledge*. Princeton: Princeton University Press.

David Rothman. 1991. *Strangers at the Bedside: How Law and Bioethics Transformed American Medicine*. New York: Basic Books.

Discussion Questions

1. What factors determine treatment protocol and decisions not to treat?

2. Some of the physicians in Bosk's study claim that "society" informs and, in some cases, makes decisions regarding infants with congenital defects. Who or what is "society" in this case?

3. What does Bosk mean when he claims that physicians need to have the "courage to fail" when making bioethical decisions?

51

The 'Do Not Resuscitate' Order as Ritual

Robert Zussman

In *this selection, Robert Zussman describes the medical notation for conflicting appraisals discussed by Bosk and for troubling judgments exemplified by Hilfiker's personal account. Organizational efforts to resolve these tensions have focused on advanced directives for care, where patients and their caregivers make decisions about care in advance of the time when the kind of care being decided upon needs to be administered. Still, many patients and caregivers alter these decisions made in advance when the actual moment for treatment arrives. Institutions and care providers have similar difficulties.*

Examining work in intensive care wards, Zussman discovers that Do Not Resuscitate orders contain a moral quality that goes beyond what staff write in patients' charts. Staff produce DNR orders for outside review. These notes cannot be taken literally by care providers. Contexts of care change, and so do decisions about care. Pay attention to the complexities of the deliberations between physicians and other health care workers. What do these deliberations suggest about advanced directives more generally? How are they related to future treatments? What are their implications for death and dying?

. . . $\mathbf{M}$ost chart notes are intended to convey information, simply and efficiently, to the rest of the medical and nursing staff. But notes about limitation of treatment are different. As one Outerboro resident explained, the Do Not Resuscitate "note itself is not writ-

ten for the other house staff. I don't think the house staff really cares what is in your note. They only care what the status of the patient is. How you word that is not really important." She suggested, moreover, that the note is written, instead, "for anyone who may review the chart," and that the "only one who would review the chart would be a lawyer or a medical review board." And another argued, about both official Do Not Resuscitate procedures in general and Do Not Resuscitate notes in particular, that, "the justification for it is legal almost exclusively, that they are worried about lawsuits being brought against the hospital." The special character of Do Not Resuscitate notes was entirely explicit in one Countryside intern's comments about a note she had written. Ann had begun her note on Mr. Novograd, a 74-year-old man with metastatic cancer, "Family (wife—Janet Novograd) & 2 daughters discussed code status requesting that ~~pt~~ patient not be resuscitated." When I ran into her later, I asked Ann why she had crossed out "pt" and replaced it with the word spelled out. I expected her to find the question strange but she surprised me. She said she was trying to get out of the habit of using abbreviations, particularly in DNR notes, because DNR notes are subject to review and lots of people, even nurses, don't always know what abbreviations stand for. Moreover, she stressed, clarity is particularly important in DNR notes, because they are likely subjects of litigation.

There is a temptation, then, to dismiss notes about the limitation of treatment as, at best, a mere formality and, at worst, obscurantist. Not only are notes written primarily for legal documentation, but they often distort the character of decision making. Yet to simply censure chart notes as obscurantist or to dismiss them as a formality would be a mistake. The distinction between form and substance is a slippery one, and forms, even obscurantist ones, often take on meanings of their own.

Formal policies about Do Not Resuscitate orders make only limited sense if we think of them as a means of making decisions. But they make considerably more sense if we think of them in a way that is less congenial to conventional modes of medical thought, as a type of medical ritual. From this point of view, the significance of Do Not Resuscitate policies is not that they shape the decisions that are made but that, in writing DNR orders, physicians are representing symbolically a set of values central to contemporary American medicine.[1]

In the case of Kelly Connors, for example, I had asked Ken just before one of his final conversations with Kelly's family why it mattered so much to him that they should agree to a DNR order, especially as Ken himself thought it highly unlikely they would be able to resuscitate her successfully. But Ken suggested that the DNR order itself was not the point: "It tells us something about the family. I might not bronch [bronchoscope] her." It would, he added, be a sign of good faith on their part. The Do Not Resuscitate order—as a formal order, appropriate for a chart note—had taken on a symbolic character.

The symbolic character of chart notes recasts their significance as legal documents. In invoking legal considerations, I would suggest—albeit speculatively—that the Outerboro and Countryside medical staffs are not expressing a concern about potential penalties, themselves something of a chimera, so much as they are searching for direction in an area that they find troubling and difficult. In invoking the law, the ICU physicians are invoking a system of symbols—a formal, codified representation of a normative order. This is not, of course, the language of physicians themselves. Yet, it is very much their meaning. The Do Not Resuscitate order, one Outerboro resident told me, is "a medical-legal decision [and] should be documented as such." Moreover, he added, "I don't think it's changed policy in any way." Still, while he groped for a way to express himself, he thought that formal procedures and formal notes had much of value: "It's just, it's made things a lot clearer for everyone, although initially there was a lot of resistance to it. . . . It makes life a lot easier for everyone, from attendings down to the nurses." Another resident made a similar point, stressing even more explicitly the importance of formal procedures in coping with the uncertainty endemic to medicine:

Without getting normal consent or a Do Not Resuscitate order, you would never not resuscitate a patient for fear of legal retaliation. . . . I've only lived in the era of a formal Do Not Resuscitate. I'm not sure what it was like before, but I think it's certainly clarified a patient's status most of the time. . . . When you're alone and you're a house officer, and you are dealing with a critically ill patient, you have to know whether to treat the patient aggressively or non-aggressively. You can't be vague about what needs to be done. It's just too difficult to manage a patient. So I think it's extremely important. I think it's very effective. I think it really helps you take care of the patient.

The symbolic character of Do Not Resuscitate and other orders is perhaps most apparent in their language.[2] If DNR orders were simply written pragmatically, we would expect their language to be prosaic and unadorned. But often it is not. One type of metaphor, in particular, recurs consistently. While some of the notes do state simply and explicitly that "no resuscitative efforts be made in the event of an arrest," that language is often supplanted by more metaphorical formulations. Consider, for example, the following Outerboro note:

Spoke to son about further use of extraordinary measures. Son expressed wish for father (patient) not to be subject to CPR or any further heroic measures should the need arise. Patient reportedly expressed this wish prior to his hospitalization. Son was fully aware & understood all that was explained. He was told of his father's critical condition & decision not to have him resuscitated was made. It was understood that pt. would be treated medically aggressively short of heroics— CPR, shock, etc.

The note does, to be sure, specify that the patient is not to be resuscitated. But the note also specifies that the patient is not to be "subject" to resuscitation, a term that suggests an evaluation. Moreover, the note refers to "heroic measures" and "extraordinary measures," terms that contain an evaluation in an implicit distinction between what is routine (and therefore can be expected of physicians) and what is not routine (and, therefore, cannot be expected). These terms suggest a moral quality that goes well beyond the mere recording of an order.

Chart notes represent a recognition of the rule of law in medicine. That recognition is not explicit so much as it is implicit in the very fact that the notes are written. But other matters are explicit.

In the first instance, chart notes acknowledge the rights of patients and their surrogates. At Countryside, responsibility for decisions is usually ascribed to the family:

> Discussed dismal prognosis [with] pt's daughter, who has decided [with] agreement of her sisters [on] a DNR status for their mother—no chest compressions, defibrillation, cardioversion—*They will further discuss options re* fluid, blood, and pressor support *and inform us* today. [Emphasis added.]

> After discussing pt's condition-prognosis [with] family *they elect* for *no code* status (no CPR, defib, chemical, or vasopressors). [Emphasis added.]

At Outerboro, responsibility is also ascribed to the family, but, in response to the stricter standards of New York state law, it is more often formulated in terms of the family's representation of the wishes of the patient himself or herself:

> Discussed status and prognosis with family. The wife and daughter feel that given his current poor state and prognosis, *that he would not want* and they do not want CPR performed should he suffer a cardiac arrest. All other therapy will be continued. [Emphasis added.]

> After detailed discussion about pts overall medical/neurological condition, his family has agreed that the use of further "heroic" measures would be meaningless. *They feel that the pt would never have wanted to be kept alive in this manner.* We will not perform CPR or resuscitate by chemical/pharmacological means. Should the pts. condition deteriorate further, we will continue supportive measures already undertaken. [Emphasis added.]

We may, of course, be rightly skeptical that the wishes of the family are always as clear and autonomous as they seem. Similarly, the formula, invoked frequently at Outerboro, that a surrogate is merely expressing the wishes of the patient is itself usually something of a fiction. Particularly in cases in which patients had not expressed wishes, the invocation of such wishes is often merely the language in which the family's preference is recorded. This the Outerboro housestaff openly admit. One intern remembered "distinctly" writing a Do Not Resuscitate order that said:

> Had a long talk with so-and-so's family, someone who was *non compos mentis*, discussed all the things about it. They feel that super human or heroic treatment at this point would not, the family thinks it . . . would not be advisable, therefore. And I say, "Oh, oh" and start all over and wrote, "The family feels that *the patient* would not want heroic measures done at this point.". . . . We sort of use the family in whatever role we want to, as either speaker for the patient or speaker for themselves or guardian or whatever.

The chart notes, then, at least in regard to the wishes of patients and their families, cannot be read as literal truth. They can, however, be read as symbolic truth—as the expression of an ideal.

Only an occasional note at Outerboro identifies either the patient or a member of the patient's family by name. More often, both are identified only as part of a general category. At Countryside, names are included, but only after they have been situated in a category. Thus, in the notes just cited, there are references to "wife," "daughter," and, without any specification, "family." Other notes refer simply to "husband," "son," "sister," or "brother." And, in some notes, even the patient is not mentioned by name. By assigning responsibility to a category of person rather than to a specific, named person, the notes move beyond the level of specific cases to the level of principle.

Thus, the Do Not Resuscitate orders and other chart notes express an ideal. Invocations of patients' or families' wishes are, in many cases, fictions. However, if they were merely fictions, we might expect the Outerboro and Countryside physicians to treat Do Not Resuscitate orders lightly, as little more than a nuisance. But they do not take the orders lightly, precisely because they approach the wishes of the patient with all due seriousness. Do Not Resuscitate orders evoke the value—if not the reality—of the patient's and family's rights. They should not be read as a statement of the patient's or family's wishes—although they may be such—but as an affirmation that those wishes *should* be assigned priority.

Beyond recognizing the rights of patients and the rule of law, Do Not Resuscitate orders and other chart notes are an affirmation that physicians have reached a decision and that they agree about that decision. This is not a trivial matter. For example, the following Outerboro note, referring to "agreement" among housestaff and attendings, was written after intense, week-long disagreements between housestaff and attendings over whether or not to continue giving transfusions to a 50-year-old man with an intractable gastrointestinal bleed.

> In discussions [with] pt's family in light of pt's condition & poor prognosis, it was their wishes that in the light of catastrophe or CVA [cerebrovascular accident] pt should have no heroic measures taken, i.e., no CPR. *The medical housestaff & attendings remained in agreement with their decision.* [Emphasis added.]

Indeed, there is often intense disagreement, among housestaff, between housestaff and attendings, and between physicians and nurses, over how aggressively to treat patients. The simple statement in the chart that a patient is not to be resuscitated is an affirmation that, in regard to at least one type of aggressive treatment, the staff has resolved its disagreements.

At the same time, the Do Not Resuscitate order affirms the sometimes complex lines of authority within medicine. The following note, written by an Outerboro resident, refers to the agreement of consultants and Dr. Taylian. It is an acknowledgment of the right of private physicians to follow the patients into the Intensive Care Unit and the priority of their responsibilities.

> Have discussed pt [with] family (husband), Dr. Taylor, & consultants fully.

Husband has asked that no further aggressive or invasive measures be taken & that the major focus be on the pt's comfort alone. Dr. Taylor agrees [with] above decisions by husband that no cardiopulmonary resuscitation or aggressive measures be done.

However, particularly at Outerboro, aside from references to private physicians, references to the agreement of named medical personnel (like references to named family) are notably absent. Thus, while Dr. Taylor is named, "consultants" are mentioned generically. Consider also the following note:

> Discussed overall situation at length w/ patient's sister, niece (closest relatives). Family understands that patient has terminal illness and prognosis is grave. They request that CPR not be initiated for cardiac arrest & that meds to support BP (pressors) not be administered. All other supportive care to continue. *The staff of the MICU supports the decision.* Therefore, the patient is do not resuscitate. [Emphasis added.]

Here, responsibility is detached from any particular person and vested, instead, in the "staff of the MICU [Medical Intensive Care Unit]" as a corporate whole. Such a formulation insists on both the agreement of the staff and the rights of that staff, regardless of the individuals involved. In this sense, the Do Not Resuscitate order is a reaffirmation of the lines of authority in medicine—whether the authority of the private physician based on a distinctive relationship to a particular patient or the collective authority of the ICU staff based on a position in the medical division of labor.

Perhaps most important of all, the Do Not Resuscitate order represents a recognition that there are limits to what medicine is required to do. This, too, is no small matter. Medicine, as I have stressed, is caught between two sometimes conflicting values: on the one hand, an ethic of intervention and treatment; on the other hand, an injunction to do no harm. The Do Not Resuscitate order expresses, symbolically and however partially, a resolution of that conflict. It is an affirmation that there are at least some instances in which potentially therapeutic intervention may be withheld. This affirmation is made, in part, to those who might review the chart and, in part, to the patient or the patient's surrogate. But more significant, it is made among physicians themselves. It is an affirmation that active treatment is not the only value of medicine but one to be balanced against concerns of comfort and humanity.

Yet, at the same time that the formal chart note ordering treatment withheld acknowledges the limits of medicine, it defies those limits. Phillippe Aries, the French social historian, has argued in his magisterial study of Western attitudes toward death that, at least in the years since World War II, we have stripped death of its moral and spiritual significance.[3] Not for us is Little Eva ascending toward heaven, or Ivan Ilyich pondering the ultimate meaning of life in the face of death, nor even family and friends gathered around the deathbed for the moment of final benediction. For us the good death has become simply the painless death, the death that comes in sleep and allows us to say, "At least he didn't suffer." We have made death, argues Aries, a technical matter, something to be managed. We can see the effort to manage death, in part, in the work of both social scientists and physicians, like Elisabeth Kubler-Ross, who lay out predictable stages of a "dying process" and subject those stages to dispassionate analysis.[4] And we can see it even more clearly in our removal of death from the home and its relocation to the hospital or the hospice, where it can be contained, postponed, and orchestrated with all the skills of contemporary medicine. "Try to make it through the night," Ken suggested to the Countryside housestaff about a 67-year-old woman who had just been made DNR: "I wouldn't like it for the family if she expired just after I talked to them. It'd be nice psychologically, for me and for them."

But death cannot be contained or postponed indefinitely. This the physicians at both Outerboro and Countryside are intensely aware of. "My feeling," one resident told me, "is that when they have made somebody DNR it hasn't really changed the outcome." Death is a nasty business which insists on its own way and its own timing despite the best efforts of contemporary medi-

cine. To contemporary medicine, insistent on an ability to manage illness, it is the ultimate reproach.

The Do Not Resuscitate order is an answer to this reproach. It represents an insistence that death is not simply something that happens, but something that is allowed to happen, something about which someone has made a decision. It is in this respect that the complex provisions of DNR policies concerning who is to decide and in what circumstances make perhaps the most sense. They are an insistence that, even in the face of death, it is possible to impose order, rationality, and technique. In this sense, then, even as it represents a recognition of medicine's limits, the Do Not Resuscitate order is also an affirmation of the powers of medicine and the powers of management.

Do Not Resuscitate orders and other formal chart notes have a dual character. They are a response to and an acknowledgment of the limits of medical discretion imposed by law and the rights of patients. But, at the same time, they are a defense of medical discretion, openly acknowledging limits in public statements only to obscure the discretion exercised in what Marcia Millman has called the "backrooms of medicine."[5] They acknowledge the limits of medical technique, while at the same time they defy those limits and are themselves an instance of the triumph of technique.

Conclusion

We are accustomed to thinking of ritual as something draped in tradition, something that grows empty or hollow—that becomes mere ritual—as the values that once animated words and gestures lose touch with current realities. We are accustomed also to thinking of ritual as something that grows crescively out of a social setting, elaborated slowly and incrementally. Neither of these images holds true for the chart note documenting a decision to limit treatment. Rather, the writing of a note is something we might think of as a ritual from above. It does not simply grow out of the values of medicine. It does not simply take values already found in medical practice and then attempt to represent them symbolically. Instead, normal policies requiring documentation of decisions to limit treatment are an attempt to shape the values of medicine—to invite the recurrent affirmation of both the appropriateness of withholding treatment and, at the same time, of patients' rights. If such policies do not exactly change the way in which anyone makes decisions, they may do something even more significant. They may require physicians to affirm a culture in which the rights of patients are included in the values of medicine. Such policies may represent the triumph of form over substance. But substance does not always matter more than form.

Notes

1. For a discussion of rituals in medicine more generally, see Charles Bosk, "Occupational Rituals in Patient Management," *New England Journal of Medicine* 303 (1980): 71-76.

2. Kathleen Nolan, "In Death's Shadow: The Meanings of Withholding Resuscitation," *Hastings Center Report* 17 (Oct.-Nov. 1987): 9-14.

3. Phillippe Aries, *The Hour of Our Death* (New York: Knopf, 1981).

4. Elisabeth Kubler-Ross, *On Death and Dying* (New York: MacMillan, 1969).

5. Marcia Millman, *The Unkindest Cut* (New York: Morrow, 1977).

Further Reading

Phillipe Aries. 1981. *The Hour of Our Death*. New York: Knopf.

Kathleen Nolan. 1987. "In Death's Shadow: The Meanings of Withholding Resuscitation." *Hastings Center Report* 17:9-14.

David Sudnow. 1967. *Passing On: The Social Organization of Dying*. Englewood Cliffs: Prentice-Hall, Inc.

Discussion Questions

1. What does Zussman mean when he claims that chart notes have a "symbolic quality"?

2. How do physicians and patients come to decide on a Do Not Resuscitate order? What do these protocols mean to institutions?

3. What effect do you believe patients' perspectives should have on end-of-life decisions and on institutional regulations regarding these decisions?

From *Intensive Care: Medical Ethics and the Medical Profession*. Pp. 161-171. Copyright © 1992 by Chicago University Press. Reprinted by permission. ✦

52

On the Ragged Edge: Needs, Endless Needs

Daniel Callahan

No doubt the United States faces an era of health care with constrained economic resources and increasingly limitless technological possibilities. Costly possibilities frame health care choices. Individual rather than social welfare is of central concern. In the United States, an underlying value of the individual and individual desires makes rationing health care a seemingly unnatural option. No one—physicians, health care organizations, or politicians—wants to restrict individual demands for health services. Yet the rising cost of meeting individual health desires has become prohibitive and unrealistic. Limitless boundaries of need will continue to grow as long as medical technology provides alternatives to current methods.

In this selection, Daniel Callahan raises the question of how the United States might address the tension between individual desires and rising costs at the national level. Limitless landscapes of need will continue to grow as long as medical technology provides advanced alternatives to current methods of treatment and care. Some states, like Oregon, have begun to address the matter of rationing care to their populations, but the process of restructuring health care is a long and difficult one. As a nation, policy decisions about quality of life, limiting access to available technology, and establishing priorities for medical treatment need to be made. Callahan claims that to make these decisions, we have to value social over individual needs. We also must determine where the frontier of medical progress will end . . . and for whom.

Two powerful ideals have in recent decades dominated the provision of healthcare in the United States. The first is that of meeting individual health needs. The second is that of doing so in a way that is economically efficient. The emphasis upon individual need has long drawn from two sources, that of the moral traditions of medicine, directed toward individual patient welfare, and that of deep-seated American traditions, placing the good of the individual at the heart of national values. Efficiency as a value has somewhat shallower historical roots, but it has nonetheless long been part of American business and institutional beliefs that waste ought to be eliminated and maximum results obtained at the lowest possible cost. With the pressures of inflationary healthcare costs, the value of efficiency has become all the more pronounced. It is the driving force behind cost-containment efforts, and the spirit invoked in most recent proposals for universal health insurance. Taken together, meeting need and promoting efficiency generate a deep conviction: If the most efficacious medicine could be provided in the most efficient way, then the health needs of each and every individual could be met at an affordable price.

That is a wonderfully bracing, but mistaken, conviction. The ideal of meeting all individual need is neither possible as a reality nor plausible as a moral goal. No level of efficiency will overcome that impossibility. Medical progress has undone it as a feasible goal and competing social demands have undercut it as a meaningful goal. We will always have to live with unfinished medical progress, an always rough line dividing past success and present failure. Yet because of the persistence of an emphasis upon individual need, we have been left with an impossible task, that of solving the social problem of allocation—how we should distribute our collective resources—with ingredients that are private and individual. The evidence that it cannot be done is all around us and grows day by day. As I will contend. . . the goal of efficiency and effective cost containment cannot be achieved unless the moral goal of meeting individual need is changed. . . .

We cannot separate health needs from health desires in our own lives, and neither can we devise a public policy that can adequately separate them. I am not referring only to the common escalation of what we want into what we need, though that will be a potent force here as elsewhere. The fundamental problem stems from uncertainty about the limits of our health potential. How long a life can we live, ought we want to live, or do we need to live? How much pain and suffering can and should we be ready to endure? How much disability can we survive, and how much fitness do we need? How much unhappiness is compatible with mental health? How much psychological stability do we require? Those are questions about the place, and extent, of health in our lives, and about the human needs that underlie our unending quest for better health. The uncertainty that such questions generate is well exploited by a technological progress whose basic purpose is ostensibly to help us meet our needs, but which in fact systematically blurs the line between need and desire. We have lost our way because we have defined our unlimited hopes to transcend our mortality as our needs, and we have created a medical enterprise that engineers the transformation.

At the heart of the public demand for good health is the insistence that life not be burdened with illness and that death be held at bay. That understandable desire has been rendered plausible by medical advances. Disease causes illness and death, and disease we now know can be conquered. What can be done ought to be done, and what began as desire ends as need. That redefined need becomes open-ended and insatiable, admitting of no boundaries. This is the transformation of health goals that lies at the root of our present problems. We cannot hope to manage the healthcare system, or our own aspirations, unless we learn how to control this transformation and the dynamic behind it.

It is a dynamic that embodies a vision of human possibility, one whose scope and elements are widely familiar if not always coherently expressed as a whole. It consists of three major ingredients: a broad, limitless definition of health; a highly subjective notion of individual need, one captivated by the diversity of personal goals and desires; and a strong view of human rights, in particular the right of individuals to have access to adequate healthcare.

It is a vision that sees health as an unbounded good, that allows the individual considerable leeway in defining, or inventing, his or her own health needs, and that allows one to make in principle as much demand on the help of fellow citizens—in the name of his or her rights and their obligations—as is required to meet those needs. It is a wonderful vision, but it is seriously flawed. It is collapsing under its own weight, and it will no longer suffice to provide the foundations for a healthcare system.

A Source of Trouble: The WHO Definition of Health

While there is no single source of our present troubles, the 1947 World Health Organization (WHO) definition of health is a good candidate, providing the first ingredient, that of an open-ended understanding of the concept of health. WHO's definition came to embody the aspirations of the developed countries of the world: "Health is a state of complete physical, mental, and social well-being and not merely the absence of disease or infirmity." The emphasis on describing health in a positive way and as something that must be "complete" is its distinctive mark.[1]

The story behind that expansionary definition is instructive. The World Health Organization came into existence between 1946 and 1948 as one of the first activities of the United Nations. The animating spirit behind the formation of the WHO was the belief that the improvement of world health would make an important contribution to world peace. Health and peace were seen as inseparable. Just why this belief gained ground is not clear from the historical record of the WHO. A lack of world health has never been advanced as a serious cause of World War II. More to the point, perhaps, was the conviction that health was intimately related to economic and cultural welfare, and they in turn to world peace.

A number of memorandums submitted to a spring 1946 Technical Preparatory Committee meeting of the WHO capture the flavor of the period. The Yugoslavian memorandum noted that "health is a prerequisite to freedom from want, to social security and happiness." France stated that "there cannot be any material security, social security, or well-being for individuals or nations without health . . . the full responsibility of a free man can only be assumed by healthy individuals." The United States contended that "international cooperation . . . in . . . all matters pertaining to health will raise the standards of living, will promote the freedom, the dignity, the happiness of all peoples of the world." But it was Dr. Brock Chisholm of Great Britain, soon to become the first director of the WHO, who personified what he called the "visionary" view of health. "The world," he argued, "is sick and the ills are due to the perversion of man: his inability to live with himself. The microbe is not the enemy: science is sufficiently advanced to cope with it were it not for the barriers of superstition. . . . The scope of the task before the Committee knows no bounds."

In Dr. Chisholm's statement are those elements of the WHO definition that gave it its power. It defined the problems of the world as a sickness, affirming that science would be sufficient to cope with the causes of physical disease, asserting that only anachronistic attitudes stood in the way of a cure of both physical and psychological ills, and declaring that the worthy cause of health can tolerate no limitations. It gave a powerful political and social mandate to the improvement of health, one that worked in tandem with the growing conviction that money invested in basic biomedical research would yield a powerful medical dividend. The rapid postwar growth of the National Institutes of Health in the United States, originally established in the late 1930s, was testimony to this belief. At the core of the WHO definition was a powerful though not self-evidently true conviction, that there is some intrinsic relationship between the good of the body and the good of the self, and between the good of the individual self and the good of the larger community, even the global community. For countries affluent enough to take it up, the basis was thereby laid for unlimited spending on health as a social good, and the health of the individual as the source of social good. . . .

Defining Our Needs

Can we define "need" in some value-neutral way, and do so in a manner sufficiently solid to use it as the foundation for the allocation of healthcare?

To get at that question, it is first necessary to specify some meaning for individual "need" in the health context.[2] Three fundamental human needs can be identified and they lend themselves to a health explication. The first need is simply to be, by which I meant, to exist, to live. That is the necessary foundation for all other human activities and that is why laws against murder are the most primary in any society. The next need is to think and to feel. We are rational, emotional, and social animals. An inability to think will mean that we have no chance to understand and manage our situation in the world or to know what sense there is to be made of things. An inability to feel cuts us off not only from the depths of our own self, but also from the richness of relationships with others; we are, as Aristotle long ago noted, social beings. While thinking and feeling can conceptually be separated, they are ordinarily joined in our actual lives. The third need is to act, to be an agent that can do something in the world. It is action that most visibly takes us out of ourselves, that extends ourselves to others and to the world around us, that changes the world in which we live or enables us to adapt our behavior to a world we cannot change.

These three needs may be spelled out in a health context as follows. We have what I will call *body needs*, corresponding to the need to be, to exist. The good health of our bodily organs is a necessary condition for our being alive at all. While the capacities of those organs can be compromised, and some even dispensed with altogether, there is a minimal level below which we cannot fall without the threat of death. The priority typically given to the saving of life in healthcare expresses the importance of our body needs. Our need to think and to feel I will call our *psychological needs*. A failure to have those needs met will mean our diminishment as human beings. We will be unable to live with ourselves or to enter into relationships with others. A mental impairment, as in Alzheimer's disease, or an emotional crisis, as in depression, will leave us crippled as a self. Our need to act I will call our *function needs*, encompassing within that term all those activities that enable us to do something, either to perceive the world (vision and hearing, for example) or to act in the world (walking and speaking, for instance). The capacity for action, mobility, and perception allows us to manage and respond actively to the world around us. . . .

As a first approximation, then, we can make some headway with the idea of human need. We can describe common features of our lives, root them in basic human needs, find their correlates in the realm of health and then determine how to apply medical means to relieve any deficiencies. We can also make a distinction of great importance between *curative medicine* (designed to restore our body and its functioning to a state of normalcy in the face of illness, or to forestall a deterioration of capacity) and *caring medicine*, which I will define as providing social, psychological, and palliative support when cure cannot be effected (or afforded, as the case may be). . . .

Is a severe depression worse than chronic arthritis? Is a life-threatening heart attack more devastating than a drawn-out struggle with Alzheimer's? Is the loss of mobility worse than the loss of sight, or the loss of psychological stability as in paranoia worse than the inability to breathe well, as in emphysema? No one can provide a definitive answer to questions of that kind. Much depends, we will ordinarily say—on the person, on the circumstances, on the extent to which the suffering can be relieved—and that seems the right answer. But answers of that kind may not be good enough for policy purposes, where we are required to make some decisions, to set some social priorities. We may simply not be able to meet all those different needs equally. Thus we must make some choices among them, as displayed in the 1987 Oregon decision to choose prenatal care over organ transplants (and its later efforts to devise a more comprehensive set of priorities). . . .

The Myth of Adequacy—Needs, Endless Needs

Yet no sooner have such levels of curative medicine been specified than they run into immediate problems, particularly death by a thousand qualifications.[3] The standard of adequacy must not be so low that many legitimate individual needs would be excluded, or so high that it would require an unavailable or ridiculously high level of medical advancement and expenditures. Nor can it be a fixed and inflexible standard, good for all times and in all places; it must be relative to the resources and expectations of different societies. . . .

The breakdown of kidney dialysis selection committees in the late 1960s, prior to Medicare coverage of dialysis, perfectly illustrates the problem. Mixed committees of laypersons and medical people were asked to decide which patients—based on unspecified personal, familial, and social criteria—should be allowed access to dialysis machines, then in short supply. The committees literally had to make life-and-death decisions. They reported themselves unable to make meaningful comparisons and choices. They could not devise appropriate moral criteria either. . . .

There is another important, and overlooked, consequence of the difficulty in defining individual needs. In recent years hope has been placed in a number of quantitative techniques meant to aid the decision-making process in allocation dilemmas. Almost all, in some way, seek to maximize a specific goal (longevity, or effective cure, or relief of pain, for instance) to arrive at a balance of some greater good. Cost-benefit analysis, the most common of these techniques, seeks to determine how to balance the cost of a treatment against its likely benefits. But the notion of a "benefit" often proves elusive, precisely because individuals will specify their needs in different ways and there is too little societal consensus on the value of having different needs met; the concept of "benefits" is rarely quantifiable.[4] The same kind of problem befalls QALYS—"quality adjusted life years."[5] Here the goal is to determine which medical expenditures will most maximize a combination of the quality of life and the length of life. But there is no agreement on what the proper ratio is, and thus no effective way to use the technique to make decisions across populations that may differ in their assessment of what it means to have their needs met.

What are we to make of the general failure to find a feasible and adequate way of giving content to the idea of meeting individual needs? Is it just an accident that all efforts to find meaningful definitions of "adequate" or "minimal" or "necessary" have failed? Is it from a lack of sufficient effort that they all turn out to be either too general to be of any practical use or too much a shopping list of diverse needs to constitute a coherent or meaningful whole? The failure, I believe, is inevitable, inherent in the project itself. Part of the problem reflects the standard difficulties of agreeing on anything about individual lives in pluralistic societies: Class, education, ethnicity, income, and the like characteristically lead people to develop different notions of what they aspire to and want, what they think they need, and what they will settle for. Thus on those grounds alone we should expect trouble.

That trouble deepens when we must make allocation decisions. We can agree on the value of setting a broken leg, but when we have to decide whether to invest in a neonatal care unit, or an expensive drug benefitting a few for a short time only (AZT for the treatment of AIDS), or bypass surgery for octogenarians, or expensive rehabilitation for auto accident victims, then consensus collapses. At that juncture, the combination of varying and individual needs, the expression of different wants and desires, the resistance to imposed solutions, and the pressure of competing societal needs renders the use of "need" as a standard all but useless. . . .

Medical Progress and Individual Need

More fundamentally, however, it is medical progress itself that has rendered the enterprise of defining individual curative need as impossible, and thus with it notions of finding some identifiable baseline of healthcare to be provided to all. That progress has created three insuperable obstacles to defining "minimal" needs or "adequate" care: (a) denying the limits of the possible; (b) widening the gap between individual needs; and (c) systematically blurring the line between desire and need by raising expectations and permitting individual choice of goals and quality of life.

Denial of the Limits of the Possible

Consider the need of the body to live. What can medicine bring to that need? It has already brought vaccines and antibiotics to deal with lethal infectious disease, respirators and dialysis units to cope with failing organ systems, transplants to provide new organs, surgery to remove tumors and repair lesions, and general biological knowledge to help us prevent potentially fatal disease. How far can all of this go? Who knows? There are no known theoretical limits. Mortality from heart disease has fallen in recent decades and continues to decline, and while cancer has yet to be conquered, there is no reason not to expect continuing progress. Organ transplantation becomes gradually more successful, and while there is a limit because of the availability of organs for transplant purposes, there is no necessary limit to the possibility of artificial organs. A gradual sharpening of the distinction between growing old (which cannot be helped) and becoming sick (which can be dealt with) does not make old age as such (in the eyes of some, at any rate) a necessarily fatal condition. Our need to live, then, admits of no discernible medical boundaries. There is no individual medical condition that does not, in principle, admit of the possibility of an eventual cure or significant amelioration. The most desperate class of patients, with the rarest of diseases, may eventually have their need to live met. It cannot be ruled out. Even now, available medical techniques can be used to gain a few hours, or days, even in the most desperate cases (which is one reason why the termination of treatment has proven so difficult even with obviously dying patients). . . .

Or consider our psychological needs. The enormous expansion of demand for mental health services in recent years reflects a widespread belief that psychological needs can be as important as physical needs, and that therapy to meet psychological needs can be as helpful, even decisive, as therapy to meet physical needs.[6] Both the research trend toward seeking a biological basis for the most serious pathologies (schizophrenia and depression, for instance) and the therapeutic trend toward short-term psychotherapies for lesser problems promise a growing ability to provide some help to most people, either now or at least in the future. The need for counseling and therapeutic help itself steadily expands, and the range of problems dealt with continues to widen, now encompassing substance abuse. This expansion is driven by a public perception of emotional and mental problems as now more socially acceptable than in the past, by the inclusion of therapy for them as part of standard packages of healthcare, and by the belief that such therapy can be efficacious. While there has been considerably less progress with the major and minor tranquilizers, as well as other psychoactive drugs, than was earlier thought possible, there remains a strong sense of optimism that the advances will eventually emerge. There is then, no discernible boundary to what people will come to define as a psychological need and to what the various health sciences can do to respond to that need.

Last, consider the need to function. At one time, the fate of someone who had suffered a devastating accident and came out of it as a paraplegic or quadriplegic was grim. A short and cruel life was likely. Now rehabilitation has progressed. The infections that would have carried him off earlier can now be controlled, and skilled rehabilitation making use of technological devices can give him the possibility of some eventual mobility. Even more can be done for the elderly stroke victim. He or she can now be helped to regain speech and the use of paralyzed arms or legs, and can often enough be restored to normalcy. A gradual improvement in hearing aids deals with a less critical malady, but one that is important and widespread among the elderly. The severely handicapped newborn can be provided with shunts to drain excess fluid in the brain, artificial assistance for malfunctioning kidneys, surgery for a defective heart, and transplants for failed organs. Improved fetal surgery will eventually be able to correct some conditions prior to birth. The gradual rejection of the term "vegetable" applied to any human being reflects not simply repugnance at the use of a demeaning term. It also signals the growing optimism that hardly any human being, no matter how handicapped or disabled, is beyond some rehabilitation.

A denial of the limits of the possible in effecting cures is thus a central part of the ideology of scientific medicine. It is sustained in part by its success in overcoming earlier obstacles and curing illnesses once thought beyond reach, and in part as an act of faith that is at one with the general faith in science. But it is a most potent faith, reaffirmed again and again by actual advances.

Widening of the Distance Between Individual Needs—Creating Vertical Gaps

If it is a part of the reigning idea of medical progress that there are no fixed limits to the therapeutic possibility of cure or amelioration, and thus no boundaries to the meeting of individual needs, that same progress widens the gap among individuals in their potential demand on the healthcare system. One person, the most lucky, may only require a shot of penicillin at a cost of a few dollars to deal with a minor infection over the course of a lifetime—and the healthcare system can meet his individual need. Another person, not so lucky, may require a kidney transplant at a cost of over $200,000 to save his life, and still others may over the course of an extended illness require treatment costing as much as $1.5 million to $2 million; their needs, with more difficulty, might also be met. One newborn child may require a few extra days in the hospital for a few thousand dollars to clear up a minor problem while another may need months in a neonatal intensive care unit at cost of over $400,000 (and perhaps additional years of extended rehabilitation once discharged); still another may require $800,000 worth of care. The possibilities of extensive rehabilitation for the teenage motorcycle victim or the elderly sufferer of a stroke—possibilities developed only recently—to mention other examples, are enormous. The chaos of state or county budgets devastated by highly extensive treatments needed by a handful of patients has become a not-uncommon story. A $2 million dollar welfare budget for an entire county consumed by only a few patients requiring extensive neonatal care poses nearly impossible dilemmas for the officials who must manage such budgets. The only perfect escape is a constantly escalating budget, one designed to keep up with medical progress.

These commonplace instances point to what I would call the increasing *vertical gap* of care; that is, the widening cost of curative and lifesaving care between the least and most expensive patients, both with the same and with different conditions. That vertical gap can take different forms. One is the gap between different patients with the same condition, a simple versus a complicated newborn case where both are, say, the result of a premature birth. Another is the gap between those with common, inexpensively treated conditions (pneumonia, for instance) and those with rare, expensively treated conditions (major organ failure). Still another is between those with common diseases for which cures (expensive or inexpensive) already exist and those with diseases that are both rare and as yet untreatable, but which might be treatable after more research. There may be what the economists call "marginal returns" in investments designed to equalize treatment for those who experience the gap, but it may just as well be that, if enough money is invested, the return for closing the gap could be a good one. But the cost of trying to do so may be enormously high.

The problem of the vertical gap is a direct consequence of attempting to meet individual needs. Those needs are diverse, but the progress of medicine in being able to do so with a widening range of patients means that there are also few boundaries here. Where death or illness would once quickly have taken the lives of those who suffered severe accidents or illnesses, they can now often be saved; but many can be saved only at great cost. Earlier, the costs would have clustered within a moderate range; now they can wildly vary. Yet if the accepted goal is the meeting of individual curative need—to give everyone a chance at, say, "normal species functioning"—then there is no logical choice but to accept the widening, and necessarily widening, vertical gap. By virtue of redefining what is "normal" and having more success at the margin, the possibilities of pursuing individual need become unlimited. It is just such situations, of course, that have occasioned a hope in cost-benefit analysis. But precisely because there is no way to quantify, or morally judge, the comparative benefits of meeting quite different individual needs, the technique must fail. . . .

Blurring the Line Between Aspiration and Need

Medical progress has meant the near-banishment of fatalism. Given enough time, money, scientific research, and clinical ingenuity—it is widely believed—no disease, no disability, no stressful psychological state is beyond care or amelioration. Our aspirations and hopes are at first made credible by medical progress; then, as they move closer to realization, they come to have the status, and the insistence, ordinarily accorded to need. This is the transformation of desire or aspiration into putative need. No one thought, a century ago, that a person suffering from heart disease "needed" a heart transplant; death was simply accepted. But the advent of heart transplants was stimulated first by hope, and that hope became concrete need as transplantation succeeded. People now "need" heart transplants. A whole new category of need has been created, a need originally thought to encompass only younger people but now coming to include older patients as well.[7]

More and more people can be cured of their illnesses, and thus more aspirations turned into needs; those who cannot be cured can be better maintained or rehabilitated, and those who can only be maintained can be given an improved quality of life. That is the faith of modern medicine. When that deeply rooted faith is combined with the high value given individual choice and self-determination, then the meeting of individual need has still another dimension added to it. It will be left to the individual to decide what constitutes need and a "quality of life. . . ."

The consequences of this widespread view can only be the blurring of the line between desire and need, particularly when combined with a belief in the indefinite possibility of medical progress. There is, above all, the problem of rising expectations, which opens the distance between aspiration for health and its actual achievement. As Dr. Arthur J. Barsky has shown with solid statistics, the actual improvement of health over recent decades has not been matched by a subjective sense of better health. Not only do people "report more frequent and longer-lasting episodes of serious, acute illness now than they did 60 years ago . . . [there is also] a progressive decline in our threshold and tolerance for mild disorders and isolated symptoms, along with a greater inclination to view uncomfortable symptoms as pathologic—as signs of disease. . . . The standard we use for judging our health appears to have been raised, so that we are more aware of—and more disturbed by—symptoms and impairments that previously we deemed less important."[8] Barsky also notes that a focus on health promotion stimulates greater attention to the body and enhanced nervousness about its condition; that can occasion still more visits to a physician. The growing acceptability of the sick role and better insurance coverage to support it also enhance a heightened social tolerance of illness and medical intervention. . . .

However we might best understand the informal logic of the transformation of desire into need, one fact seems indisputable. Healthcare expenditures rise in direct proportion to an increase in the gross national product, in the United States and elsewhere as well, but in a way much closer to the rising consumption of luxury items than to anything else. It has been observed, for instance, that there is an increase in caloric intake when there is an increase in the GNP. The ratio of that increase has been in the range of 1.5 to 1. Yet the corresponding ratio of increase in medical-care expenditures per capita has been 6 to 1, virtually the same ratio as the increase in consumption of fine wines and foreign travel. This suggests both the expansive power of health "needs" when money is available and the way in which desire can transform itself into need when money makes that possible. . . .[9]

Meeting Need: A Right to Healthcare?

Let me turn to the third part of the reigning vision. The idea of a right to healthcare, though often battered and rejected, remains

a powerful one in American life. While it sometimes takes different forms—the right of access to healthcare, or the right to a decent minimum of care—central to the notion is that the individual has a legitimate claim of access to decent healthcare regardless of an ability to pay for it. If there is a right to life, many have argued, then a right to healthcare is its political implication.[10] Health, so the argument continues, is necessary to life, and without health the pursuit of other goods and other rights is rendered impossible or severely compromised. The focal point of the right to healthcare in its most common formulations is that of individual need. . . .

Because medical progress renders individual need open-ended and subject to no intrinsic limiting principle, we are left bereft of any clear notion of what kind and scope of healthcare we actually owe each other as a society. We can give no clear meaning to terms such as "adequate care" or "minimal needs," and thus cannot establish policy in any sound way. It is not for nothing that the lesson of the dialysis experience has stuck in the craw of Congress. Established in 1973 as a universal entitlement for all who require dialysis to save their lives from kidney failure—as clear a body need as one could ask—the program grew wildly beyond all early projections and encompassed a wider and wider group of users, some 80,000 at present, including about 30 percent over the age of sixty-five (and the fastest-growing group on dialysis, increasing on average by 13 percent a year).[11]

There has proved to be no feasible way to limit claims upon that program, however sick, old, or unpromising someone might be as a candidate for it. That is the direct and inevitable outcome of making individual need the criterion for access. Moreover, when surveyed, those on dialysis would prefer to continue dialysis even at the price of a great loss of quality of life; hence, medical efficacy itself is not necessarily the only measure of its acceptability to recipients. The widespread assumption that people would prefer to be dead than live a life of low quality may be wrong. . . .

To challenge the idea of meeting individual curative need (and to suggest limits to society's obligation to meet such needs) is no less than to question some fundamental features of our entire way of life. It is to question not its failures but what are thought to be its highest ideals. It is to challenge our belief in the possibility, and virtue, of unlimited medical progress. It is to challenge the centrality we have given to the individual and his or her personal needs. It is to challenge the view that there is a special societal obligation (generating a claim on our part) to meet our individual health needs, however deep and infinite those needs turn out to be. . . .

On the Ragged Edge: Caring and Curing

Our main task as individuals, and as a society, will be to learn how to accept, and live with, what I will call the "ragged edge" of medical treatment and progress. Imagine that you are trying to tear a piece of rough cloth and want to do so in a way that leaves a smooth edge. Yet no matter how carefully you tear the cloth, or where you tear it, there is always a ragged edge. It is the roughness of the material itself that guarantees the same result; a smooth edge is impossible. No matter how far we push the frontiers of medical progress we are always left with a ragged edge—with poor outcomes, we succeeded in curing, with the inexorable decline of the body however much we seem to have arrested the process. Whether it be intensive care for the premature newborn, low-birth-weight baby, or bypass surgery for the very old, or AZT therapy for AIDS patients, the eventual outcome will not likely be good; and when, eventually, those problems are solved there will then be others to take their place. That is the ragged edge of medical progress, as much a part of that progress as its success.

The most vexing problem is not just that there is a ragged edge, however. There is bound always to be one if we are genuinely on the frontier. The inevitability of a ragged edge also makes it impossible to meet individual needs at the frontier; and individual health needs will *always* have their frontiers, most fundamentally our need to live on if we can do so. There will always be the possibility of improving the outcome with 500-gram babies (the present frontier of viability), or

ninety-five-year-old patients suffering from multi-organ failure, or the quadriplegic teenage victims of auto accidents. We thus remain dissatisfied because it is the problems of those frontiers, on those ragged edges, that capture our attention and imagination. No matter how much progress we have already made, it is the progress we have not yet achieved that galvanizes the research and clinical community. That is where the death, pain, and suffering are now located.

The offices of doctors will always be full, no matter how much progress is made. There will always be those on the edge of that progress—an office full of different patients than, say, a century ago, but still, and always, a full office. There will always be death, pain, and suffering, and there will always be a medical frontier. Fifty years ago the frontier was elsewhere. By virtue of earlier progress, however, we have raised our hopes and expectations about future progress. Why should we settle for anything less than continuing progress on this year's frontier? For most people that would be a rhetorical question, particularly if it is they, or their loved ones, who are on the frontier (or the researchers interested, as always, in the frontier conditions). The ragged edge of the frontier, moreover, has two features in medicine: the failures (most common), and the occasional successes (the rare 500-gram baby who survives and flourishes). The failures elicit our empathy, goading us forward. The successes encourage us to keep going in the face of the failures. The combination of great failure at the edge and some success is a powerful one, ever pulling us onward.

Yet the point, of course, is that we cannot win the struggle with the ragged edge. We can only move the edge somewhere else, where it will once again tear roughly, and again and again. If this is so, and if the effort to defeat the ragged edge assures ever-rising costs (for many of the easier, cleaner tears were made earlier in history), when will we know when and how to stop? Not when and how to stop because further progress cannot be made— further progress can *always* be made; we have no reason to disbelieve that. But knowing how and when to stop because further progress entails either too great an economic or social price or too little likely improvement in the human condition, or both, is a far harder decision. Yet at some point it is open to us to decide that we can live well enough with and on a ragged edge, that we need not always try to get rid of it. We can make such a decision in general about pushing back the frontiers of aging (settling, say, for our present average life span), or about particular diseases and harmful conditions (deciding, say, to stop research on how to save babies weighing less than 500 grams at birth). Or we can decide. . . . that we already have a sufficiently good level of healthcare and reduce our general efforts at still greater improvement. Why stop here and now? Because we have already come a long way and because the economic and social costs of continuing to push on have become intolerably high. . . .

The Need for Care: Changing Our Way of Life

There is an alternative. We could make the societal priority the meeting of our need for *care* rather than for cure. While the need for caring can be extensive, costly, and burdensome, it does not have about it the inherently open-ended features that mark the need for cure. If all of the needs of the body for cure cannot be met, as they can never be, the emotional and social needs of the person whose body is sick can usually be met to some minimally adequate extent. That effort does not require endless technological innovation, or constant breakthroughs on the frontiers of research. It requires that adequate provisions be made to relieve pain, to provide institutional and home care when family resources fail, and to provide counseling and support in the face of suffering. What care requires, for the most part, is concern and sympathy, time and personal attention. There will still be a ragged edge—some people will be beyond effective caring, and some forms of the relief of suffering may require technological advancement—but of much smaller, potentially manageable magnitude.

The provision of caring will become all the more important in an era increasingly dominated by chronic illness, where patients do not at once die, or necessarily show progres-

sive decline, but where their disease becomes a permanent part of their life.[12] For those in the worst condition, institutional care will be needed, or home care for those less worse off. They must be helped to live with their disease and the institutions of society must be shaped in ways that give support to these individuals in their illness. For the elderly, this kind of support will be vital. We will not be able to pursue with the elderly the cure of every condition to which the body in its aging is subject, or to provide an infinite amount of life-extending care (which is, by definition, the amount needed to meet the body needs of the elderly). What we can do, however, is to provide decent nursing-home care, and a wide range of drugs and devices which, while they will not extend life, will make life much more tolerable.

The first priority of clinical medicine and the healthcare system, therefore, should be to ensure that everyone has an adequate level of caring. For the bodily ill, this will mean the relief of pain and good nursing care. For the psychologically ill, this will mean counseling, palliative care and, when necessary, decent institutional care. For those who are disabled, handicapped, or retarded, it will mean assistance with the activities of daily living, help in adapting to their environment, and good institutional care if neither they nor their families are able to manage their care. The provision of a minimal baseline of caring, and just what it might require, will need discussion and debate—and that debate will require a recognition of limits on care. . . .

Notes

1. The discussion which follows on the definition is based on an earlier article of mine, Daniel Callahan, "The WHO Definition of Health," *Hastings Center Studies*, I:3 (1973), pp. 77-87.

2. There are a number of interesting and valuable discussions of the problems, theoretical and practical, in trying to define "needs" for policy purposes. See especially Ruth Macklin, "Equal Access to Professional Services: Medicine," *Journal of Professional and Business Ethics*, 4 (Spring/Summer 1985), pp. 1-12; "Commentary," by Bruce Jennings, *Journal of Professional and Business Ethics*, 4 (Spring/Summer 1985), pp. 13-24; Jeffrey Hadorn, "Creating a Just and Affordable Sys-

tem of National Health Insurance," unpublished M.A. thesis, 1988, University of Colorado; Gerald R. Winslow, *Triage and Justice* (Berkeley: University of California Press, 1982), pp. 41-42; Gene Outka, "Social Justice and Equal Access to Health Care," *Journal of Religious Ethics*, 2:1 (Spring 1974), pp. 11-32; Ronald Bayer et al., "Toward Justice in Health Care," *American Journal of Public Health*, 78: 5 (May 1988), esp. p. 586; Paul T. Menzel, *Medical Costs, Moral Choices: A Philosophy of Health Care Economics in America* (New Haven: Yale University Press, 1983), pp. 81-85; Earl E. Shelp, ed., *Justice and Health Care* (Dordrecht, Holland: D. Reidel Publishing Co., 1981), *passim*; David T. Ozar, "What Should Count as Basic Health Care?" *Theoretical Medicine*, 4: 2 (June 1983), pp. 129-141; Robert P. Rhodes, "Optimizing Health: Why Equality of Access to Health Care Based on Need Leads to Injustice," in David H. Smith, ed., *Respect and Care in Medical Ethics* (Lanham, Md.: University Press of America, 1984), p. 187; Jerry Avorn, "Needs, Wants, Demands, and Interests: Their Interaction in Medical Practice and Health Policy," in Ronald Bayer et al., eds., *In Search of Equity: Health Needs and the Health Care System* (New York: Plenum Press, 1983), pp. 185ff.; Robert G. Evans, *Strained Mercy: The Economics of Canadian Health Care* (Toronto: Butterworth & Co., 1984), pp. 21-26.

3. For some general writings on cost-benefit and cost-effectiveness analysis, see M.C. Weinstein and W.B. Stason, "Foundation of Cost-Effectiveness Analysis for Health and Medical Practices," *New England Journal of Medicine*, 296 (1977), pp. 716-721; E.J. Mishan, *Cost-Benefit Analysis* (New York: Praeger, 1976); Jerry Avorn has shown how a use of cost-benefit analysis could work against the elderly in "Benefit and Cost Analysis in Geriatric Care," *New England Journal of Medicine*, 310 (May 17, 1984), pp. 1294-1301.

4. An excellent analysis of the strengths and weaknesses of QALYS can be found in Paul Menzel, *Strong Medicine* (New York: Oxford University Press, forthcoming 1989), Chap. 5; see also "Logic in Medicine: An Economic Perspective," *British Medical Journal*, 295 (December 12, 1987), pp. 1537-1541; Alan Williams, "Economics of Coronary Artery Bypass Grafting," *British Medical Journal*, 291 (August 3, 1985), pp. 326-329; Michael O'Donnell, "One Man's Burden," *British Medical Journal*, 293 (July 5, 1986), p. 59; a response by Alan Williams to O'Donnell, *British Medical Journal*, 293 (August 2, 1986), pp. 337-338; John Harris, "QALYfying the Value of Life," *Journal of Medical Ethics*, 13 (1987), pp. 117-123. For a valuable discussion of the problems of selecting patients for scarce treatment in the absence of clear criteria, see Janet F. Haas, "Admission to Rehabilitation Centers: Selection of Patients," *Archives of Physical Medicine and Rehabilitation*, 69 (May 1988), pp. 1-26. One reason the British National Health Service has managed to control costs is that physicians and other experts have defined need, not patients. But this was simply a shift of power, and a political act, a point nicely made in Rudolf Klein's fascinating study of the relationship between need and demand in England, *The Politics of the National Health Service* (London: Longman, 1983), pp. 158-160.

5. Office of Disease Prevention and Health Promotion, "Mental Illness," in *Disease Prevention/Health Promotion* (Palo Alto: Bull Publishing Co., 1988), pp. 308-319.

6. See Gregory de Lissovoy, "Medicare and Heart Transplants: Will Lightning Strike Twice?" *Health Affairs*, 7 (Fall 1988), pp. 61-72; see also L. Henry Edmunds et al., "Open Heart Surgery in Octogenarians," *New England Journal of Medicine*, 319 (July 21, 1988), pp. 131-135.

7. Arthur J. Barsky, *Worried Sick: Our Troubled Quest for Wellness* (Boston: Little, Brown, 1988), p. 187.

8. See Paul Menzel, *Medical Costs, Medical Choices*, p. 82.

9. For a good discussion of the idea of a "right to health care" see James F. Childress, "Rights to Health Care in a Democratic Society," in James M. Humber and Robert Almeder, eds., *Biomedical Ethics Review, 1984* (Clifton, N.J.: Humana Press, 1984) pp. 47-70; John D. Arras, "Utility, Natural Rights, and the Right to Health Care," *Biomedical Ethics Review, 1984*, pp. 47-70; "Rights to Health Care," a special issue of *The Journal of Medicine and Philosophy*, 4 (June 1979). Also of great interest is Robert M. Veatch, *The Foundations of Justice* (New York: Oxford University Press, 1986.)

10. Health Care Financing Administration, *Special Report: Findings from the National Kidney Dialysis and Kidney Transplantation Study* (Baltimore: U.S. Department of Health and Human Services, 1987); see also Alonzo L. Plough, *Borrowed Time: Artificial Organs and the Politics of Extending Lives* (Philadelphia: Temple University Press, 1986).

11. Bruce Jennings, Daniel Callahan, and Arthur L. Caplan, "Ethical Challenges of Chronic Ill-

ness," *Hastings Center Report*, Special Supplement (February/March 1988), pp. 1-16; Anselm L. Strauss et al., *Chronic Illness and the Quality of Life* (St. Louis: C.V. Mosby Co., 2nd ed., 1984).

Further Reading

Arthur Kleinman. 1988. *The Illness Narratives: Suffering, Healing, and the Human Condition*. New York: Basic Books.

David Mechanic. 1994. *Inescapable Decisions*. New Brunswick: Tavistock Publishers.

Anselm Strauss, Juliet Corbin, Shizuko Fagerhaugh, Barney G. Glaser, David Maines, Barbara Suczek, and Carol Weiner. 1984. *Chronic Illness and the Quality of Life*. St. Louis: Mosby.

Discussion Questions

1. Explain the difference between curative medicine and caring.

2. Callahan claims a "vertical gap of care" comes from attempting to meet individual health care needs. He argues this gap is "an impossible dilemma." Why?

3. What is the "ragged edge" of health care? Does Callahan's solution for dealing with the "ragged edge" of health care make sense? Why or why not?

From *What Kind of Life: The Limits of Medical Progress.* Pp. 31-68. Copyright © 1994 by Georgetown University Press. Reprinted by permission. ✦

Directions for Health Policy

53

The Rising Costs of Health Care

David U. Himmelstein
Steffie Woolhandler

This brief selection depicts the costs of health care and insurance in the United States. Based on these national figures, Himmelstein and Woolhandler point to additional personal and social problems that emanate from the cost and structure of health care in the United States. As you read this selection, keep in mind the arguments of other authors in this section about balancing treatment and cost in health care provision.

Over the past decade, health costs have increased dramatically faster than wages. The rising portion of employee compensation devoted to health care costs constrains the expansion of wages, pensions and other benefits (Figure 53-1).

More than 37 million Americans were uninsured during an average month in 1992, according to the Census Bureau's Current Population Survey (Figure 53-2). This represented 14.7 percent of the population and was an increase of two million from the previous year. Over the past decade the number of uninsured increased by 12 million, and more people are uninsured today than at any time since the passage of Medicare and Medicaid.

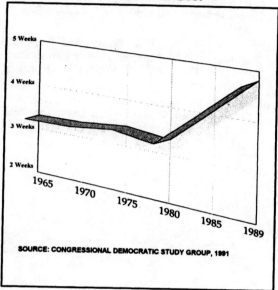

Figure 53-1
Weeks of Work at Average Wages Needed to to Meet Health Cost

SOURCE: CONGRESSIONAL DEMOCRATIC STUDY GROUP, 1991

In 1991, New England had the lowest rate of uninsurance, 10 percent of any region, while the West South Central region (Arkansas, Louisiana, Oklahoma and Texas) had the highest rate, 20.8 percent uninsured. The range for individual states was a low of 7 percent in Hawaii to a high of 25.7 percent in the District of Columbia. Hawaii, despite its employer mandate legislation, had an insurance rate only slightly lower than Connecticut (7.5 percent), North Dakota (7.6 percent) and several other states.

Men are more frequently uninsured than women; 15.8 percent versus 12.5 percent. The poor have the highest rates of uninsurance: 22.6 percent for those with family incomes below $25,000; 10.2 percent for those with family incomes between $25,000 and $50,000; and 6.9 percent for those with family incomes above $50,000 annually. Young adults are the age group most likely to be uninsured: 12.7 percent of children less than 18 years of age are uninsured; 20.9 percent of those aged 18 through 39; 12.6 percent of those aged 40 through 64; and 0.9 percent of people over the age of 64.

Further Reading

Robert J. Blendon, Robert Leitman, Ian Morrison, and Karen Donelan. 1990. "Satisfaction with Health Systems in Ten Nations." *Health Affairs* 9: 185-92.

Sally T. Burner, Daniel R. Waldo, and David R. McKusick. 1992. "National Health Expenditure Projections Through 2030." *Health Care Financing Review* 14: 1-30.

Theodore R. Marmor and Jerry L. Mashaw. 1994. "Canada's Health Insurance and Ours: The Real Lessons, the Big Choices." Pp. 470-79 in *The Sociology of Health and Illness*, edited by Peter Conrad and Rochelle Kern. New York: St. Martin's Press.

Discussion Questions

1. What sorts of individual problems come from the rising costs of health care? What kinds of social problems?

2. Making use of other readings in this section, how might you explain the rapid increase in the weeks of work needed to meet health costs?

3. Review the percentages of uninsured at the end of this selection. What do these percentages imply about the accessibility of the United States health care system?

54

The Disability Wars

Timothy Kenny

Timothy Kenny, a news manager, discloses the reality of losing his health insurance. His personal account of his struggle with Chronic Fatigue Syndrome (CFS) and maintaining health insurance indicates a global problem with the United States health care system. Layers of paper work and conflicting realities underscore claims to disability that accompany many chronic illnesses. Selections in previous sections outline accounts of illness and changes in individual conceptions of self. Kenny's account links the details of illness and altered self conceptions to larger cultural tragedies. With financial devastation just around the corner, Kenny articulates the struggle in making an illness "real" not merely for self and others but for survival. Consider some of the personal issues people with chronic illness face and think about the confounding problem of obtaining disability insurance. What macrostructural changes need to occur to alter the disability wars that Kenny describes?

"Brain mapping shows significant delta wave formation with a virtual absence of beta and alpha. Delta wave predominance is indicative of brain injury . . . [and] correlates with Tim's severe neurocognitive symptomology. . . .

"Tim's objective findings correlate with the severity of his constitutional and neurocognitive symptoms and I strongly feel he is totally disabled from any employment in the national economy, even the most sedentary, part-time position. . . ."

Paul R. Cheney, M.D., February 24, 1992, in a disability letter written on behalf of the author

My ex-employer, Diversified Communications, was supportive and helpful during my illness and the period after my disability. But even Diversified has limits; it is, after all, a business, and not a social welfare organization.

Under the terms of my company's benefits policy, I was to receive full pay and benefits for 180 days after my illness forced me out of my position. This is an extremely considerate policy and most CFS patients are not as lucky as I to have had such a great company behind them.

Wherever I go and meet with CFS patients, I almost universally hear horror stories about their disability insurance process. One executive, who was stricken with CFS before the disease even had a name, left his job still undiagnosed and walked away from hundreds of thousands of dollars in potential disability insurance payments.

I know of others whose employers had no disability insurance policy whatsoever, and still others who were self-employed and had no corporate support. There are others who may have been covered by some sort of disability policy, but the policy's underwriters refused to recognize CFS as a legitimate illness. And Social Security—well I'll get to that later.

My benefit period was to end at midnight February 15, 1992. At that moment Diversified Communications would terminate me—the "T word," Liz had called it—and I would be officially without a job for the first time since high school. Of course, I hadn't worked a single day in that six months, but I was still technically an employee, and that meant something to me. When February 15 passed, even that designation would be taken away.

I watched the calendar closely as 1991 came to an end and 1992 began, dreading the approach of the "T word."

There was nothing special about February 15. There were no calls, no letters, no papers to sign. What would happen at midnight that night would be automatic. It had been decided six months earlier. All I could do was let it happen.

. . . By eleven o'clock Hettie was asleep beside me, and I stared in the darkness toward the digital clock on the other side of our bedroom. For nearly twenty minutes, my thoughts followed no particular pattern, except that I was getting more depressed with each change on the clock. The sense of regret and dread that had been present earlier in the day were worsening as the minutes passed, and I felt the lonely world becoming colder by the second.

At 11:22, I finally came up with a more constructive plan. Rather than lie in bed and feel sorry for myself about what I'd lost, I would spend the time between then and midnight reliving the wonderful highlights of a tremendous career.

I thought of Hurricane Hugo, and how much my planning had done to make our station's coverage a success. I thought of the first time I had ever seen a President in person; the first time I ever picked up the phone to find it was the governor. I remembered flying with the Thunderbirds twice, slipping the bonds of gravity and playing in the tall clouds from the cockpit of the $20-million F-16. I remembered meeting stars in Los Angeles, slipping off to a baseball game at Dodger Stadium, jetting across the country with someone else paying the bill.

I thought of the young people whose careers I had started or shaped. I thought of the people I'd hired who had found mates after coming to work for me—an awesome feeling. (To date, my hiring has resulted in three marriages.) I remembered hard news stories, light stories, and stories of great sadness. There were investigative reports that made headlines and silly reports that made people laugh. I recalled the days of being a smiling weathercaster, of going into schools and speaking to kids, of always making the time to talk with someone interested in a career in broadcasting.

I relived the moment more than a decade earlier when I had knocked on the door at WPDE looking for work and knowing nothing about television.

I recalled staff meetings and strategy sessions, awards banquets and parades, logos on tee shirts and decals on news cars. I tried to remember it all that night and I think that I did.

And then the clock changed from 11:59 to 12:00. I was now officially unemployed. I took one final look at the clock, rolled over, and went to sleep.

When I woke up the next morning, I had one more worry to confront: paying the bills.

I had always felt young and invincible and had never even considered disability insurance before I became ill. Fortunately, Diversified Communications had included it in its benefit package for most employees, and as my 180 days wore on, I begin to learn all I could about it.

. . . In South Carolina at the time, the law allowed insurers to pay a disabled worker no more than sixty percent of his or her pre-disability salary. I knew that would be a major pay cut, but I thought Social Security would step in and pick up the balance, or at least get me close to my earlier income level. Hettie and I did not live high, but like most young couples, we needed every penny we earned.

We had a small home— our first—and a healthy mortgage payment. Hettie was an itinerant teacher, traveling up to a hundred miles a day, so she needed a full-size automobile. (South Carolina has one of the highest highway death rates in the nation; I was never comfortable with her driving so much.) I also needed a car even though I didn't work, because of my trips to Charlotte. We had student loans, a significant tax liability as a two-income, no children family, and other miscellaneous debts. And we were working hard to get Hettie through a Master's program at an expensive college in upstate South Carolina. Looking at all of that, I didn't see anywhere to cut expenses by forty percent.

I had begun the disability insurance claims process long before February 16, hoping to have everything handled in plenty of time before that date. Unfortunately, just a few days before the insurance company was to begin paying me, the company called with dreadful news: It wouldn't approve my claim. It needed more time to evaluate my case.

I was furious. I had sent the company every bit of medical information I had accumulated since my first symptoms had appeared. It had the results from every test, every office visit, every evaluation. As an Ampligen patient, I'd been put through an extensive battery of additional tests that only strengthened the case that I was disabled—

the CDC and FDA had agreed I represented an extreme CFS case—but the insurance company still balked. If the CDC and FDA agreed that I was sick, what was the problem?

At first I was told the problem was that I had "too much documentation." How can you have too much documentation of anything? I wondered. The more I called and the angrier I got, the less responsive the company became. February 16 came and went and my claim was still officially "under review." Considering house payments and car loans, I prayed this impasse wouldn't last long. Still, the insurance company offered no hope of when—or even *if*—my claim might be approved.

Then came word that I would need something called an IME—an independent medical exam. I would have to see a doctor chosen by the insurance company to screen people who'd applied for disability benefits. "Okay," I told the claims representative, "let me fax you a list of CFS specialists around the world. You pick the one I should see."

But it didn't work that way; the company didn't want me to see a CFS specialist. It wanted me to see one of its doctors. This sent me into another angry dissertation.

. . . I continued to argue this point for a few more days, and got nowhere. I would have to play by the company's rules. I called the claims representative and asked her to please rush the IME, I had bills to pay. She countered that there was no way to rush the appointment, that it could take several weeks to set up and evaluate.

This infuriated me, but I stayed calm on the phone, I would be nice and I would remain cooperative, I'd promised myself. There was simply no other way to go. My financial survival was at stake.

And then, out of the blue, my claims representative made this strange comment: "Our doctor thinks it's unusual that you haven't been examined by a psychologist. Why hasn't anyone suggested the MMPI test?"

This again! If I'd simply been disabled on the basis of clinical depression, my claim would have been settled weeks ago. But since my doctor maintained I had a physiological illness, I had gummed up the works and made everyone suspicious.

"I have taken the MMPI," I told her, and filled her in on my visits with Dr. Robertson (which had ended about a month earlier). That changed everything.

"Get us those records as soon as you can," the claims representative said. "Maybe we can clear this up after all."

In the meantime the company issued me a "conditional" check for my first month's benefit. It was money, but I really didn't consider it mine. If the company ultimately refused my claim, I'd have to repay it. I was thankful for the cash flow, but I was beginning to feel overwhelmed by the stress of fighting yet another battle.

It was at about that time, after another long and frustrating conversation with the insurance company, that I quite seriously considered just giving up. I had been abused by doctors, pharmacists, co-workers, strangers, friends, friends' doctors—and now this. I remember hanging up the telephone, slumping forward with my face in my hands, and thinking that I'd just plain had enough. "There's just no fight left in me," I told Hettie. That night was the closest I'd come to suicide in my entire CFS experience. I felt that I'd finally been beaten.

But in the coming days I bounced back, and I rushed Dr. Robertson's office along to release my records. I was concerned about how I'd scored on the MMPI, especially since I'd heard a lecture about the peculiar scores of CFS patients. Dr. Robertson told me not to worry; my scores were consistent with the "chronic pain" curve on the MMPI profile. I absolutely hated the thought that my insurance claim boiled down to how I'd scored on one simple test—I always hated being put into categories.

Dr. Robertson was training a new secretary, so typing up my results took longer than I'd expected, adding even more stress. Finally, after several days, I got the word I'd been waiting for: the records had been mailed. Now I had to once again wait for some doctor in another state to review my case.

A few days later, the call came: my claim had been officially approved. The stress mill had halted, at least for a while.

Receiving only sixty percent of your previous salary can be a pretty attractive scenario if the alternative is receiving nothing. It wasn't really sixty percent, because I now had to pay for my own health and life insurance (previously job benefits). So I was making almost half of what I had before. But considering all I had been through with the disability insurance company, that half was much appreciated. Now, I reasoned, a few weeks of dealing with Social Security and I would be financially back on track.

Not exactly.

My insurance company promptly asked me to begin the Social Security process, and it informed me that whatever amount I received from Social Security would be deducted from its monthly checks. No matter how much I got from my government disability benefits, I would still receive only that sixty percent of my previous salary. I was totally flabbergasted.

"Read your policy," the claims representative said.

But after my initial disappointment and wondering again how I would make ends meet, I finally began the lengthy process of applying for my Social Security benefits. I had paid into the program for nearly twenty years; it seemed only right that it would pick up a portion of my disability tab.

I'd heard that virtually everyone is turned down the first time he or she applies for Social Security disability payments, and that's exactly what happened to me. So, only days after the initial denial (a mere formality, I'd heard), I filed an application to have my case reviewed.

All of my records went to the South Carolina Disability Determination Office for the formal review. The state office ordered another evaluation with Dr. Cheney, paying him a whopping twenty-five dollars for his time. The office sent me piles of paperwork asking questions about how well I could kneel or crawl and whether I could stand up very long. I wrote several pages of notes about my job history, going back to the days of spending summers in a sheet metal shop or as a greenskeeper. Somehow I failed to understand what raking sand traps on a golf course had to do with my ability to be a news director,

but I knew that my only chance with the government was to respond to its every request.

Another two months passed before I heard from the Social Security Administration. Its response was priceless:

> You do have some limitations in your ability to work. You can stand and/or walk with normal breaks for a total of at least two hours in an eight-hour workday. You can sit with normal breaks for a total of about six hours in an eight-hour workday. . . . You can occasionally climb or balance, stoop or kneel, crouch or crawl. In your description of your past job as a TV news/promotion director you said that you had occasionally lifted over 100 pounds, and frequently lifted up to 25 pounds with occasional bending, and walked or stood up to eight hours a day. However, as it is described in the national economy, this job requires lifting 10 pounds maximum, walking or standing only occasionally up to two hours a day. Based on the way this job is performed in the national economy, we have concluded that you can return to your past job as a TV news and promotion director.

Thus, in the considered opinion of the Social Security Administration, I was fine. It had sagely concluded that I could do my old job, no questions asked. This was the bureaucratic crowning jewel to the miserable experience I'd endured for more than three years. Were it not so incredibly important for my long-term finances, the letter would have made me laugh for the first time in months!

I read the climactic sentence again and again: "We have concluded that you can return to your past job. . .". That was incredible! I couldn't even read a newspaper, let alone run a news department! But according to the Social Security Administration, I was healed! . . .

Fortunately, Social Security's denial had no impact on my finances, since my private disability insurance payments would have been reduced by the amount of my award anyway. But this determination had long-term consequences.

Eventually, I presumed, my disability insurance company would tire of paying me on a claim labeled "chronic fatigue syndrome." When that day came, Social Security payments would be the difference between Hettie and I and financial disaster. I prayed each month that the insurance company would continue to view my claim as the legitimate matter that it was, and I offered a prayer of thanks when every check came.

Also—though I don't completely understand the law—I would soon be unable to maintain my health insurance through my former employer's group policy. It was highly unlikely that I would be able to obtain private health coverage. Many insurance companies will not pay CFS medical claims because they say the disease is not a "real" illness. Those same companies, however, will not sell health or life insurance to CFS patients because they say the disease is a preexisting and potentially life-threatening condition. Thus, a Social Security determination of disability would mean that at least I'd have Medicare to fall back on.

There is one more thing about Social Security's denial that bothers me: For many patients, it is the only option. They have no private insurance, as I did. The delays I endured and the final determination I received would be a financial death knell to thousands of patients. I've met many of them—real people who have lost their homes, their cars, everything they've worked their entire lives to accumulate. I'm not talking about people who can't afford HBO and Cinemax; I'm talking about people a hair's breadth from being out on the street.

As I considered the ticking clock of my private disability insurance and wondered how much longer I could buy my former company's health and life insurance, there remained only one solution I could imagine for this entire mess, I had to get well again; I had to reenter the work force somehow.

. . . Two final points about the topic of disability insurance: First, there is an incredible irony to the entire Social Security process. I had paid into that fund since I was fourteen, because that was the law. Then, when I needed it most, the government turned down my request for benefits, based apparently upon my ability to kneel and crawl. The mo-

ment I would return to work, however, you can be sure of one thing: Social Security tax would be collected before I even saw my first paycheck.

Second—speaking for myself and every other CFS patient I have met who has undergone the miserable process of disability insurance claims and financial disaster—*we don't want to have to take one penny of the insurance money!* We don't want to have to rely on private insurance or Social Security. We only want one thing: to be well again. Then we can go back to work, back to making a living, back to providing for our families, back to contributing to the economy, back to saving for the future.

But until that happens, we still have to pay the bills.

Further Reading

Consumer Reports. 1990. "The Crisis in Health Insurance." 55: 533-44.

Gerben DeJong, Andrew I. Batavia, and Robert Griss. 1989. "America's Neglected Health Minority: Working-aged Persons with Disabilities." *Milbank Quarterly* 67(suppl. 2): 311-51.

Karen Seccombe and C. Amey. 1995. "Playing by the Rules and Losing: Health Insurance and the Working Poor." *Journal of Health and Social Behavior* 36(2): 168-181.

Discussion Questions

1. Have you, one of your friends, or a family member not had health insurance when you needed it? How did you/they feel? What problems did you/they have to confront?

2. Based on Kenny's account, what are the problems with the structure of health insurance in the United States?

3. Describe the link between the personal struggles of people with chronic illness and macro-structural factors associated with obtaining health insurance.

55

The Politics of Women's Health

Sally A. Shumaker
Teresa Rust Smith

On what bases do policy makers come to decisions regarding health care organization and treatment? Public and governmental decisions rest on the issues defined by social movements, as we saw in the first section of this book, and by justifications presented in scientific research. In this selection, Shumaker and Smith discuss the consequences of women's absence from the research process, giving attention to four reasons for the exclusion of women from clinical research. Through this lens, the authors examine two health issues of interest to women: childbearing and heart disease.

As you review the brief histories and research agendas of childbearing and heart disease, pay careful attention to the discussion of the contexts in which decisions about health and health care occur. Consider the relevance of these contexts for the advancement of medical science and the provision of health care more generally. As increased participation of women in the political arena has transformed women's health concerns into a political issue, will increased participation in clinical trials research and in the process of research, likewise, alter the possibilities of health care for women? Could there be adverse effects for women's health care? What impact does attention to women's health have on the health of the nation?

... Over the past few years, women's health issues have come to the fore in the United States. There are few days in which a magazine or newspaper article, scientific meeting or conference, or national televised interview does not include reference to the health needs of women, and the fact that these needs have been inadequately met by both the medical and research communities. Women's groups have been working for years to redress the imbalance that exists between research funding and medical attention for women. The recent trends in which federal agencies have both acknowledged this imbalance and instituted national policy and funding changes have been mostly heralded by these same women's groups. On the surface these changes appear to mark a positive trend toward achieving better health care for women. Yet becoming a political agenda does not guarantee optimizing health for women or men; and there are both historical and current examples of how social and political agendas have harmed rather than benefitted the health needs of women.

The major question we address in this selection is, how can those of us concerned about women's health issues leverage the fact that women's health has become a political agenda in order to maximize the benefits to all women? Factors we propose as key to achieving maximum benefits to women include broadening the definition of "benefits," involving more women in determining the hierarchy of health needs, and involving more women in both the research and clinical aspects of medicine. . . .

The Recent Political History

Several recent events at the national level regarding women's health issues in the United States have occurred that represent a marked change with respect to the attention and funding allocated to understanding health in women. These events are particularly remarkable when one realizes that most occurred within the context of a conservative trend against women's rights and various social and personal opportunities. In the past several years there has been a great deal of attention paid to the fact that women have been systematically excluded from the majority of medical research studies. The exclusion of women means that medical practitioners often do not know what recommendations to make to their female patients about the treatment and prevention of major diseases. That is, practitioners must extrapolate from data generated on primarily white male samples. Yet we know, for example, that women and some ethnic groups metabolize drugs differently than white men, and have different disease risk profiles than white men. Some reasons suggested for the systematic exclusion of women from medical research are listed below:

1. Women live longer and do not suffer "premature" deaths as frequently as men; thus, our medical dollar should be disproportionately allocated to saving men.

2. It would be exorbitantly costly to include women in clinical trials because of their lower mortality rates, their inaccessibility through existing study populations (e.g., the military, Veteran's Administration patients, physicians), and the complexity of their hormonal cycles.

3. Assumptions regarding recruitment, adherence, and dropout rates that do not favor women.

4. The androcentric view, that is, the view that white males represent the norm upon which medical facts are established and all other groups represent deviations from that norm. The frequent extrapolation of research on white males to other population groups has gone, until recently, unchallenged. However, the possibility that a clinical trial would ever be conducted on an all female or African-American population, for example, and the findings then extrapolated to white men, is unimaginable.

How is it that these imbalances in research dollars have come to be challenged? Women's groups have been actively working since the late 1960s and early 1970s to bring these concerns to the public's attention, and to empower women to take responsibility for their own bodies by learning how to detect medical needs and how to see needs. The book *Our Bodies Ourselves: A Book by and for Women* (Boston Women's Health Book Collective 1973) is an excellent example of this trend. With the election of women to both the United States House of Representatives and the Senate, and the formation of the Congressional Caucus for Women's Issues, these women's groups finally "had an ear" at the national legislative level. Documenting the disparities in women's health care was relatively easy.

The Women's Caucus, which is currently co-chaired by Patricia Schroeder and Olympia Snow, has 153 members in the House of Representatives and an additional 10 subscribers in the Senate. In July 1990, Schroeder introduced the Women's Health Equity Act—an omnibus bill that was designed to set the agenda for better health care in the 1990s and into the next century. It should be noted that women pay for over half of the money spent on health research in the United States. This bill is evidence that American women will no longer tolerate the neglect of their health care needs. Although not passed as a slate, 15 of 20 bills have been introduced independently and several passed including a breast and cervical cancers screening bill and the establishment of the Office of Research on Women's Health (ORWH) at the National Institutes of Health (NIH). Established in 1990, the ORWH promotes research that addresses gaps and inequities in research on women's health and promotes biomedical career development opportunities for women (Healy, 1991; Kirschenstein, 1991; Pinn, 1992).

In 1991 the Office of Women's Health was established for the purpose of advising the Assistant Secretary for Health on a variety of issues relating to women's health. In addition, the Office of Women's Health reviews and monitors Public Health Service activities in the area of women's health and coordinates projects in cooperation with other Public Health Services agencies whose activities include issues pertaining to women's health (United States Department of Health and Human Services, 1992).

In 1985 the Public Health Services stated that the dearth of data on women limited our understanding of women's health care needs. A 1987 report showed that the National Institutes of Health, the largest health research funding agency in the world spent only 13% of its budget on women's health care issues. Although this figure has been challenged, there is no doubt that a large gender inequity in research funding exists. That same year, the NIH indicated it would begin to encourage the inclusion of women in clinical studies by requiring a grant applicant to explain why he or she was excluding women from proposed research. In 1990, a congressional investigation of the NIH policies, through a report of the General Accounting Office, found that the NIH failed to comply with its own policies with regard to the inclusion of women in research. In August of 1990 and February of 1991, these policies were strengthened and revitalized. Also, in September 1990, with the establishment of the ORWH, these policies were reinforced by charging that ORWH ensure that research conducted and supported by the NIH appropriately address issues regarding women's health, and that women participate fully and appropriately in clinical research, including clinical trials. Applications that do not adequately address issues regarding the inclusion of women and ethnic groups are no longer considered for review.

In the spring of 1994, these policies were developed in even greater detail, and restrictions regarding the acceptability of proposed research that did not include women and ethnic diversity were made more stringent. In coming years, as studies that adhere to these restrictions come to fruition, we will begin to understand the etiology of diseases and the efficacy of various treatments for a more representative sample of Americans. It should be noted, however, that the NIH guidelines do not apply to all federal or private funding sources. For example, a large portion of medical research is funded by pharmaceutical companies and they are not required to follow the same procedures regarding representative sampling in their research. Thus, though advances have been made, we have a long way to go to ensure that medical research captures the full diversity of our population.

In April 1991, Dr. Bernadine Healy was named by then-President George Bush to head the NIH. Dr. Healy was the first woman in the history of the NIH to serve as its Director and, as a strong proponent of both research on women's health and the inclusion of women in the biomedical research community, she immediately initiated programs for women's health. She strengthened the ORWH with both personnel and funding. In addition, within one month of taking office she announced the Women's Health Initiative (WHI), which is the largest study ever undertaken with a sole focus on women's health. The budget for this complex clinical trial and observational study is over $600 million over a 14-year period.

The Institute of Medicine recently completed a study to examine issues related to the inclusion of women and minorities in clinical trials. This report concluded that although a number of recommendations, statements, and policies concerning the inclusion of women and minorities in research had come into being in recent years, adequate levels of such participation have not been attained. Recommendations of the report included the implementation of more effective recruitment and retention strategies and the inclusion of women and minorities in the research process from design to data collection. The detailed and comprehensive set of recommendations not only provides concrete measures to correct the problem but also underscores that meeting such goals is realistic and feasible (Institute of Medicine, 1994).

Dr. Healy left office on June 30, 1993, and we have yet to see whether or not the current NIH Director, Dr. Harold E. Varmus, will continue to support, as enthusiastically, research on women and the promotion of training and leadership roles for women in medicine. However, with the Women's Caucus and the current momentum, it is unlikely that ground will be lost. For example, the dissolution of the ORWH or termination of the Women's Health Initiative are unlikely. The real question is whether or not new initiatives, with input from more women, will occur or if these "quick fixes" will be perceived as sufficient to address the "political heat."

As promising as all of these recent events may appear on the surface, some questions remain regarding research priorities and whose needs are being served. For example, who is establishing the research agenda? Who are the primary individuals designing and implementing the various studies on women, including the WHI, and is this the best use of our health research dollars? Or are there other, more pressing health care issues that merit attention? Two content areas that may help address these issues are childbirth practices and heart disease.

Childbirth

The shift of childbirth from a normal human function, a private act occurring in the home, to a medical event requiring hospitalization and the supervision of physicians has been so complete that it is often surprising to learn of the recency of these changes and the circumstances under which they took place. As recently as 1900, 50% of babies born in this country were delivered by midwives (Ehrenreich & English, 1978). Noting that the continuation of midwifery was a threat to the establishment of allopathic medicine as the only legitimate healing paradigm, physicians of the mid-1800s mounted a campaign to abolish the profession (Wertz & Wertz, 1977). While their motivation was to consolidate their developing monopoly of medicine, their strategy was to discredit midwives as unqualified practitioners. By the 1970s, midwives had been virtually eliminated within the United States. The displacement of midwives by physicians occurred in two steps. First, the medical profession, which established cultural authority over definitions of health and how and where health care was to be provided, achieved close to 100% hospitalization of births by 1969. Second, along with the shift from home to hospital came a new division of tasks, assigned to those judged to have the necessary scientific background.

Although midwifery is enjoying a recent increase in this country, the practice of midwives is under continuous challenge from a range of sanctions enacted by the combined forces of the medical establishment, hospital administrators, policymakers, and ensurers. Such sanctions are illustrated by legislation to prohibit midwifery practice, prosecution of midwives, inferior treatment of laboring women transferred as emergency cases by midwives to the hospital, termination of hospital privileges of physicians who collaborate with midwives, and threatened loss of malpractice insurance to physicians providing back-up to midwives (Butter, 1993).

Since the turn of the century, there has been a decline in the mortality of the population of the United States. This decline is primarily attributable to improvements in the general health of the public as a result of improved nutrition, better sanitation, availability of birth control and the resulting reductions in the fertility rate, and other nonmedical measures. Mortality from childbirth declined during this period as well, due to many of the same factors (Oakley, 1980). Some physicians, however, claimed credit for these improvements, attributing them to advances in medicine, the superiority of medical management, and hospital birth. These dubious claims of greater safety were not sufficient to explain the success of the medical takeover of the birth process. . . .

Widespread acceptance of the medical management of childbirth meant that doctors were able to intervene in the natural process of birth with impunity. Since family members were completely excluded and the anesthetized woman was, herself, present in body only, physicians were in complete control of the birth process, now consigned to the hospital delivery room. Having been redefined as pathology, a normal human function now required active intervention. Ironically, the promised safety failed to follow and in 1925, a government researcher determined that in the nation's capital, more than three times as many women died in hospital childbirth than in giving birth at home (Edwards & Waldorf, 1984).

By the 1970s the perinatal mortality rate in the United States was 20 per thousand. Maintaining that their efforts would lower this unacceptable rate, physicians turned to increasingly higher levels of technology in the delivery room. Equipment and procedures designed for use in high-risk labor and delivery—and life-saving when applied in this population—became routine for low-risk birth as well. The findings that the benefits of many of these interventions do not outweigh the risk when applied to low-risk labors has not deterred physicians from their widespread use (Davis-Floyd, 1990). This has meant that women entering the hospital for a normal, uncomplicated birth are confronted with an imposing array of complicated medical machines and procedures, including the electronic fetal monitor, routine use of all intravenous drip drugs to hasten the progress of labor, routine episiotomy, and unsolicited pain medication. An escalating cesarean rate—from 5.5% in 1970 to 20% in 1982 (Edwards & Waldorf, 1984)—means that the specter of undergoing major surgery looms in the background. . . .

It is interesting to explore the persistence of medically managed childbirth, even in the face of evidence that such an approach to childbirth does not improve outcomes. Why do women continue to choose a method that cannot be shown to be safer and that is, in many ways, less appealing than birth without unnecessary interventions and in which respect for the natural process is maintained?

. . . In the area of medicine, technology held the potential to overcome heretofore uncontrollable and unpredictable forces of nature. While technological and scientific advances have been extremely successful in some areas of health care such as anti-biotics to treat infection and surgical advances undreamed of in the not-so-distant past, we are discovering that the promise of medical technology to conquer illness and guarantee health is not borne out in other areas such as long-term, degenerative diseases. Likewise, technology has been effective in some areas of reproductive medicine, particularly in salvaging premature infants at ever-younger gestational ages and in the treatment of infertility. . . .

Health care providers tend to promote the view that technology represents an improvement over the natural process, and consumers, having embraced this view, expect and demand medical management including all available technology. This technological imperative has meant that few births are permitted to progress without interventions and few consumers—birthing women—see any reason to object. The delicate mechanisms at work in the birth process are such that once an intervention has disrupted the process, further interventions are called for. For example, immobilization of the laboring woman for application of the fetal monitor tends to slow the progress of labor. This may result in the use of pitocin to speed the course of labor.

Remaining in one position and the use of pitocin both increase the pain of contractions and can contribute to fetal distress. This can result in the need for pain medication and can ultimately lead to a cesarean section. The greatest irony of this "cascade of interventions" (Butter, 1993) is that both the birthing woman and the physician are likely to conclude that medical technology saved this mother and baby from childbirth complications, never considering that the interventions may have been responsible for the complications in the first place. . . .

Heart Disease

. . . Heart disease is the leading cause of death of women in the United States. Yet most of the research on the natural history of the disease, risk factors, pharmacological and behavioral interventions, and rehabilitation has been conducted on men. Limited data are available on the development or treatment of heart disease that may be specific to women (Gurwitz, Col, & Avorn, 1992; Wenger, 1992). This not to say that knowledge gained from studies on men is inapplicable to women. Rather, we do not know the degree to which this information is applicable *or* if there are other risks, specific to women, that have been overlooked. With current trends in research, medical investigators are in the process of "playing catch-up" to better understand heart disease and its diagnosis and treatment in women.

In the past several years there have been over 100 articles addressing the inequity of knowledge and care for women with heart disease (see Shumaker & Czajkowski, 1993, for a review). By analyzing registry data and secondary analyses of existing clinical trial data sets, there is now ample evidence that women are less likely to seek health care for symptoms of cardiovascular disease; once seeking care, have symptoms that are less likely to be attributed to heart disease than are men presenting with the same symptoms; are less likely to be recommended for certain more sophisticated diagnostic procedures than men (for example, cardiac catheterization); are less likely than men to be aggressively treated for heart disease (for example, bypass surgery); and are less likely to be recommended for rehabilitation programs or participate and stay in such programs when referred by their health care provider.

When treated for heart disease, women do not fare as well as men. For example, women are more likely to die during bypass surgery and enjoy fewer benefits like reduced chest pain following a successful surgery, than men. Although less likely than men to initially present with an acute myocardial infarction (MI—heart attack), women are more likely to die from an MI than men (Goldberg, Gore, Yarzebski, & Alpert, 1991; Greenland, Reicher-Reiss, Goldbourt, & Behar, 1991) and are less likely to receive some of the more aggressive immediate treatments for an acute MI, such as antithrombolitic therapy (Welty, 1991; Wenger, Speroff, & Packard, 1993).

At this point let us consider several questions. First, although it is unclear how much women have been discriminated against with regard to the diagnosis and treatment of heart disease, there is little question that some level of discrimination exists. Thus, the questions are, How do we better understand the underlying causes of this discrimination, and how do we change the current situation? However, given the fact that we have evidence for *over*intervening in childbearing women, is the proper goal for women an increase in aggressive heart disease treatment? For example, is it possible that men have been intervened upon too much, rather than women being intervened upon too little? This is an approach beginning to emerge that suggests that men may, in fact, receive aggressive treatment for heart disease too often (McKinlay, Crawford, McKinlay, & Sellers, 1993). Most likely, the "truth" lies between underutilization of care for women and overutilization of care for men. The broader picture with regard to women and heart disease is not simply the underuse of high technology interventions like bypass surgery, but the apparent lack of preventive care and early diagnosis. . . .

Women Setting the Research Agenda

As noted earlier, there are a number of initiatives under way to address our knowledge about various diseases in women, and to consider optimal treatments for those diseases. However, we must question whether the fact that women's health has become a political agenda ensures better care for women. We know from the brief history we provided on midwifery that the improvement of women's health care was used as a rationale for the medicalization of birthing and virtual elimination of midwifery in this country. Women were not the primary spokespeople in that debate. How can we assure that they play a larger role in the current debate? And, perhaps more importantly, how do we ensure that the priorities they espouse are well informed and in the best interest of women, rather than reflecting the same technological imperative that has influenced medical thinking for decades in this country? The brief overview of women's roles in the evolution of high-technology childbirth and the degree to which they willingly gave up control and, in some cases, actively worked to reinforce this loss, does not bode well. Simply bringing women into the health care and research debate is not sufficient.

For example, many have argued that the lack of women at the higher levels of medical research necessarily decreases the degree to which studies are sensitive to the needs and priorities of women. However, should we assume that women as principal investigators, who have been trained and enculturated in the same medical system as their male colleagues, will necessarily produce very different solutions than their male counterparts?

It is critical that more women become involved in both the practice of medicine and biomedical research. It is not by chance that as more women came into Congress, women's needs became an agenda through the formation of the Women's Caucus. Similarly, by bringing more women into the medical arena, it is probable that the needs of women as patients will be addressed. Most of us frame our research questions by examining our own lives. Thus, it is not so surprising that a field dominated by men focuses its attention and resources on the health issues of men. At a minimum, the inclusion of women in the higher levels of our medical research and practice arenas will enlarge the scope of the questions asked. However, a broader conceptualization of health, coupled with a recognition of the limits to the technological imperative, is needed to ensure that this scope is enlightened as well as enlarged. . . .

References

Boston Women's Health Book Collective. (1973). *Our bodies, ourselves: A book by and for women.* New York: Simon and Schuster.

Butter I. H. (1993). Premature adoption and routinization of medical technology: Illustrations from childbirth technology. *Journal of Social Issues, 49*(2), 11-34.

Davis-Floyd, R. (1990). The role of obstetrical rituals in the resolution of cultural anomaly. *Social Science and Medicine, 31,* 175-189.

Edwards, M., & Waldorf, M. (1984). *Reclaiming birth: History and heroines of American childbirth reform.* New York: The Crossing Press.

Ehrenreich, B., & English, D. (1978). *For her own good: 150 years of the experts' advice to women.* Garden City, NY: Anchor.

Goldberg, R. J., Gore, J. M., Yarzebski, J., Alpert, J. S. (1991). *Sex differences in the incidents and survival rates after myocardial infarction: A community-based perspective.* Paper presented at the Conference on Women, Behavior arid Cardiovascular Disease, The National Heart, Lung and Blood Institute, Bethesda, MD.

Greenland, P., Reicher-Reiss, H. Goldbourt, U., Behar, S., & the Israeli SPRINT Investigators. (1991). In-hospital and 1-year mortality in 1,524 women after myocardial infarction. *Circulation, 83,* 484-491.

Gurwitz, J. H., Col. N. F., & Avorn, J. (1992). The exclusion of the elderly and women from clinical trials in acute myocardial infarction. *Journal of the American Medical Association, 268,* 1417-1422.

Healy, D. (1991). Women's health, public welfare. *Journal of the American Medical Association, 266,* 566-568.

Institute of Medicine. (1994). *Women and health research: Ethical and legal issues of including women in clinical studies.* Washington, DC: National Academy Press.

Kirschstein, R. L. (1991). Research on women's health. *American Journal of Public Health, 81,* 291-294.

McKinlay, J. B., Crawford, S., McKinlay, S. M.. & Sellers, D. E. (1993). *On the reported gender difference in coronary heart disease: An illustration of the social construction of epidemiologic rates.* New England Research Institute, Watertown, MA.

Oakley, A.(1980). *Women confined: Toward a sociology of childbirth.* New York: Schocken Books.

Pinn, V. (1992). Women's health research: Prescribing change and addressing the issues. *Journal of the American Medical Association, 268,* 1921-1922.

Shumaker, S. A., & Czajkowski, S. M. (1993). A review of health-related quality of life and psychosocial factors in women with cardiovascular disease. *Annals of Behavioral Medicine, 15,* 149-155.

United States Department of Health and Human Services, Public Health Service, Office of Disease Prevention and Health Promotion (1992). *Prevention 91/92.* Washington, DC: U.S. Government Printing Office.

Welty, F. K. (1991). *Gender differences in survival and recovery of cardiovascular disease diagnosis and treatment.* Paper presented at the Conference on Women, Behavior and Cardiovascular Disease, The National Heart, Lung and Blood Institute, Bethesda, MD.

Wenger, N. K., Speroff, L., & Packard, B. (1993). Cardiovascular health and disease in women. *New England Journal of Medicine, 329,* 247-256.

Wertz, R. W., & Wertz, D. C. (1977). *Lying-in: A history of childbirth in America.* New York: Schocken Books.

Further Reading

Judith D. Auerbach and Anne Figert. 1995. "Women's Health Research: Public Policy and Sociology." *Journal of Health and Social Behavior* (extra issue): 115-131.

Boston Women's Health Collective. 1973. *Our Bodies, Ourselves: A Book by and for Women.* New York: Simon and Schuster.

Institute of Medicine. 1994. *Women and Health Research: Ethical and Legal Issues of Including Women in Clinical Studies.* Washington, D.C.: National Academy Press.

Discussion Questions

1. How has women's health as a political agenda ensured better health care for women?

2. Shumaker and Smith frame their discussion in terms of the politics of women's health. Based on other readings you have done in this reader, to what extent do you believe the issues they raise are peculiar to women's health? Can you think of examples for other social groups where Shumaker

and Smith's arguments might also apply?

3. What are your feelings about the solutions that Shumaker and Smith propose for the betterment of health care? How might these solutions apply to the advancement of health care for other social groups you considered?

From *Journal of Social Issues*, Vol. 50:4. Pp. 189-202. Copyright © 1994 by Blackwell Publishers. Reprinted by permission. ✦

56

Rationing Medical Care: A Sociological Reflection

Peter Conrad
Phil Brown

All societies ration health care. Most decisions about rationing derive from a society's structure of care and its subsequent arguments for why the provision of such care is problematic. The rising costs of medical services, coupled with increased individual demand for special services, has helped define perspectives on rationing in several arenas. Take a good look at economically based, ethically based, and medical-systems responses to rationing presented in this selection. None of these models has, in fact, provided a reasonable method of organizing or rationing health care. No doubt, whether models of rationing rely upon decisions about economics, ethics, or systemic efficiency, each requires decreasing the resources available to specific subgroups of the population. Any one of these models has consequences for particular subgroups in the United States. Peter Conrad and Phil Brown argue, in fact, that particular populations are more likely to be affected by the impact of rationing strategies than others. These authors describe three sociological approaches to rationing care, pointing out the benefits and problems of each. As you read about each of these approaches, consider their applications to the current system of health care. What might these approaches to rationing suggest for particular social groups you have read about in this reader? Imagine the problems and benefits of each approach. If you were to propose a sociological approach to ra-

tioning health care, which approach or combination of approaches would you choose?

The Problems of Rising Medical Costs

. . . It is common knowledge that the costs of medical care are continually spiraling upward and are a significant health policy concern. In 1960 health care costs accounted for 5.2 percent of our Gross National Product (GNP); by 1992, health care accounted for over 13 percent of the GNP, over $800 billion, continually outstripping inflation. Assuming this continues at the same pace for the next decade, Fuchs (1990) estimates by 2002 we could be spending nearly 17 percent of our GNP on health care. Factoring in the AIDS epidemic may make this prediction conservative. Voices in medicine, government, and industry see the expansion of health costs as a threat to the nation's economic well-being, its competitiveness in the world marketplace, and its ability to deliver health services.

While a complete analysis of rising health costs is beyond the scope of this selection, a brief review of some of the most salient factors helps to situate the rationing issue. Although there may be some debate over the relative weight of each of these points, collectively they are the most significant contributors to rising medical costs.

One important factor has been population growth, which has been growing at about 1 percent a year. But more importantly, the American population is aging, hence requiring more medical care. People over 65 use services at three times the rate of those under 65 (Pagels, 1980). For example, 30 percent of Medicare expenses are spent on 6 percent of patients who are in the final year of life (Riley, Lubitz, Prihoda, and Kabb, 1987). The projected growth of the "oldest old," those aged 85 years and above, who have great medical care needs, is expected to escalate health costs significantly (Schneider and Guralnik, 1990). We have yet to feel the full effect of medical costs on our aging population; as the so called "baby boom" generation reaches older ages in the next century, health costs are expected to rise even more steeply.

Hospital costs constitute the largest portion of our health care costs (Mechanic, 1986:10). It is not unusual for hospitals to charge $500 a day for patient care (which does not include physicians' fees, tests or treatment). Hospitals' "input" costs (e.g., costs of labor, supplies, etc.) have risen faster in the health sector than in the rest of the economy (Schwartz, 1987; Fuchs, 1990), contributing to the rise in costs. The emergence and growth of corporatized and for-profit hospitals may also fuel the cost of hospital care (Relman, 1980; Starr, 1982).

Sophisticated medical technologies, including tests, treatments, and maintenance and monitoring devices have expanded enormously in the past three decades and continue to do so. While technologies can be used for diagnosis (e.g., CAT scanner), the most expensive technologies are those used for treatment or life-support maintenance. Treatments such as dialysis, organ transplantations, and coronary by-pass surgery often extend patients' lives, while adding to our health costs. For example, a liver transplant costs over $130,000 and a heart transplant over $95,000 (Kutner, 1987). Heavily technological "intensive care" services like the Cardiac Care Unit (CCU) and the Neonatal Infant Care Unit (NICU) undoubtedly save lives, but are also very expensive (e.g., more than four times a regular hospital bed). Advances in medical knowledge and continuing growth of scientific developments insure that more and more forms of medical technology will be available in the future (Schwartz, 1987).[1] Further, fear of malpractice leads to a "defensive medicine" approach which overutilizes expensive technologies.

The aging population, increasing medical technology, and hospital care are, of course, interconnected. As the population ages, there is more illness and disability, leading to greater demands for medical technology and hospital care. But other factors also contribute to rising health costs. Primary among these are third party payers and the "can-do should-do ethic."[2]

Third party payers (health insurance, Medicare, Medicaid) pay over two thirds of our health care bill. As Fuchs notes (1990:537), "without the hundreds of billions of dollars available through private and public health insurance, it seems unlikely the health sector would have grown anything close to its actual rate." Until the last 15 years or so, third party payers paid whatever the medical providers charged, so-called "reasonable and customary" charges. Patients as "consumers" were largely insulated from the direct health cost, until they faced an increased insurance premium. Thus there has been little consumer incentive to keep costs down. This is changing, since employers increasingly force employees to absorb a larger percentage of premiums, while also paying higher deductibles and copayments demanded by the insurers.

Several analysts suggest that a "can-do, should-do ethic" pervades American medicine (Fuchs, 1974). That is, there is a general belief among medical providers and the public alike that if an intervention can possibly extend the life of an individual, even for a relatively short time, then it should be done, regardless of the cost or how marginal the benefit (and often, disregarding the quality of the extended life). There has been some erosion of this ethic in the last decade, with more attention to the quality of life, "living wills" limiting heroic interventions, and more DNR (do not resuscitate) orders for the hospitalized terminally ill. Yet the can-do, should-do ethic still propels the use of life-extending medical interventions, with little regard for social or economic cost.

In the past two decades there have been numerous attempts to control rising health costs. While some of these have been successful in their own right (e.g., HMOs in delivering health services), and other innovations like second opinions and outpatient surgery have had a positive effect, overall these measures have not succeeded in slowing rising health costs. From 1975 to 1980 the percentage of GNP spent on health care rose from 8.3 to 9.1 percent, while from 1980 to 1985 it rose from 9.1 to 10.6 percent. Thus there was a 9.6 percent rise from 1975-80 compared to a 16.5 percent rise in the next five years (Reinhardt, 1987). It is hard to draw any conclusions other than the sum of cost containment efforts in the last decade has been a failure.

The Three Major Perspectives on Rationing Medical Care

The failure of cost controls and the continually increasing health care costs have made central the issue of how to allocate medical services. This issue of allocation is usually termed "rationing," or limiting medical services. Numerous health policy analysts argue that resources for medical care are not unlimited and it is inevitable that medical practitioners soon will be able to provide more medical care than society may be able to afford—indeed, some believe we have reached that point already. While the details of the rationing proposals differ, all agree that we need to begin to consider seriously what our society can afford to provide and what are the most effective and/or equitable ways to spend our health dollars. The various arguments can be differentiated as economic, bioethical, and medical perspectives on rationing. . . .

The Health Economics Perspective

Health economics centers on the financial elements of health care, especially cost-benefit analyses. For example, health economics approaches to health care access typically involve an assessment of the relative strength of incentives and barriers to utilization. The key to the health economics perspective on rationing is constraining economic resources available for medical care. This can be accomplished on three levels. At the institutional budget level, limits are placed on the amount of resources given to states, communities or hospitals. At the treatment level, restrictions are placed on specific medical interventions for particular conditions. At the individual level, queuing is used to extend the time period in which services will be made available.

The economic exemplar that has dominated the economic rationing discourse is Great Britain's National Health Service (NHS). Britain spends about 6.5 percent of its GNP on health care and, at least in terms of major health indicators, enjoys roughly the same level of health as the United States. Budget limits on the NHS have placed limitations on the amount of care that can be delivered. The NHS rations at the three levels mentioned above—budget and resource constraints, the acceptance of limits and denial of some types of treatment under certain conditions, and queuing. . . .

Treatment-level rationing is particularly well-developed. While some therapeutic procedures are as available in Britain as the United States, others are rationed. For example, few patients over 55 with kidney disease are accepted for dialysis treatment, an expensive medical intervention and the rate of coronary by-pass surgery is roughly 10 percent of the U.S. rate. British physicians and patients generally accept these limits (Aaron and Schwartz, 1984). While some have suggested that comparison of the Great Britain to the United States may be inappropriate or misleading (Marmor and Klein, 1986; Miller and Miller, 1986), the British experience remains the primary model of macro-level economic rationing. . . . .

Economists are vaguer about micro-level rationing; that is, how decisions will be made about who will receive how much medical care. Clearly if there are economically based regulations or reimbursement restrictions on types of medical care or interventions that may be delivered, this would have a direct effect on individual patient care. But when there is choice or ambiguity concerning a particular kind of available treatment (e.g., organ transplants, artificial heart), decisions on the micro-level become less clear. Do doctors or other persons make these decisions? How can doctors (or others) decide which patients should receive what care, under what circumstances, and in what priority? Short of allowing the marketplace to make the decisions—meaning those who can pay for care can receive it—or developing a system of personalized cost-benefit analysis, considered impractical by some (Relman, 1990b), it is unclear how the economic approach alone would allocate resources to individual patients.

The Bioethical Perspective

Bioethical approaches to rationing focus on issues such as justice, ethics, needs, and rights of patients and society in the context of limiting medical care. While underlying all forms of rationing is the goal of limiting economic expenditures, the bioethical approach focuses more on the justice of rationing than on cost-saving per se (Churchill, 1987).

Bioethicists seek to find a just way to ration health care. In the context of high medical costs for the elderly, age has been proposed as a criterion for rationing care (Callahan, 1987; Daniels, 1984). Callahan (1987:25, 53) urges that we halt the "compulsive effort" at longevity, arguing that "medicine should not be used for the further extension of the life of the aged, but only for the full achievement of a natural and fitting life span and thereafter for the relief of suffering." He sees individualism's good above the social good, and medicine as avidly supporting that goal. . . .

He argues that a sound health care system must combine a base level of health care (equity) with a means of limiting ineffective, marginal or too expensive procedures (efficiency) to attain some consensus on social and individual health care priorities. Only then can we meet basic health needs while living within our societal means. Although he sees medical progress as a great human achievement, he argues "that it is intrinsically limitless in its economic possibilities" and continues to create new "needs" for the wonders it produces. But the costs of unlimited medical progress are high; he argues we must begin considering "rationing medical progress" and foregoing "potentially beneficial advances in the application and development of new techniques" (Callahan, 1990), especially those that bring only marginal improvement to our already high standard of health. . . .

Medical Responses to Rationing

Although there has not been a unified or even a totally consistent response by the medical profession to the various proposals on rationing, sufficient reactions leave been articulated to allow us to speak of a medical perspective. A major spokesman of this perspective is Arnold Relman (1990a; 1990b), editor of *The New England Journal of Medicine*.

The medical perspective does not deny that health care costs are a severe problem, but doubts that either the economic or bioethical approaches to rationing are the proper solution. Rather this perspective suggests the need for a reform of the medical system, especially in terms of eliminating ineffective care, unnecessary services and general inefficiency (see also Brook and Lohr, 1986). This reflects the "growing evidence of the overuse of services, inefficient use of facilities, and excessive overhead and administrative expenses"(Relman, 1990b:911). The core of the cost problem, however, is not technology or the "insatiable" demand for it. As Relman (1990b:912) argues:

> [The medical] system has built-in incentives for waste and inflation. It is the way we organize and fund the delivery of health care that rewards the profligate use of technology and stimulates demand for nonessential services; it is the system that allows duplication and waste of resources and produces excessive overhead costs.

. . . The general theme here is that huge amounts of money in the health sector are wasted and could be saved. In this view, sufficient money is already spent in the health sector to provide decent health care for all Americans, if only the medical system is somehow reformed and the money spent more wisely and efficiently. Then rationing—which probably would not work—would not be necessary.

Toward a Sociological Approach to Rationing

. . . A sociological approach begins from the assumption that in American society rationing (or limiting or allocating) has always been a feature of the delivery of medical care, and that it can take many forms. Analysts from various perspectives acknowledge that some types of rationing already exist (Blank 1988; Churchill 1987; Fuchs 1984; Relman 1990b), but perhaps because these forms of rationing are not a result of specific policies limiting health care, they have not been placed in the center of the rationing argument. By focusing the rationing debate largely on one type of rationing (explicit rationing), analysts continue the fiction that other types of rationing are not already in effect. In this section we argue that rationing comes in at least three forms, each of which is a different way to limit health care. . . .

Allocative Rationing Allocative rationing is rationing by differential access to services and medical care. This is the most invisible form, in that it is a feature of social structural eniquities rather than a result of health policy per se. It includes the lack of availability of medical services, either general or specific. For example, if no medical facilities are available, there is a major constraint on obtaining services. More specifically, if a patient has no access to special services like an Intensive Care Unit or a Neonatal Intensive Care Unit because local or nearby facilities are lacking, this amounts to rationing by allocation. This is equally true if a hospital has only three ventilators and has five patients who require them. . . .

The cost of medical care can limit its usage. Whether we acknowledge it or not, one of the most disturbing examples of allocative rationing is the existence of roughly 37 million people without any health insurance. This includes unemployed and working people who either do not qualify for Medicaid or cannot afford private insurance premiums. This amounts to over 15% of our population to whom medical care is "rationed" because they lack adequate coverage to pay for it. There is evidence that these people may be sicker overall than the rest of the population (Davis and Rowland, 1983). These numbers have grown in recent years; between 1976 and 1984 the proportion of poor covered by Medicaid decreased 65 to 52 percent (cited in Mechanic, 1985). Not having insurance usually translates to less use of medical services. A recent Massachusetts study found that half the uninsured people with serious symptoms or chronic illness have not seen a doctor in the last year, compared to 29 percent of those with insurance (Knox, 1990). . . .

Allocative rationing of this sort has increased in the past decade; without it our medical costs would undoubtedly be still higher. It is rationing by price and availability and has a variable impact by race, class, age and employment (see Davis and Rowland, 1983), differentially affecting some of the so-

ciety's most vulnerable groups. For example, a recent study showed that between 1982 and 1986 the percentage of newborns without health insurance increased by 45 percent; newborns without health insurance had risks of adverse outcomes one-third higher than those with private insurance, and if the newborns were black, the risk was over twice as high (Braverman, Olivia, and Miller, 1989). Another recent study showed that although the rate of end-stage renal disease is higher among blacks than whites, blacks have less access to kidney transplantation and thus significantly lower rates of transplantation (Kasiske et al. 1991).

Tacit Rationing. . . . In addition to cost-containment measures, tacit rationing includes approaches which specifically limit certain services to certain groups or constrain particular categories of services. However, these are not designed as comprehensive rationing policies.

During the 1980s "cost sharing" became a popular strategy in the corporate world for reducing medical costs, especially in terms of increased coinsurance and deductibles, both of which required patients to pay more out of their own pockets. As the Rand Health Experiment showed, when patients have to pay for medical care they often use less of certain services (Newhouse et al., 1981). While the goal of cost sharing is to control health costs, it also acts as a tacit form of rationing by creating disincentives for utilization and by limiting financial resources.

DRGs (Diagnostically Related Groups), instituted in 1984 for Medicare, are also a form of tacit rationing. DRGs replace the fee-for-service system with a form of "prospective reimbursement" whereby the government pays only a specific amount for a given medical problem. The reimbursements for the 467 diagnoses are established in advance. If the hospital spends less than the set amount, it profits from the difference. While the goal is to give hospitals incentives to be efficient and save money, there is some concern that hospitals will ultimately provide fewer services. Hospitals have begun employing "case-mix management" to attract DRG-profitable patients and to discourage DRG-costly patients. DRGs have lowered the length of stay, but with some indications of premature discharge. Many hospitals have reduced ancillary services, such as physical therapy (Dolenc and Dougherty, 1985).

A variety of strategies for controlling medical costs have been included under the ideal of "managed care." Some, such as health maintenance organizations or HMOs, are also forms of prospective reimbursement. In this increasingly popular model for delivering medical care, patients pay a flat yearly fee to the organization and rely on the HMO organization for providing needed treatment. This "capitated" medical practice supplies constraints to services by creating specific budgets in which the organization must work. As Mechanic (1985:460) notes:

> HMOs are a good model of implicit rationing in that once the capitation is determined, the organization can establish its own priorities, modes of service delivery, mix of professional personnel, balance of services among prevention, acute care, and chronic disease management, and many other matters.

There is evidence that HMOs do effectively control some costs, particularly by reducing hospital admissions and total hospital days (Mechanic, 1985:461). While the ideology of HMOs is that incentives to keep people healthy will help control health costs, the reality is that they can reduce health costs by rationing services (hospital admissions, restricting use of specialists, providing extremely limited mental health coverage)....

Whenever there are limits on insurance coverage, as when Medicaid does not fund abortions or transplants, it amounts to a form of rationing. This is equally true for commercial insurance when policies specifically exclude procedures that could otherwise be available if needed. Typically this includes new treatments which are excluded while still "experimental." One recent example was lithostripsy, sonar bombardment of gallstones and kidney stones. The Blue Cross-Blue Shield National Association operates an office charged with determining when a treatment ceases to be "experimental" and becomes standard medical practice. Commercial insurance also may exclude repro-

ductive technologies, such as infertility treatment. In Massachusetts, the private carrier that insures state workers has a legislative mandate to exclude abortions.

Some of the forms of tacit rationing bear similarities to explicit rationing. For instance, we have mentioned that excluding abortions or "experimental" surgery is a way of limiting access. We do not include these as explicit forms because they are not part of the rationing discourse; these "limitations" do not enter the debate because they are neither primarily economic nor comprehensive statewide or national policies which aim at creating a rationing policy. Rather, they have a specific aim, and often a narrow scope.

Explicit Rationing The three major rationing perspectives with which we began—health economics, bioethics, and the medical perspective—are all explicit rationing strategies. They attempt to create comprehensive programs of resource allocation, usually at the national level. Most frequently mentioned is creating some type of overall financial limitations on medical services, a budget "cap" to limit expenditures on medical care, without necessarily mandating how or where the limits are set. Generally this reflects the type of rationing in place in Great Britain's NHS. This type of program requires clinicians or medical administrators to decide and implement the specific rationing policies.

A second type entails specific limitations of services, technologies or procedures. While such types of regulations often exist in public programs like Medicare or Medicaid, "such explicit limitations have most typically involved areas that were outside the conventionally defined core of covered services" (Mechanic, 1985:459). More explicit rationing would make this type of specific limitation a more dominant strategy for defining what types of care are available and for whom. Numerous proposals have suggested that specific technologies or procedures can only be rationed *before* they are introduced, since once they are introduced they become part of conventional care. This implies that these rationing decisions would be made on the health policy or administrative rather than clinical level.

Commercial insurance companies are already pursuing such administrative rationing. Using their own protocols, and often employing specialized claim processing firms, insurers are refusing coverage for treatments previously deemed medically necessary (Greer, 1991). There are apparently no legal constraints on this practice. . . .

The state of Oregon has developed an explicit rationing plan for its Medicaid program. Recognizing that the state cannot fund limitless health care, and that there are many people uncovered by Medicaid or private insurance, Oregon enacted a law that seeks to ensure that everyone in state receives health coverage. To achieve this, an "Oregon Health Decisions" project was devised, allowing for public input to decide what should be the health priorities for the 1990s. Citizens were asked to prioritize what stages of human life should get what types of health care (for details, see Crawshaw et al., 1990). Based on these responses, and using a cost-benefit formula, a state health services commission developed an extensive and specific prioritized list of services. Payment for services below a certain point on a computer-determined list would be eliminated.

This plan takes the cost of treatment, divides it by the number of years an average person would live after treatment, and divides that product by a "Quality of Well Being" rating. In all, 714 procedures were ranked according to the final figure, and this ranking was then subject to vigorous debate and lobbying. The goal of the policy was to eliminate costly procedures that benefit with health care providers is a significant feature of the problems in our current health care system. While ad hoc decisions on providing or limiting services have always been a feature of the physician's role, to put providers in the position of being explicit gatekeepers would produce further distrust.

Most rationing strategies also ignore the meso-level of institutions. Given the current organization of medical services, widespread application of rationing will leave independent practices, group practices, free-standing clinics, and even individual hospitals less capable of operating effectively. They may have a reduced capacity to influence rationing decisions, to circumvent those decisions, or to provide alternative services. On the one hand, this might hasten the spread of managed care and for-profit corporate chains to counter the new limitations. On the other hand, it could also lead to clandestine strategies to ignore or circumvent rationing policies.

Government and private insurers can use rationing plans as ways to deflect attention from their roles in creating and perpetuating the health care cost crisis. Indeed, both corporate buyers of commercial insurance and corporate self-insurers may exclude services and then proclaim themselves leaders in cost containment.

Given the nature of our current medical system, the impact of any rationing plan is likely to be inequitable. Rationing will have the greatest impact on the most vulnerable populations—the poor, the chronically ill and the elderly. These groups rely the most on government programs about which the public is increasingly ambivalent (Mechanic, 1985). Moreover, these groups have the least resources in terms of money, power, attractiveness, and access to overcome the negative impacts of limitations on services.

Rationing is more likely to come first in publicly supported medical care—as with DRGs— affecting those who can do the least about it. Just prior to Oregon's Health Decisions project, in 1987 Oregon and Arizona halted Medicaid support for organ and bone marrow transplants. National media attention focused on children in both states who died for lack of transplants (Saltus, 1988). The Oregon plan will ration expensive medical technologies while providing basic health care for all. While many praised the Oregon plan for its innovation, coverage, and democratic process, it should not escape our attention that rationing is only for Medicaid services, thus overwhelmingly affecting poor people. Although elderly, disabled and blind people are specifically exempt, people with low incomes and limited resources are particularly vulnerable under such a policy. This example highlights how, given our current health care system, well-intentioned rationing disproportionately affects those who are already medically disadvantaged. . . .

Notes

1. It is actually not medical technology per se that increases medical costs so dramatically, but the *use* of the technology. As several analysts have pointed out, Great Britain has the same medical technology as the United States, but because some technological innovations are not readily available to British patients, expenditures on technology are substantially lower (Aaron and Schwartz, 1984).

2. In a recent article, Fuchs (1990) argues that slow growth of health care productivity compared to industry or agriculture may make a contribution to the relative rise in medical costs. Fuchs also suggests that malpractice premiums and "defensive medicine" (physicians' actions to protect against charges of malpractice) appear to have a small impact on health costs.

References

Aaron, Henry J. and William B. Schwartz. 1984. *The Painful Prescription: Rationing Hospital Care.* Washington, DC: Brookings Institution.

Blank, Robert H. 1988. *Rationing Medicine.* New York: Columbia University Press.

Braveman, Paula, Geraldine Oliva, Marie Grisham Miller, Randy Reiter, and Susan Egerter. 1989. "Adverse Outcomes and Lack of Health Insurance Among Newborns in an Eight-county Area of California, 1982 to 1986." *New England Journal of Medicine* 321: 508-513.

Brook, Robert H. and Kathleen N. Lohr. 1986. "Will We Need to Ration Effective Health Care?" *Issues in Science and Technology* III (I): 68-77.

Callahan, Daniel. 1987. *Setting Limits: Medical Goals in an Aging Society.* New York: Simon and Schuster.

——. 1990. "Rationing Medical Progress: The Way to Affordable Health Care." *New England Journal of Medicine* 322: 1810-1813.

Churchill, Larry R. 1987. *Rationing Health Care in America: Perceptions and Principles of Justice.* Notre Dame, IN: University of Notre Dame Press.

Crawshaw, Ralph, Michael Garland, Brian Hines, and Barry Anderson. 1990. "Developing Principles for Prudent Health Care Allocation: The Continuing Oregon Experiment." *Western Journal of Medicine* 152: 441-446.

Daniels, Norman. 1984. "Is Rationing By Age Ever Morally Acceptable?" *Business and Health* April: 29-32.

Davis, Karen and Diane Rowland. 1983. "Uninsured and Underserved: Inequities in Health Care in the United States." *Milbank Memorial Fund Quarterly* 61: 149-176.

Dolenc, Danielle A. and Charles J. Dougherty. 1985. "DRGS: The Counterrevolution in Financing Health Care." *Hastings Center Report* 15(3): 19-29.

Fuchs, Victor. 1974. *Who Shall Live?* New York: Basic.

——. 1984. "The 'Rationing' of Medical Care." *New England Journal of Medicine* 311: 1572-1573.

——. 1990. "The Health Care Sector's Share of the Gross National Product." *Science* 247: 534-538.

Greer, David. 1991. Personal Communication to Phil Brown.

Kasiske, Bertram L., John F. Neylan, Robert Riggio, Gabriel L. Danovitch, Lawrence Kahana, Stephen R. Alexander, and Martin G. White. 1991. "The Effect of Race on Access and Outcome in Transplantation." *New England Journal of Medicine* 324: 302-307.

Knox, Richard A. 1990. "No Health Insurance Means Few Doctor Visits, Study Says." *Boston Globe* October 4: 33.

Kutner, Nancy G. 1987. "Issues in the Application of High Cost Medical Technology: The Case of Organ Transplantation." *Journal of Health and Social Behavior* 28: 23-36.

Marmor, Theodore R. and Rudolf Klein. 1986. "Cost vs. Care: American's Health Care Dilemma Wrongly Considered." *Health Matrix* IV: 19-24.

Mechanic, David. 1985. "Cost Containment and the Quality of Medical Care: Rationing Strategies in an Era of Constrained Resources." *Milbank Memorial Fund Quarterly* 63: 453-475.

Miller, Frances H. and Graham A.H. Miller. 1986. "The Painful Prescription: A Procrustean Perspective?" *New England Journal of Medicine* 314: 1383-1385.

Newhouse, J.P., W.G. Manning, C.N. Morris, L.L. Orr, N. Duan, E.B. Keeler, A. Liebowitz, K.H. Marquis, C.E. Phelps, and R.H. Brook. 1981. "Some Interim Results from a Controlled Trial of Cost-sharing in Health Insurance." *New England Journal of Medicine* 305: 1501-1507.

Pagels, D.C. 1980. *Health Care and the Elderly.* Rockville, MD: Aspen Systems.

Reinhardt, Uwe E. 1987. *Medical Economics* August 24.

Relman, Arnold. 1980. "The New Medical-Industrial Complex." *New England Journal of Medicine* 303: 963-970.

——. 1990a. "Is Rationing Inevitable?" *New England Journal of Medicine* 322: 1809-1810.

——. 1990b. "The Trouble with Rationing." *New England Journal of Medicine* 323: 911-913.

Riley, G., J. Lubitz, R. Prihoda, and E. Rabb. 1987. "The Use and Costs of Medicare Services by Cause of Death." *Inquiry* 24: 233-44.

Saltus, Richard. 1988. "Guilt in 2 States as Transplant Aid to Poor is Cut Off." *Boston Globe* June 19.

Schneider, Edward L. and Jack M. Guralnik. 1990. "The Aging of America: Impact on Health Care Costs." *Journal of the American Medical Association* 263: 2335-2340.

Schwartz, William B. 1987. "The Inevitable Failure of Current Cost-Containment Strategies: Why They Can Provide Only Temporary Relief." *Journal of American Medical Association* 257: 220-224.

Starr, Paul. 1982. *The Social Transformation of American Medicine*. New York: Basic.

Further Reading

Daniel Callahan. 1990. "Modernizing Morality: Medical Progress and the Good Society." *Hastings Center Report* 20: 28-32.

Alain C. Entoven. 1991. "International Market Reform of the British Health Service." *Health Affairs* (Fall).

Theodore Marmor. 1994. *Understanding Health Care Reform*. New Haven: Yale University Press.

Discussion Questions

1. Describe the three sociological approaches to rationing health care identified by Conrad and Brown.

2. Which of these approaches to rationing health care is the most appealing to you individually? Which do you believe best serves the social good? Is there a discrepancy between the model you selected and the one that you believed would best serve the collective good?

3. Which populations are at the biggest risk when strategies for rationing health care are considered? What factors put these subgroups at the greatest risk?

57

Why Major Reform Is Needed

Anselm L. Strauss
Juliet M. Corbin

The model of acute care based upon practitioner authority, rapid intervention, and recovery neither fits the demands of chronic care nor meets the needs of chronically ill people. The acute care model takes the individual as the unit of concern, places the patient in the passive sick role, assumes decision-making by physicians, relies on technology, and ignores problems that cannot be reduced to medical solutions. In contrast, chronic care needs to take patient and caregiver(s) into account, as Anselm Strauss and Juliet Corbin contend. Although they wrote this piece a decade ago, their position still needs to be heard. Many of the current reform proposals add piecemeal changes to the acute care model and fail to include the views of chronically ill people. For months and years, patients and families monitor symptoms, handle treatments, and follow regimens for chronic illness while the ill person remains at home. They may even do a substantial amount of work when in the hospital, as Strauss and Corbin point out. Overloading a family caregiver with arduous tasks and emotional burdens without respite only produces more patient and family conflict. Physicians must rely on patients and families for information on the patient's status. They should work with patients in handling the illness. Rather than recovery, physicians' treatment is aimed to handle symptoms and improve the quality of life. Sometimes technical interventions can help. Often they cannot. The physician's authority and control correspondingly diminish. By ignoring problems that cannot be reduced to medical solutions, practitioners may not see

the reasons why their patients fail to follow prescribed regimens.

Strauss and Corbin stress that policy-makers agree that the American health care system needs reform but do not agree on the form it should take; changing the system to a model based on chronic care that takes into account the views and circumstances of people who have chronic conditions would constitute major reform. Think about the difficulties in following a special diet when the patient cannot afford the necessary food, lacks transportation to the stores that have it, cannot prepare it independently, and when everyone else eats the forbidden food. As Strauss and Corbin imply, regimens are arduous and fraught with difficulties. Patients have their own priorities that can preclude them from attending to staff's directives. Augmenting informal care with formal home care services means costly, fragmented, and uneven assistance and ultimate impoverishment of middle-class clients. Additional problems of staff, untrained to communicate with patients and unaware of patients' actual lives and worlds, all suggest that reforming the American health care system means much more than narrow economic solutions.

The predominantly clinical or acute care approach to chronic illness seems to be only partly relevant to the many nonclinical aspects of chronic illness, and to the cluster of problems that characteristically confront the chronically ill. The inability of the ill to surmount those problems and to manage the nonclinical aspects of their lives unquestionably contributes to their specifically medical difficulties. In this chapter, we consider the prevailing acute care approach to illness—including chronic illness—and various criticisms directed against this approach. We also contrast the ways that health professionals and laypeople perceive the issues of chronic illness.

Weaknesses of the Acute Care Approach to Chronic Illness

Along with the gradual recognition by perceptive observers and researchers of the complex accompaniments of long-term illnesses, there has been evolution of a thoughtful criticism of the acute care approach to currently incurable illnesses (Brody, Poulshock, and Masciocchi 1978; Conrad 1987; Feldman 1974; La Porte and Rubin 1979). The tenor of criticism is exemplified by statements such as that of Leighton Cluff (1981), a physician and former executive vice-president of the Robert Wood Johnson Foundation. Cluff points out the efficacy of the clinical approach to illness, then faults it for what it frequently fails to do: "Medical knowledge and skill, diagnosis and treatment of disease, mortality and morbidity, pathophysiology and other similar concerns frequently dominate the interests and efforts of doctors. These concerns are important to the management of disease and contribute to functional improvement of patients. Too seldom, however, do physicians attend to the patient's ability to cope, level of discomfort, patterns of living, occupational ability or productivity, emotional status, or other functional activities" (p. 306).

It is understandable that an acute care approach should predominate in hospitals, but why should it also characterize the care of patients at clinics and in physicians' offices? Some 52 percent of those who seek help in these places suffer from chronic illness (Rice and Hodgson 1981). The answer perhaps lies in part in the overwhelming clinical emphasis of medical school faculties and, though to a rapidly lessening extent, in schools of nursing. A number of factors contribute to this clinical emphasis in the training of young physicians (Becker, Geer, Hughes, and Strauss 1964). To be accepted into a medical school, students must have undergone an undergraduate education consisting mostly of courses in science. This concentrated premed curriculum will culminate—in their eyes—in the "real thing" when they finally engage in clinical work at a teaching hospital (Becker, Geer, Hughes, and Strauss 1964). At medical school, their teachers are skilled and sometimes famous medical scientists and clinicians. The curriculum emphasizes the rigorous scientific basis ("hard science") of good medical practice, and students are trained primarily in hospitals (Becker, Geer, Hughes, and Strauss 1964). The school itself is located in a teaching hospital, most frequently devoted to the most acute kinds or phases of chronic illnesses. Students almost everywhere rank the prestige of the more socially and psychologically oriented specialties, such as psychiatry, family medicine, and rehabilitation medicine (Anderson 1978), below that of the more rigorously clinical specialties. In recent years more attention has been paid to the social and psychological aspects of patient care, yet the teaching of these is likely to be squeezed out or minimized, if only because the specialties compete so ferociously for students and the medical curriculum requires so much concentrated study. During the more intensive years of internship and residency, the postgraduate students are similarly wrapped up in clinical work and learning (Bucher and Stelling 1977; Mizrahi 1987).

Yet the clinical training of physicians cannot be the only reason that the medical-clinical perspective is so dominant at health care facilities. If medical leaders thought it was, they would do what the leaders of the nursing profession have done: emphasize the social and psychological aspects of care, even in the hospital setting, where the physicians control or influence so much of the operative policy. Perhaps, as some observers have suggested (Roth and Ruzek 1986; Strauss, Fagerhaugh, Suczek, and Wiener 1985; Wiener, Fagerhaugh, Suczek, and Strauss 1979), the very success of modern medicine in combating disease and vanquishing particular diseases, abetted by the effectiveness of an explosively evolving technology, has persuaded both physicians and laypeople that what is needed is more medical science, more high-quality medicine, and further improved technology (Strauss, Fagerhaugh, Suczek, and Wiener 1985; Wiener, Fagerhaugh, Suczek, and Strauss 1979). With these, even more disease will be conquered (Thomas 1974).

Indeed, it is difficult to talk about medical treatments without using military terminology, as several critics have pointed out (Schwartz 1987; Childress 1987; Vaisrub 1977; Sontag 1979; Warren 1987). Childress (1987 pp. 486-487), a bioethicist, makes a strong case for the physicians' use of a "metaphor of warfare." In perhaps too extreme a statement but certainly with considerable truth, he sketches out the metaphor: "The physician as the captain leads the battle against disease, orders a battery of tests, develops a plan of attack, calls on the armamentarium or arsenal of medicine, directs allied health personnel, treats aggressively and expects compliance." Good patients are those who fight vigorously and refuse to give up. Victory is sought and defeat is feared. Sometimes there is even hope for a "magic bullet" or a "silver bullet." Only professionals who stand on the firing line or in the trenches can really appreciate the moral problems of medicine. As medicine wages war against germs that invade the body and threaten its defenses, so the society itself may also declare war on cancer under the leadership of its chief medical officer—the Surgeon General. Articles and books may even herald the 'Medical-Industrial Complex: Our National Defense.'

Although the acute care approach to illness has had many victories, it also has some crucially important negative consequences that militate against the more effective management of of chronic illness—and certainly against a great success in improving the quality of life of the chronically ill. For example, the clinical approach leads directly to a faith in high-technology medicine, with its emphasis on intensive care carried out primarily in hospitals and secondarily in clinics. Hence, as noted earlier, the acute care hospital is the centerpiece of the contemporary health enterprise (Scott 1972). Funding, whether federal or through insurance, goes primarily to support acute care facilities and medical practice. Only secondarily does funding go to support home care services. Critics like Childress (1987) suggest that the acute care perspective expressed in military metaphor, leads physicians to assign "priority to *critical* care over prevention and chronic care. It tends to view health in negative rather than positive terms, as the absence of disease rather than a positive state of affairs, and concentrates on critical interventions to cure disease . . . . It tends to neglect care when the cure is impossible" (p. 486). Or it saves people without concern for the quality of their lives once they are sent home.

The acute care perspective also emphasizes technology and downplays less technological modes of care. This is true despite the great difficulty of assessing the usefulness of particular types of technology, the considerable cost of some technologies, the probable overuse of some for particular patients, and the inevitable stopgap quality or "half-way technology" (Thomas 1974, p. 16) of many. Even the funding available for medical research is skewed in the direction of "killer" illnesses; little attention is paid to less alarming but exceedingly important and widespread conditions like arthritis and disabilities derived from back trouble.

The mounting criticism of purely clinical medicine calls for an "expansion in services geared to supportive maintenance, patient management, and new kinds of preventive care" (Schwartz 1987, pp. 485-486). Supportive services "may contribute more to monitoring [patients'] functioning ability, while at the same time reducing the need for costly forms of care and assisting patients to remain or become economically independent and productive" (Cluff 1981, pp. 300-301).

These are criticisms to which we subscribe (Strauss and Glaser 1975; Strauss, Fagerhaugh, Suczek, and Wiener 1985; Corbin and Strauss 1988). In fact, we believe, as do many other researchers, that even in hospitals there should be much more focus on the social and psychological aspects of care of the chronically ill, not only to facilitate their coming to terms with their illness but also to help them learn to live with it day by day, integrating the illness into their lives. Nurses and medical social workers have been moving steadily toward that position, while developing so-called clinical "soft technologies" to supplement the more obviously "hard" technologies. Yet even these professionals do not generally understand that, because their patients usually have histories of chronic illness, they are knowledgeable about their own illness management. This inevitably leads to tensions and conflicts between the hospital staffs and the patients. . . .

If this is so for the hospital situation, consider the consequences of applying the dominant acute care approach to patients after their return home. Although patients are given a regimen and advised to adhere to it, it is anticipated that some will only partly follow these regimens. Indeed, there is a sizable research and rhetorical literature about "recalcitrance"—the professionals' term for the apparently irrational or perverse actions of patients concerning their regimens (Sackett and Snow 1979). "When this problem was first discovered, many practitioners responded with 'awestruck disbelief'" (Svarstad 1976, p. 439). Despite the probably widespread views of physicians about this matter, researchers have demonstrated that the grounds on which patients judge their regimens are quite rational; patients weigh their personal concerns, the contingencies of their lives, and the perceived seriousness of the illness or symptoms against the time and effort the regimens require and the side effects they cause (Conrad 1985; Becker and Maiman 1975; Corbin and Strauss 1985). Further, patients sometimes do not understand the regimens; staffs at the health facilities do not always explain them clearly, either because they do not realize that their explanations are unclear or because they are concentrating on problems of higher (usually clinical) priority (Levy 1979). It is possible that patients' dissatisfaction with the physician who has counseled the regimen also affects their strict adherence to it (Svarstad 1976).

Among nurses, there is an increasing emphasis on the necessity for teaching patients before their discharge from the hospital, and teaching the kin, too, if feasible. Yet the very organization of many hospital wards, especially in the intensive care units, militates against giving much priority to teaching efforts. A recent survey of practices within intensive care nurseries, combined with a careful ethnographic study of one intensive care nursery (Guillemin and Holstrom 1986), portrays vividly the staff's dedication to the work of saving the lives of infants and their great skill in doing so. This research also shows how little effort generally is made to communicate more than superficially with the parents or to attend to their psychological problems—and how little training the staff members usually have in these matters (see also Wiener, Fagerhaugh, Suczek, and Strauss 1979). (Of course, some intensive care nurs-

eries do have trained nursing care specialists who are keenly aware of such problems.) Consequently, we wonder what happens when these infants are returned to their parents who must live with and manage whatever chronic illnesses may develop despite the heroic efforts of the intensive care staff. If this is characteristic of what occurs in hospitals, consider what then happens after a hospitalized patient returns home, given both the clinical orientation at the clinics and physicians' offices and the shape of the American health care system.

. . . Home care is an undernourished child of that system. This is understandable, given that the acute care perspective so profoundly colors the thinking of the physicians who are the dominant health care professionals (Freidson 1970a), as well as that of other health professionals who work more or less under their aegis (Scott 1972). Consequently, critics can point to what seems to be a clear mismatch between the organization of health care and the requirements of managing chronic illness (Schwartz 1987; Vladeck 1983). Despite such criticism, the continued strength of the acute care perspective should not be underestimated. It is more or less shared by the legislators and executives of the federal and state governments as well as by other lay citizens. Furthermore, Freidson (1986), who has been carefully following the evolution of the medical profession, suggests there will be further evolution of new or renovated forms of organized practice (health maintenance organizations, ambulatory surgical centers, and so on); as "is the case for hospitals and medical schools, representation in such associations is institutional in character, embodied in the directors, deans, or chief executive officers responsible for the institution as a whole" (p. 76). He argues that the orientation of these personnel is principally toward protecting their institution and its interests with much consequent attention to the political and economic climate in which it operates, and with rather less concern with the everyday problems of giving patient care. Whether or not his prediction is correct—whether the officials or the physicians have the most influence—these facilities at the heart of the health care system (public health excepted) represent a very strong barrier to any radical shift of perspective on health care.

Criticisms and Suggestions

For many years, the nation's current health care arrangements have been subject to a barrage of criticism as experts and laypeople alike find fault with one or another feature of them. Indeed, with increasing acerbity and increasing numbers of players, a complex and passionately argued debate has been raging in the health care arena. It concerns the proper ways in which the health system should be organized and health care delivered. The current turmoil consequent on high medical costs and the increasingly severe regulation of hospitals and health practitioners have added to the complexity and passion of the debate. Issues of cost, quality care, bureaucratic constraints, accessibility to care, patient consent, the right to die, technological advances, and alarming technological by-products—all are now highly visible items in the news media. Moreover, it is probable that the debate will continue with unabated intensity for many years, exhibiting a further and sometimes bewildering array of panaceas, plans, programs, models, and suggestions.

The views of critics who assess the health system from the standpoint of its performance in long-term care, including their criticisms of the prevailing acute care approach, are especially pertinent to our own. We will discuss a few of their views and suggestions for improving longer-term care. While there are differences of emphasis, there seems to be a consensus that the current arrangements fall far short of what is needed. Five major points on which there is relative agreement are summarized below.

First, long-term care involves far more than is offered in acute care facilities. Second, clinical care should be supplemented by services that will meet the rehabilitative, psychological, economic, social, and other needs of the ill. Third, there should be a shift in funding patterns so that these other services can be greatly expanded. Fourth, funding for the poor requires special attention, for they bear the burden of the health care system's failings; their care is less accessible and of lower quality, although the poor are more disabled and sicker than the rest of our population. Fifth, funding arrangements to cover potential economic catastrophe for all ill or disabled Americans are imperative.

There is general agreement, too, on the list of services that would make long-term care comprehensive, continuous, flexible, responsive to what the ill and disabled require, and respectful of them and their families. As Vladeck (1983, p. 7) remarks, these requirements "are hardly radical or unfamiliar to health care professionals," at least to those especially concerned with long-term care.

On the question of how to attain these goals there is somewhat less agreement. As might be anticipated, the diversity of suggestions for changing or supplementing the present system is affected by the different perspectives associated with professional positions and experiences. We will present a few of the suggestions made by people who have been much concerned with improving long-term care.

One suggestion for reform emphasizes the necessity to raise public awareness about the long-term care issue. This emphasis is largely a political one. It has been well stated by Brody, who argues that to get maximum changes in the desired direction now, "perception of catastrophe in economic terms is the *sine qua non* for policy change" (1987, p. 135). This implies that continuity of care needs to be stated "in specific terms which then can be costed out" (p. 135). Otherwise, we cannot effectively counter the argument of legislators and others who are frightened of the bottomless pit of potential expenditures and anticipate unending demands by the aged ill and disabled. These fears are fed by memories of the haste with which legislators responded to the lobbying of kidney dialysis proponents for carte blanche aid to kidney patients. Politicians must be convinced of what research has already clearly demonstrated: the families of the ill will not abdicate their responsibilities once adequate government funding is available.

Some critics believe that Americans more or less agree on what is wrong with the health care system but disagree on what should be changed. Therefore, reform efforts are mired. "It may be that the current policy stalemate arises at root from value conflicts about the appropriate roles of government, families, and individual responsibility so profound that only creative and aggressive policy leadership, of a kind now nowhere to be found, can end it" (Vladeck 1984, p. 2). Meltzer, Farrow, and Richman (1981, p. 6) make a similar point when they assert that "the most important policy problem is a lack of consensus about the nature and extent of public responsibility for meeting long-term care needs. This results in an inability to articulate a single set of goals and directions for future policy development."

A more systematic and extended statement, based on careful research, is offered by Budrys (1986), who assesses the situation in this way: "The persistent perception of a health crisis stems from society's lack of confidence in the social control arrangements governing the activities of the health sector in recent years; what is worse the public is confused about who should be entrusted with the responsibility for planning the nation's health" (1986, p. 113). . . .

Her solution is to blow the whistle on the debate—a vain solution, we believe—buckle down to rational consideration of the inevitable strengths and weaknesses of each control system, "and develop a higher level of [political] consensus regarding the strengths and weaknesses of each before opting for changes in current health care delivery arrangements" (1986, p. 133).

A second suggestion for reform focuses on the inadequacies of current funding mechanisms and how they might be rectified to give greater financial support to those who need long-term care. When the focus is on the elderly ill and disabled or the poor elderly, then the suggestions may refer to altering Medicare or Medicaid. The tenor of such suggestions is conveyed by Davis and Rowland (1983, p. 525): "Medicaid coverage should be expanded to provide basic insurance coverage for all low-income individuals . . . implementation of coverage for the medically needy would be another step toward reduc-

ing disparities between the South and the rest of the country. . . .

When the poor or particular deprived minorities are in focus, whether they are deprived or not, a third theme colors the policy suggestions. This pertains to equity, to fairness in access to quality health care. Equity has long been a primary agenda of those who represent the poor and minorities (Wiener, Fagerhaugh, Suczek, and Strauss 1979; Davis and Rowland 1983; Fein 1986).

Other reform suggestions are more specific, centered on particular features of prevailing health care arrangements. For example, to get adequate and appropriate services, the ill have to find their way through a veritable " agency maze," with its accompanying fragmentation, lack of communication between agencies and care givers, high costs for services, and agency politics (Friedemann 1986; Harding, Heller, and Kesler 1979; Waitzkin 1983; Wheeler-Lachowycz 1983; Feder 1983). It is argued that this situation needs to be rectified by various organizational strategies. Or the rehabilitation services are believed to be inadequate in one or another regard, and this situation should be corrected (Schank 1986; Becker and Kaufman 1987; Verville 1979; Fowler 1982; Rothberg 1981; Fordyce 1976; Kaufman and Becker 1986; Roth 1984). Or the rehabilitation practitioners are viewed as typically not focused on chronic illnesses; they should be more aware of them and chronically ill patients should be referred to rehabilitation services by the physicians (Schank 1986). Or the linkage between the hospital and the home health agencies is judged to be very poor and should be greatly strengthened (Strauss, Fagerhaugh, Suczek, and Wiener 1985; Vladeck 1984, p. 11; Jillings 1987). . . .

In stating these typical positions and suggestions so baldly, we do not mean to denigrate them. In fact, each certainly deserves careful consideration, and of course some are getting that consideration rather widely.

Professional and Lay Approaches to Illness

The writings of the reform advocates cited above and others like them have a common feature, despite differences in their specific suggestions for improving long-term care. This feature is their highly professionalized view of what is wrong with organized health care arrangements. This should occasion no surprise, since the authors all have had professional training, positions, and experience (Freidson 1970a, 1970b, 1986; Hughes 1971). This does not mean they are insensitive to or disrespectful of the viewpoints or wishes of the ill and their families. Yet a professional perspective deeply colors the language even of those who advocate the most cooperative relationships with the ill. Often the ill are referred to as patients or clients, which, from a professional's standpoint, of course, they are. Therefore, we are offered suggestions for what amounts to a patient centered professional model (Cluff 1981, p. 2), a " patient centered" model (Lubkin 1986, p. 121), a "client based perspective" (Vladeck 1984, p. 1), and a "goal oriented approach" to real-life functioning, rather than a predominantly clinical approach. Programs are assessed for their matching of services with "needs" of the ill (Vladeck 1984, p. 2), and in terms of a cause-effect model of the degree to which they are effective, efficient, cost effective, and so on (Budrys 1986, pp. 51-71; Fein 1981).

This kind of terminology reflects an underlying specialist stance. It is markedly different from the attitude that can be sensed in the words and actions of some self-help groups (Maines 1984), and the more militant disabled groups (Zola 1981, 1982), as well as in writings derived from the concerns of the women's movement (Coleman, Summers, and Leonard 1982; Lewin and Olesen 1985). The perspectives of these groups surely are not those of health or rehabilitation professionals or professional gerontologists, nor of political scientists, social workers, or government administrators. Professionals and the lay disabled and ill are, of course, often able to act cooperatively in the political arena, yet their fundamental views are far from identical. We believe that the professionals' approach makes them insufficiently sensitive to some of the subtler issues involved in staying afloat when burdened with a severe chronic illness (Massie and Massie 1973). This, of course, has some negative consequences for

practitioners and policy approaches to the problems of the chronically ill. . . .

Practitioner training is highly technical, with therapies and procedures that have been carefully assessed and at least partly related to professional philosophies of treatment (Becker, Geer, Hughes, and Strauss 1964). Later experiences in the field, as practitioner, teacher, or researcher, build on a great deal of technical knowledge and skill. Further, a health professional almost always works in an organizational context. He or she inevitably must take elements of that context into account, whether they are agency requirements, intraagency and interagency relationships, legislative mandates and constraints, colleague relationships, or interdisciplinary working relationships (Scott 1972).

A somewhat intellectualized approach to illness and its accompanying social and psychological patterns is contributed to both by this organizational context and by professional training and experience (Strauss, Fagerhaugh, Suczek, and Wiener 1985; Guillemin and Holstrom 1986). (We are not saying this is bad—only different.) This can be seen in nurses, physicians, and social workers even when someone in their own family becomes chronically ill; one cannot expect them to tear their professionalized approaches from their brains, nor would it make any sense if they did. The professionalized approach, however, is at some variance with the approaches of laypeople, except those who themselves have become considerably professionalized. Their worlds are not the professional's world, and vice versa. The ill and their families are concerned with managing the vagaries of illness, and with living with it and whatever regimens and limitations it entails. They are also concerned with managing living day to day with whatever resources they have and whatever arrangements can be set up and maintained.

An essentially top-down approach is also characteristic of the professionalized policy or practitioner perspective toward the ill and their problems. Even the most sensitive of policy thinkers does not escape this top-down perspective, often expressed in administrative, economic, and political terms (see, for instance, La Porte and Rubin 1979; Meltzer,

Farrow, and Richman 1981). They fail to follow through as thoroughly as they might on their insights into the fateful situations and difficult work of the chronically ill, and, for that matter, on their knowledge of the inadequacies of health services and health personnel (see Vladeck 1984). The language of many professionals shows the basic stance. There are people who "deliver" health care and people who "receive" health care. Sometimes health professionals talk about "consumers" and "providers," thinking about health services in market or even industrial terms. Clients and caretakers are supposed—or at least hoped—to act rationally and sensibly. Appropriate behavior includes their adhering to regimens faithfully, monitoring themselves or the ill person carefully, and reporting accurately to responsible practitioners. All of this presumably makes sense to most professionals, as it does in part, to many clients. Yet it is far from the whole story. Laypeople see the regimens, services, practitioners, and so on as fitting or not fitting into the flow of illness-affected life (Corbin and Strauss 1985, 1988). There is not necessarily a conflict between lay and professional views, but they are certainly not mirror images of each other.

One probable consequence is the professionals' inevitable piecemeal approach to the endemic problems of the chronically ill. Practitioners at clinics or physicians' offices or who visit the ill in their homes see many of them, but can see individuals only at intervals. They must necessarily monitor or assess ill people in their current state only. The temporal perspective of the ill person and kin is quite otherwise. Moreover, the problems of the ill and their kin are unquestionably theirs; they are not the problems of aggregates of ill persons, as the policy researchers and advocates are almost always likely to consider them owing to the very nature of policy research and advocacy. Also, as we have indicated, professionals are likely to see these problems from the standpoint of their own specialties and professional positions, however broad a perspective they have on chronic illness issues. Indeed, it is striking how specialized the literature that they tend to cite is, whether they are medical sociologists (Conrad 1987), social worker-gerontologists (Brody

1987), economists (Fein 1986), or political scientists (Vladeck 1983) with an eye on the pertinent governmental legislation. And, it is rare to find in the literature written by these otherwise astute critics as candid a statement as the following: "We are going to have to find better ways of making our care system more responsible to the expressed and implicit desires of clients and informal caretakers. How to do this in a systematic way is not something about which I have a lot to say" (Vladeck 1983, p. 3).

The prevailing acute care approach to illness has proven to be inadequate to the task of providing care for the chronically ill. Strong criticisms of the acute care perspective and proposals for reform have been made by many critics, especially those professionally involved with rehabilitation or gerontology. Their suggestions, however, also suffer from a number of weaknesses, in part because of the inevitable difference between the professional attitude of the critics toward the ill and the concerns of the ill and their families themselves.

References

Anderson, T. "Educational Frame of Reference: An Additional Model for Rehabilitation Medicine." *Archives of Physical Medicine and Rehabilitation*, 1978, 59 203-206.

Becker, G., and S. Kaufman. "Old Age, Rehabilitation and Research: A Review of the Issues." Unpublished paper, Department of Social and Behavioral Sciences, University of California, San Francisco, 1987.

Becker, H. , B. Geer, E. Hughes, and A. Strauss, *Boys in White*. Chicago: University of Chicago Press, 1964.

Becker, M., and I. Maiman. "Sociobehavioral Determinants of Compliance with Health and Medical Care Recommendations." *Medical Care*, 1975, *13*, 10-24.

Brody, E. " 'Women in the Middle' and Family Help to Older People." *The Gerontologist*, 1981, *21*, 471-480.

Brody, S. "Strategic Planning: The Catastrophic Approach." *The Gerontologist*, 1987, 27, 131-138.

Brody, S., S. Poulshock, and C. Masciocchi. "The Family Caring Unit: A Major Consideration in the Long-Term Care Support System." *The Gerontologist*, 1978, *18*, 555-561.

Bucher, R., and J. Stelling. *Becoming Professional*. Newbury Park, CA: Sage, 1977.

Budrys, G. *Planning the Nation's Health.* New York: Greenwood, 1986.

Childress, J. "Sociocultural Metaphors." In H. Schwartz (ed.), *Dominant Issues in Medical Sociology.* (2nd ed.) New York: Random House, 1987.

Cluff, L. "Chronic Disease, Function and the Quality of Care." *Social Science and Medicine,* 1981, *34*; 299-304.

Coleman, V., T. Summers, and F. Leonard, "Till Death Do Us Part: Caregiving Wives of Severely Disabled Husbands." Gray Paper no. 7. Washington, D.C.: Older Women's League, 1982.

Conrad, P. "The Meaning of Medication: Another Look at Compliance." *Social Science and Medicine,* 1985, *20,* 29-37.

Conrad, P. "The Experience of Illness: Recent and New Directions." In J. Roth and P. Conrad (eds.), *Research in the Sociology of Health Care.* Vol. 6: *The Experience and Management of Chronic Illness.* Greenwich, Conn.: JAI Press, 1987.

Corbin, J., and A. Strauss. "Issues Concerning Regimen Managing in the Home." *Ageing and Society,* 1985, *5,* 249-265.

Corbin, J., and A. Strauss. *Unending Work and Care: Managing Chronic Illness at Home.* San Francisco: Jossey-Bass, 1988.

Crossman, L., C. London, and C. Barry. "Older Women Caring for Disabled Spouses: A Model for Supportive Services." *The Gerontologist,* 1981, *21,* 464-470.

Davis, K., and D. Rowland. "Uninsured and Underserved: Inequities in Health Care in the United States." In H. Schwartz (ed.), *Dominant Issues in Medical Sociology.* (2nd ed.) New York: Random House, 1983.

Fagerhaugh, S., and A. Strauss. *The Politics of Pain Management: Staff-Patient Interaction.* Reading, MA: Atherton, 1977.

Feder, J. "Effects of Changing Federal Health Policies on the General Public, the Aged and the Disabled." *Bulletin of the New York Academy of Medicine,* 1983, *59,* 41-49.

Fein, R. (ed.). *Health Planning in the United States.* Vol. 1. Washington, D.C.: National Academy Press, 1981.

Fein, R. *Medical Care, Medical Costs: The Search for a Health Insurance Policy.* Cambridge, Mass.: Harvard University Press, 1986.

Feldman, D. "Chronic Disabling Illness: A Holistic View." *Journal of Chronic Disease,* 1974, *27,* 287-291.

Fengler, A., and N. Goodrich. "Wives of Elderly Disabled Men: The Hidden Patients." *The Gerontologist,* 1979, *19,* 175-183.

Fordyce, W. "A Behavioral Perspective in Rehabilitation." In G. Albrecht (ed.), *The Sociology of Physical Disability and Rehabilitation.* Pittsburgh, Pa.: University of Pittsburgh Press, 1976.

Fowler, W. "Viability of Physical Medicine and Rehabilitation in the 1980s." *Archives of Physical Medicine and Rehabilitation,* 1982, *63* 1-5.

Freidson, E. *Profession of Medicine.* New York: Dodd, Mead, 1970a.

Freidson, E. *Professional Dominance.* Chicago: Aldine, 1970b.

Freidson, E. *Professional Powers.* Chicago: University of Chicago Press, 1986.

Friedemann M.L. "The Agency Maze." In I. Lubkin (ed.), *Chronic Illness: Impact and Interventions.* Boston: Jones and Bartlett, 1986.

Guillemin, J. and Holstrom, L. *Mixed Blessings: Intensive Care for Newborns.* New York: Oxford University Press, 1986.

Harding, R., J. Heller, and R. Kesler. "The Critically Ill Child in the Primary Care Setting." *Primary Care,* 1979, *62,* 322-329.

Hughes, E. "Professions." In E. Hughes, *The Sociological Eye.* Vol. 2. Chicago: Aldine-Atherton, 1971.

Jillings, C. "Is Chronic Illness a Relevant Topic for the Critical Care Nurse?" *Critical Care Nurse,* 1987, 7; 14-17.

Kaufman, S. and G. Becker. "Stroke: Health Care on the Periphery." *Social Science and Medicine,* 1986, *22,* 983-989.

La Porte, V. and J. Rubin. (eds.). *Reform and Regulation in Long-Term Care.* New York: Praeger, 1979.

Levy, N. "The Chronically Ill Patient." *Psychiatric Quarterly,* 1979 *51,* 189-197.

Lewin, E., and O. Olesen. *Women, Health and Healing: A New Perspective.* New York: Tavistock-Methuen, 1985.

Lubkin, I. (ed.). *Chronic Illness: Impact and Interventions.* Boston: Jones and Bartlett, 1986.

Maines, D. "The Social Arrangements of Diabetic Self-Help Groups." In A. Strauss and others, *Chronic Illness and the Quality of Life.* (2nd ed.) St. Louis, Mo.: Mosby, 1984.

Massie, R., and S. Massie. *Journey.* New York: Knopf, 1973.

Meltzer, J., F. Farrow, and H. Richman (eds.): *Policy Options and Long-Term Care.* Chicago: University of Chicago Press, 1981.

Mizrahi T. *Getting Rid of Patients: Contradictions in the Training of Internists.* New Brunswick, N.J.: Rutgers University Press, 1987.

Rice, D. and T. Hodgson. "Social and Economic Implications in the United States." In U.S. Public Health Service, *Vital and Health Statistics.* Series 3, no. 20. Department of Health and Human Services publication no. PHS-81-1404. Washington, D.C.: U.S. Government Printing Office, 1981.

Roth, J. "The Public Hospital: Refuge for Damaged Humans." In A. Strauss (ed.), *Where Medicine Fails.* New Brunswick, NJ: Transaction, 1984.

Roth, J., and S. Ruzek. (eds.). *Research in the Sociology of Health Care.* Vol. 4: *The Adoption and Social Consequences of Medical Technologies.* Greenwich, Conn.: JAI Press, 1986.

Rothberg, J. "The Rehabilitation Team: Future Direction." *Archives of Physical Medicine and Rehabilitation,* 1981 *62,* 407-410.

Sackett, D., and J. Snow. "The Magnitude of Compliance and Noncompliance." In R. Haynes, D. Taylor, and D. Sackett (eds.), *Compliance in Health Care.* Baltimore, MD: Johns Hopkins University Press, 1979.

Schank, A. "Rehabilitation." In I. Lubkin (ed.), *Chronic Illness: Impact and Interventions.* Boston: Jones and Bartlett, 1986.

Schwartz, H. "Irrationality as a Feature of Health Care in the United States." In H. Schwartz (ed.), *Dominant Issues in Medical Sociology.* (2nd ed.) New York: Random House, 1987.

Scott, R. "Professionals in Hospitals: Technology and the Organization of Work." In B. Georgepoulos (ed.), *Organization Research on Health Institutions.* Ann Arbor: Institute for Social Research, University of Michigan Press, 1972.

Sontag, S. *Illness as Metaphor.* New York: Farrar, Straus & Giroux, 1979.

Strauss, A., S. Fagerhaugh, B. Suczek, and C. Wiener. *The Social Organization of Medical Work.* Chicago: University of Chicago Press, 1985.

Strauss, A. and B. Glaser. *Chronic Illness and the Quality of Life.* St. Louis, MO: Mosby, 1975.

Strauss, A. and others. *Chronic Illness and the Quality of Life.* (2nd ed.) St. Louis, MO: Mosby, 1984.

Svarstad, B. "Physician-Patient Communication and Patient Conformity with Medical Advice." In D. Mechanic (ed.), *Growth of Bureaucratic Medicine.* New York: Wiley, 1976.

Thomas, L. *The Living Cell.* New York: Bantam Books, 1974.

Vaisrub, S. *Medicine's Metaphors: Messages and Menaces.* Oradell, N.J.: Medical Economics, 1977.

Verville, R. "The Rehabilitation Amendments of 1978: What Do They Mean for Comprehensive Rehabilitation?" *Archives of Physical Medicine and Rehabilitation,* 1979, *60,* 141-144.

Vladeck, B. "Two Steps Forward, One Back: The Changing Agenda of Long-Term Home Care Reform." *Pride Institute Journal of Long-Term Home Care,* 1983, *2* 1-7.

Vladeck, B. "Meeting the Needs of the Elderly: A Client-Based Approach." Paper presented at the Conference on Strategies, Services Structures—Quality Care for the Elderly: Meeting the Financial Challenge, San Diego, Calif., Feb. 13, 1984.

Waitzkin, H. "Community-Based Health Care: Contradictions and Challenges." *Annals of Internal Medicine,* 1983, *98,* 235-242.

Warren, V. "A Powerful Metaphor: Medicine as War." Unpublished paper, cited in H. Schwartz (ed.), *Dominant Issues in Medical Sociology.* (2nd ed.) New York: Random House, 1987.

Wheeler-Lacowycz, J. "How to Use Your VNA." American Journal of Nursing," 1983, *83* 1164-1167.

Wiener, C., S. Fagerhaugh, B. Suczek, and A. Strauss. "Trajectories, Biographies and the Evolving Medical Technology Scene: Labor and Delivery and the Intensive Care Nursery." *Sociology of Health and Illness,* 1979, *1,* 261-283.

Zola, I. "Structural Constraints in the Doctor-Patient Relationships: The Case of Non-Compliance." In L. Eisenberg and A. Kleinman (eds.), *The Relevance of Social Science for Medicine.* Dordrecht, The Netherlands: Reidel, 1981.

Zola, I. *Missing Pieces: A Chronicle of Living with a Disability.* Philadelphia: Temple University Press, 1982.

Further Reading

David Himmelstein and Steffie Woolhandler. 1994. *The National Health Program Book: A Source Guide for Advocates.* Monroe, ME: Common Courage.

Nancy F. McKenzie (ed.). 1994. *Beyond Crisis: Confronting Health Care in the United States.* New York: Penguin.

Vicente Navarro. 1995. "Why Congress Did Not Enact Health Care Reform." *Journal of Health, Politics, Policy and Law.* 20: 455-462.

Discussion Questions

1. Why would people with chronic illnesses hold different perspectives and policy objectives than professionals who state that their policy proposals are patient oriented?

2. What do you see as the main obstacles to a better health care system? Why?

3. How do you account for the persistence of the acute care model in today's health care system?

CPSIA information can be obtained
at www.ICGtesting.com
Printed in the USA
FFOW01n0737060818
47655659-51265FF